HANDBOOK OF ANESTHESIA

Karen Conniks
7/99

~£60.-

For Churchill Livingstone:

Project Editor: Gavin Smith
Project Controller: Mark Sanderson
Text Design: Charles Simpson
Indexer: June Morrison
Cover Design: Carole Thomas

HANDBOOK OF CLINICAL ANESTHESIA

EDITED BY

J. C. Goldstone
MB BS MD FRCA
Senior Lecturer;
Consultant, Intensive Care Medicine,
UCL Medical School,
The Middlesex Hospital,
London, UK

B. J. Pollard
BPharm MB ChB MD FRCA
Senior Lecturer in Anaesthesia;
Consultant Anaesthetist,
University Department of Anaesthesia,
Manchester Royal Infirmary,
Manchester, UK

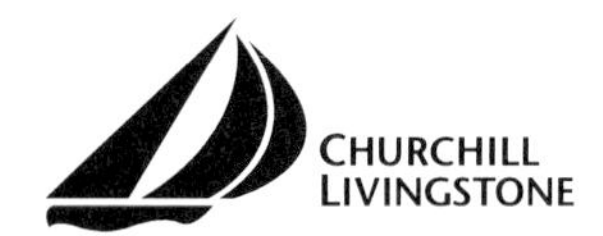

NEW YORK EDINBURGH LONDON MADRID
MELBOURNE SAN FRANCISCO TOKYO 1996

CHURCHILL LIVINGSTONE
Medical Division of Pearson Professional Limited

Distributed in the United States of America by Churchill Livingstone Inc., 650 Avenue of the Americas, New York, N.Y. 10011, and by associated companies, branches and representatives throughout the world.

First published 1996

ISBN 0-443-04984X

British Library Cataloguing in Publication Data
A catalogue record for this book is available from the British Library.

Library of Congress Cataloging in Publication Data
A catalog record for this book is available from the Library of Congress.

Medical knowledge is constantly changing. As new information becomes available, changes in treatment, procedures, equipment and the use of drugs become necessary. The editors, contributors and publishers have, as far as possible, taken care to ensure that the information given in this text is accurate and up to date. However, readers are strongly advised to confirm that the information, especially with regard to drug usage, complies with latest legislation and standards of practice.

The publisher's policy is to use **paper manufactured from sustainable forest**

Printed in Hong Kong

NPC/01

CONTENTS

PART 1: PATIENT CONDITIONS

CONTRIBUTORS

M. Y. Aglan MD FRCA FFARCSI DEAA
Senior Registrar in Anaesthesia,
Manchester Royal Infirmary,
Department of Anaesthesia,
Manchester, UK

T. Ainley FRCA
Senior Registrar,
St Mary's Hospital,
Department of Anaesthesia,
London, UK

Quentin Ainsworth
Consultant Anaesthetist,
Nuffield Department of Anaesthesia,
John Radcliffe Hospital,
Oxford, UK

Baha Al-Shaikh MB ChB FFARCSI
Consultant Anaesthetist,
William Harvey Hospital,
Willesborough,
Ashford, UK

R. J. Alcock MB BS FRCA
Senior Registrar in Anaesthesia,
Royal Free Hospital,
London, UK

Peter Amoroso FRCA
Consultant Anaesthetist,
St Bartholomew's Hospital,
Directorate of Anaesthesia,
London, UK

J. M. Anderson FRCA
Senior Registrar,
Middlesex Hospital,
London, UK

J. M. Anderton MB ChB DObstRCOG FRCA
Consultant Anaesthetist,
Manchester Royal Infirmary,
Manchester, UK

J. Appleby MB BS FRCA
Consultant Anaesthetist,
Kent and Sussex Weald NHS Trust,
Tunbridge Wells,
Kent, UK

W. Aveling MB BChir FRCA
Consultant Anaesthetist,
Department of Anaesthesia,
University College London Hospitals,
The Middlesex Hospital,
London, UK

I. Banks MB BS FRCA
Senior Registrar in Anaesthesia,
Department of Anaestheisa,
Manchester Royal Infirmary,
Manchester, UK

Mathew Barnard
Senior Registrar,
University College London Hospitals,
The Middlesex Hospital,
London, UK

J. Barrie
Consultant Anaesthetist,
Royal Oldham Hospitals,
Oldham,
Lancashire, UK

A. Batchelor MB ChB FRCA
Consultant Anaesthetist,
Department of Anaesthesia,
Royal Victoria Infirmary,
Newcastle Upon Tyne, UK

M. J. Beech FRCA
Consultant Anaesthetist(Late),
University Hospitals of South Manchester,
Manchester, UK

M. Bellman MB ChB FRCA
Consultant Anaesthetist and Honorary
Lecturer in Anaesthesia,
University Hospitals of South Manchester,
Manchester, UK

Jonathan P. Benson MB ChB FRCA
Senior Registrar in Anaesthesia,
Department of Anaesthesia,
University of Birmingham,
Birmingham, UK

S. Berg BSc FRCA
Consultant Paediatric Anaesthetist,
John Radcliffe Hospital,
Oxford, UK

S. A. Bew MA MB BS FRCA
Senior Registrar in Neuroanaesthesia,
The National Hospital for Neurology and
Nerosurgery,
Queen Square,
London, UK

P. Bickford-Smith FRCA
Senior Registrar in Anaesthesia,
Bradford Royal Infirmary,
Directorate of Anaesthesia,
Bradford, UK

R. Bingham MB BS
Consultant Paediatric Anaesthetist,
Department of Anaesthesia,
National Hospital for Sick Children,
London, UK

J. F. Bion MB BS MRCP FRCA MD
Senior Lecturer and Honorary Consultant in
Intensive Care Medicine,
Queen Elizabeth Hospital,
University of Birmingham,
Birmingham, UK

D. Bogod MB BS FFA RCS
Consultant Anaesthetist,
City Hospital,
Nottingham, UK

M. J. Boscoe FRCA
Consultant Anaesthetist,
Harefield Hospital,
Harefield,
Middlesex, UK

D. Brighouse BM FRCA
Consultant Obstetric Anaesthetist,
Department of Anaesthesia,
Southampton University Hospitals,
Southampton, UK

J. Broadfield
Consultant Anaesthetist,
Kings College Hospital,
London, UK

P. M. Brodrick MB BS FRCA
Consultant Anaesthetist,
Mount Vernon and Watford Hospitals NHS
Trust,
Mount Vernon Hospital,
Northwood, UK

L. M. Bromley FRCA
Senior Lecturer and Consultant Anaesthetist,
University College School of Medicine,
The Middlesex Hospital,
London, UK

H. E. Brunner
Senior Registrar in Anaesthesia & Intensive
Care,
Queen Elizabeth Hospital,
University of Birmingham,
Birmingham, UK

P. Bunting MB ChB FRCA
Consultant Anaesthetist,
Royal Preston Hospital,
Preston, UK

I. Calder FRCA
Consultant Anaesthetist,
National Hospital for Neurology and Neurosurgery,
Department of Anaesthesia,
Queen Square,
London, UK

I. T. Campbell MD FRCA
Honorary Senior Lecturer and Consultant Anaesthetist,
Department of Anaesthesia,
University of Manchester,
Withington Hospital,
Manchester, UK

L. E. S. Carrie MB ChB FRCA
Consultant Anaesthetist,
Nuffield Department of Anaesthetics,
John Radcliffe Hospital;
Clinical Lecturer,
Maternity Department,
Oxford University,
Headington,
Oxford, UK

I. S. Chadwick MB ChB DCH FRCA
Consultant Anaesthetist,
North Manchester General Hospital,
Manchester, UK

A. J. Charlton MB ChBFRCA
Consultant Anaesthetist,
Department of Anaesthesia,
Manchester Royal Infirmary,
Manchester, UK

E. Cheetham FRCA
Research Fellow in Anaesthesia,
Manchester Royal Infirmary,
Manchester, UK

M. S. Chetty BSc MB ChB MRCP FRCA
Consultant Anaesthetist,
Hope Hospital,
Salford, UK

T. H. Clutton-Brock MB ChB MRCP
Semior Lecturer in Anaesthesia & Intensive Care,
Queen Elizabeth Hospital,
University of Birmingham,
Birmingham, UK

R. Collis MB BS FRCA
Senior Registrar,
Royal London Hospital,
Whitechapel,
London, UK

A. Corbett FRCA
Registrar in Anaesthesia,
Department of Anaesthesia,
Manchester Royal Infirmary,
Manchester, UK

S. Cottam MB ChB FRCA
Consultant Anaesthetist,
King's College Hospital,
London, UK

I. J. Crabb MB BS FRCA DA(UK)
Finsbury Park,
London, UK

Peter D. Curry BSc MB BS FFA RCSI DA
Senior Registrar in Anaesthetics,
University of Birmingham,
Queen Elizabeth Hospital,
Birmingham, UK

N. Curzen BM(Hons) MRCP
MRC Fellow in Anaesthesia,
Honorary Registrar in Cardiology and Intensive Care,
Unit of Clinical Care,
Royal Brompton Hospital,
London, UK

A. Dash MB BS FRCA
Consultant Anaesthetist,
Department of Anaesthesia,
Northampton General Hospital,
Northampton, UK

D. W. L Davies MB ChB DRCOG DCH FRCA
Consultant Anaesthetist,
Department of Anaesthesia,
University College London Hospitals,
The Middlesex Hospital,
London, UK

A. G. Davis MB ChB FRCA
Consultant Anaesthetist,
Department of Anaesthesia,
Southern General Hospital NHS Trust,
Glasgow, UK

S. Deegan FDSRCSED. FRCA
Senior Registrar Anaesthetics,
Queen Elizabeth Hospital,
Birmingham, UK

N. Denny FRCA
Department of Anaesthesia,
Queen Elizabeth Hospital,
King's Lynn, UK

J. P. Desborough MD FRCA
Senior Lecturer and Consultant,
Department of Anaesthesia,
St George's Hospital Medical School,
London, UK

A. Devine BSc MB ChB FRCA
Lecturer in Anaesthesia,
University Department of Anaesthesia,
Manchester Royal Infirmary,
Manchester, UK

J. Dinsmore MB BS FCAnaesth
Department of Anaesthesia,
St George's Hospital Medical School,
London, UK

H. Dodsworth MB FRCP FRCPath
Haemotologist (Retired);Senior Lecturer in Haemotology,
St Mary's Hospital Medical School,
London, UK

N. Duncan
Head of Communications;
Member of the Institute of Public Relations,
BMA Public Affairs Division,
London, UK

J. Dziersk FRCA
Registrar in Neuroanaesthesia,
The National Hospital for Neurology and Neurosurgery,
Queen Square,
London, UK

J. Eddleston FRCA
Consultant Anaesthetist,
Department of Anaesthesia,
Manchester Royal Infirmary,
Manchester, UK

W. G. Edge MB ChB FFA RCS DA
Consultant Anaesthetist,
Stoke Mandeville Hospital,
Aylesbury,
Bucks, UK

R. Edwards FRCA
Senior Registrar Anaesthesia,
Department of Anaesthesia,
St Georges's Hospital Medical School,
London, UK

J. M. Elliot MB BS FRCA DipIMC RCS(Ed)
Senior Registrar in Anaesthesia,
Queen Elizabeth Hospital,
Birmingham, UK

J. G. Farrimond MRCP FFA RCS
Consultant Anaesthetist,
Harefield Hospital,
Harefield, UK

W. J. Fawcett FRCA
Consultant Anaesthetist,
Royal Surrey County Hospital,
Guildford,
Surrey, UK

T. Freeley
Stanford University School of Medicine,
Stanford, USA

J. M. Freeman
Queen Elizabeth Hospital,
University of Birmingham,
Birmingham, UK

J. Frossard FRCA
Consultant in Anaesthesia,
University College School of Medicine,
The Middlesex Hospital,
London, UK

J. H. Gaston MB FRCA FRCPC
Clinical Director and Constultant Anaesthetist,
Department of Anaesthetics,
Royal Hospitals Trust Belfast,
Whitla Medical Building,
Belfast, UK

J. Goddard FRCA
Consultant Anaesthetist,
Shackleton Department of Anaesthesia,
Southampton General Hospital,
Southampton, UK

C. Goldsack MB ChB BSc MRCP
Lecturer in Neuroanaethesia,
The National Hospital for Neurology and Neurosurgery,
Queen Square,
London, UK

J. C. Goldstone MB BS MD FRCA
Senior Lecturer;
Consultant, Intensive Care Medicine,
University College London Hospitals School of Medicine,
The Middlesex Hospital,
London, UK

C. Gomersall FRCA
Department of Anaesthesia,
St Mary's Hospital,
London, UK

A. Goodwin
Department of Anaesthesia,
University College London Hospitals,
Middlesex Hospital,
London, UK

J. W. W. Gothard MB BS FRCA
Consultant Anaesthetist,
Royal Brompton National Heart & Lung Hospital,
London, UK

H. StJ. Gray MB BS MRCP FRCA
Consultant Anaesthetist,
Wythenshawe Hospital,
Wythenshawe,
Manchester, UK

R. Greenbaum MB ChB DObstRCOG FRCA
Consultant Anaesthetist,
University College London Hospitals,
London, UK

D. Greenhalgh MB ChB FRCA
Consultant Anaesthetist,
Wythenshawe Hospital,
Wythenshawe,
Manchester, UK

S. G. Greenhough BSc MB ChB FRCA
Consultant Anaesthetist,
Manchester Royal Infirmary,
Manchester, UK

E. M. Grundy BSc MB ChB MRCP MRCS LRCP FFA RCS DObstRCOG
Consultant Anaesthetist,
University College London Hospitals and Royal National Orthopaedic Hospital Trust,
London, UK

C. Gwinnutt MB BS FRCA
Consultant Anaesthetist,
Hope Hospital,
Salford, UK

G. M. Hall PhD MB BS MRCS LRCP(Lon) FFA RCS
Professor of Anaesthesia,
St George's Hospital Medical School,
London, UK

P. A. Hall MB BS FRCA
Senior Registrar,
University Hospital Birmingham NHS Trust,
University of Birmingham,
Edgbaston,
Birmingham, UK

C. Hamilton-Davies MB BS
Kingston Upon Thames,
Surrey, UK

M. R. Hamilton-Farrell BSc MB BS MRCP FRCA
Whipps Cross Hospital,
London, UK

J. S. Hammond MB BS FRCA
Senior Registrar in Anaesthesia,
Department of Anaesthesia,
Withington Hospital,
Manchester, UK

R. C. M. Hanley MB BCh BAO MRCP(Ireland) FRCA
Registrar in Anaesthesia,
Department of Anaesthesia,
Manchester Royal Infirmary,
Manchester, UK

M. Harmer MB BS FRCA
Senior Lecturer,
Department of Anaesthetics and Intensive Care Medicine,
University of Wales College of Medicine,
Cardiff, UK

W. Harrop-Griffiths MA FRCA
Consultant Anaesthetist,
Department of Anaesthesia,
St Mary's Hospital,
London, UK

T. E. J. Healey
Professor of Anaesthesia,
University of Manchester,
Manchester Royal Infirmary,
Manchester, UK

M. Heining MD FRCA
Consultant Anaesthetist,
Nottingham City Hospital,
Nottingham, UK

D. Higgins
Consultant Anaesthetist,
Department of Anaesthesia,
Southend Hospital,
Westcliff-on-Sea,
Essex, UK

A. T. Hindle MB ChB Bsc(Hons) FRCA
Lecturer in Anaesthesia,
Academic Unit of Anaesthesia,
Leeds General Infirmary,
Leeds, UK

N. P. Hirsch MB BS FRCA
Consultant in Neuroanaesthesia,
The National Hospital for Neurology and Neurosurgery,
Queen Square,
London, UK

U. M. Hodges BSc(Hons) MB BS FRCA
Consultant Anaesthetist,
St Andrews Centre for Plastic Surgery,
Billericay, UK

B. Holt FRCA
Department of Anaesthesia,
Manchester Royal Infirmary,
Manchester, UK

P. M. Hopkins MB BS MD FRCA
Senior Lecturer in Anaesthesia;
Honorary Consultant Anaesthetist,
Academic Unit of Aanaesthesia,
St James's University Hospital,
University of Leeds,
Leeds, UK

J. M. Hopkinson FRCA
Senior Registrar in Anaesthesia,
Department of Anaesthesia,
University Hospital of South Manchester,
Manchester, UK

E. Lesley Horsman FRCA
Consultant Anaesthetist,
Department of Anaesthesia,
Central Manchester Healthcare Trust,
Manchester, UK

C. J. Hull MB BS MRCS LRCP(Lon) FFA RCS DA
Honorary Consultant Anaesthetist,
Royal Victoria Infirmary,
Newcastle-Upon-Tyne;
Professor of Anaesthesia,
University of Newcastle,
Newcastle-Upon-Tyne, UK

J. M. Hull FRCA
Consultant Anaesthetist,
Good Hope Hospital NHS Trust,
Sutton Coldfield,
W. Midlands, UK

P. Hutton PhD FRCA
Professor of Anaesthesia,
Queen Elizabeth Hospital,
University of Birmingham,
Birmingham, UK

G. S.Ingram MB BS FRCA
Consultant in Neuroanaesthesia,
The National Hospital for Neurology and Neurosurgery,
Queen Square,
London, UK

A. P. Jackson FRCA
Consultant Cardiac Anaesthetist;
Honorary Clinical Lecturer,
Queen Elizabeth Hospital,
University of Birmingham,
Birmingham, UK

C. Jerwood
Queen Elizabeth Hospital,
University of Birmingham,
Birmingham, UK

M. J. Jones FRCA
Department of Anaesthesia,
Manchester Royal Infirmary,
Manchester, UK

J. Jones Bsc FRCP FFARCS
Consultant Anaesthetist,
Department of Anaesthesia,
St. Mary's Hospital,
London, UK

M. J. Jordan FRCA
Consultant Anaesthetist,
St Peter's Hospital,
Chertsey,
Surrey, UK

B. Keogh
Consultant Anaesthetist,
Royal Brompton Hospital,
London, UK

A. A. Khan FRCOG FRCS FFARCS
Consultant Anaesthetist;
Honorary Clinical Lecturer,
Department of Anaesthesia,
Manchester Royal Infirmary,
Manchester, UK

D. Knights
Clinical Research Fellow,
Queens Medical Centre,
Nottingham, UK

G. Krishnakumar MD MRCP
Assistant Intensivist
King Faisal Specialist Hospital and Research Centre
Riyadh, Saudi Arabia

P. F. S. Lee MB BS DA
Consultant Anaesthetist,
Royal Preston Hospital,
Preston, UK

C. Littler
Senior Resistrar in Anaesthesia,
Manchester Royal Infirmary,
Manchester, UK

A. Loach MA MB BChir FRCA
Consultant Anaesthetist;
Honorary Clinical Lecturer,
Nuffield Department of Anaesthetics,
University of Oxford,
Oxford, UK

C. Lorenzini
Queen Elizabeth Hospital,
University of Birmingham,
Birmingham, UK

A. T. Lovell
Wellcome Training Fellow,
Department of Anaesthesia,
University College London Hospitals,
The Middlesex Hospital,
London, UK

A. Lumb
South Ealing,
London, UK

J. Mackay
Magill Department of Anaesthesia,
Westminster and Chelsea Hospital,
London, UK

S. Mallett
Consultant Anaesthetist,
Royal Free Hospital,
London, UK

A. McCluskey BSc MB ChB FRCA
Senior Registrar in Anaesthesia,
University Hospital of South Manchester,
Manchester, UK

I. McConachie MB ChB FRCA
Consultant Anaesthetist,
Victoria Hospital,
Blackpool, UK

P. J. McKenzie MD FRCA
Consultant Anaesthetist,
John Radcliffe Hospital,
Oxford, UK

T. J. McLeod MB BS FRCA
Senior Registrar,
Queen Elizabeth Hospital,
University of Birmingham,
Birmingham, UK

P. J. McQuillan FRCA FFICANZCA
Consultant in Anaesthesia and Intensive Care Medicine,
Portsmouth Hospitals NHS Trust,
Portsmouth, UK

G. Meakin MD FRCA DA
Senior Lecturer in Paediatric Anaesthesia,
University of Manchester;
Honorary Consultant Paediatric Anaesthetist,
Royal Manchester Children's Hospital,
Manchester, UK

K. Merrett FRCA
Department of Anaesthesia,
St Mary's Hospital,
London, UK

I. M. Mettam MA FRCA
Consultant Anaesthetist,
Shackleton Department of Anaesthesia,
Southampton General Hospital,
Southampton, UK

N. El Mikatti MD FRCA
Consultant Anaesthetist,
South Manchester University Hospitals NHS Trust,
Manchester, UK

R. Milaszkiewicz MB BS FRCA
Consultant Anaesthetist,
Edgeware General Hospital,
Edgeware,
Middlesex, UK

J. P. Millns FRCA
Consultant Anaesthetist,
Birmingham Women's Healthcare NHS Trust,
Edgbaston,
Birmingham, UK

R. K. Mirakhur MD PhD FRCA
Senior Lecturer;
Consultant Anaesthetist,
Department of Anaesthetics,
The Queen's University of Belfast,
Whitla Medical Building,
Belfast, UK

C. Morgan
Consultant Anaesthetist,
Department of Anaesthesia,
Royal Brompton Hospital,
London, UK

A. J. Mortimer BSc MD FRCA
Consultant Anaesthetist,
Department of Anaesthesia,
South Manchester University Hospitals NHS Trust,
Manchester, UK

I. Munday FRCA
Department of Anaesthesia,
St. Mary's Hospital,
London, UK

L. Murdoch
Consultant Anaesthetist,
Royal Brompton National Heart & Lung Hospital,
London, UK

P. Newman FRCA
Senior Registrar in Intensive Care,
Department of Anaesthesia,
St George's Hospital Medical School,
London, UK

N. Newton MB ChB FRCA DA
Consultant Anaesthetist,
Department of Anaesthesia,
Guy's Hospital,
London, UK

M. E. Nicol FRCA
Consultant Anaesthetist,
Department of Anaesthesia,
Southend Healthcare NHS Trust,
Southend-on-Sea, UK

P. Nightingale FRCA MRCP
Consultant in Anaesthesia and Intensive Care,
Intensive Care Unit,
University Hospitals of South Manchester NHS Trust,
Manchester, UK

D. Nolan FRCA
Consultant Anaesthetist,
University Hospitals of South Manchester NHS Trust,
Manchester, UK

D. O'Malley RGN
Acute Pain Service,
Department of Anaesthesia,
Manchester Royal Infirmary,
Manchester, UK

G. O'Sullivan MD FRCA
Consultant Anaesthetist,
St. Thomas' Hospital,
London, UK

D. Ostergaard MD
Consultant Anaesthetist,
Department of Anaesthesiology,
Gentofte Hospital,
Hellerup, Denmark

H. Owen-Reece BSc FRCA
Registrar in Anaesthesia
University College London Hospitals
Middlesex Hospital
London, UK

J. H. McG. Palmer
Senior Registrar in Anaesthesia,
Manchester Royal Infirmary,
Manchester, UK

D. K. Patel MB ChB FFARCS
Consultant Anaesthetist,
Mount Vernon Hospital,
Northwood,
Middlesex, UK

V. Patla
Queen Elizabeth Hospital,
University of Birmingham,
Birmingham, UK

J. Payne
Queen Elizabeth Hospital,
University of Birmingham,
Birmingham, UK

T. Peachey
Consultant Anaesthetist,
Royal Free Hospital,
London, UK

A. Pearce
Department of Anaesthesia,
Guy's Hospital,
London, UK

D. Phillips MB ChB FRCA
Consultant Anaesthetist,
Lincoln County Hospital,
Lincoln, UK

S. Piggott FRCA
Consultant Anaesthetist,
Derby City General Hospital,
Derby, UK

B. J. Pollard B.Pharm MD FRCA
Senior Lecturer in Anaesthesia,
University Department of Anaesthesia,
Manchester Royal Infirmary,
Manchester, UK

C. J. D. Pomfrett BSc PhD
Lecturer in Neurophysiology,
University Department of Anaesthesia,
Manchester Royal Infirmary,
Manchester, UK

S. Porter
The National Hospital for Neurology and Neurosurgery,
Department of Neuroanaesthesia,
Queen Square,
London, UK

D. Potter MB BS FRCA
Consultant Anaesthetist,
Liver Transplantation Anaesthetic Service,
Kings College Hospital,
London, UK

J. Powell MB BS FRCA
Senior Registrar in Anaesthesia,
Cambridge University Teaching Hospitals NHS Trust,
Cambridge, UK

M. L. Price BSc MB BS FRCA
Consultant Anaesthetist,
Department of Anaesthesia,
St. Mary's Hospital,
London, UK

A. C. Quinn MB ChB FFARCSI
Lecturer in Anaesthesia,
Academic Unit of Anaesthesia,
St George's Hospital Medical School,
Leeds General Infirmary,
Leeds, UK

P. C. Randall BM FRCA
Consultant in Anaesthesia and Intensive Care,
Department of Anaesthesia,
Victoria Hospital,
Blackpool, UK

N. Redfern FRCA BSc
Consultant Obstetric Anaesthetist,
Royal Victoria Infirmary,
Newcastle-Upon-Tyne, UK

H. O. Reece
Registrar in Anaesthesia,
University College London Hospitals School of Medicine,
Middlesex Hospital,
London, UK

M. Rela MS FRCS
Consultant Surgeon Liver Transplant Surgery,
Kings College Hospital,
London, UK

D. W. Riddington FRCA
Lecturer in Anaesthesia and Intensive Care,
University of Birmingham Medical School,
Queen Elizabeth Hospital,
Birmingham, UK

S. P. Roberts MA FRCA
Consultant Anaesthetist,
South Manchester University Hospitals NHS Trust,
Withington Hospital,
Manchester, UK

E. J. Roberts FRCA
Shackleton Department of Anaesthesia,
Southampton General Hospital,
Southampton, UK

G. Robson FRCA
Consultant Anaesthetist,
North Manchester General Hospital,
Manchester, UK

S. C. Robson
Senior Lecturer in Obstetrics and Gynaecology,
Department of Obstetrics and Gynaecology,
Royal Victoria Infirmary,
Newcastle-upon-Tyne, UK

R. G. Rowlands MB ChB FRCA
Registrar in Anaesthesia,
Royal Lancaster Infirmary,
Lancaster, UK

I. F. Russell FRCA BMedBiol
Consultant Anaesthetist;
Honorary Senior Fellow,
Department of Psychology,
Hull Royal Infirmary,
Hull, UK

A. Sanchez-Capuchino LMC FRCA FFARCSI
Consultant Anaesthetist,
Stepping Hill Hospital,
Stockport,
Cheshire, UK

P. Saunders MB BS FFA RCS
Consultant Anaesthetist,
Royal Surrey County Hospital,
Guildford,
Surrey, UK

M. Scanlan FRCA
Consultant Anaesthetist,
Royal Brompton Hospital,
London, UK

S. M. Scuplak
The National Hospital for Neurology and Neurosurgery,
Department of Neuroanaethesia,
Queen Square,
London, UK

R. F. Seal MD FRCPC
Assistant Clinical Professor;
Chief of Paediatric Anesthesia,
Children's Health Centre of Northern Alberta,
Edmonton,
Alberta, Canada

A. Severn MA FRCA
Consultant Anaesthetist,
East Cheshire NHS Trust,
Macclesfield, UK

R. M. Sharpe
The National Hospital for Neurology and Neurosurgery,
Queen Square,
London, UK

J. Shaw FRCA
Consultant Anaesthetist,
Department of Anaesthesia,
Manchester Royal Infirmary,
Manchester, UK

A. C. Shukla FRCA
Research Fellow,
Department of Anaesthetics,
The Middlesex Hospital,
London, UK

M. Simpson FRCA
Consultant Anaesthetist,
Department of Anaesthesia,
Manchester Royal Infirmary,
Manchester, UK

R. M. Slater FRCA
Consultant Anaesthetist,
Department of Anaesthesia,
Manchester Royal Infirmary,
Manchester, UK

G. Smith BM FRCA
Consultant Anaesthetist,
Intensive Care Unit,
Queen Alexandra Hospital,
Portsmouth Hospitals NHS Trust,
Cosham,
Portsmouth, UK

M. Smith MB BS FRCA
Consultant Neuro Anaesthetist,
Surgical ITU,
The National Hospital For Neurology &
Neurosurgery,
Queen Square,
London, UK

N. Soni MD FANZCA FRICANZCA FRCA
Senior Lecturer,
Magill Department of Anaesthesia,
Westminster and Chelsea Hospital,
London, UK

S. Stainthorpe
Consultant Anaesthetist,
Booth Hall Children's Hospital,
Manchester, UK

J. C. Stanley FFARCS(I)
Consultant Anaesthetist,
Royal Victoria Hospital,
Whitla Medical Building,
Lisburn Road,
Belfast, UK

M. Stokes FRCA
Queen Elizabeth Hospital,
University of Birmingham,
Birmingham, UK

D. Stott FRCA
Consultant Anaesthetist,
University Hospital of South Manchester,
Manchester, UK

T. Strang MB ChB FRCA DCH
Consultant Anaesthetist,
Department of Anaesthesia,
Manchester Royal Infirmary,
Manchester, UK

B. L. Taylor Bsc FRCA FFICANZCA
Consultant in Anaesthesia and Intensive Care
Medicine,
Portsmouth Hospitals NHS Trust,
Portsmouth, UK

V. Taylor
Royal National Orthopaedic Hospital,
Stanmore,
Middlesex, UK

D. Thomas
Department of Obstetrics and Gynaecology,
Leazes Wing,
Royal Victoria Infirmary,
Newcastle-upon-Tyne, UK

E. A. Thornberry FRCA
Consultant Anaesthetist,
Queen Alexandra Hospital,
Cosham,
Portsmouth, UK

N. M. Tierney BSc MB ChB FRCA
Consultant Anaesthetist,
Department of Anaesthesia,
Bury General Hospital,
Bury, UK

D. Tupper-Carey FRCA
Senior Registrar in Anaesthesia,
Department of Anaesthesia,
Manchester Royal Infirmary,
Manchester, UK

N. M. Turner
Queen Elizabeth Hospital,
University of Birmingham,
Birmingham, UK

R. Vanner FRCA
Consultant Anaesthetist,
Gloucestershire Royal Hospital,
Gloucester, UK

S. Varley FRCA
Senior Registrar in Anaesthesia,
North Western Regional Health Authority, UK

J. Viby-Mogensen MD DMSc
Professor and Chairman,
Department of Anaethesia and Intensive Care,
The National University Hospital,
Rigshospitalet,
Blegdamsvej, Denmark

A. Vohra MB ChB DA FRCA
Consultant Anaesthetist,
Department of Anaesthesia,
Manchester Royal Infirmary,
Manchester, UK

R. Walker FRCA
Consultant Paediatric Anaesthetist,
Royal Manchester Childrenís Hospital,
Pendlesbury,
Manchester, UK

M. Wall
Stanford University School of Medicine,
Stanford, USA

P. Ward
St Mary's Hospital,
Department of Anaesthesia,
London, UK

N. Watson FRCA
Department of Anaesthetics,
St Mary's Hospital,
London, UK

M. Weisz FRCA
Department of Anaesthesia,
St Mary's Hospital,
London, UK

D. M. Weston
Department of Neuroanaesthesia,
The National Hospital for Neurology and
Neurosurgery,
Queen Square,
London, UK

R. S. Wheatly FRCA
Consultant Anaesthetist,
Wythershaw Hospital,
Manchester, UK

M. P. Wilkes
Queen Elizabeth Hospital,
University of Birmingham,
Birmingham, UK

S. Wilson MB BS FRCA
Consultant in Neuroanaesthesia,
The National Hospital for Neurology and
Neurosurgery,
Queen Square,
London, UK

W. Wooldrige
Consultant Anaesthetist,
Wythershaw Hospital,
Manchester, UK

J. D. Young DM FRCA
Clinical Reader in Anaesthetics,
Nuffield Department of Anaesthetics,
The Radcliffe Infirmary,
Oxford, UK

PREFACE

Conventional wisdom orders textbooks into large chapters which logically begin with the basic science and then the clinical information follows. This approach enables many readers to begin the task of understanding new information but demands time of those who are already informed; additional information on any given subject may need to be sought from other areas of the book or possibly other textbooks. An alternative approach is to gather information from journals and monographs. Although review articles offer a definitive overview these may not be available within a department to a clinician at the appropriate time. For many, a more rapid access to relevant facts is desirable.

We have approached this problem by producing this comprehensive guide. Each article is designed to present all necessary information in a concise form written by individual clinicians who appreciate the difficulty of assimilating knowledge during the busy working day. Each article has a consistent format, beginning with pathophysiology and continuing through the anaesthetic sequence in the form of headline information and bullet lists. This format is repeated throughout the text.

The way in which the articles are collected together is problem oriented and has been arranged in the same way as problems appear clinically. Thus a surgical list is often the starting point and many simply mention a hernia repair, thyroidectomy or varicose vein excision. At the preoperative visit the problems may become apparent. The patient in whom a simple hernia repair is proposed may also have an underlying medical condition; for example, decompensated lung disease. Further problems may relate to the surgical procedure itself. Thyroidectomy demands access to the neck and the airway may be compromised. Finally, the last patient undergoing a simple surgical procedure may require a particular anaesthetic technique; for example total intravenous anaesthesia. This textbook is therefore divided into these three areas or sections. Firstly, the *Patient Condition* which deals with coexisting disease and the anaesthetic implications. The next section is *Surgical Procedures*, which considers individual operations which have a direct impact on anaesthetic technique. Lastly, *Anaesthetic Factors*, describes how an anaesthetic is performed from assessment through to predicting outcome. The interrelations between subjects within these three areas is emphasised and can be easily illustrated (Figure 1).

In this problem oriented system there will be patients where the pre-existing medical condition overlaps with the proposed surgery and anaesthetic technique. Such a patient represents the overlap between the three elements which order this textbook. In order to facilitate the movement between the three sections and to emphasise this overlap we have included a cross referencing dialogue box at the end of each article.

The three major sections are further divided into Subsections which are ordered

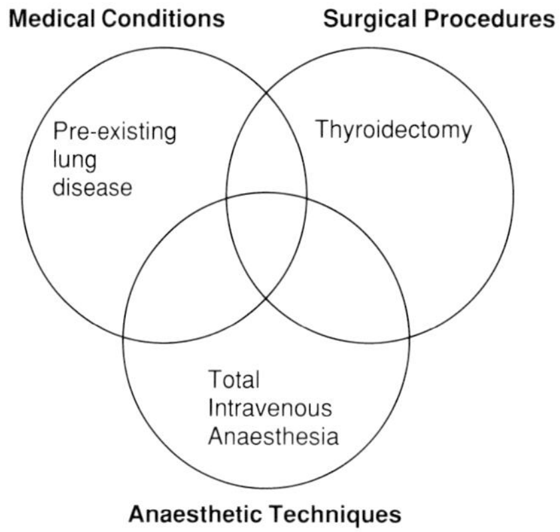

Figure 1
An anaesthetist may be presented with different types of preoperative problems and these are divided between the sections Medical Conditions, Surgical Procedures and Anaesthetic Techniques.

systematically (cardiovascular, respiratory etc). In order to find the relevant article, one must first decide which is the relevant section. For example, for the anaesthetic considerations of a patient with hypothyroidism, the article would be found in the Patient Conditions section and the Endocrine subsection. Thyroidectomy appears in the Surgical Procedures section, Head and Neck subsection etc.

There will be many ways of using this textbook and we hope that there will be an easy method of finding the headline details in any given situation. Inevitably, our ordering system will not encompass every clinical scenario, yet we believe that many half remembered facts will be quickly found and the less common case or unfamiliar technique remembered. We feel that these articles are the beginning of the story. For additional details, the reader will still need to consult the major texts in the subject. Some of the links between the individual articles are in place and as such they represent islands in a vast sea of knowledge. The approach may in the future be electronic in format and at that stage all the islands will be linked together. For the time being, we feel that this text will serve to guide clinicians during the busy clinical day.

London J.C.G.
Manchester B.J.P.
1996

PART 1

PATIENT CONDITIONS

1

CENTRAL NERVOUS SYSTEM

N. P. Hirsch
M. Smith

AUTONOMIC DYSFUNCTION

N. P. Hirsch

Autonomic dysfunction (dysautonomia) may be either a result of a central nervous disorder or, more commonly, a disorder of the peripheral nervous system (Table 1).

Table 1.
Classification of clinically important autonomic neuropathies

Central nervous system disorders
Pure autonomic failure
Autonomic failure with multisystem atrophy (Shy–Drager syndrome)
Autonomic failure with Parkinson's disease
Peripheral nervous system disorders
Diabetes
Primary amyloidosis
Porphyria
Guillain–Barré syndrome
Familial dysautonomia (Riley–Day syndrome)

PATHOPHYSIOLOGY

Although the pathophysiological mechanisms causing the autonomic dysfunction vary depending on the aetiology, the symptoms that result are remarkably similar.

Cardiovascular

In normal individuals, assumption of the erect position from the supine position results in a transient fall in arterial blood pressure due to a decrease in the venous return to the heart. Compensatory mechanisms involving aortic and carotid baroreceptors and the vasomotor and cardioinhibitory centres result in an increase in vasomotor tone and heart rate. Arterial blood pressure is rapidly returned to normal levels. In patients with autonomic dysfunction, the compensatory mechanisms are impaired, and on standing a sustained period of hypotension follows (orthostatic hypotension). Similarly, the response to the Valsalva manoeuvre is abnormal.

Respiratory system

Heart rate normally increases during inspiration (sinus arrhythmia) due to inhibition of the cardioinhibitory vasomotor centres by the central inspiratory drive centres. This response is lost in some forms of autonomic dysfunction.

In the Shy–Drager syndrome, abductor vocal cord paralysis may result in problems with phonation and in inspiratory stridor. Poor central respiratory control, weakness of respiratory muscles and recurrent aspiration pneumonia are common features of familial dysautonomia.

Gut

Disorders of oesophageal and gastric motility may occur, as may poor sphincter control. Gastric emptying may be delayed, resulting in greater than normal resting gastric volume. Constipation may be a feature.

Genitourinary system

Urinary retention is common, as is impotence.

Other

The normal sweating response may be impaired.

PREOPERATIVE ASSESSMENT AND TREATMENT

History

- Of underlying disorder if present (e.g. diabetes mellitus) and any coexisting disorder (e.g. ischaemic heart disease)
- Of postural hypotension, syncope, intestinal stasis and disorders of sweating
- In the case of the Shy–Drager syndrome, look for history of problems with phonation associated with vocal-cord paralysis.

Investigations

- Assessment of the underlying medical disorder

- Response of heart rate (using R–R interval of ECG) to altered posture and to the Valsalva manoeuvre
- More specialized investigations, including sympathetic skin response testing, sweat tests and plasma catecholamine levels.

Preoperative treatment

In most cases, autonomic disturbances are not of sufficient severity to warrant specific preoperative therapy. If postural hypotension is causing symptoms, treatment is directed to increasing blood volume by increasing dietary intake of salt, and by the use of fludrocortisone. Simple measures such as the wearing of graded elastic stockings may help.

In the period leading up to surgery, attention should be directed towards ensuring adequate hydration, using intravenous crystalloid if necessary.

PERIOPERATIVE MANAGEMENT

Premedication

Drugs which have major effects on the autonomic system (e.g. anticholinergic drugs, the phenothiazines and butyrophenones) should be avoided. If premedication is necessary, a benzodiazepine should be given.

H_2 receptor antagonists should be given to patients with delayed gastric emptying.

Monitoring

- Should start in the anaesthetic room
- ECG (CM_5)
- Blood pressure measurement (via indwelling arterial cannula if autonomic dysfunction is severe)
- Spo_2
- Central venous pressure or pulmonary capillary wedge pressure measurement, if indicated
- Temperature measurement (poor temperature homeostasis may result in hypothermia if procedure is prolonged).

Induction and maintenance of anaesthesia

Induction of anaesthesia and the maintenance of anaesthesia with volatile anaesthetic agents may cause precipitous falls in arterial blood pressure in this group of patients. Such agents must therefore be used with great care and in the lowest doses possible. Similarly, the introduction of IPPV may cause hypotension.

A rapid sequence induction may be indicated in those patients with delayed gastric emptying and those with a history of recurrent aspiration.

If hypotension occurs, treat initially with a fluid challenge. If this proves unsuccessful, give a small dose of an α receptor agonist (e.g. methoxamine). Be aware that this may result in a large rise in arterial blood pressure. If bradycardia is present, this is readily treated with an anticholinergic drug.

Regional anaesthesia

The hypotensive effect of extradural and spinal anaesthesia may be exaggerated in these patients.

POSTOPERATIVE CARE

- Maintain adequate hydration.
- Adequate postoperative pain relief is essential. Apnoea following narcotic administration is common.
- Stridor may occur in the postoperative period in the Shy–Drager syndrome.

BIBLIOGRAPHY

Axelrod F B, Donenfield R F, Danzier F, Turndorf H. Anaesthesia in familial dysautonomia. Anesthesiology 1988; 68: 631–635

Drury P M E, Williams E G N. Vocal cord paralysis in the Shy–Drager syndrome. Anaesthesia 1991; 46: 466–468

Hutchinson R C, Sugden J C. Anaesthesia for Shy–Drager syndrome. Anaesthesia 1984; 39: 1229–1231

CROSS REFERENCES

Diabetes mellitus (IDDM)
Patient Conditions 2: 42
Intraoperative hypotension
Anaesthetic Factors 33: 638

1

EPILEPSY

Martin Smith

Epilepsy is a common disorder occurring in approximately 1 in 200 of the general population. It is the manifestation of an underlying disorder of neuronal activity. Although there has been considerable progress in the medical treatment of epilepsy in recent years, some patients remain refractory or intolerant to therapy. Surgery may now be considered in this group of patients if there is a discrete seizure focus which may be resected without producing neurological deficits.

PATHOPHYSIOLOGY

Electrical activity in the brain is normally well controlled, but in epileptogenic disorders normal brain regulatory functions are altered. Sudden and disordered neuronal activity is responsible for the clinical manifestations of epilepsy. In epilepsy there is:

- Loss of postsynaptic inhibition
- Introduction of significant excitatory synaptic connections
- The appearance of pacemaker neurones.

Pacemaker neurones appear to be the centre of the epileptic focus and have the capacity to spontaneously produce burst discharges. Interictal EEG spikes, pathognomonic of certain classes of epilepsy, originate in this area. Increase in cellular activity and loss of inhibitory tone in the pacemaker zone lead to frank seizure activity, as uncontrolled neuronal firing spreads to surrounding areas. Spread of epileptic discharge from the pacemaker zone occurs because of:

- Membrane changes and alteration in ion flux
- Impaired GABA-mediated synaptic inhibition
- Local alteration in neurotransmitter levels.

CLASSIFICATION

Epilepsy may be generalized or partial (Table 1). Generalized epilepsies occur in 20% of patients with epilepsy, involve both hemispheres and are associated with an initial impairment of consciousness. Partial epilepsies have clinical signs and EEG findings reflecting initial discharge limited to a discrete area of one hemisphere. The typical EEG finding is the interictal spike. In simple partial epilepsy, the seizure remains a focal discharge and there is no impairment of consciousness. Complex partial seizures are the most common seizure disorder and are associated with secondary loss of consciousness. This latter group includes temporal lobe epilepsy.

Table 1.
Classification of the epilepsies

Classification of the epilepsies
Generalized epilepsies
Generalized absence (petit mal)
Generalized tonic–clonic (grand mal)
Myoclonic
Atonic/tonic (drop attacks)
Partial epilepsies
Simple partial
Complex partial (includes psychomotor/temporal lobe)

ANTICONVULSANT THERAPY

The aim of medical treatment in epilepsy is a seizure-free patient with minimal side-effects. Correct choice of anticonvulsant involves consideration of seizure type (Table 2), seizure history, patient age and side-effects.

Therapy is initiated with a single agent given in a dose sufficient to produce adequate plasma levels. If seizures continue, or if unacceptable side-effects develop, a second agent is substituted for the first. Should single therapy remain insufficient, combination therapy is initiated, with attention being paid to drug interactions.

Anticonvulsant agents have side-effects which

Table 2.
Toxicities, first-line indications and therapeutic levels of anticonvulsants drugs

Drug	Therapeutic level (μmol.l^{-1})	First-line therapy for seizure type	Side-effects
Phenytoin	25–80	Complex Grand mal Tonic–clonic	Rash, hypersensitivity, gingival hyperplasia, ataxia, megaloblastic anaemia, neuropathy, encephalopathy, Stevens–Johnson syndrome
Sodium valproate	350–700	Grand mal Tonic–clonic	Tremor, weight gain, alopecia, thrombocytopenia, raised hepatic transaminase, hepatic failure
Carbamezapine	34–50	Complex	Rash, diplopia, sedation, thrombocytopenia, leukopenia, cholestatic jaundice, hyponatraemia
Phenobarbitone	65–170	Complex	Rash, hypersensitivity, sedation, megaloblastic anaemia, folate deficiency, osteomalacia
Ethosuxamide	280–700	Petit mal	Nausea, vomiting, sedation, confusion, ataxia, photophobia, thrombocytopenia
Primidone	23–60	Complex	Ataxia, nystagmus, sedation, thrombocytopenia, leukopenia
Vigabatrin	39–271	Not first-line therapy	Sedation, irritability, aggression, psychosis, weight gain, mild anaemia
Lamotrigine	4–16	Not first-line therapy	Rash, diplopia, dizziness, sedation, headache, ataxia, irritability, gastrointestinal disturbance, Stevens–Johnson syndrome

are of interest to the anaesthetist; these and their therapeutic levels are shown in Table 2.

PREOPERATIVE ASSESSMENT

The patient's history should be evaluated in relation to the epilepsy and other coexisting medical problems. Particular attention should be paid to:

- Seizure frequency
- Seizure type and pattern
- Current anticonvulsant therapy (including plasma levels)
- Complications of anticonvulsant therapy (Table 3)
- IQ (poorly controlled, chronic epilepsy may be associated with low IQ).

Anticonvulsant therapy must be continued up to and including the day of surgery. Plasma anticonvulsant levels must be checked and the dose adjusted to ensure adequate levels. Premedication may be prescribed as required, and benzodiazepines are appropriate.

ANAESTHETIC AGENTS AND THE EEG

Anaesthetic agents affect the EEG to varying degrees. Some have minimal EEG effects, others have an anticonvulsant action, whilst others may activate the EEG and precipitate seizures.

Barbiturates

Most barbiturates are anticonvulsants at normal clinical doses, and thiopentone may be used to control seizures. Thiopentone infusion has also been used in the treatment of status epilepticus. Methohexitone, however, activates the EEG, especially in those with temporal lobe epilepsy.

Propofol

There have been varying reports of the effects of propofol on the EEG. Activation in temporal lobe epilepsy has been described, as well as seizures and opisthotonos in patients with no history of seizures. Conversely, however, anticonvulsant effects have also been reported and propofol has been successfully used in the treatment of status epilepticus resistant to other therapies. Recent work suggests that the effect of propofol is dose related, with EEG activation occurring at small doses and anticonvulsant activity (ultimately burst suppression) at normal clinical doses. Further elucidation of the effects of propofol on the normal and pathological EEG is awaited.

Table 3.
Complications of anticonvulsant therapy with implications for the anaesthetist

Gingival hypertrophy/poor dentition
Phenytoin
Anaemia
Phenytoin
Phenobarbitone
Vigabatrin
Thrombocytopenia
Sodium valproate
Carbamezapine
Ethosuxamide
Primidone
Leukopenia
Carbamezapine
Primidone
Hyopnatraemia
Carbamezapine
Abnormal liver function tests
Sodium valproate
Carbamezapine
Sedation
Phenobarbitone
Ethosuxamide
Primidone
Vigabatrin
Lamotrigine

1

Benzodiazepines

Diazepam and other benzodiazepines have anticonvulsant EEG effects and are widely used in the treatment of seizures.

Inhalational anaesthetics

The EEG effects of inhalational anaesthetic agents are dose dependent. EEG activity is maintained with isoflurane levels below 1 MAC, although background epileptiform activity may be suppressed. Low-dose isoflurane has been used in the treatment of resistant status epilepticus. Higher inspired levels of isoflurane have profound effects on the EEG and at levels of >2 MAC the EEG becomes isoelectric. The effects of halothane are similar to isoflurane, with background epileptic activity being suppressed at clinically useful concentrations. Enflurane, in high concentration, has a convulsant activity which is more marked in the presence of hypocarbia. Dose-dependent EEG changes occur secondary to nitrous oxide, with anticonvulsant effects at higher inspired concentrations.

Opiates

Opiates in usual clinical dosage have minimal effect on the EEG. Fentanyl at moderate doses ($25\ \mu g\ kg^{-1}$) causes activation of the EEG, whereas high-dose opiate techniques result in EEG slowing.

Local anaesthetics

Lignocaine has a biphasic effect on the EEG. At low plasma levels it has anticonvulsant-like actions, whilst at high levels it causes excitation of the central nervous system, including the provocation of seizures.

ANAESTHETIC TECHNIQUE

Patients with epilepsy may present for surgery for incidental conditions, following injury during a seizure or for neurosurgery for medically intractable epilepsy. General or local anaesthesia may be provided using standard techniques which avoid factors known to precipitate seizures (Table 4). Anaesthetic agents which are proconvulsant at usual clinical doses should be avoided (see above). The side-effects of anticonvulsant therapy should also be considered when planning the anaesthetic technique (Table 3).

Table 4.
Causes of seizures in the perioperative period

Cause
Pre-existing epilepsy
Hypoxia
Hypercarbia
Proconvulsant drugs/anaesthetic agents
Electrolyte disturbances
Hyponatraemia
Hypoglycaemia
Uraemia
Related disorders
Head injury
Eclampsia

POSTOPERATIVE CARE

Postoperative care is directed towards the nature of the surgery. It is essential to continue anticonvulsant therapy into the postoperative period, and anticonvulsant levels must be checked postoperatively. Some anticonvulsants (e.g. carbamezapine) have no parenteral preparation and in a sedated patient should be administered via a nasogastric tube or as a suppository.

Recurrent seizures, leading to status epilepticus, are more common in the postoperative period. They may be precipitated by use of proconvulsant drugs or anaesthetic agents, hypoxia or electrolyte disturbances (Table 4). Treatment of seizures in the postoperative period must be rapid and aggressive and precipitating factors should be corrected. Seizures should be rapidly terminated with a short-acting anticonvulsant such as thiopentone or a benzodiazapine. A top-up dose of the long-acting anticonvulsant should be added if plasma levels are low. Recurrent seizures or status epilepticus should be treated with infusion of chlormethiazole and the patient monitored in a HDU. Ventilatory support may be required. Muscle relaxants will prevent acidosis from the intense muscle activity associated with seizures. Continuous EEG monitoring is mandatory under such circumstances. Problematic seizures in the postoperative period must be investigated with formal 16-lead EEG and continuously monitored with processed EEG techniques such as the CFAM.

BIBLIOGRAPHY

Modica P A, Tempelhoff R, White P F. Pro- and anti-convulsant effects of anaesthetics (part 1). Anesthesia and Analgesia 1990; 70: 303–315

Modica P A, Tempelhoff R, White P F. Pro- and anti-convulsant effects of anaesthetics (part 2). Anesthesia and Analgesia 1990; 70: 433–443

Smith M. Anaesthesia in epilepsy surgery. In: Shorvon S, Dreifus F, Fish D, Thomas D (eds). The treatment of epilepsy. Blackwells Science, Oxford, Ch 62, p 794–804

Smith M. Anaesthesia for epilepsy and stereotactic surgery. In: Walters F J M, Ingram G S, Jenkinson J L (eds). Anaesthesia and intensive care for the neurosurgical patient. Blackwell Scientific Publications, London, ch 12, p 318–344

GUILLAIN–BARRÉ SYNDROME

N. P. Hirsch

Guillain–Barré syndrome (GBS) is an acute infective neuropathy characterized by progressive neuropathic weakness of more than one limb and areflexia. Criteria necessary for diagnosis may be divided into essential and supportive criteria (Table 1).

Table 1.
Diagnostic criteria for Guillain–Barré syndrome

Essential criteria
- Progressive weakness of more than one limb due to neuropathy
- Areflexia
- Duration of progression less than 4 weeks

Supportive criteria
Clinical features:
- Weakness is usually symmetrical
- Sensory signs are mild
- Cranial nerve involvement common
- Autonomic dysfunction common

Laboratory features:
- CSF – after first week, total protein content increased (in 80%); white cell count near normal (in 90%)
- EMG – nerve conduction slowed, suggesting demyelination

PATHOPHYSIOLOGY

Incidence is 1–2 per 100 000 of the population. In 60% of cases of GBS, the condition is preceded (usually 1–2 weeks before) by a viral infection (often affecting the respiratory or gastrointestinal tract). Commonly implicated organisms include cytomegalovirus, Epstein–Barr and human immunodeficiency viruses as well as *Mycoplasma pneumoniae* and *Campylobacter jejuni* bacteria. Antibody mediated demyelination following infection has been proposed as the pathogenesis of GBS.

CLINICAL FEATURES

Neurological

GBS starts with pain, mild sensory symptoms and weakness. Weakness is usually symmetrical and is more pronounced proximally. Cranial nerves (especially facial and bulbar nerves) are commonly affected. Areflexia occurs early and urinary retention is common. The Miller–Fisher variant of GBS is characterized by external ophthalmoplegia, diminished pupillary reflexes, ataxia and areflexia.

Respiratory system

Respiratory muscle weakness requiring positive pressure ventilation occurs in 25–30% of patients. Bulbar dysfunction occurs in a similar proportion and may require tracheal intubation for airway protection.

Autonomic dysfunction

Approximately 70% of patients show a persistent tachycardia with or without accompanying paroxysmal hypertension. Postural hypotension occurs in 20% of patients. Cardiac arrhythmias may include bradycardia and asystole. ECG changes include T-wave inversion. Excessive sweating occurs in 30% of patients.

Metabolic derangements

Hyponatraemia occurs commonly and may be related to excessive ADH secretion.

TREATMENT

Mortality is in the range 2–13%, depending on severity, where nursed, etc.

General care

- Good general medical and nursing care (including monitoring) are essential
- Early tracheal intubation is indicated if respiratory muscle weakness occurs (i.e. if vital capacity falls) or bulbar function is compromised
- Tracheostomy should be performed early if it is obvious that a prolonged period of artificial ventilation is necessary
- Measures to prevent deep venous thrombosis and pulmonary embolus (e.g. subcutaneous heparin therapy, graded elastic stocking, etc.) are mandatory.

Plasma exchange

Accelerates recovery if performed within 2 weeks of onset of the disease. Patients likely to benefit most are those exchanged within 1 week of onset of symptoms and those with rapid deterioration of limb power.

Immunoglobulin

High dose intravenous immunoglobulin (Ig) therapy appears to be effective in accelerating recovery in GBS. The relative efficacy of plasma exchange and intravenous Ig (or a combination of the two) has yet to be determined.

Steroids

A number of series have failed to show any benefit of steroid therapy.

ANAESTHETIC CONSIDERATIONS

Patients usually present for elective tracheostomy and are already intubated.

Preoperative assessment:

- If unintubated, assess airway, mouth, dentition, neck. Special examination of bulbar function to assess risk of pulmonary aspiration at induction.
- Assess respiratory muscle function – vital capacity, mouth occlusion pressures, cough.
- Assess automonic function – ECG, postural hypotension, excessive sweating.

Investigations

Electrolyte determination for signs of dehydration or hyponatraemia.

Perioperative management:

- Monitoring should include ECG, noninvasive/invasive BP monitoring, oxygen saturation
- If bulbar function is poor or if a full stomach is suspected, a rapid sequence induction is indicated
- Suxamethonium should be avoided in the chronic stages of the condition, as widespread denervation may result in hyperkalaemia

- If respiratory muscle weakness is present, the patient's lungs should be ventilated during surgery
- Nondepolarizing muscle relaxants should be used sparingly, and with neuromuscular monitoring.

Postoperative management

- Adequate pain relief must be administered, even if this means a period of postoperative ventilation is necessary
- Monitoring of postoperative respiratory function should ideally be carried out in an intensive care setting.

BIBLIOGRAPHY

Guillain–Barré Syndrome Study Group. Plasmapheresis for acute Guillain–Barré syndrome. Neurology 1985; 35: 1096–1104

Hughes R A C. Guillain–Barré syndrome. Springer-Verlag, London, 1990

Van der Merche F G A, Schmitz P I M, Dutch Guillain–Barré Study Group. A randomized trial comparing intravenous immunoglobulin and plasma exchange in Guillain–Barré syndrome. New England Journal of Medicine 1992; 326: 1123–1129

CROSS REFERENCES

Autonomic dysfunction
Patient Conditions 1: 4

Weaning from mechanical ventilation
Anaesthetic Factors 33: 677

HEAD INJURY

R. M. Sharpe and M. Smith

The anaesthetist plays a key role in the management of head injured patients during initial resuscitation, interhospital transfer and anaesthesia for both neurosurgical and non-neurosurgical trauma. Early aggressive resuscitation results in improved outcome.

PATHOPHYSIOLOGY

This is divided into primary and secondary brain injury.

Primary brain damage occurs at the time of injury as a direct result of impact or acceleration/deceleration forces on the brain. Primary brain damage may be due to skull fracture, diffuse axonal injury and intracranial haematoma.

Secondary brain damage occurs some time after the initial insult and is a cause of significant morbidity and mortality. It is caused by a reduction in cerebral perfusion and oxygenation. This results in inadequate oxygen delivery, build up of toxic metabolites and neuronal swelling and death.

The commonest causes of secondary brain damage are:

- Hypoxaemia
- Hypotension
- Raised intracranial pressure (ICP).

Autoregulation may be lost following head injury and cerebral perfusion pressure (CPP) becomes dependent on mean arterial pressure (MAP):

$$CPP = MAP - ICP$$

It is necessary to maintain MAP at supranormal levels in the presence of an elevated ICP. Of head injuries in coma, 70% have a raised ICP. *Secondary cerebral injury is preventable by prompt and adequate resuscitation.* The clinical causes of secondary brain damage are listed in Table 1.

Table 1.
Causes of secondary brain damage

Hypotension
Hypoxaemia
Raised ICP secondary to:
  Haematoma
  Hypercapnia
  Cerebral oedema
Seizures
Meningitis

PRIMARY TREATMENT/RESUSCITATION

Airway

This must be cleared of blood, teeth and foreign bodies and protected if necessary. Table 2 lists the indications for tracheal intubation. If intubation is necessary, a sleep dose of thiopentone or propofol should be used to attenuate the rise in ICP associated with laryngoscopy. Hypotension should, however, be avoided. A full stomach must be assumed and suxamethonium used to facilitate intubation during a rapid sequence induction.

Table 2.
Indications for intubating the head-injured patient

Airway protection:
- Loss of protective laryngeal reflexes
- Unconscious patient (GCS <8)
- Copious bleeding into the mouth
- Facial injuries compromising the airway

Hypoventilation:
- Hypoxaemia (P_aO_2 <9 kPa on air)
- Hypercapnia (P_aCO_2 >6 kPa)
- Spontaneous hyperventilation (P_aCO_2, <3.5 kPa)
- Associated chest injury

In preparation for transfer:
- If neurological deterioration is likely in transit
- If seizures have occurred
- Unconscious patient (GCS <8)

The neck must be immobilized by in line cervical stabilization or a stiff neck collar, as there is a high association between head injury and cervical spine fracture.

Breathing

Inadequate ventilation may be central or peripheral in origin. Central causes result from cerebral damage or cervical cord injury, whereas peripheral causes include airway obstruction, aspiration, and chest injuries such as pneumothorax.

Rapid correction of hypoventilation is essential to prevent secondary brain damage due to hypoxaemia and a rise in ICP secondary to hypercapnia. Moderate hyperventilation (P_aCO_2 3.8–4.2) is a useful means of emergency control of ICP.

Circulation

Hypotension results in reduced cerebral perfusion. *Closed head injury is never a cause of hypotension in adults*, and other injuries should be sought. Volume replacement may be achieved with 0.9% saline, colloid and/or blood. Dextrose solutions are best avoided, as glucose is metabolized to lactate in the ischaemic brain and high lactate levels adversely affect outcome.

Dysfunction (neurological)

Initial consciousness level is assessed using the Glasgow Coma Scale (GCS) (Table 3). In addition, localizing signs and pupillary reaction are noted.

Examine

A full examination should be performed looking for other injuries. Treatment of life-threatening chest and abdominal injuries and control of bleeding take priority over head injury.

SECONDARY MANAGEMENT

- *Mannitol* 20%. (0.5 g kg^{-1}) may be used as a temporary means of reducing ICP (following consultation with the neurosurgical centre)
- *Anticonvulsants* are used following seizures, and prophylactically if indicated
- *Antibiotics* are given prophylactically to patients with basal skull and other compound skull fractures.

Table 3.
The Glasgow Coma Scale

Best motor response (observed in the upper limb)	Score
Obeys commands	6
Withdraws from painful stimuli	5
Localizes to painful stimuli	4
Flexes to painful stimuli	3
Extends to painful stimuli	2
No response	1
Best verbal response	
Orientated	5
Confused speech	4
Inappropriate words	3
Incomprehensible sounds	2
None	1
Eye-opening response	
Spontaneously	4
To speech	3
To pain	2
None	1

Table 4.
Guidelines for transfer of head-injured patients

- *The patient must be stabilized prior to transfer*
- The doctor escorting the patient should be of appropriate seniority and have sufficient skill to recognize and treat deteriorations that may occur during transfer
- All equipment and drugs, including oxygen, should be checked prior to departure
- All intubated patients require:
  - Sedation, to prevent increases in ICP
  - Paralysis, to prevent coughing and to facilitate hyperventilation
  - Analgesia, if indicated
- Short-acting agents such as propofol, vecuronium and fentanyl, can be rapidly withdrawn at the neurosurgical centre to allow further assessment
- Monitoring should be of the same standard as in the operating theatre and ECG, BP and Sao_2 are the minimum acceptable

TRANSFER

Many head-injured patients require interhospital transfer for CT scanning and/or neurosurgical management. This is a critical time. Table 4 lists the considerations before transfer.

ANAESTHETIC CONSIDERATIONS

Preoperative:

- Treatment of expanding intracranial haematoma may require urgent surgical intervention
- The timing of surgery for non-neurological injuries should ideally allow time for a period of stable neurological observation
- In addition to minimum monitoring, $ETco_2$ and direct BP measurement are necessary; temperature and urinary output monitoring are desirable
- A nasogastric tube will decompress acute gastric dilatation which occurs commonly following head injury and may be used for the administration of drugs and enteral nutrition in the postoperative period.

Intraoperative:

- The patient should be positioned on the table with moderate head-up tilt and unobstructed venous drainage from the head
- IPPV with neuromuscular paralysis allows moderate hyperventilation
- Isoflurane at <1 MAC is not associated with a significant increase in cerebral blood flow; alternatively, TIVA with propofol may be used, provided that BP is maintained.

Postoperative:

- Neurological observation should be continued into the postoperative period
- Fluid balance should be tailored to avoid precipitating cerebral oedema; 30 ml kg^{-1} per 24 h of 0.9% saline is usually adequate
- Admission to ITU for postoperative ventilation or observation may be necessary; intracranial pressure monitoring is desirable if the patient requires sedation.

OUTCOME

This depends on the patient's age, GCS score on admission, and the pupillary state. Long-term outcome may be significantly improved by aggressive treatment in the first few hours after injury.

BIBLIOGRAPHY

Briggs M, Clarke P, Crockard A et al. Guidelines for the initial management after head injury in adults. British Medical Journal 1984; 288: 983–985

Bullock R, Teasdale G. Head injuries I. British Medical Journal 1990; 300: 1515–1518

Bullock R, Teasdale G. Head injuries II. British Medical Journal 1990; 300: 1576–1579

Gentleman D, Dearden M, Midgley S, Maclean D. Guidelines for resuscitation and transfer of patients with serious head injury. British Medical Journal 1993; 307: 547–552

Mayberg T S, Lam A M. Management of central nervous system trauma. Current Opinion in Anaesthesiology 1993; 6: 764–771

CROSS REFERENCES

Anaesthesia for supratentorial surgery
Surgical Procedures 12: 275

Raised ICP/CBF control
Anaesthetic Factors 33: 662

MOTOR NEURONE DISEASE

N. P. Hirsch

This condition is characterized by degeneration of motor neurones within the motor cortex, the brainstem motor nuclei of the cranial nerves and the anterior horn cells of the spinal cord. It therefore produces:

- Amyotrophic lateral sclerosis – due to an upper motor neurone lesion with pyramidal tract damage due to neuronal loss in the motor cortex. This results in spastic limb weakness. Bulbar motor neurone lesions cause a pseudobulbar palsy.
- Progressive bulbar palsy – due to lower motor neurone lesions of the brainstem motor nuclei of the cranial nerves.
- Progressive muscular atrophy due to a lower motor neurone lesion of the anterior horn cells.

The majority of patients exhibit a combination of these defects.

Prevalence is 5 in 100 000 of the population, with men more commonly affected than women. The peak age of onset is 50–70 years. In 5–10% of cases there is an autosomal dominant inheritance, these patients presenting at an earlier age.

The spinal muscular atrophies are a group of rare inherited conditions (including Werdnig–Hoffmann and Wohlfart–Kugelberg–Welander diseases) that are characterized by degeneration of motor neurones. They occur in infancy, childhood or adolescence.

CLINICAL FEATURES

Nervous system

Presentation is variable, depending on which part of the nervous system is predominantly affected. If the picture is one of a lower motor neurone deficit, patients may present with weakness and wasting of the small muscles of the hand or with wasting of the distal leg muscles and foot drop. Fasciculation is a characteristic feature. Other patients may present with an upper motor neurone picture with spastic weakness of the limbs. Reflexes are characteristically brisk. In a high proportion of patients, bulbar symptoms may be present with difficulty in phonation, chewing and swallowing. As bulbar dysfunction becomes more impaired, pulmonary aspiration may occur during swallowing. These patients characteristically have poor tongue and palatal movements with accompanying fasciculation and atrophy of the tongue.

Distressingly, there is no impairment of intellect. The sensory system is unaffected.

Respiratory system

The respiratory muscles are usually affected late in the disease process. Progressive respiratory muscle failure leads to breathlessness (especially when lying flat), poor cough, recurrent pneumonia, and respiratory failure. Nocturnal hypoventilation may lead to characteristic symptoms, e.g. morning headaches, daytime hypersomnolence, etc. The poor bulbar function results in recurrent pulmonary aspiration which further compromises respiratory function. Most patients die within 3 years of diagnosis due to the associated pulmonary problems.

PREOPERATIVE ASSESSMENT

History and examination:

- General details of disease and any associated conditions.
- Bulbar function – ask whether patient has problem with phonation, chewing and swallowing. Does food or liquid 'go the wrong way'. Examine palatal movement while testing the gag reflex. Look for pooling of saliva in the pyriform fossae.
- Respiratory function – ask about recurrent chest infections. Measure vital capacity both standing and lying. A drop of more than 30% on lying suggests significant diaphragmatic weakness. Breathlessness on lying flat, especially when associated with paradoxical abdominal movement on inspiration, will confirm the suspicion. Ask about symptoms of nocturnal hypoventilation.

Investigations:

- To confirm diagnosis, e.g. electromyographic and nerve conduction studies
- Routine haematological and biochemical investigations
- Chest X-ray, pulmonary function tests, arterial blood gases, tests of diaphragmatic function (e.g. mouth occlusion pressures)
- Videoflouroscopy to investigate the swallowing mechanism may be indicated.

PERIOPERATIVE MANAGEMENT

Premedication

Opioid premedication should be avoided because of its respiratory depressant action. If premedication is required, a small dose of a benzodiazepine is appropriate.

If bulbar function is poor, prophylaxis against pulmonary aspiration (i.e. an H_2 receptor antagonist) should be administered.

Monitoring:

- Should start in the anaesthetic room
- ECG (CM_5)
- Blood pressure measurement
- Spo_2
- $ETco_2$ (maintain patient at normocarbia as defined by preoperative arterial blood gases)
- Neuromuscular function monitoring.

Induction and maintenance of anaesthesia

Patients are very sensitive to the respiratory depressant effects of anaesthetic induction agents. These should be carefully titrated against response.

Poor bulbar function dictates that the patient is intubated in order to protect the airway. Although a rapid sequence induction may be indicated, suxamethonium is contraindicated in motor neurone disease, and therefore tracheal intubation must be effected without this agent.

The administration of suxamethonium may result in dangerous hyperkalaemia in the presence of the widespread denervation found in motor neurone disease.

Because of increased sensitivity to the nondepolarizing neuromuscular blocking drugs, these agents should be used in the lowest possible doses and neuromuscular blockade should be continuously monitored.

During anaesthesia controlled ventilation is recommended.

Tracheal extubation should be performed with the patient fully awake to ensure maximal function of the laryngeal reflexes.

Regional anaesthesia
If appropriate, this would appear to have distinct advantages over general anaesthesia. However, if extradural or spinal anaesthesia is planned, care must be taken to ensure that the level of block does not compromise an already weak respiratory musculature.

POSTOPERATIVE MANAGEMENT

Effective postoperative pain relief must be administered without the use of agents which depress respiratory function. The use of regional analgesia should be considered.

Postoperative ventilation may be required and weaning may be prolonged.

BIBLIOGRAPHY

Gronert G A, Lambert E M, Theye R A. The response of denervated skeletal muscle to succinylcholine. Anesthesiology 1973; 39: 13–22

Rosenbaum K J, Neigh J T, Strobel G E. Sensitivity to non-depolarizing muscle relaxants in amylotrophic lateral sclerosis: report of two cases. Anesthesiology 1971; 35: 638–641

CROSS REFERENCES

Restrictive lung disease
Patient Conditions 3: 80

MOVEMENT DISORDERS

A. Severn

Parkinsonism is a clinical syndrome with features of tremor, rigidity, bradykinesia and autonomic instability. Not all signs are required for a diagnosis.

CLINICAL FEATURES

Cardinal features:

- Tremor
- Rigidity
- Bradykinesia
- Autonomic instability.

Secondary features relevant to anaesthesia:

- Sweating disorders
- Excessive salivation and bronchial secretion
- Disorders of oesophageal motility
- Sleep disturbance
- Dementia
- Depression.

AETIOLOGY

- Parkinson's disease – the commonest cause, affecting over 1% of people over 65 years
- Secondary Parkinsonism:
  - Drugs, e.g. phenothiazines, metoclopramide
  - Toxic substances, e.g. carbon monoxide
  - As a late consequence of encephalitis
  - In degenerative CNS disease, e.g. Alzheimer's disease.

PATHOPHYSIOLOGY

The defect in parkinsonism is a failure of the dopaminergic neurones projecting to D1 and D2 receptors in the striatum from the substantia nigra and important in the initiation of movement. The striatum itself contains cholinergic nerves, and to some extent the two neurotransmitters have antagonistic actions.

In Parkinson's disease a loss of nigral cell bodies can be detected at autopsy. Noninvasive techniques such as magnetic resonance imaging and positron emission spectroscopy may in future be used for screening of asymptomatic patients. A neurotoxin, a by-product of illicit pethidine synthesis, has enabled researchers to develop a primate model for parkinsonism. Inactivation of this toxin, achieved by inhibition of brain (type B) monoamine oxidase, may in future prove to slow the progression of the disease.

MANAGEMENT

Dopamine is replaced as oral L-dopa, which is decarboxylated to dopamine in the brain and liver. Dopamine itself does not cross the blood–brain barrier. Liver decarboxylase is inhibited by benzserazide or carbidopa which together with L-dopa respectively constitute the preparations Madopar (Roche) and Sinemet (Dupont). Signs of systemic dopamine administration are not found in Parkinsonism treated in this way.

On the other hand, direct D1 and D2 stimulation with pergolide and bromocriptine can cause arrhythmias and postural hypotension, as can intravenous L-dopa, which is supplied by Roche on a named-patient basis without a decarboxylase inhibitor. Intravenous L-dopa can be used on patients who are not absorbing oral medication after major surgery.

Inhibition of brain monoamine oxidation with selegiline improves the availability of dopamine. At 10 mg day^{-1} it has a specific effect on the type B isoenzyme. The 'cheese reaction', due to monoaminergic activity after tyramine ingestion and a complication of irreversible inhibition of the type A isoenzyme, does not occur.

Summary of treatments:
- Reduce central cholinergic activity
- Increase the availability of dopamine
- Stimulate dopamine receptors
- Avoid drugs with antidopaminergic actions
- Measures to improve mobility and social function.

ANAESTHESIA

Give antiparkinsonian medication up to the time of surgery: previous advice on discontinuation of L-dopa predates the use of decarboxylase inhibitors and is no longer relevant. Sudden withdrawal of L-dopa or use of antidopaminergic drugs may result in a life-threatening centrally mediated pyrexia (neuroleptic malignant syndrome) and may impair the patient's postoperative mobility.

Beware of oesophageal reflux, and even achalasia, but beware also of a case report of hyperkalaemia with suxamethonium.

Bronchial secretions and sialorrhoea may make the airway difficult to manage.

Autonomic failure and postencephalitic parkinsonism predispose to episodes of obstructive and central sleep apnoea. Specific postoperative requirements e.g. oxygen therapy and oximetry, or even nasal continuous positive airways pressure (CPAP) may be needed for such patients.

It is theoretically possible that opioid induced rigidity may be a form of Parkinsonism, and a case of reversible Parkinsonism apparently induced by pethidine has been reported. Caution is therefore advised with opioids. Pethidine in particular, because of its specific interraction with serotonin uptake, may be hazardous in patients on selegiline.

Regional anaesthesia may be difficult because of tremor or poor cooperation, but at least avoids some of the hazards noted above. If an indirectly acting amine such as ephedrine is used to counteract hypotension, it should be used with care in a patient on selegiline.

Ondansetron is a logical antiemetic, being a specific inhibitor of serotonin type-3 receptors, and devoid of extrapyramidal actions.

PREOPERATIVE PREPARATION

History:

- Is there a tendency to recurrent chest problems?
- Is there a history of dysphagia?
- Is there a history of postural hypotension?
- Is the patient confused?
- If so, has this state arisen as a result of illness and hospitalization, or is there a pre-existing dementia?
- Has all appropriate medication been continued since admission?
- Has inappropriate medication, e.g. phenothiazine, been used?
- What is the likely aetiology of the parkinsonism?

Examination:

- Assume an active mind trapped in a disabled body
- Assess ability to cooperate with instructions to breathe deeply, cough and expectorate
- Assess postural blood pressure changes if mobile
- Assess likely impact of resting posture and tremor on transfer to theatre and cooperation with anaesthetic room routine (including local anaesthetic procedures)
- Confirm that the patient is not pyrexial.

Investigations:

- Spirometry may confirm a restrictive pattern
- Chest X-ray will establish a baseline against which postoperative atelectasis can be compared
- ECG performed during a Valsalva manoeuvre may show changes of autonomic neuropathy.

BIBLIOGRAPHY

Hill S, Yau K, Whitwam J. MAOIs to RIMAs in anaesthesia – a literature review. Psychopharmacology 1992; 106: S41–S43

Severn A M. Parkinsonism and the anaesthetist. British Journal of Anaesthesia 1988; 61: 761–770

Tojo K, Iizuka K, Honda H, Shimojo S, Miyahara T. A case of neuroleptic malignant syndrome due to levodopa withdrawal. Jikeikai Medical Journal 1989; 36: 195–202

CROSS REFERENCES

The elderly patient
Patient Conditions 11: 252

MULTIPLE SCLEROSIS

M. D. Weston

Multiple sclerosis (MS) is a slowly progressive disease affecting the brain and spinal cord in which the myelin sheaths of nerve fibres are destroyed.

INCIDENCE

Varies from 1 in 100 000 in equatorial areas to 30–80 in 100 000 in the Northern hemisphere. More common in Caucasians. A genetic factor is suggested by a high incidence in monozygotic twins born to parents with MS and also by the frequent occurrence of certain histocompatibility antigens in patients with the disease. In approximately 65% onset is between the ages of 20 and 40 years.

PATHOPHYSIOLOGY

- Aetiology remains unknown, but involves genetic, immunological and infective factors. Whatever the precipitating cause, evidence suggests an aberrant autoimmune reaction to myelin antigens.
- Precipitating events occurring before the initial symptoms or exacerbations of the disease include infection, trauma and pregnancy.
- Myelin sheaths are destroyed by perivascular inflammation resulting in sclerotic plaque formation in the brain and spinal cord white matter.
- Most commonly affected areas are the optic nerves and chiasm, periventricular regions and the subpial regions of the spinal cord.

SYMPTOMS

- Characterized by periods of exacerbation and remission; neurological dysfunction often develops over hours or days and resolves over weeks or months.
- 20–30% of cases follow a benign course.
- 5% exhibit a rapid progression with the remainder accumulating disability over 10–20 years.
- Classic features include motor weakness and spasticity, paraesthesiae, impaired vision, nystagmus, diplopia, dysarthria, ataxia, bladder dysfunction, trigeminal neuralgia, cognitive impairment and mood disturbance.

DIAGNOSIS

History

- Clinical manifestations suggesting multiple lesions in different regions of the CNS
- History of exacerbations and remissions.

Investigations

- Abnormal cerebrospinal fluid:
  - Increased white cell count
  - Increased total protein content (in 40% of patients)
  - Oligoclonal bands seen on electrophoresis (in 90% of cases)
- Imaging: plaques seen on MRI or enhanced CT scan
- Evoked potentials: abnormal visual, auditory or somatosensory evoked potentials.

TREATMENT

- No treatment predictably slows the course of MS
- Immunosuppressive agents may have marginal benefit
- Methylprednisolone may speed recovery (or alter course of) acute optic neuritis
- β Interferon may reduce rate of exacerbation
- Monoclonal antibodies may be a future avenue of treatment.

ANAESTHETIC MANAGEMENT

The stress of surgery and anaesthesia has been implicated in subsequent exacerbation of symptoms, although there is no evidence to support this.

PREOPERATIVE ASSESSMENT

Routine assessment should include:

- Evidence of infection – a 0.5–1.0°C rise in temperature exacerbates the conduction block in demyelinated neurones. It is therefore essential that the patient is infection free.
- Respiratory function – respiratory reserve may be poor. Respiratory function tests and arterial blood gas analysis should be performed if indicated.
- Bulbar function – should be examined. There may be evidence of recurrent pulmonary aspiration.
- Autonomic hyperreflexia may be present in patients with extensive spinal cord demyelination.
- The presence of contractures and pressure sores.
- Mental state.
- Steroid medication.

PREMEDICATION

- Sedative premedication is acceptable
- Steroid supplementation, if indicated
- Deep venous thrombosis prophylaxis
- H_2 receptor antagonists
- Atropine should be avoided as it may increase body temperature.

GENERAL ANAESTHESIA

- Suxamethonium should be avoided – it may produce a profound increase in serum potassium in patients with extensive demyelination
- Response to nondepolarizing neuromuscular blocking agents appears to be normal but neuromuscular monitoring is advisable
- Central temperature should be monitored and steps taken to maintain normothermia
- Tracheal intubation is indicated in those patients with poor bulbar function
- Positioning of the patient must be performed extremely carefully in those patients with contractures or pressure sores.

REGIONAL ANAESTHESIA

- There is no absolute contraindication to regional blockade in patients with MS, although patients may attribute subsequent relapse or exacerbation to the local anaesthetic procedure.
- The merits of local and general anaesthesia should be discussed with the patient and a suitably worded consent form may be used for medicolegal protection.

POSTOPERATIVE CARE

- Intensive physiotherapy to remove pulmonary secretions and prevent contractures may be needed
- The methods of providing postoperative pain relief should take preoperative respiratory function into account
- If the patient becomes febrile, an antipyretic drug (e.g. aspirin) should be considered.

BIBLIOGRAPHY

Jones R M, Healey T E J. Anaesthesia and demyelinating disease. Anaesthesia 1980; 35: 879–884

Nosworthy J H. Clinical trials in multiple sclerosis. Current Opinions in Neurology and Neurosurgery 1993; 6: 209–215

CROSS REFERENCES

Autonomic dysfunction
Patient Conditions 1: 4
Antacid prophylaxis
Surgical Procedures 20: 400
Preoperative assessment of pulmonary risk
Anaesthetic Factors 34: 697

NEUROFIBROMATOSIS

S. M. Scuplak

Neurofibromatosis is a heterogeneous group of disorders characterized by cutaneous pigmentation and tumour formation. Von Recklinghausen or type 1 neurofibromatosis is the only common form in clinical practice (Table 1). It is inherited as an autosomal dominant trait with a prevalence of 1 in 5000; half of cases represent new mutations.

Table 1.
Clinical features of von Recklinghausen neurofibromatosis

Major defining features
- Café au lait spots, usually more than six >1.5 cm in diameter
- Peripheral neurofibromas
- Iris hamartomas (Lisch nodules)

Minor features
- Short stature
- Macrocephaly

Disease complications
- Intellectual handicap
- Epilepsy
- CNS tumours
- Bone dysplasias, scoliosis
- Hypertension
- Pulmonary fibrosis

PATHOPHYSIOLOGY

The severity of disease and the occurrence of complications cannot be predicted due to variable gene expression. Neurofibromas virtually always involve the skin, but can also affect visceral tissue innervated by the autonomic nervous system. Involvement of the pharynx, larynx, trachea, spinal cord and ventricular outflow has been reported.

Cardiovascular
Neurofibromas developing in blood vessel walls can produce vascular obstruction or aneurysmal dilatation. Renal artery stenosis occurs in approximately 2% of cases giving rise to hypertension, most commonly in children. Hypertension occurring in adults is generally due to phaeochromocytoma.

Respiratory
Restrictive lung disorders are common. Diffuse pulmonary fibrosis associated with bullous emphysema can result in arterial hypoxaemia and cor pulmonale; it may also present as pneumothorax. Lung volumes are further reduced by chest wall abnormalities such as scoliosis and intrathoracic neurofibromas. Obstructive disorders may be produced by neurofibromas within the airway.

Endocrine
Phaeochromocytoma develops in approximately 1% of patients and may be part of the multiple endocrine neoplasia syndrome which includes medullary carcinoma of the thyroid.

Central nervous system
Epilepsy occurs in at least 4% of patients, although no underlying abnormality is usually found. Occasionally it may signal the presence of an intracranial tumour, especially gliomas.

PREOPERATIVE ASSESSMENT

History:
- Review of cardiovascular and respiratory systems.
- Symptoms of airway obstruction:
  - Dyspnoea
  - Dysphagia
  - Dysphonia.
- Phaeochromocytoma:
  - Paroxysmal tachycardia
  - Sweating.

Examination:
- Assess distribution of neurofibromas
- Posture and presence of scoliosis
- CNS deficits indicative of intracranial or spinal neurofibromas.

Investigations:
- Chest X-ray to detect intrathoracic abnormalities and assess thoracic spine
- Lung function tests for obstructive and restrictive disease
- Arterial blood gases
- CT/MRI imaging of the airway in the presence of obstructive symptoms
- The investigation of hypertension should include plasma catecholamine levels or urinary metabolites.

PERIOPERATIVE MANAGEMENT

Premedication
Respiratory depressant drugs are only contraindicated in the presence of severe respiratory insufficiency. Anticholinergic agents should be given if difficulty in intubation is anticipated.

Monitoring
This should commence in the anaesthetic room.

- ECG
- Spo_2
- Arterial cannula, if hypertensive
- Peripheral nerve stimulator
- Airway pressure monitor.

General anaesthesia
No particular anaesthetic technique or drug has advantages over another. Evidence of airway obstruction is an indication for awake fibreoptic intubation. If muscle atrophy is present succinylcholine should be avoided. Succinylcholine, pancuronium and D-tubocurarine have been reported to produce prolonged neuromuscular blockade and monitoring of blockade and the use of shorter acting drugs is recommended. Positioning must be carried out with care to avoid undue pressure on large cutaneous neurofibromas. Severe kyphoscoliosis can hinder positioning. High airway pressures can be achieved in patients with severe restrictive lung disease, and the possibility of pneumothorax must be considered.

Regional anaesthesia
Regional anaesthesia has been used successfully. The presence of cutaneous neurofibromas overlying the site of injection can hinder successful placement of the needle and this can be further complicated by bony abnormalities such as scoliosis.

POSTOPERATIVE CARE

- Position with adequate padding; cutaneous neurofibromas can be tender
- Continuous oxygen therapy
- Chest physiotherapy.

BIBLIOGRAPHY

Huson S M, Harper P, Compston D A S. Von Recklinghausen neurofibromatosis: a clinical and population study in south-east Wales. Brain 1988; 111: 1355

McD Fisher M. Anaesthetic difficulties in neurofibromatosis. Anaesthesia 1975; 30: 648–650

Van Aken H, Scherer R, Lawin P. A rare intra-operative complication in a child with Von Recklinghausen's neurofibromatosis. Anaesthesia 1982; 37: 827–829

CROSS REFERENCES

Epilepsy
Patient Conditions 1: 6
Restrictive lung disease
Patient Conditions 3: 80
Hypertension
Patient Conditions 4: 11

SPINAL CORD INJURY (ACUTE)

J. S. Porter and M. Smith

AETIOLOGY

The incidence of spinal trauma is about 50 per million of the population per year. The cervical spine is the most susceptible to injury as it is the least supported; C5–C6 is the commonest level affected. Injuries may involve fracture of bony elements, disruption of intervertebral discs or ligamentous/soft tissue injury. Other injuries occur in 60% of cases, with head injury being a common association. Road traffic accidents account for about 70% of all cervical spine injuries.

PATHOPHYSIOLOGY

The primary injury is caused by stretching or direct trauma to the spinal cord and is characterized by vasodilatation and disruption of the microvasculature and marked oedema in the grey matter. Local hypoxia sets up a chain of events culminating in neuronal death. Rises in intracellular calcium, synthesis of vasoactive peptides, free radical production and lipid peroxidation are all implicated in this process. Secondary ischaemic injury may follow because of hypotension, hypoxaemia and progressive cord oedema. Treatment is directed at respiratory and cardiovascular support to minimize secondary injury.

Nervous system

'Spinal shock' occurs due to interruption of visceral and somatic sensation with flaccid paralysis and absent autonomic and somatic reflexes following spinal cord injury. It may last up to 6 weeks followed by progressive spasticity of the affected levels (see chronic spinal cord injury, p 1.1.26). Interruption of the spinal cord outflow has major effects on other physiological systems.

Cardiovascular system:

- Hypertension occurs at the time of the injury
- Hypotension follows within minutes due to loss of sympathetic (autonomic) tone, with intense cutaneous vasodilatation
- Hypotension may be exacerbated by bleeding from other injuries
- Loss of compensatory reflexes for changes in cardiac output and blood pressure if lesion above T1
- Severe bradycardia may ensue due to unopposed vagal activity.

Respiratory system:

- Respiratory insufficiency is common, although the degree depends upon the level of cord damage. Respiratory impairment may also result from associated injuries.
- *Lesion above C4:* diaphragmatic paralysis, loss of intercostal function and paralysis of all four limbs occurs. Such patients require ventilatory support. If the lesion extends to the upper cervical levels and lower cranial nerves, accessory muscle function is also lost.
- *Lesion at C4–C5:* voluntary control of breathing is maintained under cervical control at 20–25% of normal vital capacities. Such patients often require ventilatory assistance, especially in the early stages.
- *Lesion below C5:* diaphragmatic sparing occurs but the intercostal muscles are affected to varying degrees. There is a decrease in alveolar ventilation and paradoxical respiration. A decreased cough occurs due to loss of intercostal function and paralysed abdominal musculature.
- In the early stages of injury, during the phase of spinal cord oedema, the level of the lesion may ascend and a patient requiring minimal respiratory support may become entirely ventilator dependent.
- Pulmonary oedema is common after spinal cord injury and is a common cause of death – it may be neurogenic in origin or due to the inability to cope with fluid overload.

Gastrointestinal tract:
- Acute gastric dilatation and paralytic ileus
- Increased risk of regurgitation and pulmonary aspiration.

Temperature
Temperature regulation is impaired due to the inability to sweat and cutaneous vasodilatation.

Genitourinary tract
Bladder atony and urinary retention occur.

1

ACUTE MANAGEMENT

The resuscitation of patients with spinal cord injuries should follow guidelines for any patient with major trauma.

Airway
The airway should be secured and supplemental oxygen delivered to prevent hypoxaemia. Tracheal intubation may be necessary (Table 1). Airway control is dealt with below.

Table 1.
Indications for tracheal intubation after acute spinal cord injury

$P_{a}O_2$ <10.0 kPa
$P_{a}CO_2$ >6.5 kPa
Vital capacity <20 ml kg^{-1}
Pulmonary aspiration
Pulmonary oedema
Associated chest/lung injuries

Breathing
Artificial ventilation may be necessary to maintain oxygenation and normocapnia (see above).

Circulation
Bradycardia should be treated with atropine. Hypovolaemia due to vasodilatation/venodilatation requires aggressive filling to ensure adequate cardiac output and blood pressure. Central venous pressure (CVP) monitoring is mandatory, and because of the inability to deal with fluid overload monitoring of pulmonary artery capillary wedge pressure (PCWP) is required in many cases. Vasoconstrictors or inotropes may be required if blood pressure fails to respond to adequate filling.

Drugs
Steroids and naloxone have been used in an attempt to block the cascade of neuronal damage after spinal cord injury. Steroids should be given in high dosage and within 8 h of the injury.

Other
A nasogastric tube and urinary catheter should be inserted.

DEFINITIVE SURGICAL TREATMENT

Aim
Reduction and stabilization of unstable spinal fractures may prevent further spinal cord damage.

Conservative management
The spine can be immobilized with traction to the cervical spine applied using skull tongs. This entails prolonged bedrest with an increased incidence of decubitus ulcers and thromboembolic episodes. A halo body jacket device allows early mobilization.

Surgical management
Open reduction and internal fixation allows early mobilization. Cord decompression in the acute phase is gaining in popularity.

ANAESTHESIA FOR ACUTE SPINAL CORD INJURY

Preoperative assessment:
- Careful attention must be paid to the respiratory and cardiovascular systems (see above)
- Other injuries should be dealt with as appropriate
- Respiratory depressant drugs should be avoided in patients who are self-ventilating
- An antisialogue may be useful in those in whom fibre-optic nasal intubation (FNI) is required
- Atropine should be given prior to intubation if the patient is bradycardic.

Airway control
There is much debate over the safest method of endotracheal intubation in patients with an unstable cervical spine. Secondary damage to the spinal cord is common if precautions are not taken. No difference in neurological outcome has been shown between the different intubation methods.

- Awake FNI using topical anaesthesia. In skilled hands this may be the method of choice.
- Oral or nasal intubation under direct laryngoscopy. The neck should be immobilized by either a hard collar, external fixation device or manual in-line stabilization (MILS) by an assistant.
- Tracheostomy under local anaesthesia.

Problems associated with tracheal intubation in patients with spinal cord injury include:

- Unable to extend neck
- Cervical spine fixation devices
- Associated facial injuries
- Full stomach/gastric dilatation
- Cricoid pressure difficult – may exacerbate cervical spine subluxation.

Monitoring:

- ECG, invasive BP, CVP, temperature and urine output, as a minimum
- PCWP and cardiac output may aid fluid therapy
- Somatosensory evoked potentials during procedures involving spinal cord manipulation.

Anaesthetic technique

- No specific technique is better than another
- Falls in blood pressure should be avoided by cautious use of intravenous induction agents, minimum airway pressures, maintenance of normovolaemia and careful positioning
- Suxamethonium should be avoided beyond day 3 after injury.

Postoperative considerations

- Continuation of respiratory support may require full ventilation or assisted ventilation with CPAP
- Maintenance of adequate circulating volume and urinary output
- Skilled physiotherapy is essential
- Adequate analgesia
- Careful positioning to avoid decubitus ulcers
- Deep vein thrombosis prophylaxis (TED stockings, intermittent calf compression and subcutaneous heparin should all be considered)
- Gastrointestinal protection with H_2 receptor antagonists or sucralfate
- Adequate nutrition should be maintained; enteral feeding is usually possible.

BIBLIOGRAPHY

Durret J M. The early management of spinal injuries. Current Anaesthesia and Critical Care 1994; 5: 17–22

Johnston R A. The management of acute spinal cord compression (review). Journal of Neurology, Neurosurgery and Psychiatry 1993; 56: 1046–1054

MacKenzie C F, Shin B, Krishnaprasad D, McCormack F, Illingworth W. Assessment of cardiac and respiratory function during surgery on patients with acute quadriplegia. Journal of Neurosurgery 1985; 62: 843–849

Mansel J K, Norman J R. Respiratory complications and management of spinal cord injuries. Chest 1990; 97: 1446–1451

Mendoza N D, Bradford R, Middleton F. Spinal injury. In: Greenwood R, Barnes M, Macmillan T, Ward C (eds) Neurological rehabilitation. Churchill Livingstone, Edinburgh, ch 47, p 545–560

CROSS REFERENCES

The failing heart
Patient Conditions 4: 129
Intraoperative hypotension
Anaesthetic Factors 33: 638

SPINAL CORD INJURY (CHRONIC)

J. S. Porter and M. Smith

1

Chronic spinal cord injury is characterized by reflex somatic and autonomic overactivity which develops approximately 6 weeks after spinal cord injury and follows the acute phase of spinal shock.

PATHOPHYSIOLOGY

Central nervous system

Supraspinal inhibitory influences are lost below the level of injury. This results in:

- Spastic motor paralysis
- Hyperactive tendon reflexes
- Muscle spasms
- Autonomic hyper-reflexia.

Severe overactivity of somatic and autonomic function can be precipitated by even minor stimuli.

Cardiovascular system

Autonomic hyper-reflexia

Somatic or visceral stimulation below the level of cord injury (e.g. bladder distension, surgical incision) may result in uncontrolled sympathetic discharge. This leads to intense vasoconstriction below the level of injury with compensatory vasodilatation above. The clinical features of autonomic hyper-reflexia are shown in Table 1. This condition is rarely seen with lesions below T10.

Table 1.
Clinical features of autonomic hyper-reflexia

Hypertension
Bradycardia and other arrhythmias
Headache
Cerebral haemorrhage
Flushing and sweating above level of injury
Piloerrection and pallor below level of injury

Postural hypotension

Venous return may be reduced because of venodilatation. Relative hypovolaemia may occur. Cardioaccelerator influences may be lost, resulting in unopposed vagal activity.

Respiratory system

Respiratory impairment is common, but the degree depends upon the level of spinal cord injury (see acute spinal cord injury, p 1.1.23). Abnormal respiratory muscle function may result in:

- Decreased functional residual capacity
- Decreased expiratory reserve volume
- Kyphoscoliosis
- Chest infection (which is common).

Genitourinary system

Loss of bladder function necessitates an in-dwelling urinary catheter or intermittent self-catheterization. The bladder may empty involuntary, but often incompletely, by means of a spinal reflex which can be initiated by skin stimulation.

Problems include:

- Recurrent urinary tract infection
- Hydronephrosis
- Bladder/renal calculi
- Renal parenchymal infection
- Renal failure (the commonest cause of death).

Gastrointestinal system

Bowel function may be lost, requiring frequent enemas and manual evacuation of faeces. Some patients may develop regular emptying via a spinal reflex. Weight loss and poor nutritional status are common.

Other systems:

- Thromboembolic disease is common
- Decubitus ulcers occur and may become infected
- Osteoporosis and hypercalcaemia rapidly develop in non weight-bearing patients.

PREOPERATIVE ASSESSMENT

Frequent surgery is required, in particular

urological, orthopaedic, plastic and neurosurgical procedures.

Attention must be paid to assessing:

- Level of cord injury
- Respiratory status
- Presence of autonomic hyper-reflexia
- Presence of infection
- Renal impairment
- Suitability for regional anaesthesia.

Preoperative investigations are listed in Table 2. Particular care must be paid to assessing respiratory status in relation to the level of cord injury. Premedication should be avoided in those with decreased respiratory reserve.

Table 2.
Preoperative investigations

Investigation	Common finding
Full blood count	Anaemia, raised white cell count
Biochemistry	Electrolyte disturbances, low albumin
Renal function tests	Renal impairment, chronic/ acute renal failure
ECG	Bradycardia, other arrhythmias
Chest X-ray	Infection, kyphoscoliosis
Microbiology	Infected sputum/urine
Arterial blood gases	Hypoxaemia/hypercarbia
Pulmonary function tests	Reduced VC, ERV and FRC

PERIOPERATIVE PROBLEMS

Cardiovascular system:

Autonomic hyper-reflexia

Deep general anaesthesia and regional techniques are equally effective in obtunding autonomic hyper-reflexia secondary to surgical stimulation. Treatment of perioperative autonomic hyperactivity includes cessation of stimulus, deepening of anaesthesia and the use of antihypertensive agents.

Arrhythmias

These may be associated with autonomic hyper-reflexia. Bradycardia may occur due to unopposed vagal activity, and can exacerbate hypotension during regional anaesthesia.

Hypotension

Absent cardiovascular reflexes predispose to falls in BP during anaesthesia. Hypotension may develop during induction of anaesthesia, initiation of positive pressure ventilation, changes in posture and following regional anaesthesia. Adequate preoperative and perioperative hydration, minimum airway pressures and careful patient positioning are essential.

Other

- Temperature control – quadraplegics are poikilothermic, and aggressive measures must be undertaken to maintain normothermia
- Posture – careful positioning is essential to avoid fracturing osteoporotic bones, to avoid pressure areas and to prevent hypotension
- Thromboembolic disease – thromboembolic prophylaxis should be continued into the perioperative period.

ANAESTHESIA FOR CHRONIC SPINAL CORD INJURY

Even if sensory loss is complete below the level of injury, anaesthesia is required for surgical procedures to minimize the effects of autonomic and somatic hyper-reflexia. This is particularly important in patients with high lesions.

Monitoring:

- ECG
- Spo_2
- $ETco_2$
- Invasive BP
- Central venous pressure (essential for patients with lesions above T10)
- Pulmonary artery capillary wedge pressure (PCWP) (in those with cardiovascular instability)
- Urinary output
- Temperature
- Somatosensory evoked potentials (during spinal cord surgery).

General anaesthesia:

- Adequate depth of anaesthesia can be maintained with either inhalational agents or total intravenous anaesthesia with propofol
- Intubation and controlled ventilation to ensure maintenance of oxygenation and minimize development of atelectasis
- Fibre-optic nasal intubation may be required if difficult intubation is anticipated in those with cervical spine injury (see

acute spinal cord injury, p 1.1.23) or previous spinal fixation
- Suxamethonium must be avoided because of the risk of hyperkalaemia due to widespread denervation.

Regional anaesthesia
Spinal and epidural blockade prevent autonomic hyperactivity by inhibition of visceral afferent pathways. They provide good conditions for surgery below midthoracic level. Potential problems include:

- Difficulty in testing sensory levels
- Difficulty in interpreting epidural test doses
- Risk of hypotension – postural hypotension is common in this group of patients and adequate fluid loading is essential
- Bradycardia – atropine may be required prior to initiation of regional anaesthesia.

POSTOPERATIVE MANAGEMENT

- Postoperative ventilation or respiratory support may be required
- Chest physiotherapy is essential to minimize risk of chest infection
- Adequate analgesia
- Careful attention to pressure areas
- Thromboembolic prophylaxis
- Maintenance of adequate nutrition.

BIBLIOGRAPHY

Mendoza N D, Bradford R, Middleton F. Spinal injury. In: Greenwood R, Barnes M, MacMillan T, Ward C (eds) Neurological rehabilitation. Churchill Livingstone, Edinburgh, ch 47, p 545–560

Schonwald G, Fish K J, Perkash I. Cardiovascular complications during anaesthesia in chronic spinal cord injured patients. Anaesthesiology 1981; 55: 550–558

CROSS REFERENCES

Autonomic dysfunction
Patient Conditions 1: 4
Chronic renal failure
Patient Conditions 6: 158
Complications of position
Anaesthetic Factors 33: 618
Thrombotic embolism
Anaesthetic Factors 33: 664

TETANUS

M. D Weston and
N. P. Hirsch

Tetanus is a clinical condition characterized by either local or generalized muscle spasm. It is caused by infection with *Clostridium tetani*, a Gram-positive, obligate anaerobic organism. Although *C. tetani* spores are ubiquitous in soil and the gastrointestinal tracts of humans and other animals, under certain conditions multiplication of the organism and production of a neurotoxin occurs.

EPIDEMIOLOGY

- Tetanus remains a common (and uncontrolled) disease in the developing world, especially in unimmunized rural communities
- An estimated 500 000 cases occur world-wide annually
- More common in the elderly who have failed to be immunized with tetanus toxoid during childhood or military service
- Tetanus may follow surgery, burns, otitis media, dental infection or abortion; the practice of 'skin popping' amongst narcotic addicts accounts for a proportion of cases in urban centres.

PATHOPHYSIOLOGY

- Incubation period 4–10 days.
- Symptoms of muscle spasm are due to a toxic neurotoxin, tetanospasm (MW 56 000), which is released by the organism.
- The mechanism by which the toxin acts is obscure, but it binds to peripheral nerve endings and then travels in a retrograde

fashion to reach central inhibitory interneurones. At this point it inhibits inhibitory neurotransmitters.

CLINICAL FEATURES

- Rarely, tetanus may be localized to the site of inoculation
- More usually it is generalized (Table 1).

Table 1.
Clinical features of tetanus

Early manifestations
- Muscle stiffness
- Spasm of masseter muscle (trismus or lockjaw)

Later manifestations
- Tetanospasms occur causing:
  - Clenching of the jaw (risus sardonicus)
  - Arching of the back (opisthotonos)
  - Flexion of arms, extension of legs
- Autonomic involvement: hypo/hypertension, arrhythmias
- Respiratory failure, aspiration pneumonia
- Fractures, especially of thoracic vertebrae

PROGNOSIS

- Poor prognosis is associated with short incubation period, rapid progression from local spasm to generalized tetanospasm, an injury close to the head, extremes of age and frequency and severity of convulsions
- Overall mortality 50%.

TREATMENT

Prevention is with tetanus toxoid.

In established cases:
- Debridement of wound and drainage of abscess.
- Human tetanus immunoglobulin.
- Penicillin G, 1–10 million units for 10 days (erythromycin or tetracycline if history of penicillin allergy).
- Close monitoring of patient in a quiet environment.
- Diazepam or chlorpromazine useful for mild spasm.
- Early use of dantrolene (1 mg kg^{-1} over 3 h) may control spasm and help avoid tracheal intubation.
- If, despite these measures, laryngospasm, respiratory muscle spasm or pulmonary aspiration occurs, tracheal intubation should be performed and the patient mechanically ventilated. Sedation and muscle relaxants are required to allow effective IPPV.
- Autonomic overactivity may be treated with β adrenergic receptor blockers (e.g. propanolol, labetalol).
- After recovery, patient should receive tetanus toxoid immunization, as previous infection does not confer future immunity.

GENERAL ITU CARE

- Ensure adequate fluid balance
- Patients should receive thromboembolic prophylaxis
- Enteral (or parenteral) feeding should be established early
- Full recovery usually occurs within 2–4 weeks.

BIBLIOGRAPHY

Checketts M R, White R J. Avoidance of intermittent pressure ventilation in tetanus with dantrolene therapy. Anaesthesia 1993; 48: 969–971

Edmondson R S, Flowers M W. Intensive care in tetanus: management, complications and mortality in 100 cases. British Medical Journal 1979; 1: 1401–1404

CROSS REFERENCES

Autonomic dysfunction
Patient Conditions 1: 4

2

ENDOCRINE SYSTEM

G. Hall

ACROMEGALY

W. Fawcett

2

Acromegaly results from increased growth hormone (GH) secretion, leading to an overgrowth of bone, connective tissue and viscera.

PATHOPHYSIOLOGY

Acromegaly usually results from a pituitary adenoma, and rarely from ectopic growth hormone producing tumours. In addition to the effects of hypersecretion of GH, there may also be clinical features arising from local pressure effects (visual field defects) and/or from damage to normal pituitary tissue causing hypopituitarism. There is a higher mortality from malignancy, and also respiratory, cardiovascular and cerebro-vascular disease in patients with acromegaly. The diagnosis may be confirmed by the failure of GH to fall in response to an oral glucose tolerance test.

Cardiovascular system:
- Hypertension
- Cardiomyopathy
- Complications of diabetes mellitus.

Neuromuscular system
Proximal myopathy and nerve entrapment syndromes.

Respiratory system:
- Somnolence and sleep apnoea
- Partial upper respiratory tract obstruction resulting from soft tissue hypertrophy of the pharyngeal and nasal mucosa
- Voice changes, from vocal cord involvement (glottic stenosis, calcification or vocal cord paresis)
- Macroglossia and prognathism.

Endocrine system:
- Overgrowth of soft tissues and skeleton, particularly head, tongue, jaw, hands and feet
- Impaired glucose tolerance
- Hypercalcaemia and hypercalcuria
- Other related endocrine problems include
  - Nodular goitre
  - Hyper- and hypo-thyroidism
  - Hypopituitarism
  - Diabetes insipidus.

PREOPERATIVE ASSESSMENT

Careful assessment of the upper airway (stridor, snoring, sleep apnoea). Associated cardiovascular, neuromuscular and endocrine involvement is sought.

Investigations:
- Blood tests: urea and electrolytes, glucose, calcium, thyroid function tests.
- Neck X-rays (for glottic involvement, pharyngeal tissue overgrowth).
- Indirect laryngoscopy may characterize vocal cord involvement.
- Cardiovascular investigations should include:
  - Chest X-Ray
  - ECG
  - Echocardiography.
- Consider a baseline arterial blood gas estimation.

Preparation should be made for a difficult intubation, including fibre-optic broncho-scopy. Arrangements should be made for postoperative respiratory monitoring in the ITU.

Premedication should avoid respiratory depressant drugs in patients with upper airway involvement. A drying agent (glycopyrrolate) is useful if a fibre-optic intubation is contemplated. If glucose intolerance is present, a glucose and insulin infusion may be required.

PERIOPERATIVE MANAGEMENT

Airway
If intubation is required (particularly if there is upper airway involvement) then skilled

assistance is mandatory. A selection of long armoured tracheal tubes should be available. Awake fibre-optic intubation is probably safest in experienced hands. The oral route is preferred as the nasal mucosa may be thickened considerably. There may be difficulties obtaining an air-tight fit with a face-mask. Without serious upper airway involvement, intravenous induction and intubation avoiding the pressor response to laryngoscopy (e.g. alfentail 10 μg kg^{-1}) should be undertaken, ensuring that the patient can be ventilated before administering nondepolarizing neuromuscular blocking drugs. Some would advocate elective tracheostomy in those with sleep apnoea or if there is vocal cord involvement.

Monitoring

- Full monitoring in the anaesthetic room is necessary (including ECG, blood pressure and Sa_{O_2})
- An arterial cannula for those undergoing prolonged surgery, or who need respiratory care in the ITU afterwards
- Central venous or pulmonary arterial catheterization may be useful in those with significant cardiac disease
- A peripheral nerve stimulator (there may be altered sensitivity to nondepolarizing neuromuscular blocking drugs, e.g. neuromuscular abnormalities, hypercalcaemia)
- Serum glucose.

POSTOPERATIVE MANAGEMENT

Those with airway involvement should be admitted to the ITU. Although extubation at the end of the procedure is normal, those with serious upper airway problems may require a period of postoperative intubation or tracheostomy. Patients should receive humidified oxygen, with monitoring of arterial blood gases, and Sa_{O_2}. Caution is required in the use of opioid analgesics in the extubated patient.

In addition, patients undergoing hypophysectomy will also have a marked reduction in insulin requirements in the postoperative period. They may develop diabetes insipidus (permanent or temporary) needing treatment with DDAVP, and in the longer term need replacement with ACTH and thyroid stimulating hormone (TSH) (see hypopituitarism, p 1.2.50).

BIBLIOGRAPHY

Goldhill D R, Dalgleish J G, Lake R H N. Respiratory problems and acromegaly. Anaesthesia 1982; 37: 1200–1203

Kitahata L M. Airway difficulties associated with anaesthesia and acromegaly. British Journal of Anaesthesia 1971; 43: 1187–1190

Southwick J P, Katz J. Unusual airway difficulty in the acromegalic patient: indications for tracheostomy. Anaesthesiology 1979; 51: 72–73

CROSS REFERENCES

Diabetes mellitus (IDDM)
Patient Conditions 2: 42

Cardiomyopathy
Patient Conditions 4: 103

Hypertension
Patient Conditions 4: 111

Difficult and failed intubation
Surgical Procedures 20: 408

ADRENOCORTICAL INSUFFICIENCY

A. Quinn

Primary adrenocortical insufficiency (Addison's disease), is a rare condition in which there is destruction of the adrenal cortex. Secondary insufficiency is due to inadequate ACTH production by any disease affecting the hypothalamus or pituitary. However, the commonest cause of this disorder results from exogenous steroid administration. The usual cause of primary insufficiency is an autoimmune disorder, and the patient may exhibit signs of other autoimmune diseases, e.g. pernicious anaemia, hypothyroidism, diabetes. Other causes are listed in Table 1.

Table 1.
Causes of primary hypoadrenalism

Causes
Autoimmune disease
Tuberculosis
Surgical removal
Haemorrhage/infarction:
Meningococcal septicaemia
Venography
Infiltration:
Malignant destruction
Amyloid
Schilder's disease (adrenal leukodystrophy)

PATHOPHYSIOLOGY

Cardiovascular system

Mineralocorticoids act on the distal tubule to increase sodium reabsorption. Loss of this function leads to sodium and secondary fluid loss resulting in hypovolaemia and hypotension. Glucocorticoids facilitate the action of noradrenaline on the arterioles; in their absence, vasodilation exacerbates hypotension.

Skin

ACTH is a pigmentary hormone. High levels present in Addison's disease may cause abnormal pigmentation in the mouth, on the hands, flexural regions or on recent scars.

Biochemical/metabolic:

- Hyponatraemia and high urinary sodium
- Hyperkalaemia (moderate)
- Hyperuricaemia
- Symptomatic hypoglycaemia as cortisol antagonizes the effects of insulin; reduced gluconeogenesis and glycogenolysis
- Hypercalcaemia.

Haematological:

- Raised haematocrit
- Normochromic normocytic anaemia (after rehydration)
- Eosinophilia, leucocytosis.

PREOPERATIVE ASSESSMENT

History

The history is often insidious and includes anorexia, weight loss, nausea and vomiting, abdominal pain, diarrhoea or constipation, weakness and dizziness. The addisonian crisis is usually associated with the stresses of illness, infection, surgery or trauma, and the patient may present in a moribund state.

Investigations:

- Urea and electrolytes, blood glucose
- Full blood count
- ECG (peaked T waves, widened QRS)
- Chest X-ray for evidence of TB
- Abdominal X-ray (TB may cause calcified adrenals).

A patient presenting with an addisonian crisis who requires emergency surgery should be managed in an ITU. Central venous, pulmonary artery and arterial cannulation enable rapid fluid replacement and frequent blood electrolyte sampling. A urinary catheter may be required to monitor urine output.

Fluid replacement:

- Sodium chloride 0.9%, 1 l rapidly, then more slowly

- Dextrose (50% i.v.) to correct hypoglycaemia
- Plasma volume expanders, e.g. gelofusine
- Treat hyperkalaemia with insulin (added to the dextrose) and calcium gluconate (10 mmol).

Hyponatraemia
Chronic hyponatraemia should be corrected with a 0.9% sodium chloride infusion. Correction of hyponatraemia in Addison's disease using hypertonic saline has been documented before emergency surgery. However, this treatment is controversial as 'osmotic demyelination' may occur, associated with sudden deterioration, brain damage and death.

Adrenal hormone replacement

Acute presentation, cardiovascular collapse
Hydrocortisone hemisuccinate or phosphate (200 mg i.v.) followed by an infusion of 100 mg hydrocortisone in 0.9% saline over 24 h.

After the initial acute presentation
- *Major surgery*: 25 mg hydrocortisone i.v. at induction of anaesthesia and thereafter an intravenous infusion of hydrocortisone (100 mg over 24 h) and then reduced to 50 mg over 24 h and tapered until oral replacement is possible. (The hydrocortisone phosphate preparation causes perineal discomfort on rapid intravenous administration and should be given slowly.)
- *Minor surgery*: 25 mg hydrocortisone i.v. at induction only.

Oral maintenance for Addison's disease is cortisone 20–30 (mg day^{-1} in divided doses) plus fludrocortisone (0.1 mg once a day).

PERIOPERATIVE MANAGEMENT

Monitoring:
- Central venous pressure
- Pulmonary artery flotation catheter
- Arterial cannula (sodium, potassium, blood glucose)
- ECG (arrythmias)
- Capnography (hypocapnia will lower extracellular potassium)
- Urine output.

General anaesthesia
Induction of anaesthesia should be in theatre with full monitoring. There are no particular indications for any one anaesthetic technique: a careful conventional anaesthetic is appropriate. These patients are susceptible to the depressant effects of many induction agents, narcotic analgesics and general anaesthetics. Ketamine was successfully used in a previously documented case. The induction agent etomidate inhibits the release of cortisol and is contraindicated. The importance of the adrenocortical responses to anaesthetic and surgical stress is unclear, particularly in view of the finding that patients may withstand surgery after the adrenocortical responses have been pharmacologically inhibited. Inadequate replacement of fluid and electrolytes is the more usual cause of perioperative hypotension.

Local anaesthesia
Inadequate fluid replacement may lead to cardiovascular instability.

POSTOPERATIVE MANAGEMENT

The patient should be monitored in the ITU:

- Fluid balance
- Electrolyte abnormalities (may have postoperative hypokalaemia)
- Renal function
- Steroid replacement.

BIBLIOGRAPHY

Herzberg L, Shulman M S. Acute adrenal insufficiency in a patient with acute appendicitis during anaesthesia. Anesthesiology 1985; 62: 517–518
Smith M G, Byrne A J. An Addison crisis complicating anaesthesia. Anaesthesia 1981; 361: 681
Weatherill D, Spence A A. Anaesthesia and disorders of the adrenal cortex. British Journal of Anaesthesia 1984; 56: 741–749

CROSS REFERENCES

Water and electrolyte disturbances
Patient Conditions 10: 246

APUDOMAS

J. Desborough

2

APUD describes groups of cells characterized by amine precursor uptake and decarboxylation, which results in the synthesis of biologically active amines and peptides. APUDomas are tumours of cells with APUD properties. The clinical manifestations of the tumour are characterized by overproduction of particular hormones and peptides. APUD cells are found in the pituitary, adrenal medulla, peripheral autonomic ganglia, gastrointestinal tract, pancreas, lung, gonads and thymus. Tumours may occur as part of multiple endocrine neoplasia (MEN). The management of patients with phaeochromocytoma, insulinoma and carcinoid tumours is dealt with elsewhere.

GASTRINOMA

A rare gastrin-producing tumour. Incidence is one case per million population per year. Manifests as Zollinger–Ellison syndrome characterized by gastric acid oversecretion with peptic ulceration and diarrhoea. One-third occur as part of MEN associated with other endocrine tumours.

Perioperative management

Elective surgery is considered if medical therapy does not suppress gastric acid oversecretion Therapy includes:

- Proton pump antagonists, e.g. omeprazole
- H_2 receptor antagonists, e.g. ranitidine
- Octreotide (octapeptide analogue of somatostatin).

Patients may present acutely with gastrointestinal bleeding and perforation. Diarrhoea and vomiting secondary to pyloric stenosis may cause electrolyte disturbances, volume depletion, arrhythmias.

Invasive cardiovascular monitoring is generally required.

Surgery is likely to be prolonged.

Postoperative management:

- Continue monitoring
- Provide analgesia
- Mortality is high during emergency procedures.

VIPomas

Extremely rare tumour releasing vasoactive intestinal peptide (VIP). Most arise from the pancreas, but may occur in other tissues. The syndrome is associated with watery diarrhoea, hypokalaemia and achlorhydria (WDHA syndrome). Also called Verner–Morrison syndrome.

Preoperative assessment

Symptoms should be controlled prior to elective surgery using drugs to stabilize the tumour:

- Ocreotide
- Glucocorticoids may also be used.

Assess for hypovolaemia, metabolic acidosis, electrolyte abnormalities.

Perioperative management

- Invasive cardiovascular monitoring
- Frequent blood sampling to check acid–base status, electrolytes.

BIBLIOGRAPHY

Owen R. Anaesthetic considerations in endocrine surgery. In: Lynn J, Bloom S R (eds) Surgical endocrinology. Butterworth-Heinemann, Oxford, 1993, p 71–84

Philippe J. Apudomas: acute complications and their medical management. Baillière's Clinics in Endocrinology and Metabolism 1992; 6: 217–228

Thakker R V. Multiple endocrine neoplasia and molecular genetics. In: Lynn J, Bloom S R (eds) Surgical endocrinology. Butterworth-Heinemann, Oxford, 1993, p 34–46

CROSS REFERENCES

Multiple endocrine neoplasia
Patient Conditions 2: 59

CONN'S SYNDROME

A. Quinn

Aldosterone, the mineralocorticoid secreted by the zona glomerulosa of the adrenal cortex promotes sodium reabsorption and potassium exchange in the renal tubules. Excess aldosterone production may be due to an adrenal adenoma (60%), bilateral adrenal hyperplasia (30%) or to a carcinoma. Conn's syndrome is rare, accounting for <1% of hypertension.

PATHOPHYSIOLOGY

Biochemical/renal

Plasma renin levels are low, plasma aldosterone levels are high. Urinary potassium is high despite a low total body potassium, and serum sodium may be elevated. Renal function may be abnormal, and this is related to chronic potassium depletion and hypertension.

Cardiovascular system:

- Hypertension may be severe, associated with renal and retinal damage.
- The ECG may show arrythmias or T wave flattening and U waves.

Metabolic:

- Hypokalaemic alkalosis
- Abnormal glucose tolerance test in up to 50% of patients.

PREOPERATIVE ASSESSMENT

Adrenal pathology

Differentiation of adenoma from hyperplasia involves adrenal CT or MRI, complex biochemical testing and venous sampling. In Conn's syndrome, aldosterone levels are high only in the adrenal vein draining the tumour and suppressed on the contralateral side. Surgical removal is recommended for unilateral adenoma only; bilateral hyperplasia responds better to medical treatment.

History

The common symptoms are weakness, nocturia, polyuria and polydipsia. Hypokalaemia may result in tetany; quadriparesis has been described which was reversed by potassium.

Investigations:

- Urea, electrolytes and blood glucose
- Arterial blood gases
- ECG for arrythmias, signs of hypokalaemia, left ventricular hypertrophy
- Chest X-ray may show cardiomegaly
- Blood cross-matching.

PREOPERATIVE MANAGEMENT

- Potassium infusion, e.g. 6–20 mmol h^{-1} (at least 24 h may be required to restore potassium equilibrium)
- ECG (hypokalaemia causes ST depression, flattened T waves, U waves)
- Aldosterone antagonist, e.g. spironolactone (100 mg t.d.s.)
- Insulin infusion.

PERIOPERATIVE MANAGEMENT

Premedication

Moderate sedation with opioids or hypnotics.

Induction and maintenance

The anaesthetic technique should be tailored to avoid hypotensive or hypertensive events:

- Preoxygenate
- Slow intravenous induction and intubation with direct arterial pressure monitoring, e.g. alfentanyl (20–30 μg kg^{-1}), thiopentone (2–5 mg kg^{-1}), atracurium (0.5 mg kg^{-1})
- IPPV.

Special points for adrenalectomy

There may be marked intraoperative blood loss from nearby major blood vessels. Good muscle relaxation is important as surgical access may be difficult. Postoperative pneumothorax may occur.

Monitoring:

- Arterial cannula to monitor acid–base

balance, blood glucose, haematocrit and direct arterial pressure
- Central venous line for monitoring fluid requirements
- ECG monitoring during induction and intubation; high risk of arrhythmia, ischaemia
- Capnography; hyperventilation exacerbates alkalosis
- Urinary catheter, as risk of renal failure
- Peripheral nerve stimulation; increased sensitivity to myoneural blocking agents (hypokalaemia and alkalosis)
- May have hypertensive surges during surgical manipulation; treat with, e.g. labetalol (10–50 mg i.v.) or phentolamine (2.5–5 mg) every 5 min.

POSTOPERATIVE CARE

- HDU/ITU
- Postoperative respiratory support; there may be a compensatory respiratory acidosis for the metabolic alkalosis and increased sensitivity to respiratory depressant drugs and muscle relaxants that the patient may require
- Postoperative arrhythmias
- Renal function
- Beware pneumothorax
- Following surgery, it may take a week for sodium and potassium to return to normal values, and hypertension may persist even longer
- Glucocorticoid therapy should only be required if both adrenal glands are mobilized or removed.

BIBLIOGRAPHY

Brown B. Clinical report: primary aldosteronism with uncommon complications. Anesthesiology 1976; 45: 542–544

Shipton E A, Hugo J M. An aldosterone-producing adrenal cortical adenoma. Anaesthesia 1982; 37: 933–936

Weatherill D, Spence A A. Anaesthesia and disorders of the adrenal cortex. British Journal of Anaesthesia 1984; 56: 741–749

CROSS REFERENCES

Hypertension
Patient Conditions 4: 111
Assessment of renal function
Patient Conditions 6: 155

CUSHING'S SYNDROME

A. Quinn

This is the term used to describe the clinical state of increased free circulating glucocorticoid. It occurs most frequently as a result of exogenous corticosteroid administration; all the spontaneous forms are rare.

Causes of Cushing's syndrome

ACTH-dependent disease (60–70%):
- Pituitary-dependent (Cushing's disease) producing bilateral adrenal hyperplasia
- Ectopic ACTH-producing tumours (bronchial, pancreatic carcinoma)
- ACTH administration

Non-ACTH-dependent causes:
- Adrenal adenomas
- Adrenal carcinomas
- Glucocorticoid administration

Other:
- Alcohol-induced pseudo-Cushing's syndrome

PATHOPHYSIOLOGY

The main actions of glucocorticoids are:

- Suppression of pituitary ACTH secretion
- Glycogen deposition, increased gluconeogenesis, fat deposition
- Increased protein catabolism and decreased synthesis
- Potassium loss, sodium retention, increased free water clearance and uric acid production

- Immunosuppression and increased circulating neutrophils.

PREOPERATIVE ASSESSMENT

Some patients will require perioperative intensive care management for optimal treatment of diabetes, hypertension/cardiac failure, restrictive lung disease, fluid and electrolyte abnormalities (low potassium, especially if diuretic therapy) and steroid requirements.

Morphological:
- Assessment of airway in obese patient
- Careful positioning (osteoporosis and pathological fractures, obesity, easy bruising)
- Assessment of fragile veins/arteries
- Assessment of ease of local anaesthetic technique.

History
The following history may be elicited:

- *Metabolic*: diabetes
- *Cardiovascular*: hypertension, oedema
- *Skin and subcutaneous tissue*: centripetal obesity, acne, hirsutism, bruising, striae, pigmentation, thin skin, poor wound healing, skin infection, frontal balding pattern, moon face, plethora, buffalo hump
- *Bone*: osteoporosis, rib fractures, pathological fractures, vertebral collapse, kyphosis
- *Muscle*: proximal muscle wasting, proximal myopathy, weakness
- *CNS*: depression/psychosis
- *Children*: growth arrest.

Investigations:
- Full blood count
- Urea and electrolytes, blood glucose
- ECG (ischaemia, hypokalaemia)
- Chest X-ray (kyphoscoliosis, osteoporosis, cardiac enlargement, left ventricular failure, lower lobe collapse, carcinoma of the bronchus)
- Lung function tests.

PERIOPERATIVE MANAGEMENT

The patient may present for adrenalectomy (see Conn's syndrome, 1.2.37), but more commonly for routine emergency or elective surgery.

The mortality after bilateral adrenalectomy in Cushing's syndrome is 5–10%.

Premedication
Preoperative apprehension has little effect on plasma cortisol. Conventional premedication is used. May require steroid cover (see Iatrogenic adrenocortical insufficiency, 1.2.34). Concomitant medication commonly includes: antihypertensives, diuretics (e.g. spironolactone), insulin, antibiotics, antacids, inhibitors of cortisol synthesis (e.g. metyrapone, glutethimide, bromocriptine), H_2 antagonists and deep venous thrombosis (DVT) prophylaxis.

Monitoring
This should commence in the anaesthetic room and includes:

- Central venous pressure (CVP) and pulmonary artery pressure measurement (patients with Cushing's syndrome tend to have a bleeding tendency and a raised CVP)
- Arterial pressure monitoring
- Blood sampling for arterial blood gases, blood glucose, haematocrit
- ECG (CM_5 to detect myocardial ischaemia)
- Capnography, Sp_{O_2}
- Peripheral nerve stimulator
- Urine output.

INTRAOPERATIVE MANAGEMENT

No particular anaesthetic technique is indicated. However, anaesthetic agents should be administered slowly and carefully as these patients are sensitive to any cardiodepressant effects.

General anaesthesia:
- Rapid sequence induction for obese patient
- Prepare equipment for difficult intubation
- IPPV
- May require high $F_{I}O_2$
- Careful patient positioning is essential.

Local anaesthesia
This may lessen the stress response to surgery, e.g. epidural anaesthesia. This may be technically difficult, but the advantages are that it produces good analgesia and enables minimal administration of opioids and rapid mobilization. It may also reduce the incidence of thromboembolism.

POSTOPERATIVE MANAGEMENT

Patients should be admitted to the ITU postoperatively. Muscle weakness, obesity, kyphosis and frequent rib fractures make respiratory complications common. There is delayed wound healing and increased incidence of postoperative CVA, myocardial infarction, stress ulceration and pulmonary thromboembolism.

- Electrolyte abnormalities: avoid excessive administration of sodium-containing intravenous fluids because of the mineralocorticoid effect of excess cortisol
- Continuous humidified oxygen therapy
- Analgesia: opioid infusion, patient-controlled analgesia, epidural opioid/local anaesthetic
- Steroids: maintenance therapy following surgery may be necessary for rest of life
- Insulin infusion
- Physiotherapy/early mobilization
- DVT prophylaxis
- Vitamin D (treatment prior to surgery may lead to hypercalcaemia and renal stones)
- Pancreatitis (after adrenalectomy).

BIBLIOGRAPHY

Pender J W, Basso L V. Diseases of the endocrine system. In: Katz J, Benumof J, Kadis L B (eds) Anaesthesia and uncommon diseases. W B Saunders, Philadelphia, 1981, p 155–221

Weatherill D, Spence A A. Anaesthesia and disorders of the adrenal cortex. British Journal of Anaesthesia 1984; 56: 741–749

CROSS REFERENCES

Hypertension
Patient Conditions 4: 111
Anaemia
Patient Conditions 7: 168
Metabolic and degenerative bone disease
Patient Conditions 8: 200

DIABETES INSIPIDUS

W. Fawcett

Diabetes insipidus (DI) is a syndrome in which there is either failure of arginine vasopressin (AVP) production (neurogenic or cranial DI) or of the kidneys to respond to AVP (nephrogenic DI). AVP is usually released in response to increased serum osmolality or a reduction in plasma volume. Thus there is failure to conserve water, leading to polydypsia and polyuria.

PATHOPHYSIOLOGY

Cranial DI
- Primary
- Secondary
  - Trauma
  - Tumour (primary or secondary)
  - Infection
  - Vascular causes

Nephrogenic DI
- Primary
- Secondary
  - Hypercalcaemia
  - Hypokalaemia
  - Drugs (lithium, demeclocycline, glibenclamide, amphotericin B, methoxyflurane)

The hallmarks of the syndrome are large urine volumes (up to $1\ l\ h^{-1}$) with low urine osmolality ($50–100\ mOsm\ kg^{-1}$). However, plasma osmolalities and sodium concentrations may be in the normal range if there is access to free water. If this is not the case then hypovolaemia and hypernatraemia may rapidly follow. There is a wide range of severity, depending on whether or not there is a complete loss of osmoregulation, and whether or not the response to volume stimuli is intact. The syndrome is be diagnosed by the inability to concentrate urine (>800 mOsm l^{-1}) following fluid deprivation. The ability to correct this defect is next tested by giving DDAVP: in cranial DI there is a response, in nephrogenic DI there is no response.

PREOPERATIVE ASSESSMENT

The preoperative assessment will be directed principally towards the assessment of fluid balance and serum osmolality. Thus attention should be directed towards the quantities the patient is drinking, and the fluid balance status. Look for signs of dehydration suggested by:

- Dry mouth, loss of skin turgor.
- Tachycardia, low venous pressure, and eventually hypotension. In addition, in secondary DI, there may be other problems, e.g. lung carcinoma.

Investigations:
- Serum urea, electrolytes and osmolality
- Serum calcium
- Urinary volumes and osmolality; the aim should be to have a serum osmolality of less than 290 mOsm l^{-1}.

No patient with uncontrolled DI should undergo surgery until it is corrected. This should be done in conjunction with an endocrinologist, and would usually include intranasal DDAVP (5–20 μg b.d.) for cranial DI. Other treatments for cranial DI include chlorpro-pramide and carbamazepine which augrnent AVP release. Nephrogenic DI is treated with thiazides. Acute treatment of hypovolaemia should be to gradually reduce serum sodium and osmolalities (over 48 h). Rapid correction with large amounts of hypotonic fluids is to be condemned as there is a substantial risk of cerebral oedema, and haemorrhage.

The patient should not undergo prolonged fasting without intravenous fluids. Patients will need to be monitored postoperatively in an ITU/HDU environment.

PERIOPERATIVE MANAGEMENT

The principal aim is to maintain the patient's fluid balance. Thus meticulous care is required to ensure that urine loss and other losses from surgery (insensible/blood) are accurately replaced.

Monitoring should include:

- Urine output
- Arterial cannula for major surgery
- Central venous pressure
- Serum osmolalities need to be checked regularly (i.e. 2–4 hourly) in the acute situation.

In cranial DI, DDAVP would normally be given immediately preoperatively, and further amounts given if the serum osmolalitiy exceeds 290 mOsm l^{-1}. In patients with some AVP production, the 'stress' response of surgery may produce adequate amounts of AVP, but this cannot be relied upon.

POSTOPERATIVE MANAGEMENT

The patient will require continued management of fluid balance in the postoperative period, particularly following major surgery, or whilst blood loss is a problem.

CROSS REFERENCES

Water and electrolyte disturbances
Patient Conditions 10: 246

DIABETES MELLITUS (IDDM)

R. Milaszkiewicz

An autoimmune disorder of the pancreas characterized by islet cell destruction.

Characteristics:
- Age of onset usually less than 30 years
- Absolute insulin deficiency
- Abrupt onset of symptoms
- Tendency to ketosis.

Complications
Long term:
- Retinopathy
- Ischaemic heart disease
- Hypertension
- Nephropathy
- Neuropathy – peripheral and autonomic
- Stiff joint syndrome.

Short term:
- Hypoglycaemia
- Hyperglycaemia with metabolic disturbance; may be exacerbated by the 'stress response' during surgery
- Gastric stasis is common, especially with ketoacidosis.

In the long term, good control of blood glucose decreases the risk of developing microvascular, but not macrovascular, complications.

PREOPERATIVE ASSESSMENT

History
- Diabetes:
  - Duration
  - Control
  - Type, quantity and timing of insulin dosage.
- Kidneys: nephropathy (mild-severe).
- CVS:
  - Coronary artery disease
  - Hypertension.
- CNS: peripheral and autonomic neuropathy.
- Other drugs.

Examination
Full physical examination, including lying and standing blood pressure, and heart rate during deep breaths or Valsalva manoeuvre to exclude autonomic neuropathy. Airway assessment: the stiff joint syndrome (SJS) may cause difficulty with intubation.

Investigations
- Short-term glycaemic control: fasting blood glucose
- Long-term glycaemic control:
  - Glycosylated haemoglobin (HbA_1C), or fructosamine
  - Full blood count.
- Renal function:
  - Urinalysis, plasma urea, creatinine and electrolyte concentration
  - Chest X-ray, if clinically indicated.
- ECG: silent ischaemia.

AIMS OF PERIOPERATIVE MANAGEMENT

Maintenance of normoglycaemia
Blood glucose should stay within the range 6–12 mmol l^{-1}. Hyperglycaemia causes dehydration, electrolyte disturbance, acidosis, poor tissue perfusion and organ ischaemia, impaired wound healing and increased susceptibility to infection. Any cerebral or myocardial ischaemia will be aggravated by hyperglycaemia. Hypoglycaemia may cause cerebral damage.

Appropriate management of coexisting disease
This is a greater cause of morbidity than the diabetes itself. In patients with, or at risk of, coronary artery disease, diabetes is a factor in the development of postoperative ischaemia; valvular disease and cardiac failure are predictors of serious cardiac morbidity or death. Autonomic neuropathy may cause cardiovascular instability during anaesthesia.

GENERAL PRINCIPLES OF MANAGEMENT

Major surgery
Ideally, the patient is admitted 24–48 h preoperatively. Following assessment, the

insulin regimen is adjusted to optimize glycaemic control. In practice, many patients are admitted late on the day before surgery. It is usually impractical to alter their existing therapy. Diabetic patients should be operated on at the beginning of morning lists.

Glucose

Sufficient glucose is supplied to prevent hypoglycaemia and to provide basal energy requirements. It is recommended that 5–10 g h^{-1} of glucose is given, as either 5% or 10% dextrose. For longer term infusions, 0.9% sodium chloride is also needed to prevent hyponatraemia.

Insulin

The morning dose of insulin should be omitted. However, if the patient is due to have surgery in the afternoon, either set up infusions of insulin and glucose in the morning, or give half the usual dose of insulin with a light breakfast, then set up an infusion midmorning.

Insulin is given with glucose to prevent gluconeogenesis, glycogenolysis, ketosis and protein break-down. It should be given by an intravenous infusion, as absorption of subcutaneous insulin is variable, especially in the perioperative period. Intravenous boluses are unphysiological, and may cause deterioration of metabolic control. Infusions may be given with glucose (the Alberti regimen, see Table 1) or as a separate infusion by sliding scale (Table 2). The usual requirements are 0.25–0.35 units per gram of glucose.

Insulin requirements are increased with: steroid therapy, sepsis, liver disease, obesity and during cardiopulmonary bypass.

Table 1.
The Alberti regimen

Glucose 10%	500 ml
Insulin (soluble)	15 units
Potassium	10 mmol

- Add together
- Infuse this at 100 ml h^{-1}
- Blood glucose is monitored 2 hourly and the insulin content of a bag adjusted by 5 units if the blood glucose falls outside the range 6–12 mmol l^{-1}.

Table 2.
Sliding scale for insulin

Blood glucose (mmol l^{-1})	Insulin infusion* (units h^{-1})
0–5	0–1
6–10	1–2
11–15	2–3
16–20	3–4
>20	4–6

*Infusion: make up 50 units insulin to 50 ml with saline (1 unit ml^{-1}). No need to add colloid, provided the first few millilitres are flushed through the giving set.

Potassium

Potassium should be added as required. Usually, 10 mmol l^{-1} of glucose, however this may need adjusting, according to plasma concentrations.

Minor surgery/day-cases

The safety of anaesthetizing IDDM patients as day-cases is not yet established, but is becoming increasingly common. Facilities must exist to admit these patients postoperatively, if necessary. Ideally, the operation should be performed in the morning, it should be short, and unlikely to prevent the patient from returning to a normal diet soon after surgery.

There is no consensus regarding management. Starting a glucose and insulin infusion is safe.

Either:
Omit the morning dose of insulin (except for long-acting insulins such as ultralente, which will not affect or be affected by the fasting in the perioperative period), and give a partial dose before the next meal.

Or:
Omit the morning dose of insulin and start glucose and insulin infusions.

A glucose and insulin infusion should be started if the fasting glucose is low, or if there is any delay to the start of surgery, and should be started if the patient suffers from nausea and vomiting postoperatively, until eating normally. Nausea and vomiting may indicate the development of ketoacidaemia.

Monitoring

Both hypoglycaemia and hyperglycaemia are

harmful. Under anaesthesia symptoms of hypoglycaemia are masked.

- *Blood glucose* should be checked 0.5–1 hourly in theatre, both using stick tests, and periodically confirming with laboratory blood glucose. Postoperatively, check hourly until normal eating established.
- *Plasma potassium* should be monitored 3–4 hourly, or more frequently if clinically indicated.

The insulin and glucose infusions are continued until the patient has resumed a normal diet.

Anaesthesia
Regional techniques, where appropriate, are preferable to general anaesthesia, as they usually allow a swifter return to normal eating patterns. They may partially decrease the 'stress response' associated with surgery.

CROSS REFERENCES

Assessment of renal function
Patient Conditions 6: 155
Carotid endarterectomy
Surgical Procedures 22: 451
Leg revascularization and amputation
Surgical Procedures 22: 453
Coronary artery bypass grafting
Surgical Procedures 27: 511

DIABETES MELLITUS (NIDDM)

R. Milaszkiewicz

Characterized by both hepatic and extrahepatic insulin resistance. Insulin secretion and insulin action are thought to be deficient with excessive hepatic glucose production.

Characteristics:
- Variable age of onset; usually >30 years
- Slower onset
- Unlikely to develop ketoacidosis.

Complications:
- Increased incidence of macrovascular disease, especially peripheral vascular and cardiovascular disease, irrespective of age at diagnosis
- Nephropathy is common and is associated with cardiovascular disease.

Unlike IDDM, glycaemic control has less influence on the development of complications. In younger patients the aim is to maintain fasting blood glucose at <7 mmol l^{-1}. In the elderly patient, <10 mmol l^{-1} is more realistic.

Management
- *Diet.*
- *Sulphonylureas*: increase pancreatic β-cell sensitivity to glucose. Thereby enhance insulin release. Highly protein bound. Metabolized by liver; metabolites have some activity. Excreted by kidneys.
- *Biguanides*: several possible modes of action. Most likely reduce hepatic glucose production. Metformin only available drug.

Not protein bound. Not metabolized by liver. Excreted unchanged by kidneys.
- *Acarbose*: inhibits α-glucosidases in the brush border of small intestinal mucosa. Delays absorption of glucose.

PREOPERATIVE ASSESSMENT

Should follow the same lines as for IDDM.

PERIOPERATIVE MANAGEMENT

These patients are still able to secrete some insulin; however, they are insulin resistant.

Minor surgery/Day surgery

Well-controlled, diet-treated patients do not need special treatment apart from monitoring of the blood glucose. For those on oral hypoglycaemic agents there is controversy. If on long-acting agents, such as chlorpropramide, ideally this should be changed to a shorter acting drug a few days before surgery. Omit the morning dose of any hypoglycaemic agent. If the fasting blood glucose is >12 mmol l^{-1}, start an infusion of glucose and insulin. If blood glucose is <12 mmol l^{-1} it may be sufficient to just monitor the blood glucose. The most important feature is careful, frequent monitoring of blood glucose and early corrective measures if the blood glucose goes outside the range 6–12 mmol l^{-1}.

Major surgery

Treat as IDDM patients. Hyperosmolar, hyperglycaemic, nonketotic coma may occur postoperatively.

Fluids

There is some evidence against the use of Hartmann's solution, and at present it is better avoided.

Anaesthesia

Many of these patients will be presenting for surgery for complications of their diabetes. Anaesthesia should cause minimal metabolic disturbance. Regional techniques are usually preferable to general anaesthesia, unless there is severe cardiovascular disturbance.

BIBLIOGRAPHY

Hirsch I B, McGill J B, Cryer P E, White P F. Perioperative management of surgical patients with diabetes mellitus. Anesthesiology 1991; 74: 346–359

2

HYPERPARATHYROIDISM

R. Edwards

Hyperparathyroidism is a syndrome due to increased secretion of parathyroid hormone (PTH) from the parathyroid glands. Parathyroid hormone acts both directly and indirectly to increase serum calcium (normal total serum calcium 2.3–2.8 mmol l^{-1}).

Hyperparathyroidism may be classified as primary, secondary or tertiary hyperparathyroidism.

Causes of hyperparathyroidism

Primary hyperparathyroidism:
- Adenoma (85%) or hyperplasia (10–15%) of parathyroid glands
- Adenoma may be part of MEA syndrome
- Carcinoma (1–3%)
- Ectopic PTH produced by carcinoma lung/kidney.

Secondary hyperparathyroidism:
- Physiological response to hypocalcaemia produced by another disease, e.g. chronic renal failure.

Tertiary hyperparathyroidism:
- Chronic secondary hyperparathyroidism has led to an autonomous adenoma.

Actions of PTH:
- Directly increases renal tubular reabsorption of calcium and decreases tubular reabsorption of phosphate
- Increases calcium reabsorption from bone
- Controls hydroxylation of 25-hydroxycholecalciferol in the kidney, and therefore promotes the synthesis of 1,25-dihydroxycholecalciferol and increases calcium absorption from the gut.

Metabolic abnormalities

Primary and tertiary hyperparathyroidism
- Serum calcium high
- Low serum phosphate
- PTH high
- Raised alkaline phosphatase
- Mild hyperchloraemic acidosis.

Secondary hyperparathyroidism
- Serum calcium low
- High serum phosphate.

PATHOPHYSIOLOGY

Most of the signs and symptoms of hyperparathyroidism are due to hypercalcaemia, and their severity is related to the level of serum calcium. Patients with mild hypercalcaemia (serum calcium <3.0 mmol l^{-1}) are often asymptomatic.

General:
- Muscle fatigue and hypotonicity
- Psychosis and depression with severe, prolonged hypercalcaemia
- Calcium deposition in conjuntiva, usually medical limbus of eye
- X-rays of hands, feet and teeth may show subperiosteal resorption, bone cysts and loss of lamina dura of teeth.

Renal system:
- Polyuria
- Polydipsia
- Dehydration
- Renal calculi, nephrocalcinosis and later renal failure.

Gastrointestinal tract:
- Anorexia
- Nausea
- Vomiting
- Abdominal pain
- Constipation
- Dyspepsia
- Peptic ulceration.

Cardiovascular system:
- Tachycardia
- Arrhythmias
- Hypertension.

PREOPERATIVE ASSESSMENT

History

Review of symptoms associated with hypercalcaemia.

Investigations:

- Serum calcium serum electrolytes and urea for renal failure
- ECG (shortened PR or QT interval).

Patients with severe hypercalcaemia may present with hypovolaemia and coma. Emergency treatment comprises: hydration; diuresis and phosphate repletion; emergency parathyroidectomy.

PERIOPERATIVE MANAGEMENT

- No special monitoring is required
- Care should be taken to protect the eyes from pressure or abrasion during surgery
- An armoured orotracheal tube avoids airway obstruction due to kinking of the tube
- All airway connections should be secured prior to draping the patient, as access to the head and neck is limited when surgery has commenced
- No advantage of any one anaesthetic agent over another has been demonstrated in these patients.

POSTOPERATIVE COMPLICATIONS

Nerve damage

Bilateral recurrent laryngeal nerve injury (due to trauma or oedema) leads to stridor and laryngeal obstruction due to unopposed adduction of vocal cords. Requires immediate intubation and tracheostomy until recovery occurs. Unilateral damage is often unnoticed due to compensatory overadduction of the opposite cord.

Oedema of the glottis and pharynx may occasionally follow parathyroid surgery.

Metabolic abnormalities

Hypocalcaemia may occur due to insufficient residual parathyroid tissue, delay in recovery of normal tissue, operative trauma/ischaemia. Causes laryngeal spasm, convulsions. Chvostek's/Trousseau's signs positive.

Hypomagnesaemia/hypophosphataemia may also occur postoperatively. Correction of serum magnesium concentration is important, as a low level inhibits the secretion of parathyroid hormone.

Serial determinations of serum calcium, phosphate, magnesium and parathyroid hormone are required for several days postoperatively. These investigations may be difficult to obtain in a District General Hospital.

BIBLIOGRAPHY

Roizen M F. Diseases of the endocrine system. In: Katz J, Benumof J L, Kadis L B (eds) Anesthesia and uncommon diseases. W B Saunders, Philadelphia, 1990, p 245–292

Sebel P S. Thyroid and parathyroid disease. In: Nimmo W S, Smith G (eds) Anaesthesia. Blackwell Scientific, Oxford, 1989, p 771–778

CROSS REFERENCES

Bronchogenic carcinoma
Patient Conditions 3: 73
Water and electrolyte disturbances
Patient Conditions 10: 246

HYPERTHYROIDISM

R. Edwards

2

This is a clinical syndrome due to excessive production of the thyroid hormones triiodothyronine (T3) and thyroxine (T4). The production of these hormones from the thyroid gland is regulated by thyroid stimulating hormone (TSH) from the anterior pituitary, which is in turn influenced by thyrotrophin releasing factor (TRF) from the hypothalamus. Diagnosis is confirmed by elevated serum concentrations of free and total T4 and T3 and undetectable serum TSH.

PATHOPHYSIOLOGY

In 90% of cases there is multinodular diffuse enlargement of the thyroid gland. In Graves' disease there is a toxic nodular goitre.

Rarer causes include:
- Thyroid adenoma
- Choriocarcinoma
- Thyroiditis
- Pituitary adenoma.

CLINICAL FEATURES

General:
- Weight loss
- Heat intolerance
- Fatigue
- Anxiety.

Cardiovascular
- Tachycardia
- Atrial fibrillation
- Increased cardiac output
- Cardiac failure
- Increased myocardial sensitivity to catecholamines (thyroid hormones increase the number of myocardial B receptors)
- Elderly patients may present with heart failure.

Gastrointestinal
Diarrhoea.

Neuromuscular
Muscle weakness, proximal myopathy.

Haematological
Anaemia, thrombocytopoenia.

PREOPERATIVE ASSESSMENT

It is essential that patients are rendered euthyroid prior to surgery as the operative risk is greater in the untreated patient. This is achieved with antithyroid drugs for 2–3 months followed by iodine for 10 days to reduce the vascularity of the gland. Propanolol alone or in combination with the above regimen may be used and is associated with rapid relief of symptoms and perioperative cardiovascular stability.

History and examination
Preoperative assessment should include a systematic review of symptoms or signs to determine adequate control of thyroid function. A resting heart rate of less than 80 beats min^{-1} and the absence of tremor indicates that the patient is euthyroid. The neck should be examined and position of the trachea noted. A history of stridor suggests tracheal compression by a goitre.

Investigations:
- Full blood count
- Thoracic inlet X-ray – allows evaluation of the extent of compression or deviation of the trachea by a thyroid goitre
- Chest X-ray – to exclude retrosternal extension which may impair respiration
- ECG
- Cross-matched blood available.

PERIOPERATIVE MANAGEMENT

- Premedication
- Higher doses of premedicant drugs are necessary to reduce anxiety
- Atropine should be avoided due to tachycardia
- Antithyroid drugs, including beta blockers should be administered prior to surgery.

Monitoring
- Prior to induction, continuous ECG monitoring should be instituted and maintained throughout

- Indirect arterial pressure measurements are adequate in the absence of cardiovascular instability, pulse oximetry
- An oesophageal stethoscope is useful as patient access is limited during surgery
- Core temperature.

Airway management
If preoperative assessment suggests tracheal involvement, equipment for difficult intubation is required:

- Suxamethonium should be administered after it is ensured that the patient's lungs can be ventilated manually. Alternatively, awake intubation may be considered.
- A smaller orotracheal tube than usual may be required, although the trachea is usually distensible.
- The tip of the tube should be advanced beyond any area of compression. An armoured tube is advisable to avoid kinking during surgical dissection.
- The tube should be firmly taped in position and all connections secured, as access to the airway is limited during surgery.

There is no evidence that the choice of anaesthetic agent is important, although studies in rodents treated with T3 have demonstrated a higher incidence of hepatic necrosis with halothane anaesthesia. The patient is positioned with the neck fully extended and a head-up tilt to reduce venous bleeding. Many surgeons infiltrate the site of incision with adrenaline-containing local anaesthetic solutions. Care should be taken that the accepted dose of adrenaline is not exceeded and in this circumstance isoflurane is the volatile agent of choice. The eyes should be adequately protected and taped shut, especially in patients with the proptosis and lid retraction associated with Graves' disease. Bradycardia and hypotension is a complication of carotid sinus manipulation. This usually ceases with cessation of surgery and administration of atropine. Infiltration of the area with lignocaine prevents recurrence.

Venous air embolism may occur, especially if the patient is in the head-up position.

POSTOPERATIVE COMPLICATIONS

Thyroid storm:

- Low incidence but high mortality
- Occurs in untreated or partially treated patients, or those with intercurrent infection
- May occur up to 18 h postoperatively
- Symptoms are fever, tachycardia, cardiac failure, coma
- May be confused with malignant hyperthermia
- Treatment comprises intravenous propanolol, steroids, sodium iodide and fluids and surface cooling.

Nerve injury
Recurrent laryngeal nerve:

- Unilateral nerve injury is well tolerated due to compensation by the unaffected cord. Bilateral nerve injury causes airway obstruction and requires reintubation.
- Superior laryngeal nerve (sensory innervation to larynx and piriform fossa); may remain undetected until the patient takes their first drink, when aspiration occurs.

Other complications

- Haematoma formation: some advocate extubation while the patient is asleep to reduce the incidence of coughing and, therefore, the risk of haematoma formation. Stitch cutters or clip removers must be immediately available.
- Tracheal collapse.
- Tracheal laceration.
- Tracheo-oesophageal fistula.
- Pneumothorax.
- Phrenic nerve injury.
- Pneumomediastinum.
- Parathyroid damage leading to postoperative hypocalcaemia.

BIBLIOGRAPHY

Mercer D M, Eltringham R J. Anaesthesia for thyroid surgery. Ear, Nose and Throat Journal 1985; 64: 375–378

Roizen M F. Diseases of the endocrine system. In: Katz J, Benumof J L, Kadis L B (eds) Anesthesia and Uncommon Diseases. W B Saunders, Philadelphia, 1990, p 245–292

Sebel P S. Thyroid and parathyroid disease. In: Nimmo W S, Smith G (eds) Anaesthesia. Blackwell Scientific, Oxford, 1989, p 771–778

CROSS REFERENCES

Thyroidectomy
Surgical Procedures 15: 326
Artificial airways
Anaesthetic Factors 30: 554

HYPOPITUITARISM

W. Fawcett

There are six major anterior pituitary hormones:

- Growth hormone (GH)
- Prolactin
- Thyroid stimulating hormone (TSH)
- Follicle stimulating hormone (FSH)
- Leuteinizing hormone (LH)
- ACTH (and related peptides such as lipoproteins, endorphins and melanocyte stimulating hormone (MSH)).

Deficiency of the posterior lobe hormones (AVP and oxytocin) is rare in lesions confined to the pituitary fossa, but occurs more commonly with hypothalamic disease and/or suprasellar extension of a pituitary tumour.

PATHOPHYSIOLOGY

Hypopituitarism commonly arises from a primary pituitary tumour (e.g. prolactinoma in adults, and craniopharyngioma in children). Other causes include trauma, secondary tumours, infection, vascular causes (malformations, massive blood loss), postoperative/postradiation. The clinical features depend on the degree of disruption of the various hormones. Of major relevance to anaesthesia are ACTH and TSH deficiency from the anterior pituitary, and AVP deficiency from the posterior pituitary (to be considered elsewhere). It is noteworthy that when cortisol and AVP deficiency coexist, there may not be any features of diabetes insipidus as cortisol deficiency reduces free water excretion. Diagnosis may be confirmed by no response of GH to hypoglycaemia, and no response of TSH to thyrotrophin releasing factor (TRH).

TSH deficiency

Thyrotrophin is the principal regulator of thyroid function. The patient will therefore be hypothyroid, and there will be low circulating serum thyroxine (T4) and TSH, and impaired response to TRH. The clinical features may include:

- A reduced cardiac output (secondary to reduced stroke volume and bradycardia); ischaemic heart disease
- Reduced respiratory reserve (due to a reduction in maximum breathing capacity and carbon monoxide transfer factor, and pleural effusions)
- Hoarseness, sleep apnoea and respiratory obstruction (related to mucopolysaccharide deposition on the vocal cords)
- Reduced response to both hypoxia and hypercarbia
- A reduction in plasma volume, anaemia and coagulopathy.

ACTH deficiency

This will cause adrenal cortisol hyposecretion, but mineralocorticoid secretion should be normal (although not always). The classical picture is that of:

- Hypovolaemia, hyponatraemia, hyperkalaemia and hypoglycaemia
- Normochromic, normocytic anaemia may coexist
- There will be low serum cortisol and ACTH, but a response to synacthen.

PREOPERATIVE ASSESSMENT

A thorough cardiovascular and respiratory system evaluation is required, looking for airway obstruction (snoring, sleep apnoea), cardiac failure and hypotension. In addition, the underlying cause for hypopituitarism should be known, and other systems evaluated as necessary, such as neurological assessment in patients with head injuries.

Investigations

Investigations include:

- Full blood count
- Clotting screen
- Serum urea and electrolytes, glucose, T4 and cortisol levels

- A chest X-ray, ECG and echocardiography should all be considered.

Patients must have normal circulating T4 and cortisol values before undergoing elective surgery and, if necessary, surgery should be postponed until this is so. Treatment should be carried out in conjunction with an endocrinologist. Very great care is required in the use of intravenous T4 which may precipitate myocardial ischaemia. Replacement hormones should be continued throughout the perioperative period. Those patients requiring steroid hormones would conventionally receive extra steroid 'cover'. Sedative premedication should be used sparingly, if at all, in patients with hypothyroidism.

PERIOPERATIVE MANAGEMENT

Patients with normal hormone levels but with no other problems (such as raised intracranial pressure) require no special treatment. However, it is sometimes necessary to operate on patients who do not have a normal hormone profile. There may be a number of problems:

- Those who are hypothyroid will be very sensitive to all sedative agents (opioids, benzodiazepines and anaesthetic agents) and, in addition, they will have reduced metabolism and excretion of these agents
- Induction must be undertaken with extreme care: cardiac arrest has been reported at induction for both hypothyroidism and hypoadrenalism
- Avoid etomidate in those with impaired cortisol secretion
- Hypothermia may be a problem, and active measures should be taken to reduce heat loss (warming of intravenous fluids, warming mattress).

Those patients who are cortisol deficient will need cortisol to cover surgery (hydrocortisone 25 mg i.v. at induction, followed by 100 mg per 24 h). In addition they are likely to be dehydrated, and will require careful titration of both saline and glucose to maintain serum sodium and glucose within normal limits.

Monitoring

In addition to standard monitoring:

- Arterial and central venous cannulae (or pulmonary artery catheters) in patients with cardiac impairment and/or fluid balance problems
- Temperature
- Urine output
- Serum glucose should be monitored and if low (<4 mmol l^{-1}), 50% glucose given.

If unexplained hypotension occurs, then cardiac filling pressures should be checked first. Fluids, and/or hydrocortisone (which has a permissive effect on endogenous catecholamines) and occasionally fludrocortisone (which is usually for primary adrenocortical insufficiency) may be required.

POSTOPERATIVE MANAGEMENT

Patients with hypopituitarism following major surgery warrant ITU/HDU treatment postoperatively. Particular emphasis should be placed on:

- The airway (in those with vocal cord involvement)
- Cardiovascular status
- Temperature control
- Urine output
- Biochemistry, such as electrolytes and glucose.

Maintenance hormones should be continued into the postoperative period, as should steroid cover if used. Many cases of postoperative collapse in patients with a disrupted hypophyseal–adrenal–pituitary axis are probably not related to insufficient steroids, but to other factors, particularly hypovolaemia or, more rarely, sepsis. This should be borne in mind as they have very little physiological reserve, and tolerate these conditions very poorly.

CROSS REFERENCES

Diabetes insipidus
Patient Conditions 2: 40
Hypothyroidism
Patient Conditions 2: 48
Anaesthesia for trans-sphenoidal hypophysectomy
Surgical Procedures 12: 270

HYPOTHYROIDISM

R. Edwards

2

This is a clinical syndrome resulting from a deficiency of the thyroid hormones, triiodothyronine (T3) and thyroxine (T4). The diagnosis is confirmed by demonstrating a low serum concentration of T4 and elevated thyroid stimulating hormone (TSH) (unless the hypothyroidism is secondary to TSH deficiency).

PATHOPHYSIOLOGY

Causes of hypothyroidism:

- Autoimmune thyroiditis (Hashimoto's disease)
- Iatrogenic: surgical/medical radioiodine therapy for thyrotoxicosis
- Iodine deficiency
- Drugs, e.g. lithium, amiodarone
- Congenital
- Secondary hypothyroidism: pituitary disease, idiopathic TRH deficiency.

CLINICAL FEATURES

General:

- There is a reduction in the basal metabolic rate leading to lethargy, reduced mental function, weight gain and cold intolerance
- Hypothermia is a risk, especially in the elderly
- There is increased sensitivity to narcotics and anaesthetic agents.

Cardiovascular system:

- There is both bradycardia and reduced stroke volume and, therefore, reduced cardiac output
- Pericardial effusion may occur.

Respiratory system:

- There is a reduction in the ventilatory response to hypoxia and hypercapnia
- Maximum breathing capacity and carbon monoxide transfer factor may be reduced
- Pleural effusions may occur, further reducing ventilatory capacity.

Skin:

- There is dryness, alopecia and vitiligo
- Mucopolysaccharide deposition beneath the skin causes nonpitting oedema ('myxoedema'), and in the vocal cords causes hoarseness and even acute respiratory obstruction.

Haematological:

- Anaemia (normochromic normocytic or macrocytic)
- There is an association with pernicious anaemia.

Gastrointestinal tract:

- Constipation
- Ileus
- Ascites.

Untreated hypothyroidism culminates in myxoedema coma which is characterized by hypothermia, shock, acidosis, hyponatraemia, hypoglycaemia and, finally, coma and death.

PREOPERATIVE ASSESSMENT

History and examination

Symptoms and signs of hypothyroidism should be sought. Patients should be rendered euthyroid prior to surgery with thyroxine (50–200 μg daily). In the previously undiagnosed patient triiodothyronine is effective in a few hours and may be given intravenously in an emergency. This must be done in the intensive care setting with full monitoring, including ECG.

History of hoarseness is important, indicating vocal cord involvement. Assessment of goitre should be thorough, as for hyperthyroidism.

Investigations:

- Haemoglobin
- Serum urea and electrolyte concentrations
- ECG – slow voltage with flattened or inverted T waves in untreated hypothyroidism

- Chest X-ray – look for cardiomegaly, pleural effusion
- X-ray of thoracic inlet for tracheal involvement by goitre.

PERIOPERATIVE MANAGEMENT

Hypothyroidism is usually coincidental to surgery, unlike hyperthyroidism. The treated hypothyroid patient does not usually present a particular problem for anaesthesia and surgery. Untreated hypothyroidism is associated with adrenocortical insufficiency, and steroid supplements should be given prior to surgery.

Premedication

Narcotics and sedatives should be used with care due to increased sensitivity and the risk of respiratory depression. Cardiac output is decreased due to a reduction both in heart rate and stroke volume. Blood volume is also reduced, therefore myocardial depression and blood loss is poorly tolerated. Induction agents should be administered cautiously, with ECG and arterial pressure monitoring.

Airway management in the presence of a goitre is the same as for the hyperthyroid patient. Arterial pressure, ECG, respiratory parameters and temperature should be closely monitored from induction through to the postoperative period. Controlled ventilation should be employed as the respiratory response to hypoxia and hypercarbia is reduced. A reduction in thyroid hormone secretion results in a reduction in basal metabolic rate and a reduced ability to increase core temperature. Facilities for warming the patient should be employed to avoid intra- and post-operative hypothermia. Intravenous fluids and inhaled gases should be warmed.

POSTOPERATIVE MANAGEMENT

Opioids are associated with prolonged respiratory depression and there is the possibility of delayed recovery, whatever technique is employed. Intensive care facilities should therefore be available for these patients postoperatively.

Hyponatraemia can occur postoperatively due to reduced free water excretion.

BIBLIOGRAPHY

Ladenson P W, Levin A A, Ridgeway E C, Daniels G H. Complications of surgery in hypothyroid patients. The American Journal of Medicine 1984; 77: 261–266

Murkin J M. Anaesthesia and hypothyroidism: a review of thyroxine physiology, pharmacology and anaesthetic implications. Anaesthesia and anaesthetic implications. Anaesthesia and Analgesia 1982; 61: 371–383

IATROGENIC ADRENOCORTICAL INSUFFICIENCY

A. Quinn

Synthetic glucocorticoids are used for many non-endocrine conditions:

- Respiratory disease:
  - Asthma, chronic bronchitis and emphysema
  - Sarcoidosis
  - Hay fever (usually topical).
- Gastrointestinal disease:
  - Ulcerative colitis
  - Crohn's disease.
- Neurological disease:
  - Cerebral oedema.
- Tumours:
  - Hodgkin's lymphoma
  - Other lymphomas.
- Renal disease:
  - Some nephrotic syndromes
  - Glomerulonephritis.
- Rheumatological disease
  - Rheumatoid arthritis
  - Systemic lupus erythematosus
  - Polymyalgia rheumatica.
- Skin disease.
- Transplantation:
  - Immunosuppression.

Short-term use carries little risk of adrenal suppression. However, daily oral doses of prednisolone (7.5 mg) or the equivalent of an alternative steroid, for a period of greater than 1 month will suppress the hypothalamic–pituitary–adrenal (HPA) axis, as may lower doses in chronic diseases, e.g. rheumatoid arthritis. Suppression may also occur after topical, oral, parenteral, nebulized or inhaled preparations.

Steroid	Glucocorticoid	Mineralo-corticoid
Cortisol (hydrocortisone)	1	1
Prednisolone	4	0.7
Dexamethasone	40	2
Aldosterone	0.1	400
Fludrocortisone	10	400

PATHOPHYSIOLOGY

The patient receiving exogenous glucocorticoid may exhibit many of the signs and symptoms of Cushing's syndrome and have suppression of the HPA axis. The adverse effects of particular importance to the anaesthetist are diabetes, obesity and hypertension.

Adverse effects of corticosteroid therapy

- *Cardiovascular system*: hypertension
- *Renal*: polyuria, nocturia
- *CNS*: depression, euphoria, psychosis, insomnia
- *Gastrointestinal tract*: peptic ulcer, pancreatitis
- *Eyes*: cataracts
- *Increased susceptibility to infection*: septicaemia, tuberculosis, skin (e.g. fungi)
- *Skin*: thinning, easy bruising
- *Endocrine*: weight gain, diabetes, impaired growth, amenorrhoea
- *Bone and muscle*: osteoporosis, proximal myopathy and wasting, aseptic necrosis of the hip, pathological fractures.

PREOPERATIVE ASSESSMENT

History

See appropriate sections on the assessment of problems associated with obesity (p 1.5.148), hypertension (p 1.4.111), diabetes (p 1.2.40) and Cushing's syndrome (p 1.2.38).

Degree of adrenal suppression

Perioperative steroid requirements are difficult to assess. The adverse sequelae of excessive corticosteroid therapy include retardation of healing, increased susceptibility to infection and gastrointestinal haemorrhage, and attempts should be made to rationalize steroid supplementation for surgical patients at risk of having adrenocortical insufficiency. In some cases, however, it may be imperative to continue high dose steroid treatment, e.g. severe immunological conditions such as SLE or glomerulonephritis.

The following tests may be useful in assessing adrenal suppression:

- *Plasma cortisol level* >500 nmol l^{-1} indicates the adrenal to be free from significant suppression.
- *The insulin tolerance test* measures the cortisol response to hypoglycaemia. This is the gold-standard diagnostic test, but is difficult and potentially dangerous to perform.

PERIOPERATIVE MANAGEMENT

Premedication:

- Steroid cover: 25 mg of hydrocortisone intravenously at induction of anaesthesia, then 100 mg infused over the following 24 h
- Concomitant medication commonly includes: antihypertensives, diuretics, insulin, antibiotics, antacids, H_2 antagonists and deep venous thrombosis (DVT) prophylaxis.

Monitoring:

- Arterial cannula
- Blood glucose
- Capnography, Spo_2
- Urine output.

Intraoperative anaesthesia

There are no particular indications for any one anaesthetic technique for this disorder. However, anaesthetic agents should be administered slowly and carefully as these patients are sensitive to any cardiodepressant effects.

General anaesthesia

Induction and maintenance:

- Rapid sequence induction for obese patient
- Prepare equipment for difficult intubation
- IPPV
- May require high F_IO_2
- Careful positioning, as susceptibility to bruising and fractures
- Hypotension, usually reflects inadequate fluid replacement.

Local anaesthesia

Subarachnoid, epidural block, regional blocks, etc. These may be technically difficult but have the advantages of good analgesia and enable minimal administration of opioids and rapid mobilization. May also reduce the incidence of thromboembolism.

POSTOPERATIVE MANAGEMENT

These patients may require postoperative ventilatory support and there are often problems with delayed wound healing.

- High dependency unit
- Continuous humidified oxygen therapy
- Analgesia: opioid infusion, patient-controlled analgesia, epidural opioid/local anaesthetic
- Steroids: start on oral steroids once gastrointestinal function resumed
- Insulin infusion, DVT prophylaxis
- Renal function
- Physiotherapy/early mobilization.

BIBLIOGRAPHY

Kehlet H, Binder C. Adrenocortical function and clinical course during and after surgery in unsupplemented glucocorticoid-treated patients. British Journal of Anaesthesia 1973; 45: 1043–1048

Symreng T, Karlberg B E, Kagedal, Schildt B. Physiological cortisol substitution of long-term steroid-treated patients undergoing major surgery. British Journal of Anaesthesia. 1981; 53: 949–953

CROSS REFERENCES

Asthma
Patient Conditions 3: 68
Rheumatoid disease
Patient Conditions 8: 202

INSULINOMA

J. Desborough

An insulin secreting tumour of pancreatic B cells. More than 80% are solitary and benign; 7–10% are multiple, some of which are associated with multiple endocrine neoplasia (MEN). Approximately 8% are malignant. Incidence is up to 4 cases per million population per year.

PREOPERATIVE ASSESSMENT

The diagnosis will have been made and the patient prepared for elective surgery. However, endocrine abnormalities may occur in patients presenting for emergency surgery.

- Fasting insulin and glucose concentrations should be checked.
- Inappropriate insulin and/or proinsulin secretion leads to hypoglycaemia, which causes a variety of symptoms and signs:
  - Cerebral dysfunction, focal neurological deficits
  - Abnormal behaviour, confusion
  - Blurred vision, weakness, sweating.
- Document concurrent medical therapy:

Drug therapy	Main effect
Diazoxide	Maintain blood sugar
Octreotide	Maintains blood sugar
Cytotoxic drugs (5-FU)	
Beta blockers, calcium channel blockers	Antihypertensives

- The patient should be assessed for symptoms/signs of other endocrine neoplasia (MEN).
- Patients may be obese and hypertensive.

Premedication

Should be generous; these patients are often very anxious.

PERIOPERATIVE MANAGEMENT

Direct arterial and central venous pressure monitoring. Diazoxide is a vasodilator and hypotension on induction of anaesthesia has been reported in patients on diazoxide infusions.

Blood glucose management

A separate line is required for blood sampling. Frequent intermittent sampling for glucose and potassium (15 min has been suggested) or on-line glucose estimation with feedback glucose/insulin infusion (artificial pancreas) is required. An infusion of glucose (10%) and potassium (20 mmol l^{-1}) should be continued throughout surgery.

50% glucose should be available in case hypoglycaemia occurs in response to manipulation of the insulinoma.

Ultrasound

At laparotomy, intraoperative ultrasound may be required to localize small nonpalpable tumours or to identify the relation of pancreatic ducts to the tumour.

POSTOPERATIVE MANAGEMENT

Immediate

The effects of insulin may persist. However, hyperglycaemia may occur in the first few days because of persistent secretion of counter-regulatory hormones. Blood sampling for glucose and potassium should continue until stable.

Later

Surgery carries low postoperative morbidity and mortality if performed by a skilled pancreatic surgeon. Normal life-span can be predicted after surgical removal of benign tumours. Risk of noninsulin-dependent diabetes mellitus, peptic ulceration and psychiatric disturbances has been reported.

BIBLIOGRAPHY

Marks V, Teale J D. Hypoglycaemia in the adult. Baillière's Clinical Endocrinology and Metabolism 1993; 7: 705–729

Owen R. Anaesthetic considerations in endocrine surgery. In: Lynn J, Bloom S R (eds) Surgical endocrinology. Butterworth-Heinemann, Oxford, 1993, p 71–84

MALIGNANT HYPERTHERMIA

J. Dinsmore

Malignant hyperthermia (MH) is a pharmacogenetic disorder of skeletal muscle which is triggered in susceptible individuals by all volatile anaesthetic agents and suxamethonium. It is potentially fatal unless promptly recognized and treated. The reported incidence varies between 1 in 12 000 anaesthetics in children and 1 in 40 000 anaesthetics in adults. The exact aetiology is unknown, but the primary defect is believed to lie in calcium regulation. A gene mutation on the short arm of chromosome 19 is thought to be responsible for MH in about 50% of families. This is expressed in skeletal muscle as a calcium release channel of the sarcoplasmic reticulum (ryanodine receptor). However, human MH is a heterogeneous disorder and mutations in other proteins participating in the regulation of myoplasmic calcium will probably be found. MH is a hypermetabolic state with increased skeletal muscle metabolism. The clinical features are shown in Table 1.

PREOPERATIVE ASSESSMENT

Identification of susceptible individuals is difficult, as they appear entirely normal until exposed to triggering agents. Also, susceptible individuals may have undergone uneventful anaesthesia previously. Patients with a history of a MH-like reaction, or a family history of MH, need to be investigated prior to anaesthesia. Diagnosis depends on in vitro muscle contracture responses to caffeine and halothane. This is invasive, but it is the most accurate test available at present. Testing based on DNA markers can only be offered to families where linkage with chromosome 19 mutations has been shown to exist.

Various other neuromuscular disorders and stress syndromes have been linked to MH. The association appears fairly strong in the case of central core disease and both Duchenne's muscular dystrophy and King–Denborough syndrome are possibly associated. The evidence for an association with other disorders (e.g. myotonia congenita, sudden infant death syndrome, neuroleptic malignant syndrome) is scarce.

PREMEDICATION

Opinion is divided regarding prophylaxis with dantrolene, but there is little evidence to support its routine use. MH reactions are reputed to have occurred despite pre-treatment, and dantrolene may be associated

Table 1.
Clinical features of MH

Signs	Investigations
Masseter spasm* and muscle rigidity	Decreased pH, raised P_aCO_2, increased base deficit and decreased P_aCO_2
Rising P_aCO_2 and tachypnoea	Hyperkalaemia
Tachycardia and cardiac arrhythmias	Increased creature kinase
Hypertension	Myoglobinuria
Increasing body temperature	

*Only 50% of those who develop masseter spasm will be MH susceptible by contracture testing. The safest course of action is to abandon surgery and monitor for other signs of MH. There is a reluctance to investigate by muscle biopsy everyone who reacts idiosyncratically to suxamethonium, but the patient should be referred for further investigation, especially if there is corroborative evidence.

with significant side-effects. Otherwise, choice of drugs for premedication depends on personal preference.

THEATRE PREPARATION

If a general anaesthetic is to be given, a volatile-free anaesthetic machine is needed. A machine can be decontaminated by removal of the vaporizers, flushing with oxygen at $8\,l\,min^{-1}$ for 20 min, and the use of new tubing. Dantrolene should be available, along with facilities for resuscitation.

MONITORING

This should be commenced in the anaesthetic room and include:

- Arterial cannula for invasive monitoring and ABGs
- ECG
- Sao_2
- P_aco_2
- Temperature.

When appropriate for state of patient or operation:

- Central venous pressure
- Urine output.

ANAESTHETIC TECHNIQUE

Many drugs have been implicated but the only agents proven to trigger MH are suxamethonium and volatile agents. All other drugs may be presumed safe. Provided a volatile-free anaesthetic machine is used and trigger agents are avoided, general anaesthesia should pose no problem. All local anaesthetics are considered safe. However, it has been proposed on theoretical grounds that amide local anaesthetics and sympathetic vasoconstrictors should be avoided during an acute MH episode.

POSTOPERATIVE MANAGEMENT

MH can present in the recovery room or even later postoperatively. Cases should be monitored on the HDU for 24 h. There have been suggestions recently that straightforward cases might be done as day-cases. All suspected cases should be followed up and family members screened.

MANAGEMENT OF AN ACUTE MH REACTION

- Stop trigger agents and terminate surgery as soon as possible. Maintain anaesthesia with nontriggering drugs such as midazolam and fentanyl. Establish monitoring as recommended, and ventilate with 100% oxygen (up to three times the minute volume may be necessary).
- Dantrolene ($1–10\ mg\ kg^{-1}$). Most MH reactions are reversed by dosages of $2–3\ mg\ kg^{-1}$.
- Correct acidosis with sodium bicarbonate, as necessary.
- Correct hyperkalaemia with insulin and glucose. Consider early haemodiafiltration.
- Vigorous rehydration with intravenous fluids (Hartmann's solution is best avoided due to its lactate).
- Treat dysrhythmias as appropriate.
- Encourage diuresis after fluid loading.
- Cooling, if required (surface cooling is largely ineffective).
- Admit to ITU for further management.

OUTCOME

With better early recognition of the clinical signs and prompt treatment the mortality of MH has fallen from more than 80% to less than 7% in recent years. However, this is still regarded as unacceptably high. The reasons for this clinical discrepancy include pre-occupation with the name hyperthermia, leading to delays in diagnosis and pre-occupation with nonspecific therapy such as cooling. Neurological and renal damage contribute to the morbidity resulting from the acute episode in survivors, particularly if body temperature exceeds 43°C.

BIBLIOGRAPHY

Ellis F R. The diagnosis of MH: its social implications. British Medical Journal 1988; 60: 251–252

Ellis F R, Heffron J J A. Clinical and biochemical aspects of MH. In: Atkinson R S, Adams A P (eds) Recent advances in anaesthesia and analgesia. Churchill Livingstone, Edinburgh, 1985; 15: 173–207

Maclennan D H, Phillips. Malignant hyperthermia. Science 1992; 256: 789–793

Sims C. Masseter spasm after suxamethonium in children. British Journal of Hospital Medicine 1992; 47: 139–143

Wedel D J. Malignant hyperthermia and neuromuscular disease. Neuromuscular Disorders, 1992; 2: 157–164

CROSS REFERENCES

Muscular dystrophies
Patient Conditions 2: 60
Strabismus correction
Surgical Procedures 13: 298
Total intravenous anaesthesia
Anaesthetic Factors 32: 606
Masseter muscle spasm
Anaesthetic Factors 33: 646

MULTIPLE ENDOCRINE NEOPLASIA

J. Desborough

This condition occurs when tumours involve two or more endocrine organs. Multiple endocrine neoplasia (MEN) may occur without a family history or by autosomal dominant inheritance. Two major forms are characterized by tumours in specific endocrine tissue.

Type of MEN	Tumour site
MEN 1 (Werner's syndrome)	Parathyroids Pancreatic islets Anterior pituitary
MEN 2 (Sipple's syndrome)	Medullary thyroid carcinoma (MTC) Phaeochromocytoma
Three further groups are recognized:	
MEN 2a	MTC Phaeochromocytoma Parathyroid tumours
MEN 2b	MTC Phaeochromocytoma with marfanoid habitus Mucosal neuromas Medullated corneal fibres Megacolon
MTC only	

PREOPERATIVE ASSESSMENT

The anaesthetic management of patients with MEN depends on the clinical syndrome resulting from the particular tumours involved. Patients will have been diagnosed and prepared for elective surgery. In patients presenting for emergency surgery, the possibility of endocrine abnormalities should not be forgotten.

MEN 1

Primary hyperparathyroidism in 95% patients. Pancreatic islet tumours (30–80% of patients) may produce:

- Gastrin
- Insulin
- Glucagon
- Vasoactive intestinal polypeptide (VIP)

PERIOPERATIVE MANAGEMENT

- Generous premedication
- Invasive cardiovascular system monitoring
- Separate line for blood sampling
- Sample frequently for electrolytes, calcium, glucose, depending on tumour.

POSTOPERATIVE MANAGEMENT

- Continue monitoring
- Provide analgesia.

BIBLIOGRAPHY

Owen R. Anaesthetic considerations in endocrine surgery. In: Lynn J, Bloom S R (eds) Surgical endocrinology, Butterworth-Heinemann, Oxford, 1993, p 71–84

Thakker R V. Multiple endocrine neoplasia and molecular genetics. In: Lynn J, Bloom S R (eds) Surgical endocrinology, Butterworth-Heinemann, Oxford, 1993, p 34–46

MUSCULAR DYSTROPHIES

P. Newman

The muscular dystrophies are a group of genetically determined primary degenerative myopathies. They are best classified by their mode of inheritance.

- *X-linked:*
  - Duchenne's (most common and most severe)
  - Becker's.
- *Autosomal recessive:*
  - Limb-girdle
  - Childhood
  - Congenital (? associated with arthrogryposis).
- *Autosomal dominant:*
  - Facioscapulohumeral
  - Oculopharyngeal.

All the above show atrophy and weakness of muscle to differing degrees. The onset and groups of muscles involved vary according to the specific dystrophy; fortunately, their names often define the muscles involved. Involvement of organs other than muscles is uncommon except in Duchenne's, which is by far the most common and severe. In view of this, the information given below refers mainly to Duchenne's dystrophy.

PATHOPHYSIOLOGY

Duchenne's dystrophy affects striated, smooth and cardiac muscle fibres.

Respiratory system

Respiratory failure is common due to:

- Muscle weakness
- Oropharyngeal muscle weakness allowing repeated aspiration
- Spinal deformities, causing restrictive lung disease.

Cardiovascular system

Obstructive cardiomyopathy occurs, but failure is often masked due to immobility.

Arrhythmias are common; tachycardia and ventricular fibrillation have been reported on induction. Severe bradycardia may occur in the facioscapulohumeral variant. There is a particular ECG pattern with Duchenne's dystrophy:

- Sinus tachycardia
- Tall R in V1
- Deep Q in lateral leads
- Short P–R interval.

Gut
Hypomotility of the gastrointestinal tract and weak pharyngeal muscles predispose to aspiration. Acute gastric dilatation has been reported.

Musculoskeletal
Pseudohypertrophy of affected muscles occurs and contractures can be problematic. Kyphoscoliosis occurs early on in the disease and further diminishes respiratory reserve. There may be an association with malignant hyperthermia; a malignant-hypothermia (MH) like syndrome has been reported following suxamethonium and halothane.

PREOPERATIVE ASSESSMENT

History:
- Review of respiratory function
- Previous anaesthetic history (MH)
- Swallowing difficulties.

Investigations:
- Respiratory function tests
- Arterial blood gases
- ECG
- Echocardiography if significant cardiovascular (CVS) disease
- Chest X-ray (aspiration, cardiac failure).

Premedication:
- Avoid respiratory depressants
- Acid aspiration prophylaxis and at least 6 h starvation
- If positive history of MH-type reaction, use nontriggering anaesthetic agents.

PERIOPERATIVE MANAGEMENT

Monitoring:
- ECG
- $ETco_2$
- Temperature
- Peripheral nerve stimulator (PNS).

Induction and maintenance
Positioning may be difficult due to contractures and kyphoscoliosis.

The association with MH is by no means proven, and suxamethonium and volatile agents have been given uneventfully. However, suxamethonium has been associated with hyperkalaemia, cardiac arrest, muscle rigidity and rhabdomyolosis and should be avoided. If there is significant CVS disease then the minimum of volatile agent should be used with opioids. Total intravenous anaesthesia provides a safe alternative to a volatile anaesthetic technique. Sensitivity to nondepolarizing muscle relaxants has been reported; small doses of vecuronium seem to be safe with continued monitoring with a PNS. Watch $ETco_2$, ECG and temperature for early signs of MH, and have dantrolene readily available in theatre.

Local or regional techniques will avoid the risks of general anaesthesia, but may be difficult due to contractures and kyphoscoliosis.

A nasogastric tube should be passed as a precaution against gastric dilatation.

POSTOPERATIVE MANAGEMENT

- Observation on ITU/HDU for at least 24 h
- Ventilate prophylactically if any doubt about respiratory function
- Physiotherapy will reduce postoperative respiratory complications
- Acute gastric dilatation occurs up to 48 h postoperatively, so leave nasogastric tube in situ.

2

BIBLIOGRAPHY

Sethna N F, Rockoff M A, Worthen H M, Rosnow J M. Anesthesia related complications in children with Duchenne's muscular dystrophy. Anesthesiology 1988; 68: 462–465
Smith C L, Bush G H. Anaesthesia and progressive muscular dystrophy. British Journal of Anaesthesia, 1985; 57: 1113–1118

CROSS REFERENCES

Cardiomyopathy
Patient Conditions 4: 103

MYASTHENIA GRAVIS AND EATON–LAMBERT SYNDROME

P. Newman

Myasthenia gravis is an autoimmune disease of the neuromuscular junction, resulting from the production of antibodies against the postjunctional acetylcholine (ACh) receptors. Clinically there is muscle weakness and fatiguability on repeated muscle use. The incidence is 1 in 20 000 adults with a 2:1 female/male ratio. The Eaton–Lambert syndrome is an acquired myasthenic disorder associated with cancer, particularly small cell cancer of the lung. Muscle weakness improves with exercise.

PATHOPHYSIOLOGY

There may be respiratory complications due to weakness of muscles of respiration and bulbar muscles, leading to aspiration. It may be associated with other autoimmune diseases:

- Thyroid hypofunction
- Rheumatoid arthritis
- SLE.

Patients presenting for surgery due to lung cancer may have Eaton–Lambert syndrome.

PREOPERATIVE ASSESSMENT

Treatment

- *Anticholinesterase drugs*: neostigmine and pyridostigmine. These provide symptomatic relief only; may need atropine concurrently to block muscarinic effects. Useful for diagnosis.
- *Plasmapheresis*: short term but effective and useful in myasthenic crisis or for preoperative preparation.
- *Immune suppression*: azathioprine, cyclosporin and steroids eliminate the antibodies. Now first-line treatment.
- *Thymectomy*: complete removal of thymus leads to remission in many patients. This is best performed via the trans-sternal route for more complete removal, but the transcervical route is less invasive. Thymectomy is increasingly the early method of treatment, even for the less severe cases (see sternotomy/thymectomy).

History:

- Involvement of bulbar and respiratory muscle
- Drug treatment.

Investigations and preparation:

- Preoperative optimization regimen prior to thymectomy. This may mean an increase in or addition of any of the above treatments
- Respiratory function tests, including arterial blood gases
- Preoperative chest physiotherapy.

Premedication:

- Continue steroids (see iatrogenic adrenocortical insufficiency, p 1.2.54)
- Minimal sedative premedication due to lack of respiratory reserve
- Acid aspiration prophylaxis if bulbar involvement
- Intramuscular atropine guards against potentiated vagal responses
- Discussion of possibility of postoperative ventilation is wise.

There remains controversy as to the timing of discontinuation of anticholinesterase therapy. A recent review suggests continuing until the evening of surgery. Respiratory monitoring will reveal impending respiratory failure due to myasthenic crisis.

PERIOPERATIVE MANAGEMENT

Monitoring

Peripheral nerve stimulator.

Induction and maintenance

The major problem with myasthenic patients is the unpredictable response to suxamethonium and sensitivity to nondepolarizing relaxants. In view of the problems with muscle relaxants, intubation and muscle relaxation with inhalational anaesthesia is the preferred anaesthetic technique for some anaesthetists. If this is employed CVS/RS depression may be a problem.

Resistance to suxamethonium occurs due to blockade of ACh receptors, so increased doses are often needed for rapid sequence induction (N.B. bulbar weakness). Extreme sensitivity to nondepolarizing relaxants occurs due to reduced numbers of ACh receptors; one-tenth the normal dose will provide adequate relaxation. Atracurium and vecuronium have both been used safely in myasthenics and can be completely reversed. Neuromuscular monitoring is mandatory for titration of relaxants. Reversal of residual block with neostigmine and atropine is safe, but excessive doses above those that the patient is taking orally may precipitate cholinergic crisis.

30 mg p.o. = 1 mg i.v. neostigmine
120 mg p.o. = 4 mg i.v. pyridostigmine

High thoracic epidural anaesthesia with opioid and local anaesthetic block and light inhalational anaesthesia have been used for thymectomy, and is particularly good for postoperative pain relief.

POSTOPERATIVE MANAGEMENT

- Ensure adequate respiratory function before extubation
  - FVC >15 ml/kg
  - Peak occlusion pressure >30 cmH_2O
- If any doubt about respiratory function, ventilate postoperatively
- Chest physiotherapy to clear secretions
- Monitoring on ITU/HDU for 24 h
- Restart anticholinesterases in reduced doses; intravenous or intramuscular doses may need to be given if oral medication is difficult
- Myasthenic or cholinergic crises may occur
- Pain relief is important after thymectomy; opioids must be administered with care and with constant respiratory monitoring.

BIBLIOGRAPHY

Baraka A. Anaesthesia and myasthenia gravis. Canadian Journal of Anaesthesiology 1992; 39: 476–486

Redfern N, Mcquillan P J, Conacher I D, Pearson D T. Anaesthesia for trans-sternal thymectomy in myasthenia gravis. Annals of the Royal College of Surgeons of England 1987; 68: 289–292

Saito Y, Sakura S, Takatori T, Kosaka Y. Epidural anesthesia in a patient with myasthenia gravis. Acta Anaesthesiologica Scandinavica 1993; 37: 513–515

CROSS REFERENCES

Hypothyroidism
Patient Conditions 2: 52
Bronchogenic carcinoma
Patient Conditions 3: 73
Rheumatoid disease
Patient Conditions 8: 202

MYOTONIA

P. Newman

Myotonia is the sustained contraction of a muscle which persists after the cessation of voluntary effort or stimulation. It is an abnormality of muscle rather than the neuromuscular junction. It appears in three hereditary syndromes, all of which are of autosomal dominant inheritance:

- Dystrophia myotonica
- Myotonia congenita
- Paramyotonia.

The latter two are essentially benign myotonic disorders of skeletal muscle only, which do not shorten life. Dystrophia myotonica (myotonic muscular dystrophy or myotonia atrophica) is a form of muscular dystrophy with myotonic symptoms which *precede* atrophy and weakness. However, atrophy and weakness, particularly of facial, sternomastoid and distal muscles, are the major complaints. Incidence is 1 in 20 000, with onset between the second and fourth decades. The diagnosis is often made late in the clinical course.

PATHOPHYSIOLOGY

Respiratory

Respiratory failure is common due to:

- Muscle weakness and myotonia
- Central nervous system mediated respiratory failure
- Oropharyngeal muscle weakness allowing repeated aspiration.

There is a reduced response to carbon dioxide.

Gut

Smooth muscle involvement leads to difficulty in swallowing and decreased gastric motility, both predisposing to aspiration. There is a high incidence of gallstones.

Eyes

Pre-senile cataracts can be the earliest presenting feature.

Cardiovascular system:

- Rhythm and conduction abnormalities both occur; first-degree heart block is the commonest, leading to Stokes–Adams attacks
- Cardiomyopathy has been noted and arterial pressure is usually low but rises with worsening congestive heart failure
- Cor pulmonale may occur due to respiratory failure.

Endocrine system:

Abnormal glucose tolerance tests are common.

PREOPERATIVE ASSESSMENT

History:

- Review of respiratory disease
- Swallowing difficulties
- Cardiovascular history (pacemaker for heart block?)
- Drugs for myotonia: quinine, procainamide, phenytoin, steroids.

Investigations:

- Respiratory function tests and arterial blood gases
- Chest X-ray (bronchiectasis/infection from aspiration)
- Fluoroscopy will detect diaphragmatic myotonia
- ECG and 24 h tape if rhythm disorder suspected
- Echocardiography if significant cardiovascular system (CVS) involvement.

Premedication:

- Avoid respiratory depressants
- Acid aspiration prophylaxis is advisable.

PERIOPERATIVE MANAGEMENT

Monitoring

This must commence in the anaesthetic room:

- ECG
- Arterial cannula for pressure and blood gas monitoring is desirable

- Invasive CVS monitoring is advisable if there is significant CVS impairment
- Peripheral nerve stimulator (N.B. may give false sense of security regarding muscle power)
- Temperature.

Induction and maintenance

Cardiovascular and respiratory depression may be profound with the induction of anaesthesia. A minimal dose of induction agent should be used. Gaseous induction may be preferable, but may lead to CVS/respiratory system depression.

Positive pressure ventilation is usually required and endotracheal intubation will also protect the airway. Due to muscle atrophy, intubation can usually be performed without muscle relaxation. Suxamethonium should be avoided as widespread myotonia may occur, making intubation very difficult. Short-acting nondepolarizing muscle relaxants may provide relaxation but often do not; minimal doses with close monitoring should be used. Reversal of nondepolarizing block with neostigmine may increase myotonia; therefore it is safest to allow the block to wear off spontaneously. Opioids should be restricted due to respiratory depression.

Normothermia should be maintained to decrease postoperative shivering which will increase myotonia.

Myotonia may be treated with intravenous procainamide (N.B. heart block) or phenytoin.

Regional techniques

These avoid general anaesthesia and its complications; unfortunately myotonia is not abolished and paralysis of the abdominal muscles may precipitate respiratory failure. Epidural block may be helpful for pain relief, particularly after upper abdominal surgery, and avoids opioids postoperatively.

Local anaesthetic injected directly into the muscle will relieve myotonia and may be used at the surgical site.

POSTOPERATIVE MANAGEMENT

- Patients should be closely monitored in the ITU/HDU
- Postoperative ventilation is advisable
- Controlled oxygen therapy should be used in those with chronic hypoxic drive
- Early physiotherapy
- Tracheostomy/minitrachoestomy may be required if bronchial secretions are troublesome
- ECG monitoring should be continued, as arrhythmias and sudden death have been reported.

BIBLIOGRAPHY

Aldridge L M. Anaesthetic problems in myotonic dystrophy. British Journal of Anaesthesia 1985; 57: 1119–1130

Moore J K, Moore A P. Postoperative complications of dystrophia myotonica. Anaesthesia 1987; 42: 529–533

CROSS REFERENCES

Cardiomyopathy
Patient Conditions 4: 103
Disorders of the oesophagus and of swallowing
Patient Conditions 5: 138
Laparascopic cholecystectomy
Surgical Procedures 18: 370
Pacing and anaesthesia
Anaesthetic Factors 33: 651

3

RESPIRATORY SYSTEM

R. Armstrong

ASTHMA

Neil Soni and
John Mackay

3

Asthma is a respiratory disorder which may be defined as recurrent attacks of paroxysmal dyspnoea, characterized by variable airflow obstruction and increased bronchial hyper-responsiveness to a range of stimuli. Aetiology, pathology and clinical presentation are all heterogenous, but an underlying inflammatory response is usually present. There is an immense range of clinical pathology from children with reversible bronchospasm through to elderly patients in whom the bronchospasm is superimposed on chronic respiratory disease.

EPIDEMIOLOGY

Variable geographical distribution, affecting about 5% of the population as a whole but up to 10% of children.

MORBIDITY

Increased risk of postoperative respiratory complications, especially in the older patient with chronic airways disease in whom cardiac problems may also be present.

PATHOPHYSIOLOGY

Nonspecific hyper-responsiveness is a common feature. This may be demonstrated by increased response to methacholine, exercise, histamine, cold-air challenge or hyperventilation. Airway obstruction is due to constriction of airway smooth muscle, mucus secretion and oedema of the airway wall. Mechanisms include neural and cellular pathway activation. The neural pathway involves afferent irritant receptors in airways, causing reflex stimulation of postganglionic parasympathetic fibres, resulting in smooth muscle constriction and mucus secretion. C fibre stimulation releases local neuropeptides; substance P changes membrane permeability and mucus secretion, while neurokinin A causes bronchoconstriction. Cellular pathway activation is known to involve immunoglobin E mediated histamine release from mast cells, but eosinophils, neutrophils, macrophages and lymphocytes may also release mediators. An early acute phase leads into a late-phase reaction which is associated with cellular infiltration and may be sustained for several days.

At a cellular level, smooth muscle tone is controlled by intracellular levels of cAMP and possibly cGMP, low levels leading to bronchoconstriction. The effect on ventilatory function is V/Q mismatch leading to hypoxia, and air trapping leading to hypercapnia.

PREOPERATIVE ASSESSMENT

If asthma is known to be present, the severity in terms of frequency of attacks, hospital admissions, exercise tolerance, current medication required, as well as any trigger factors must be established. A history of atopy or a family history of asthma should also alert the anaesthetist to the possibility of intra-operative bronchospasm. Patients with COAD may have a significant reversible or asthmatic

Mediator	Bronchospasm	Oedema	Mucus secretion
Histamine	+	+	+
Prostaglandin	+		+
Leukotrienes C4, D4, E4	+	+	+
Thromboxane	+		+
Platelet activating factor		+	+

component to their chest problems. On physical examination the presence of wheezes might indicate inadequate control and that current medication requires review. The presence of a respiratory-tract infection is a relative contraindication to anaesthesia.

Investigations:

- Chest X-ray may show elements of hyperinflation. In the older patient chronic lung changes or concomitant cardiac problems may be identified. Look for evidence of right ventricular predominance, suggesting long-standing and major problems.
- An ECG may also provide evidence of long-standing right ventricular hypertrophy or cor pulmonale in patients with chronic disease, these patients constitute a very high-risk group.
- Lung function tests: FEV_1 reduced more then FVC (FEV_1 normally 50 ml kg^{-1}, and 70–80% FVC).
- Blood gases: baseline blood gases on asthmatics with COAD may be of value in postoperative management.

MAINTENANCE DRUGS

The most significant change in the management of asthmatics over the last few years is the range of agents which can maintain control of the asthma (Table 1). Many of these are now long acting. Patients should continue on their maintenance therapy throughout their hospital stay if possible.

Table 1.
Agents used to maintain control of asthma

Stabilizing agents	
Sodium chromoglycate	
Bronchodilators	
Salbutamol	β_2 Agonist
Terbutaline	β_2 Agonist
Salmeterol	Long-acting β_2 agonist
Aminophylline	Phosphodiesterase inhibitor
Ipratropium	Anticholinergic agent
Steroids	
Becotide	Beclamethasone Diproprionate
Flixotide	Fluticasone high potency, low toxicity (pit axis)
Budesonide	Beclamethasone (can be nebulized)
Prednisolone	

PREMEDICATION

Sedation is often useful as anxiety may provoke an attack in some patients. Atropine will inhibit vagally mediated spasm. If an intramuscular opioid is required, pethidine is probably the least undesirable. An additional dose of bronchodilator may be given by inhaler or nebulizer with the premedicant drugs. Patients taking high-dose steroids (>1500 μg day^{-1} in adults less in children) may have adrenal suppression and will require perioperative replacement.

CHOICE OF ANAESTHESIA

Regional anaesthesia may be both feasible and acceptable to the patient, but anxiety can trigger bronchospasm and so patient acceptance is important. If general anaesthesia is necessary, avoid stimulation of the respiratory tract and, where possible, drugs known to cause bronchospasm.

Induction

Theoretically, induction agents which may release histamine should be avoided. Methohexitone and thiopentone can release histamine and fail to block airway reflexes, but are usually safe agents to use. Propofol has been used in asthma and its apparent effect on airway reflexes may be beneficial. Etomidate is safe to use. Ketamine has been used to treat status asthmaticus and is unlikely to trigger bronchospasm. It is not an ideal induction agent, but has a place in the asthmatic patient with bronchospasm requiring emergency anaesthesia.

Intubation

Although spraying the larynx with lignocaine, prior to intubation, has its advocates, some reports and studies confirm the ability of sprayed lignocaine to stimulate bronchospasm (not histamine mediated). The place of the laryngeal mask has yet to be established.

Maintenance

The volatile agents halothane, enflurane and isoflurane are all potent bronchodilators and have been used in the treatment of refractory asthma. Sevoflurane has been used in asthmatics and appears to have bronchodilator properties. Light anaesthesia, however, with volatile agents, particularly sevoflurane, can result in bronchospasm.

MUSCLE RELAXANTS

Suxamethonium is a potent histamine releaser and should be avoided if possible. Older relaxants such as curare with potent histamine-releasing properties are contra-indicated. Pancuronium is devoid of such problems, but is long acting and generally requires an anticholinesterase for reversal and these may induce spasm. Atracrurium can cause histamine release, but does have the advantage of Hofmann degradation which reduces the need for anticholinesterases. With its short duration of action and low histamine-releasing potency, vecuronium is probably the relaxant of choice.

ANALGESIA

Local and regional techniques are recommended, but are not always feasible. Morphine and diamorphine release histamine and so should be avoided. There is controversy as to the histamine-releasing potential of pethidine, but it has been widely used. Fentanyl and alfentanil are probably the safest of the opioids commonly used. Aspirin is known to cause bronchospasm in one group of asthmatic patients and is best avoided. The place of other NSAIDs is less clear.

Reversal anticholinesterases can induce bronchospasm, although the atropine given concurrently should inhibit this.

POSTOPERATIVE MANAGEMENT

Analgesia must be effective, whether using systemic drugs or regional techniques. The problems of chronic asthmatics refer to the problems of chronic lung disease. Effective analgesia and the ability to tolerate physiotherapy and cough adequately prevents the development of atelectasis. Warm, humidified air and the use of bronchodilators should minimize the impact of mucus retention and plugging.

THE EMERGENCY CASE WITH SYMPTOMATIC BRONCHOSPASM

This is a potentially disastrous situation, but fortunately is rare. Surgery must be absolutely essential. The normal methods for treating bronchospasm should be employed aggressively, with the use of steroids if indicated. The induction agent of choice is probably ketamine. Suxamethonium does release histamine in some patients but its use may be difficult to avoid. An opiate such as fentanyl can be used. Inhalational agents such as isoflurane or halothane are effective in treating bronchospasm and should assist induction. Once induced and deep on these agents, the patient may be better controlled than prior to induction. Continued bronchospasm with high airway pressure may require the use of β agonists and, if required, adrenaline (either by nebulizer or intravenously).

Ventilation may pose problems, as airway pressures are likely to be high. Manipulation of tidal volume rate and I/E ratios can be used to minimize peak airway pressure with due attention to the maintenance of an adequate minute ventilation. The possibility of a pneumothorax must be considered throughout the case. Postoperative management should be in an ITU.

DEVELOPMENT OF INTRAOPERATIVE ASTHMA

It must be remembered that not all wheezing is necessarily asthma. Tube placement at the carina or in a main bronchus can produce wheezing. Airway obstruction may result from tube blockage, secretions or blood, while aspiration, tension pneumothorax or an anaphylactic or anaphylactoid reaction may all produce spasm. Treatment consists of eliminating these possibilities and the use of deep inhalational anaesthesia and bronchodilators to gain relief of the problem.

Salbutamol (2–5 μg kg^{-1} slowly i.v.) or aminophylline (5 mg kg^{-1}). Steroids, or hydrocortisone (100 mg) will not have immediate effect but may assist in gaining control. Airway pressures may have been very high (see above), so beware of pneumothorax developing.

DRUGS TO AVOID

- Curare
- Morphine, diamorphine and other histamine-releasing opiates
- Beta blockers
- Aspirin, and probably other NSAIDs which are prostaglandin mediated.

BIBLIOGRAPHY

Busse W. Asthma in the 1990s. Postgraduate Medicine 1992; 92: 177–190

Hirshman C A. Perioperative management of the athmatic patient. Canadian Journal of Anaesthesia 1991; 38: R26–R32

CROSS REFERENCES

Iatrogenic adrenocortical insufficiency
Patient Conditions 2: 54

Pulmonary hypertension
Patient Conditions 4: 118

Intraoperative bronchospasm
Anaesthetic Factors 33: 632

BRONCHIECTASIS

J. D. Young

Bronchiectasis is a chronic lung disease characterized by permanent abnormal dilatation of the bronchi, accompanied by chronic inflammation and expectoration of purulent sputum. The prevalence of bronchiectasis has been declining since the advent of antibiotics and the life-expectancy of bronchiectatic patients has improved considerably. Bronchiectasis is now diagnosed by high-resolution CT of the lung rather than bronchography under general anaesthesia, and treatment by surgical resection of the affected lobes has been replaced by medical management, so anaesthesia for investigation or treatment of the primary condition is uncommon.

PATHOPHYSIOLOGY

Many cases of bronchiectasis are the long-term sequelae of childhood pulmonary infections, but there are several congenital conditions predisposing to bronchiectasis.

Causes of bronchiectasis

- Following childhood pneumonia
- Congenital causes:
  - cystic fibrosis
  - bronchial cartilage deficiency
  - abnormal ciliary motility
  - hypogammaglobulinaemia
- Distal to bronchial obstruction:
  - inhaled foreign body
  - tumour.

Bronchiectasis usually affects only part of the lung. The clinical features and severity of symptoms vary with the cause and extent of the disease. Severe bronchiectatics produce up to 500 ml of purulent sputum per day, with worse exacerbations. Self-limiting haemoptases occur because of extensive collateral circulation from bronchial and intercostal arteries. In severe cases, pulmonary hypertension and cor pulmonale may occur due to destruction of lung tissue and systemic–pulmonary collateral circulation. Amyloidosis and lung or distant abscess formation are rare complications.

The conservative treatment of bronchiectasis is based on percussive chest physiotherapy and postural drainage, with either prophylaxis or early treatment of exacerbations with antibiotics. *Haemophilus influenzae* or *Pseudomonas aeroginosa* are common infecting organisms.

PREOPERATIVE ASSESSMENT

Lung function

Helpful:

- History, especially the patient's assessment of how they are compared with their 'best'
- Arterial blood gases as a baseline for postoperative management
- High-resolution CT to define the extent of the disease.

Not helpful:

- Spirometry
- Plain chest radiography.

Cardiovascular system

Clinical examination and an ECG will elicit signs of cor pulmonale. Right ventricular function can be examined with echocardiography.

PERIOPERATIVE MANAGEMENT

Preparation of the patient

Admit the patient to hospital several days prior to operation for extensive chest physiotherapy with postural drainage. Give amoxycillin (3 g day^{-1}) if needed to control bronchial sepsis.

Premedication

Avoid anticholinergics as they may make bronchial secretions more viscid.

Respiratory depressant drugs should be used with caution.

Monitoring

Monitoring should be started in the anaesthetic room and should include pulse oximetry and ECG. In severe cases an arterial line will assist intra- and post-operative management.

Anaesthetic management

The choice of anaesthetic will be determined by the type and site of surgery. In general, regional or local anaesthetic techniques are preferred. If general anaesthesia is used, artificial ventilation should be used.

Respiratory management during anaesthesia

- Maintain adequate gas exchange:
  - Adjust oxygen to maintain 90% or greater $Sa{O_2}$.
  - The $ETCO_2$:P_aCO_2 difference may be widened, as in all chronic lung disease.
- Avoid retention of sputum and infected material:
  - Use humidified anaesthetic gases, either a heater/humidifier or a passive heat and moisture exchanger
  - Frequent tracheal suction (catheters that can be directed into the left or right bronchi are useful)
  - On-table positioning to assist postural drainage, if possible
  - Perioperative flexible bronchoscopy to help clear sputum.
- Avoid contamination of nonbronchiectatic areas with infected sputum: in severe cases the bronchiectatic area must be isolated from the unaffected lung using a left endobronchial tube or a bronchial blocker placed under rigid bronchoscopy.

POSTOPERATIVE MANAGEMENT

- Give immediate postural drainage and physiotherapy; this will require good analgesia with patient controlled devices, epidural analgesia or NSAIDs
- Entonox may be useful during physiotherapy
- Humidified oxygen should be used
- Intravenous antibiotics may be required for exacerbations
- There is no place for elective postoperative ventilation, except for rewarming.

BIBLIOGRAPHY

Hopkin J M. The suppurative lung diseases. In: Weatherall D J, Ledingham J G G, Warrell D A (eds) Oxford textbook of medicine, 2nd edn. Oxford University Press, Oxford, 1987, p 15.100–15.103

Katz J. Anaesthesia and uncommon paediatric diseases. W B Saunders, Philadelphia, 1987, p 83–84

CROSS REFERENCES

Pulmonary hypertension
Patient Conditions 4: 118
Lobectomy
Surgical Procedures 17: 349

BRONCHOGENIC CARCINOMA

J. Farrimond

Cancer of the lung now kills more people than any other tumour. The most common tumour is bronchogenic carcinoma.

Table 1.
Lung cancer and its incidence

Tumour	Incidence
Bronchogenic carcinoma	90% Squamous-cell carcinoma 63% Adenocarcinoma 9% Undifferentiated carcinoma 18% of which large-cell = 11% oat- or small-cell = 7%
Alveolar-cell carcinoma	2%
Bronchial adenoma	5%
Mesenchymal and other tumours	3%

Bronchogenic carcinoma is almost unknown among non-smokers. Peak incidence is in men aged 50–60 years. It is a tumour of the bronchial epithelium, 75% occurring at the carina or the first-, second- or third-order bronchus. The tumour may break through the epithelium into the bronchial lumen, ultimately causing obstruction and lung collapse, or it may spread along peribronchial tissues invading other mediastinal organs.

Lymphatic involvement and haematological spread to distant organs is common. Adrenal glands, brain and bone are frequently involved.

PRE-OPERATIVE ASSESSMENT

Presenting symptoms

- Cough
- Haemoptysis
- Chest pain

- Dyspnoea (pleural effusion)
- Metastases
- Hoarseness
- Ectopic hormonal activity.

Physical examination of the chest may well be unremarkable. Grossly abnormal physical signs such as lobar collapse, consolidation, pleural effusion or superior vena caval obstruction indicate late presentation. Signs of coincident obstructive airways disease are common. It is worthwhile assessing general muscle mass and strength as peripheral neuropathy and neuromuscular transmission problems (Eaton Lambert Syndrome) are sequelae of bronchial carcinoma.

Physical examination may reveal ectopic hormone activity by bronchogenic cancer. Virtually any polypeptide hormone may be produced, usually by the histologically small-cell variety of tumour. These hormones, of anaesthetic importance, include ADH, ACTH, PTH, insulin and glucagon. Bronchial adenomas are usually carcinoid tumours capable of 5HT secretion, clinically manifest as the carcinoid syndrome.

Investigations

- Chest X-ray, PA and lateral. May or may not reveal the tumour. However, it will be helpful in assessing coincident disease such as the increased anterior–posterior diameter and flattened diaphragms of chronic obstructive airways disease. Pleural effusion will be obvious. Enlarged heart shadow may mean pericardial effusion and mediastinal invasion.
- ECG. May be useful as atrial fibrillation commonly complicates thoracic surgery.
- Serum electrolytes. Ectopic antidiuretic hormone may cause a remarkably low serum sodium, clinically expressed as confusion and weakness.

  Ectopic adrenocorticotrophic hormone can lead to features of hypercortisolaemia, particularly hypokalaemia. Clinical features of Cushing's syndrome rarely develop as overall 5-year survival is 9% and for small-(oat)-cell tumours 2-year survival is only 6%.

  Adrenocortical failure (Addison's disease) may occur with metastatic carcinoma invasion of the gland, and hyperkalaemia – with or without hyponatraemia – can be a clue.

  Ectopic parathyroid hormone can cause elevated serum calcium, resulting in renal problems and shortening of the PR interval on the ECG. Widespread bony metastases will have similar consequences.

  Ectopic ACTH, glucagon and insulin may cause glucose metabolism problems.
- Lung function tests. These are mandatory if lung resection is considered. FEVI and FVC are most commonly available and useful. Arterial blood gases on air are essential as a pre-operative baseline.
- Thoracic cavity tomographic scan. Routinely performed to help assess operability of lung tumours, particularly mediastinal lymph-gland enlargement.

Signs of inoperability in advanced disease:

- SVC obstruction
- Left recurrent laryngeal nerve palsy
- Carinal or tracheal involvement
- Phrenic nerve palsy
- Oesophageal mucosal invasion
- Cardiac and great vessel involvement
- Pancoast's syndrome
  - apical carcinoma invading 8th cervical and first thoracic nerves, causing pain and wasting in the upper limb plus stellate ganglion involvement giving features of Horner's syndrome:
    - Ptosis
    - Enophthalmos
    - Miosis
    - Impaired sweating on face
- Vertebral involvement.

PERI-OPERATIVE PREPARATION

- Optimize respiratory function
- Physiotherapy
- Bronchodilators
- Pleural effusion drainage
- Correct anaemia or electrolyte disturbance
- Antibiotic cover and treatment of respiratory infections.

Although all patients should be cross-matched prior to surgery the use of blood transfusion in cancer patients has recently been reviewed. Several investigators have described an adverse outcome in those patients who have received peri-operative transfusion; this has led to consideration of anaesthetic techniques designed to reduce the requirement of transfusion.

Premedication

Any premedication including a drying agent will be suitable.

Anaesthetic technique

Mechanical ventilation is preferable in all but the briefest of procedures.

Neuromuscular monitoring is essential, and short- to medium-acting agents, which do not accumulate, should be used.

Bronchodilating anaesthetic techniques including volatile anaesthetic agents avoid possible intra-operative bronchoconstriction.

Postoperative care

Although many patients are treated in a higher dependency area in the initial postoperative phase, more intensive treatment, especially postoperative ventilation, often implies a much greater severity of respiratory disease. Although postoperative respiratory failure is not common, these patients frequently do not survive the initial postoperative period.

Analgesia

Respiratory function will be enhanced when diaphragmatic splinting due to pain is reduced to a minimum, and the use of epidural analgesia is common in patients with respiratory disease.

BIBLIOGRAPHY

Mechanical ventilation for acute postoperative respiratory failure after surgery for bronchial carcinoma. Thorax 1985; 40: 387–390

The possible immunosuppressive effects of perioperative blood transfusion in cancer patients. Anesthesiology 1988; 68: 422–428

O'Neill Lambert–Eaton Syndrome. Brain 1988; III: 577–96

Anesthesia for an unsuspected Lambert–Eaton myasthenic syndrome with autoantibodies and occult small cell lung carcinoma. Anesthesiology 1992; 76: 142–145

CROSS REFERENCES

Lobectomy
Surgical Procedures 17: 349
Pneumonectomy
Surgical Procedures 17: 355
One lung anaesthesia
Anaesthetic Factors 32: 602
Intraoperative bronchospasm
Anaesthetic Factors 33: 632
Preoperative assessment of pulmonary risk
Anaesthetic Factors 34: 697

COPD AND ANAESTHESIA

J. C. Goldstone

PATHOPHYSIOLOGY

Obstruction to airflow is the hallmark of this common respiratory disease which affects thousands of patients and is responsible for 10% of absence from work and 10% of bed occupancy in general hospitals. Airflow obstruction results in:

- raised residual volume
- hyperinflation of the thorax
- decrease in inspiratory capacity (respiratory muscle shortening).

Clinically, two patterns of disease often present (Table 1).

It is common that these clinical extremes overlap. In general, oxygen therapy, general anaesthesia and the effect of sleeping are more problematic in the 'blue bloater' type. The presence of cor pulmonale is an insidious sign, especially in emphysema.

PRE-OPERATIVE ASSESSMENT

The necessity for pre-operative pulmonary function tests may be assessed in part from the preoperative history of

- Breathlessness
- Cough
- Sputum production
- Exercise limitation.

In the presence of symptomatology, peak flow, FEV_1 and mid-expiratory flow rate can be assessed. This can be performed at the

Table 1.
Patterns of disease

Chronic bronchitis ('blue bloaters')	Emphysema ('pink puffers')
Thickening of bronchial wall and excessive mucous production leading to: increased airways resistance reduced expiratory airflow	Destruction of lung tissue: decrease in elastic recoil narrowing and collapse of airways during expiration
Severe hypoxaemia	Severe breathlessness
Hypercapnia	Normoxaemic or slightly hypoxaemic
Cor pulmonalae	Normocapnic

Table 2.
FEV_1 and MEFR

	FEV_1 (% predicted)	$MEFR_{25-75}$ (% predicted)
Asymptomatic	65–80	60–75
Moderate	50–64	45–59
Marked	35–49	30–44

bedside with hand-held spirometers or calculated from a Vitalograph tracing.

In chronicity, poor pulmonary function leads to hypercapnia and this should be excluded by performing arterial blood gas analysis while breathing room air. Additionally, the degree of hypoxaemia can be assessed as well as any acute decompensation.

Table 3.
Investigations on sequelae of airflow obstruction

Important further sequelae of airflow obstruction	Investigations
Cor pulmonale	ECG Echocardiography
Sleep apnoea	Overnight oximetry in obstructive lesions Formal sleep study if central apnoea present
Polycythaemia	FBC

The development of heart failure is ominous with a 30% 5-year survival. The likelihood of postoperative ventilation is related to the severity of disease; those patients with hypercapnia are a particular at-risk group. Some attention should be given to the feasibility of postoperative oxygen therapy.

PERI-OPERATIVE MANAGEMENT

- Cessation of cigarette smoking
- Pre-operative physiotherapy
- Optimization of bronchodilator therapy
- Additional bronchodilator therapy if persistent wheezing
- Caution with sedative drugs in patients with hypercapnia/severe obstruction.

Cessation of smoking may be helpful acutely by reducing carboxyhaemaglobin levels. A reduction in postoperative morbidity occurs if abstinence is greater than 8 weeks. In all but those patients who have a fixed, non-reversible obstruction, pre-operative broncho-dilation with nebulized β_2 agonist is a usual preparation.

ANAESTHETIC TECHNIQUE

The maintenance of spontaneous breathing and an awake patient unaffected by centrally acting drugs is an attractive feature of regional anaesthesia and this is the preferred technique in many peripheral procedures. Of practical significance is the effect of dyspnoea on patient position and the duration of surgery. Obstructive lung disease is characterized by expiratory muscle hypertrophy and prolongation of expiratory flow. Extensive regional techniques which reduce expiratory muscle strength are likely to decompensate patients and motor loss above T8 may not be tolerated.

General anaesthesia

General anaesthesia may be indicated when neuromuscular paralysis is required or when a procedure is not likely to be tolerated, e.g. in the severely dysnoeic. A spontaneously breathing technique has many advantages:

- avoids excessive positive intrathoracic pressure
- avoids auto-peep induced by mechanical ventilation
- may avoid endotracheal intubation.

Bronchodilatation is enhanced by volatile anaesthetic agents, and experimentally halothane and isoflurane are of equal efficacy. Recently, little difference was found between volatile and propofol-based general anaesthesia in COPD in terms of intra-operative lung mechanics or outcome, suggesting an alternative to this traditional approach. It is suggested that propofol may have bronchodilating properties in addition to its sedating effects.

Mechanical ventilation

Airway control, avoidance of respiratory depression and further hypercapnia and difficulties with volatile uptake are all advantages of mechanical ventilation. Of particular note is:

- Auto-peep
- Barotrauma.

POSTOPERATIVE CARE

Analgesia

Effective analgesia without respiratory depression is the indication for postoperative epidural analgesia for abdominal or thoracic surgery. This should be monitored in the setting of a high dependency area which allows further monitoring of ventilatory status. Peripheral nerve blocks, especially as a continuous technique via a catheter may also be advantageous.

Respiratory monitoring

Although oxygenation may be monitored by pulse oximetry, an indwelling arterial cannulae allows frequent ABG analysis. Rapid shallow breathing may indicate decompensation. Knowledge of pre-operative ABG status is essential when interpreting postoperative changes.

Postoperative ventilation

Hypercapnic patients with severe airflow obstruction may not easily resume spontaneous ventilation and difficulties with weaning may be anticipated. Continuance of mechanical ventilation into the postoperative ventilation merely postpones trials of weaning and is seldom beneficial, contrasting to maintenance of mechanical ventilation in patients with decompensated cardiovascular disease. In order to breathe, such patients require an adequate central drive, no reduction in respiratory muscle strength and an optimized load:strength ratio. It may not be possible to achieve this immediately post-operatively, although this should be the goal.

OUTCOME

Hypercapnia denotes decompensation and distinguishes a more severely affected group of patients, and this group is likely to require postoperative support and ITU admission. Postoperative complications are common when FEV_1 is low. Unfortunately, pre-operative pulmonary function testing alone does not select those patients at risk; rather, general indicators such as ASA and duration of surgery are significant factors.

BIBLIOGRAPHY

DeSouza G, DeLisser E A, Turry P, Gold M I. Comparison of propofol with isoflurane for maintenance of anaesthesia in patients with chronic obstructive pulmonary disease; use of pulmonary mechanics, peak flow rates and blood gases. Journal of Cardiothoracic and Vascular Anaesthesia 1995; 9: 24–28

Wong D H, Weber E G, Schell M J, Wong A B, Anderson C T, Barker S J. Factors associated with postoperative pulmonary complications in patients with severe chronic obstructive pulmonary disease. Anaesthesia and Analgesia 1995; 80: 276–284

Conti G, DellUtri D, Vilardi V, De Blasi R A, Pelaia P, Antonelli M, Bufi M, Rosa G, Gasparetto A. Propofol induces bronchodilation in mechanically ventilated chronic obstructive pulmonary disease (COPD) patients. Acta Anaesthesiologica Scandinavica 1993; 37: 105–109

CROSS REFERENCES

Polycythaemia
Patient Conditions 7: 186
Intraoperative bronchospasm
Anaesthetic Factors 33: 632
Weaning from mechanical ventilation
Anaesthetic Factors 33: 677
Preoperative assessment of pulmonary risk
Anaesthetic Factors 34: 697

CYSTIC FIBROSIS

A. Lumb

Cystic fibrosis (CF) is a congenital disease of Caucasians affecting 1 in 1500 births, with currently an estimated 5200 patients in England and Wales. It presents between birth and early infancy and, despite advances in treatment, still progresses to multisystem failure and death during early adult life. Patients with CF require surgery more frequently than normal (Table 1) and involvement of the cardiorespiratory system renders anaesthesia hazardous. However, mortality associated with surgery in CF patients has decreased from 27% in the 1950s to 0.5% in 1987 (Figure 1).

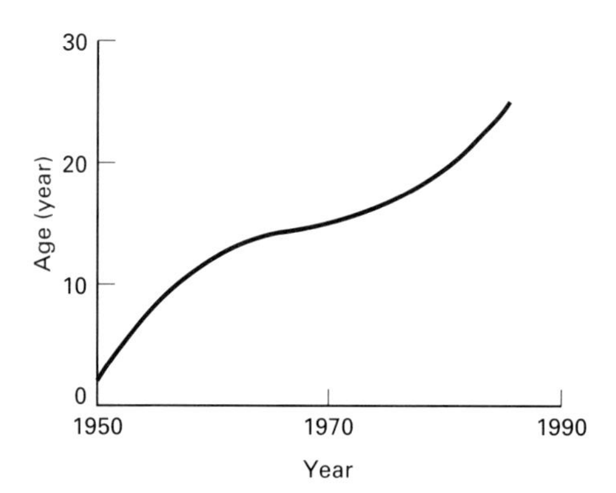

Figure 1
Average survival of CF patients.

Table 1.
Operative procedures associated with CF

Age group	Procedures
Neonates/infants	Meconium ileus/obstruction
Teenagers	Nasal polyps, bronchoscopy
Over 20 years	Pleurodesis, lobectomy, gastrostomy, feeding lines, lung or heart–lung transplant

PATHOPHYSIOLOGY

The CF gene and the protein for which it codes have both been identified, which may possibly lead to a gene therapy cure for CF. Chloride and sodium transport in mucosal cells is defective, causing the production of abnormal mucus resulting in impaired ciliary function, infection and, ultimately, organ damage (Table 2).

Table 2.
Organ pathology resulting from CF

Organ system	Disease process
Lung	Obstruction, emphysema, bronchiectasis, fibrosis
Heart	Pulmonary hypertension, right heart failure
Liver	Obstructive jaundice, biliary cirrhosis, coagulopathy
Pancreas	Diabetes mellitus, malabsorption (vitamins A, E, K)
Bowel	Obstruction, malabsorption and cachexia

In the lung the pathological process leads to:

- Type 1 respiratory failure (normal or low $P_{a}CO_2$)
- Low V/Q ratios
- Increased alveolar to arterial oxygen difference
- Hypoxic respiratory drive
- Hyper-reactive bronchioles.

PREOPERATIVE MANAGEMENT

Assessment

Clinical evaluation to assess the various disease processes involved in CF is essential. The usual preoperative investigations are performed. Reduced forced vital capacity (FVC), hypoxaemia and dyspnoea at rest are associated with postoperative ventilation.

Preparation

Before surgery, vigorous efforts are required to optimize the patient's condition, including:

- Physiotherapy
- Bronchodilators
- Hydration (consider intravenous fluids)
- Antibiotics for respiratory infections
- Parenteral vitamin K (if not on oral treatment).

Premedication

Opioids are not advisable and drying agents should not be given prior to theatre. Benzodiazepines may be used for particularly anxious patients.

PERIOPERATIVE MANAGEMENT

Regional anaesthesia

Regional anaesthesia is preferable to general anaesthesia for both respiratory function and postoperative analgesia. Unfortunately, the age of CF patients and the likely surgery performed are not ideal for regional techniques.

Induction

Preoxygenation followed by intravenous induction is preferable in all age groups, with an anticholinergic given at this time if required.

Maintenance

A high $F_{I}O_2$ may be needed and nitrous oxide is contraindicated in pneumothorax, bullous pulmonary disease, or neonatal obstruction; a volatile agent technique is therefore preferable to opioid/nitrous oxide for maintenance. The following measures should be considered throughout the procedure, but particularly before extubation:

- Effective humidification
- Frequent tracheal suctioning
- Tracheal normal-saline instillation
- Chest physiotherapy.

Airway

Tracheal intubation with paralysis and IPPV is advisable in almost all cases. This allows control of the airway and respiration as well as facilitating effective tracheobronchial toilet and preventing coughing during surgery.

Monitoring

In addition to the usual monitoring the following are useful in CF patients:

- Airway pressure (to detect pneumothorax, bronchospasm or mucous plugs)
- $ETCO_2$
- Arterial blood gases (keep $P_{a}CO_2$ at the preoperative value)
- Blood glucose
- Transcutaneous oxygen in neonates.

POSTOPERATIVE CARE

Respiratory care

Before return to the recovery area, patients should have normal neuromuscular function and be able to cough well. Humidified oxygen of controlled $F_{I}O_2$ should be given and intensive chest physiotherapy must begin in the recovery area and continue until the patient is discharged. Following major surgery, monitoring of the respiratory system (e.g. pulse oximetry) should continue for a few days, particularly at night, and oxygen given as necessary.

Facial or nasal CPAP may be useful postoperatively. If possible IPPV should be avoided in CF patients because of the risk of barotrauma. Weaning from ventilation may be prolonged due to uncompliant lungs and chronic malnutrition.

Analgesia

When feasible, regional analgesia is the method of choice even in small children (caudal injections) and thoracic procedures (thoracic epidurals or intercostal nerve blocks). Provided that renal and pulmonary function allow, NSAIDs may be used and should be commenced before or during surgery. Finally, in many cases opioids are still required and should be used in carefully titrated doses with close monitoring of the patient, e.g. in a HDU.

BIBLIOGRAPHY

Cole R R, Cotton R T. Preventing postoperative complications in the cystic fibrosis patient. International Journal of Pediatric Otorhinolaryngology 1990; 18: 263–269

Lamberty J M, Rubin B K. The management of anaesthesia for patients with cystic fibrosis. Anaesthesia 1985; 40: 448–459

Nunn J F, Milledge J S, Chen D, Dore C. Respiratory criteria for fitness for surgery and anaesthesia. Anaesthesia 1988; 43: 543–551

CROSS REFERENCES

Bronchiectasis
Patient Conditions 3: 71
Pulmonary hypertension
Patient Conditions 4: 118
The jaundiced patient
Patient Conditions 5: 142
Mediastinal operations
Surgical Procedures 17: 351
Rigid bronchoscopy
Surgical Procedures 17: 360
Lung and heart–lung transplantation
Surgical Procedures 23: 467
One lung anaesthesia
Anaesthetic Factors 32: 602

RESTRICTIVE LUNG DISEASE

M. R. Hamilton-Farrell

INTRODUCTION

Restrictive lung disease is characterized by a reduced vital capacity, usually with a small resting volume and normal airway resistance. Relevant conditions include:

- Chest wall or respiratory muscle disease
  - Kyphoscoliosis
  - Myasthenia gravis, Guillain–Barré syndrome, polio
- Pleural thickening
  - Tumour, Inflammation
- Space-occupying lesions
  - Tumour, pleural effusion, pneumothorax
- Lung resection
- Pulmonary infiltration
  - Known causes: asbestos, radiation, drugs (chemotherapy etc.)
  - Unknown causes: idiopathic infiltration, collagen vascular disease, amyloidosis, sarcoidosis.

This section will discuss mainly pulmonary infiltration. Although symptoms and signs of the other conditions are different, relevant investigations are similar.

Restrictive and obstructive lung disease commonly co-exist.

PATHOPHYSIOLOGY

- Thickened alveolar interstitium and irregular fibrosis
- 'Honeycomb' destruction of alveoli
- Desquamation of macrophages in alveolar spaces.

Anaesthetic risk presented by:

- Limited alveolar gas transfer
- Variable ventilation/perfusion mismatch
- Inability to respond to stress/exercise
- Superadded lung infection.

Co-existent medical conditions present their own risks.

PRE-OPERATIVE PREPARATION

- *History.* Dyspnoea, with rapid shallow breathing; early dyspnoea on exertion; dry irritating cough; ankle oedema and other evidence of cor pulmonale; recurrent chest infections may also occur.
- *Examination.* Cyanosis, especially on exertion; fine crackles on auscultation (without oedema); finger clubbing may be seen in long-standing cases; signs of cor pulmonale; signs of superadded chest infection.
- *Investigations.* Evidence of specific conditions as above; chest X-ray may show a ground glass haziness, small lung fields, basal collapse, and raised diaphragm(s); chest infection may be visible; spirometry reveals decreased vital capacity, decreased FEV_{1sec}, but perhaps increased FEV_{1sec}/FVC ratio; the spirogram may show a square initial wave form; total lung volume, functional residual capacity and residual volume may fall; pressure/volume curves are flattened and displaced downwards; lung diffusion capacity reduced. Arterial blood gas analysis:
  - reduced Pa_{O_2} and Pa_{CO_2}
  - normal pH
  - Pa_{O_2} falls early in stress conditions
  - Pa_{CO_2} rises with progressing disease

  Cardiac output is limited by raised pulmonary vascular resistance; raised cardiac output may not increase oxygen uptake, because of V/Q mismatch.

Pre-operative preparation

- Drainage of interpleural fluid and/or air
- Treatment of co-incident reversible airflow limitation: bronchodilators, steroids if indicated
- Attention to superadded chest infection: antibiotics, physiotherapy for sputum clearance
- Optimization of cardiac failure: diuretics, anti-hypertensives, vasodilators
- Preparation for recovery: respiratory exercises.

PERI-OPERATIVE MANAGEMENT

Premedication

Respiratory depressant drugs should be used with caution. Anticholinergic agents should be given if intubation is anticipated as difficult.

Airway

Boney chest wall deformity may pose problems with tracheal intubation. Pre-oxygenation and rapid sequence induction may be necessary.

Mechanical ventilation

Assisted ventilation is advisable, because the work of breathing is increased, and airway recruitment may be useful. Nevertheless, positive pressure ventilation may not improve oxygen uptake beyond pre-operative levels owing to impaired alveolar diffusion and irregular ventilation/perfusion mismatch. There is a risk of pneumothorax with positive airway pressure in interstitial lung disease; attention to high inflation pressures and oxygen desaturation is necessary.

Regional anaesthesia

Respiratory failure may occur if extradural anaesthesia reaches levels higher than the T10 segment. Head-down positioning contraindicates spontaneous breathing.

Intra-operative monitoring

ECG
BP
Sa_{O_2}
ET_{CO_2}
Fluid balance.

Post-operative care

These patients are at risk of basal lung collapse and sputum retention. Late extubation is advisable, and at least a brief period of ventilation in a recovery/high-dependency area should be considered to optimize weaning from support. Analgesia with drugs non-depressant to ventilation is preferable. Monitoring of Sa_{O_2} during recovery is essential, and supplementary oxygen is required.

LATER POSTOPERATIVE CARE

Respiratory physiotherapy and close attention to post-operative chest infection are most important.

BIBLIOGRAPHY

Hughes J M, Lockwood D N, Jones H A, Clark R J. DLCO/QAM diffusion limitation at rest and on exercise in patients with interstitial fibrosis. Respiratory Physiology 1983; 2: 155–166

West J B. Restrictive diseases in pulmonary pathophysiology – the essentials, 3rd edn. Williams & Wilkins, Baltimore, 1987, pp 92–111

SARCOIDOSIS

A. Shukla

INTRODUCTION

Sarcoidosis is a systemic granulomatous disease characterized by spontaneous and complete remissions in the early stages and by a slowly progressive course if the disease persists. Its aetiology is unknown and it occurs in almost all races and all regions of the world. There is a slightly higher prevalence among females between the ages of 20 and 40 years.

The diagnosis is usually made by a combination of clinical, radiographic and histological findings. The Kveim–Siltzbach skin test is an intradermal injection of a heat-treated suspension of a sarcoidosis spleen extract which is then biopsied 4–6 weeks later. This yields sarcoidosis-like lesions in 70–80% of individuals with sarcoidosis, with less than 5% false-positives. Angiotensin-converting enzyme is elevated in the serum in approximately two-thirds of patients with sarcoidosis, but false-positives and false-negatives are common. An elevated 24-hour urine calcium level is consistent with the diagnosis, but is not specific.

PATHOPHYSIOLOGY

Although sarcoidosis can affect almost every system in the body, the areas of most concern to anaesthetists are the respiratory, cardio-vascular, renal, neurological and metabolic systems.

Respiratory system

Some 90% of patients with sarcoidosis will have an abnormal chest X-ray at some time during their illness (bilateral hilar lymphadenopathy being the most common abnormality). Overall, approximately 50% develop permanent pulmonary abnormalities and 5–15% have progressive fibrosis of the lung parenchyma. Sarcoidosis of the lung is primarily an interstitial lung disease leading to a restrictive defect with an associated fall in diffusing capacity. Occasionally, the large airways may be involved to a degree sufficient to cause an obstructive defect. Rarely, the larynx may be involved, usually presenting as hoarseness and dyspnoea but may possibly cause complete obstruction.

Cardiovascular system

The incidence of clinical cardiac sarcoid is low (1.5%). The common patterns of presentation in order of frequency are complete heart block, ventricular extrasystoles or ventricular tachycardia, myocardial disease with failure, supraventricular arrythmias, mitral valve dysfunction and pericarditis.

Once the clinical symptoms of cardiac sarcoid become evident, the risk of sudden death increases. Additionally, over 25% of patients with sarcoidosis have clinically silent myocardial involvement.

Renal system

Renal impairment in sarcoidosis is often nephrocalcinosis, due to prolonged hypercalcaemia. This occurs in about 1% of cases and is a late and serious problem because it can lead to pyelonephritis, fibrosis and intractable chronic renal failure. Rarely, massive granulomatous infiltration may occur, also resulting in renal failure.

Neurological system

Any part of the nervous system may be affected and overall 7% of patients show evidence of neurological involvement. Peripheral neuropathies tend to occur with acute-onset sarcoidosis. Dysphagia may complicate sarcoidosis due to involvement of the glossopharyngeal and vagus nerves. Chronic sarcoidosis can be involved with granulomatous changes or space-occupying nodular lesions in the brain, spinal cord and meninges. This may present with signs of raised intracranial pressure, obstructive hydrocephalus or focal epilepsy.

PRE-OPERATIVE MANAGEMENT

Respiratory system

Chest X-ray and arterial blood gases are advisable in patients with or without clinical respiratory involvement. If abnormal, additional formal pulmonary function tests should be requested.

The larynx should be assessed formally if involvement is suspected. Late-onset respiratory tract involvement may occur up to 36 hours post-extubation. This may require treatment with steroids and nebulized adrenalin.

Cardiovascular system

A pre-operative ECG should be obtained in all cases. However, as more than 25% of patients with sarcoidosis have silent myocardial involvement, continuous observation is required. If any signs of conduction defects are present, pre-operative pacing should be considered. Heart block may occur during anaesthesia as the first sign of cardiac involvement, requiring permanent pacing. Echocardiography for mitral valve dysfunction may be required if sudden signs of failure occur.

Renal/metabolic system

Electrolytes should be checked pre-operatively. Calcium is often raised but usually responds to simple measures such as rehydration. Patients with renal impairment should be treated according to the degree of impairment.

Neurological system

The extent of involvement needs to be evaluated. The presence of neuropathies/space-occupying lesions would dictate the use/avoidance of depolarizing blockers/spinal anaesthesia respectively.

PERI-OPERATIVE MANAGEMENT

Respiratory premedication may worsen subclinical hypoxaemia and should be used judiciously. Supplementary oxygen should be prescribed post-premedication. Steroids may already be prescribed. However, if not, they should be discussed, as respiratory and cardiovascular symptoms and signs are often ameliorated.

Anaesthetic technique

The technique is dependent on the degree of involvement of the various systems, e.g.

Table 1.
Investigations and results

Investigations	Results (if system involved)
Chest X-ray	Bilateral hilar lymphadenopathy, reticulonodular shadowing, pleural effusions, cardiomegaly, atelectasis
Electrocardiogram	Conduction defects, ventricular hypertrophy
Arterial blood gases	Reduced Po_2 in room air
Lung function tests	Restrictive/obstructive defects
Electrolytes	Raised calcium/potassium
Echocardiography	Ventricular hypokinesis, mitral valve involvement, septal thickening and bright echoes (consistent with fibrogranulomatous infiltration)

awake intubation in the presence of laryngeal involvement.

In general, intubation and ventilation are preferable to spontaneous respiration. Higher inspiratory oxygen concentration should be administered. It should be remembered that respiratory function, especially diffusing capacity, is usually worse than clinically apparent and that conduction defects may become apparent for the first time during anaesthesia.

POSTOPERATIVE MANAGEMENT

Supplementary oxygen postoperatively. Close monitoring is required for 24–36 hours postoperatively if upper respiratory tract involvement is suspected.

BIBLIOGRAPHY

Silverman K J, Grover G M, Buckley B H. Cardiac sarcoid: a clinicopathological study of 84 unselected patients with systemic sarcoidosis. Circulation 1978; 58: 1204–1211

Miller A, Brown L K, Sloane M F et al. Cardiorespiratory responses to incremental exercise in sarcoidosis patients with normal spirometry. Chest 1995; 107: 2

Thomas D W, Mason R A. Complete heart block during anaesthesia in a patient with sarcoidosis. Anaesthesia 1988; 43: 578–580

Wills M H, Harris M M. An unusual airway complication with sarcoidosis. Anaesthesiology 1987; 66: 554–555

Valentine H, McKenna W J, Nihoyannapoulos P. Sarcoidosis: a pattern of clinical and morphological presentation. British Heart Journal 1987; 57: 256–263

CROSS REFERENCES

Restrictive lung disease
Patient Conditions 3: 80
Cardiac conduction defects
Patient Conditions 4: 99
Difficult airway – difficult mask anaesthesia/ventilation
Anaesthetic Factors 30: 565
Pacing and anaesthesia
Anaesthetic Factors 33: 651

SMOKING AND ANAESTHESIA

P. Amoroso

Smoking has been described as a dangerous addiction. It is one of the many factors that predispose to postoperative complications. This risk is lessened the longer that smoking is stopped before surgery. A history of smoking is a standard part of any preoperative assessment.

PATHOPHYSIOLOGY

Respiratory system:

- Mucus hypersecretion
- Impairment of mucociliary clearance
- Small airway narrowing
- Increased bronchial reactivity and epithelial permeability
- Reduced pulmonary surfactant and compliance
- Ventilation–perfusion mismatch.

Cardiovascular system:

- Nicotine produces a pressor response resulting in increased levels of catecholamines, tachycardia and vasoconstriction with raised systolic and diastolic blood pressure at blood levels of 15–50 ng l^{-1} found in smokers
- Carbon monoxide has a great affinity for haemoglobin, reducing the oxygen supply to tissues by up to 15% in smokers
- Oxygen dissociation curve shifted to the left by carboxyhaemoglobin
- Carbon monoxide exerts a negative inotropic effect.

Haematological system:

- Increased red blood cell mass to compensate for chronic tissue hypoxia (overall oxygen content may be equal to nonsmokers)
- Increased incidence of arterial thromboembolism
- Decreased platelet survival time and increased aggregability.

Immune system:

- Tobacco smoke attracts alveolar macrophages causing excessive proteolysis with resulting damage to alveolar interstitium (N.B. emphysema); exhaustion of supply means the patient is unable to combat infection
- IgE levels increased
- Altered T-cell activity.

PREOPERATIVE ASSESSMENT

- Discourage smoking, even on the day of the operation (the perioperative period is in many ways an ideal time to abandon the smoking habit permanently)
- Exclusion of commonly associated medical conditions
- Systematic review of likely chronic diseases; excessive alcohol consumption is often associated with heavy smoking
- Chest physiotherapy is recommended together with deep-breathing exercises (postoperative respiratory complications are commoner in the smoker.)

Investigations

See Table 1.

Table 1.
Preoperative investigations in smokers

Investigation	Result
Full blood count	Increased red cell mass. Increased haematocrit. Raised white cell count
ECG	Ischaemic heart disease
Chest X-ray	Chronic airways limitation. Malignancy
Arterial blood gases	Hypoxaemia
Lung function tests	Decreased FEV_1. Diminished FVC. Decreased PEFR

3

PREMEDICATION

Withdrawal syndrome from smoking is a potential hazard. This may manifest itself as irritability, headache, nausea, sleep disturbance and anxiety. However, there can be no case for continuation of smoking up to the time of surgery.

- Consider an anxiolytic, bronchodilator, anticholinergic agent, anticoagulant and antibiotics.
- Avoid histamine-releasing drugs.

PERIOPERATIVE MANAGEMENT

Preoxygenation and increased inspired oxygen concentration throughout surgery.

- The combined effects of carbon monoxide and nicotine on the cardiovascular system result in less oxygen being available when more is demanded (N.B. ischaemic heart disease and/or acute blood loss perioperatively)
- Altered drug handling due to liver enzyme induction (e.g. opiates, lignocaine, propranolol, theophylline, warfarin); dosage and frequency of drugs administered may need to be increased because of accelerated metabolism
- Antacids and H_2 blockers are less effective in smokers.

Regional anaesthesia

Ideal for the prevention of coughing and to encourage deep breathing postoperatively.

Airway

Intubation may show an exaggerated pressor response in the presence of nicotine, but an endotracheal tube allows bronchial toilet to be performed. Lignocaine spray to the glottis and carina reduces coughing.

Mechanical ventilation may be preferred to avoid deep anaesthesia in the spontaneously breathing patient and to prevent coughing.

Monitoring

- ECG
- Noninvasive BP
- $ETCO_2$
- SaO_2 (an overestimation of saturation by pulse oximetry of the order of several per cent is possible because of the effect of carbon monoxide).

Table 2.
Benefits of stopping smoking in the perioperative period

Time before surgery (approx)	Benefit
2 h	Nicotine blood levels fall
12 h	Carbon monoxide blood levels fall
Days	Sputum volume reduced; haematocrit falls
Weeks	Ciliary activity restored towards normal; epithelial permeability returns towards normal
Months	Immune system recovery; drug metabolism restored towards normal

POSTOPERATIVE MANAGEMENT

- Stop smoking – the benefits from giving up smoking are both immediate and long term (Table 2)
- Physiotherapy
- Humidified oxygen by mask for up to 24 h
- Analgesic requirements may be increased because of liver enzyme induction and anxiety through not smoking.

OUTCOME

In 1944, Morton reported a six-fold increase in the incidence of postoperative respiratory morbidity in smokers over non-smokers. These findings have been confirmed in several other studies more recently. Every opportunity should be taken to discourage smoking in the perioperative period.

BIBLIOGRAPHY

Chodoff P, Margand P M S, Knowles C L. Short term abstinence from smoking: its place in preoperative preparation. Critical Care Medicine 1975; 3: 131–133

Egan T D, Wong K C. Perioperative smoking cessation and anesthesia: a review. Journal of Clinical Anesthesia 1992; 4: 63–72

Forrest J B, Rehder K, Cahalan M K, Goldsmith C H. Multicentre study of general anaesthesia. III. Predictors of severe perioperative adverse outcomes. Anesthesiology 1992; 76: 3–15

Pearce A C, Jones R M. Smoking and anaesthesia: preoperative abstinence and peroperative morbidity. Anesthesiology 1984; 61: 576–584

CROSS REFERENCES

COPD and anaesthesia
Patient Conditions 3: 75

4

CARDIOVASCULAR SYSTEM

C. Morgan

GENERAL CONSIDERATIONS

C. Morgan

Goldman in his classic work of 1977, identified nine risk factors associated with life-threatening or fatal postoperative cardiac complications (Table 1). Important valvular aortic stenosis was the only valve lesion found to be a significant risk factor. Mitral valve disease in itself was not an independent risk factor. However, advanced mitral valve disease is invariably associated with some of the identified risk factors. Not infrequently, a third heart sound or an elevated jugular venous pressure is present in patients with mitral valve disease. Surprisingly variables such as smoking, diabetes mellitus, hypertension, stable angina and cardiomegaly were not found to be significant risk factors. Of the nine risk factors, four are potentially treatable or controllable. Heart failure can be treated, the patient who has had a recent infarct can have his or her operation delayed, abnormal rhythms can be treated and the general medical condition of a patient can be improved.

Table 1.
Cardiac complications – risk factors

- Signs of heart failure
- Recent myocardial infarction
- Atrial arrhythmia
- Premature ventricular contractions
- Major surgery planned
- Age >70 years
- Aortic stenosis
- Emergency
- Poor general condition

More recently, Jackson et al reviewed risk factors in valvular heart disease (VHD) and came to broadly the same conclusions as Goldman. They noted that there is a correlation between the severity of the patient's preoperative symptoms and the perioperative risk of cardiac morbidity and mortality. Thus in VHD an accurate assessment of risk can be made without resorting to expensive invasive and noninvasive investigations.

While, in general, the severity of symptoms in patients with VHD helps to quantify the underlying inotropic state of the myocardium, heart failure may imply an imbalance between the inotropic state of the myocardium and the pressure and volume loads on the heart. An example of this is seen in pregnancy in a patient who, with previously well-compensated mitral stenosis, presents in heart failure. A second example of this may be seen in a patient with an acute septic condition, e.g. cholecystitis, who develops heart failure.

One in five patients with VHD will show new or increased heart failure following surgery.

PATHOPHYSIOLOGY

Valvular heart disease causes either abnormal volume or abnormal pressure loads on the heart.

Pressure loads (e.g. aortic stenosis) cause concentric hypertrophy of the myocardium with a greatly increased ventricular wall thickness. While there is a considerable increase in the myocardial muscle mass, the overall size of the heart is not increased. This type of hypertrophy imposes an increased demand on the systolic function of the heart.

In contrast, volume loads cause an eccentric hypertrophy when the heart becomes grossly dilated (e.g. aortic regurgitation, mitral regurgitation). During diastole an increased volume of blood flows through the regurgitant valves. This imposes an increased demand on diastolic function.

Both the systolic and diastolic functions of the myocardium consume energy. In all varieties of VHD there are increased energy demands. Therefore, patients with ischaemic heart disease and VHD are more prone to cardiac decompensation.

ANAESTHETIC MANAGEMENT

Premedication

In all cases of VHD one should avoid heavy premedication. This will ensure that the balance between preload and afterload is maintained and that myocardial function is not depressed. Premedication which causes undue respiratory depression may precipitate respiratory failure or, in susceptible patients, aggravate pulmonary hypertension.

Temazepam (10 mg orally) or morphine (5–10 mg) combined with Hyoscine (0.2–0.3 mg intramuscularly) will be effective and safe in most adults.

Anaesthesia

A full range of resuscitation drugs including both vasopressors and vasodilators should be readily available.

Appropriate monitoring is essential in every case. In general, this should be at a higher level than in patients without VHD and in major cases may include invasive systemic arterial pressure monitoring, central venous pressure monitoring and pulmonary artery and wedge pressure monitoring.

Agents which depress the myocardium should be avoided. Of all the commonly used intravenous induction agents, etomidate is least likely to depress the myocardium.

Conclusion

Safe anaesthesia depends on an understanding of:

- The abnormal volume and pressure loads caused by abnormal valves
- The secondary effects, both on the heart and other organs, particularly the lungs
- The compensatory mechanisms adopted by the heart.

If risk factors are present which can be treated, anaesthesia and surgery should be delayed unless the indications for surgery are life-threatening.

BIBLIOGRAPHY

Braunwald E. Valvular heart disease. In: Braunwald E (ed) Heart disease. W B Saunders, Philadelphia, 1988

Goldman L, Caldera D L, Nussbaum S R et al. Multifactorial index of cardiac risk in non-cardiac surgical procedures. *N Engl J Med* 1977; 297: 845

Jackson J M, Klein P S, Thomas S J. Preoperative assessment of the patient with valvular heart disease. In: Mangano D T (ed) Preoperative cardiac assessment. J B Lippincott, Philadelphia, 1990, p 57–83

GOALS

	HR	SVR
aortic stenosis	60-80	
incompetence	80-100	avoid ↑
mitral stenosis	60-80	
incompetence	80-100	avoid ↑
tricuspid stenosis		
incompetence		

	preload	diastolic
aortic stenosis	avoid ↓	avoid ↓
incompetence		
mitral stenosis		
incompetence		

ADULT CONGENITAL HEART DISEASE: SPECIFIC EXAMPLES

B. Keogh

This article is not designed to encompass all the possibilities which may be encountered, but rather to consider some of the likely or troublesome conditions which may present for noncardiac anaesthesia. Principles in therapy discussed in the previous chapter are obviously relevant to the management of these individual conditions.

EBSTEIN'S ANOMALY

The most common form of congenital tricuspid regurgitation, representing 0.5% of congenital heart disease. Clinical relevance includes potential for profound hypoxia but also late presentation in adult life. Such patients may present undiagnosed for surgical procedures.

Anatomy

The tricuspid valve is displaced downwards into the right ventricle and the effective right ventricular chamber is small. The degree of tricuspid regurgitation is variable, as is the often associated tricuspid stenosis. Most patients have an atrial septal defect with potential for right-to-left shunt.

Clinical spectrum

Patients may be essentially asymptomatic or severely cyanosed. Many present late in life with dyspnoea, fatigue, palpitations and cyanosis. Some are unrecognized and diagnosed at autopsy.

Pathophysiology

Tricuspid regurgitation and variable degree of tricuspid stenosis result in reduced cardiac output. Dilatation of the right atrium predisposes to wide variety of arrhythmias. Up to 10% incidence of Wolff–Parkinson–White accessory pathway. Recurrent cyanotic attacks suggest paroxysmal tachycardia.

Anaesthetic implications

Limited cardiac output which may be difficult to manipulate. Tachyarrhythmias are common and badly tolerated due to decrease in diastolic filling time. Right ventricular function may be poor – if inotropic support is required, consider phosphodiesterase inhibitors. Avoid excess chronotropy with inotropes. Pulmonary vasodilatation (e.g. prostocyclin) should be useful, but *not* in decompensated patients.

Assessment of preload is difficult. Such patients require an adequate preload, but central venous pressure is misleading. Pulmonary artery catheters are only useful for assessing flow (pulmonary arterial and left atrial pressures should be low) and their use is ill-advised due to arrhythmia potential and exacerbation of tricuspid valve dysfunction. Volume titration with fluid challenges is the appropriate method of establishing adequate preload.

Aim for CVS stability, e.g. give etomidate, fentanyl or alfentanil and vecuronium. Patients with Ebstein's anomaly also tolerate bradycardia badly, so with deep anaesthesia there may be a need for rate support, either with intermittent low doses of atropine or very low dose isoprenaline ($<0.01\ \mu g\ kg^{-1}\ min^{-1}$).

EISENMENGER'S SYNDROME

This rare condition, characterized by pulmonary hypertension and a significant intracardiac right-to-left shunt, has substantial and grave implications for the anaesthetist. Its incidence is decreasing with improved neonatal and paediatric intervention, but such patients continue to present for general procedures.

Anatomy

Eisenmenger's syndrome is a functional rather than purely anatomical diagnosis, occurring after the unprotected pulmonary circulation is exposed to high blood flow. Pulmonary hypertension develops and results either in a reversal of shunt to right-to-left, or a decrease in pulmonary blood flow and increasing cyanosis. Common associations include untreated VSD and complex anomalies, but it can occur with large ASD and even PDA.

Pathophysiology

Patients with Eisenmenger's syndrome who previously had left-to-right shunts become cyanotic as the PVR increases and bi-directional shunt occurs through intracardiac connections. Changes in PVR and SVR can then influence the relative degree of each directional shunt, but in reality PVR in these patients is essentially fixed. The most common event witnessed clinically is an increase in cyanosis associated with a decrease in SVR.

Anaesthetic implications

These patients represent a very high-risk group. They may present at any stage, including in cardiac decompensation. The fundamental principle of management is maintaining the balance of PVR and SVR. Since PVR is essentially fixed, agents which avoid systemic vasodilatation are preferable, and vasoconstrictor infusions are commonly necessary.

Induction

Aim for CVS stability, e.g. give etomidate, vecuronium or narcotics. Ketamine has been used in such patients, even though there is a potential risk of increased PVR. In practice, the benefits of SVR maintenance may outweigh any small increase in PVR.

Maintenance

Inhalational and intravenous techniques are appropriate. Vasodilatory effects of isoflurane may be undesirable, hence consider halothane. Pulmonary vasodilators tend not to work, but nebulized prostacyclin or nitric oxide are worth trying. Intravenous prostacyclin may increase cyanosis due to predominant effects on SVR. Vasoconstrictor infusions (e.g. noradrenaline 0.01–0.1 $\mu g\ kg^{-1}\ min^{-1}$) should be used to counteract SVR fall. High $F_{I}O_2$ and hyperventilation are appropriate.

Monitoring

SaO_2 monitoring is mandatory, as is an arterial line in any but the shortest procedures. It must be possible to identify haemodynamic trends rapidly before spiral deterioration occurs. CVP access is required for vasoactive drugs and volume titration. A pulmonary artery catheter may be impossible to insert and provides little useful information, depending on the anatomy. Even if correctly sited such catheters are notoriously difficult to wedge in severe pulmonary hypertension. $ETCO_2$ monitoring, although an inaccurate indicator of $P_{a}CO_2$, provides a useful indication of changes in pulmonary blood flow.

Eisenmenger's syndrome in obstetrics

This is an extremely difficult area when fetal requirements are added to the equation. Discussions relating to the advisability of allowing labour as opposed to Caesarean section are ongoing in the literature. Success has been reported with both general and epidural anaesthesia for Caesarean section. To the cardiac anaesthetist a narcotic-based general anaesthetic, with its favourable haemodynamic profile and appropriate environment for aggressive cardiovascular manipulation, along with elective ventilation of the neonate would appear the best option. An obstetric anaesthetist may take the view that a carefully managed, elective Caesarean under epidural with appropriate intravascular monitoring and low-dose vasoconstrictors, if necessary, may provide a better option. To the author's knowledge, this controversy remains unresolved. Certainly, improved understanding of the haemodynamic manifestations of Eisenmenger's syndrome should improve outcome, and it is not unreasonable to suggest that such patients should be managed in units with access to the expertise of both cardiac and obstetric anaesthetists.

SPECIFIC TREATED CONDITIONS

It is impossible to consider all the possibilities which may be encountered. However, several conditions will be encountered regularly and deserve consideration.

Surgical procedures for transposition of the great arteries

The therapy of choice is complete correction in the neonatal period with transection and appropriate reconnection of the great arteries (arterial switch). Such patients should, with a good surgical result, have normal life expectancy. The Mustard procedure, an intra-atrial baffle to redirect systemic and pulmonary venous return at atrial level, is undertaken if patients present late or the anatomy is unsuitable for switch. These patients have a morphologically right systemic ventricle, are prone to obstruction of either venous return and to arrhythmias, have a shortened life-span and may present in cardiac failure. The morphological right ventricle is likely to require inotropic support.

Procedures for tricuspid atresia or univentricular heart

The ideal is to separate the systemic and pulmonary blood flow. This is achieved by the Fontan operation or total cavopulmonary anastomosis (TCPA), where the systemic venous return is connected directly to pulmonary arteries without a pumping ('right') ventricle. An increasing number of such patients will be encountered in the community. The Glenn procedure, anastomosis of SVC to pulmonary artery, may be an early stage of this approach. Pulmonary blood flow in both situations is passive and requires adequate preload. CVP measurement is mandatory in all but the simplest procedures, remembering that this represents pulmonary artery pressure. An ideal level of CVP is 18 mmHg, although a lower level is acceptable if systemic output is maintained. Higher levels lead to systemic venous congestion with ascites and pleural effusions, but may be necessary in the short term. Glenn procedure and some fenestrated TCPA patients are cyanosed, although complete TCPA patients are not. These patients, however, have limited cardiac output and tolerate tachyarrhythmias poorly. Manipulation of the circulation involves adequate preload and pulmonary vasodilatation. Inotropes tend to be ineffective and their effect on the underfilled, hypertrophied systemic ventricle may be adverse. If inotropes are required, the phosphodiesterase inhibitors with their positive lusitropic effects are probably those of choice. Such patients are physiologically at an advantage with spontaneous respiration, but if IPPV is necessary it should be performed with a view to limiting the retard of venous return and pulmonary blood flow.

Because of the particular anatomy, such patients are greatly advantaged by the maintenance of sinus rhythm. This may be because the right atrium is incorporated as a pumping chamber in the pulmonary circuit. If the right atrium is not in circuit, sinus rhythm is still favourable for systemic cardiac function and decreasing systemic atrial pressure (hence enhancing the hydrostatic gradient for pulmonary blood flow). Loss of sinus rhythm under anaesthesia should be treated with cardioversion. If the rhythm proves refractory, consider amiodarone. Usual loading dose is 5 mg kg^{-1} over at least 20 min followed by an infusion of approximately 10 mg kg^{-1} day^{-1}. If more rapid injection is required, beware the substantial negative inotropic effects.

BIBLIOGRAPHY

Cohen A M, Mulvein J. Obstetric anaesthetic management in a patient with the Fontan circulation. British Journal of Anaesthesia 1994; 73: 252–255

Lowe D A. Abnormalities of the atriventricular valves. In: Lake C L (ed) Paediatric cardiac anaesthesia. Appleton and Lange, Norwalk, 1988, p 310–314

Pollack K L, Chestnut D H, Wenstrom K D. Anaesthetic management of a parturient with Eisenmenger's syndrome. Anaesthesia and Analgesia 1990; 70: 212–215

Wilton N C T, Traber K B, Deschner L S. Anaesthetic management for Caesarian section in a patient with uncorrected truncus arteriosus. British Journal of Anaesthesia 1989; 62: 434–438

CROSS REFERENCES

Cardiac conduction defects
Patient Conditions 4: 99
Pulmonary hypertension
Patient Conditions 4: 118

AORTIC VALVE DISEASE

Mike Scallan

AORTIC STENOSIS

concentric

Pathophysiology

Systolic function is affected by the increase in pressure load and leads to hypertrophy of the left ventricle. With progression of the disease, the ventricle becomes stiff and diastolic function is impaired. There is a decrease in diastolic compliance.

Clinical features

Patients with aortic stenosis may remain asymptomatic for 30 or 40 years. However, when symptoms develop there is a rapid deterioration over the next 1–2 years.

The symptoms of aortic stenosis are angina (Table 1), syncope and heart failure. Heart failure is a late symptom in this disease. Any of these symptoms are contraindications for noncardiac surgery unless the indications for surgery are life-threatening.

Anaesthesia

It is essential that the balance between preload and afterload is maintained. A decrease in the preload may impair filling of the poorly compliant left ventricle.

If the systemic diastolic pressure is allowed to fall, coronary perfusion will be impaired. For this reason an alpha agonist should be available in the event of a fall in the diastolic pressure. Both metaraminol and phenylephrine, which must be given *cautiously*, are effective in this situation.

Table 1.
Causes of angina in aortic stenosis

- A greatly increased muscle mass of the left ventricular wall has an increased basic oxygen requirement
- To overcome the obstruction caused by the aortic valve, the wall tension of the left ventricle is increased.
- Systolic emptying is prolonged. This shortens the diastolic time and, therefore, the time available for coronary artery blood flow. It is during diastole that most coronary blood flow takes place.
- Due to the poor ventricular compliance, the left ventricular end-diastolic pressure is elevated. This impairs coronary blood flow through the subendocardial region of the myocardium.
- There is an increased incidence of coronary artery disease in patients with aortic stenosis.
- A jet of blood passing through the stenotic aortic valve may cause a Venturi effect in the proximal aorta. Since this is where the coronary arteries are sited, this may impair coronary blood flow during systole.

Because of the risk of myocardial ischaemia, glyceryl trinitrate should be available. However, it should be used with caution because it may decrease the diastolic pressure and adversely affect myocardial oxygen supply.

Because of the poor compliance of the left ventricle, atrial contraction contributes 40% of left ventricular filling. The normal contribution is 20%. For this reason the anaesthetist should avoid agents which may cause arrhythmias. If they arise they should be treated. DC conversion may be necessary.

Tachycardias should be avoided in that they will aggravate myocardial ischaemia. In addition, the shorter diastole seen in tachycardias will decrease the filling of the stiff left ventricle.

AORTIC REGURGITATION

Pathophysiology:

- There is both a systolic and diastolic volume overload of the left ventricle.
- There is eccentric enlargement of the left ventricle with an increase in size of the left ventricular cavity and some thickening of the wall.
- Left ventricular stroke volume is increased

and cardiac output is well maintained in the early years of the disease. Peripheral vasodilatation is common and this aids cardiac output.

- Although the left ventricular end-diastolic volume is increased, in the early phase of the disease the left ventricular end-diastolic pressure remains normal.
- In the latter phase of the disease when cardiac decompensation is near, the left ventricular end-diastolic pressure is increased, the cardiac output falls and an increase in the peripheral vascular resistance is seen.
- Due to stretching of the mitral valve orifice by the dilated left ventricle, mitral regurgitation may arise.

Clinical features

Patients with aortic regurgitation may remain asymptomatic for 20 years. Symptoms are not usually seen until the regurgitant fraction is greater than 40%. Dyspnoea and tiredness are the usual presenting features.

Unlike aortic stenosis, angina is not a feature of aortic regurgitation. This is in spite of the low systemic diastolic pressure. Relatively little energy is required for the fibre shortening of the volume overloaded ventricle. This is in contrast to the considerable energy required for pressure generation in aortic stenosis.

Tachycardia may develop as a late sign. The short diastole associated with tachycardia will decrease the regurgitation.

Anaesthesia

Vasodilators should be used with caution because they may decrease the diastolic pressure. However, if the systemic vascular resistance is elevated, regurgitation would be aggravated. In this situation, afterload reduction would be of benefit. Thus a balance must be maintained.

Bradycardia increases regurgitation. A heart rate between 80 and 100 beats/min is beneficial.

BIBLIOGRAPHY

Grayboys T B, Cohn P F. The prevalence of angina pectoris and abnormal coronary arteriograms in severe aortic valvular disease. Am Heart J 1977; 93: 683

Rappaport E. Natural history of aortic and mitral valve disease. Am J Cardiol 1975; 35: 221

ATRIAL SEPTAL DEFECT

M. Barnard

EMBRYOLOGY

The atrial septum is derived from the septum primum and the septum secundum. The septum primum develops initially and joins the endocardial cushions inferiorly. The ostium primum is formed by its lower free edge. Perforations form superiorly in the septum and coalesce to form the ostium secundum. The septum secundum then arises from an infolding of the right atrial wall following its incorporation of the left sinus horn. The septum secundum forms the valve of the foramen ovale by covering the ostium secundum. Persistence of the ostium primum is due to faulty fusion of the anterior and posterior endocardial cushions, and is often associated with a cleft in the anterior leaflet of the mitral valve. An unusually large ostium secundum or failure of the septum secundum to approximate with the septum primum results in a secundum defect. A sinus venosus defect results from abnormal fusion of the sinus horn (the primitive venous collecting chamber) with the right atrium.

ANATOMIC TYPES

Ostium primum forms of ASD occur early and may be associated with defects of the heart valves.

Defects of the septum secundum can be classified into

- Patent foramen ovale
- Ostium secundum
- Sinus venosus.

Table 1.
Atrial septal defects

Ostium primum	Usually large and lead to early manifestation of symptoms. The atrial septum may be entirely absent, which results in a single atrial chamber. This lesion is associated with endocardial cushion defects and is a type of partial atrioventricular canal defect.
Patent foramen ovale	Frequent other cardiac defects; 40% of patients with a ventricular septal defect have an associated patent foramen ovale.
Ostium secundum	Accounts for 80% of all atrial defects. They comprise an opening in the atrial wall (which may be fenestrated) due to resorption of the septum primum, defective septum secundum development, or a short septum primum that fails to close the foramen ovale.
Sinus venosus	The defect is rare, and occurs high in the septal wall above the fossa ovalis close to the junction of the right atrium with the superior vena cava. Commonly associated with anomalous pulmonary venous drainage.

PATHOPHYSIOLOGY

The degree of shunting of blood across an atrial septal defect is related to the relative compliance of the two ventricles and the cross-sectional area of the defect. In the neonate right- and left-sided cardiac pressures are approximately equal, and little or no shunting occurs. As pulmonary vascular resistance falls, left-to-right shunting develops. Symptoms are related to the ratio of the pulmonary:systemic flow (Qp/Qs). A ratio of less than 1.5 is well tolerated with minimal symptoms, whereas a ratio greater than 3 results in fatigue, dyspnoea and heart failure. An increase in pulmonary blood flow leads to increased pulmonary artery pressures and pulmonary vascular resistance. This, in turn, results in right ventricular hypertrophy and further elevations in pulmonary artery pressures. Eventually the ventricular pressures may equalize, which causes bidirectional shunting across the defect. Uncommonly in severe cases the raised pulmonary vascular resistance can cause right to left shunting. This manifests as cyanosis, and is a type of Eisenmenger syndrome. Surgery will halt the progression to cyanotic disease, but if it is delayed until pulmonary vascular resistance is fixed and irreversible, closure can precipitate acute right heart failure.

NATURAL HISTORY

Atrial septal defects do not often close spontaneously.

Small, haemodynamically insignificant defects have no effect on life span, although there is a small increase in infective endocarditis and paradoxical embolism.

Moderate defects are usually well tolerated into adulthood, when left-to-right shunt and right ventricular volume overload may manifest in the third or fourth decade.

- 14% of adults with large atrial septal defects manifest signs of congestive heart failure
- 20% exhibit dysrythmias.

Large defects cause pulmonary vascular disease and decrease life expectancy.

Operative closure of atrial septal defects prevents late complications and increases life expectancy. Closure is preferably carried out at 4–5 years of age. Patients who have defects repaired after 40 years of age have decreased survival compared with controls.

DIAGNOSIS AND PRE-OPERATIVE EVALUATION

Uncomplicated defects are asymptomatic and are detected by auscultation of pulmonary flow murmurs and echocardiography. Significant defects are associated with frequent respiratory infections in children and fatigue and dyspnoea in adults. Patients with large defects present in early infancy with symptoms of increased pulmonary flow and heart failure, whereas smaller defects may remain undetected until adulthood. Examination reveals a pulmonary systolic murmur and fixed splitting of the second heart sound. There may be a tricuspid flow murmur.

Cardiac catheterization is not necessary for the pre-operative evaluation of atrial septal

Table 2.
Investigations used for evaluation

ECG	Right ventricular hypertrophy and incomplete right bundle-branch block
CXR	Increased peripheral vascularity and heart size
Transthoracic echocardiography	Detects primum and secundum defects with 89% sensitivity
Transoesophageal echocardiography	Necessary for identification of sinus venosus defects

defect repair, and is rarely carried out before other surgery. If it has been performed, an increase in oxygen saturation will be apparent at the atrial level. There may be a small systolic gradient in the right ventricular outflow tract due to increased blood flow.

ASD and Eisenmengers

Patients with right-to-left shunts will appear cyanosed and have finger clubbing. Auscultation reveals an increased pulmonic component to the second heart sound. Pulmonary regurgitation, if present will cause a decrescendo diastolic murmur. Chest radiography shows right ventricular hypertrophy, prominent pulmonary arteries and increased lung markings. Cardiac catheterization will confirm increased right ventricular and pulmonary artery pressures.

ANAESTHETIC TECHNIQUE

Choice of premedication assumes importance only in those patients with significant heart failure, low cardiac output and right-to-left shunting. In these patients caution with sedatives is necessary as profound decompensation may occur with small doses.

The alveolar concentration of moderately soluble agents (e.g. halothane) increases more rapidly in patients with left-to-right shunts during induction. Insoluble agents, such as nitrous oxide, are little influenced by the shunt.

Intravenous induction is relatively slower due to the additional dilution by recirculating blood. An increased dose of induction agent may be necessary, with attention paid to the risks of overdosage. However, these theoretical concerns on the rate of induction are of relatively minor clinical importance compared with the nature of premedication and the adequacy of alveolar ventilation. Standard hypnotic agents (thiopentone, propofol) are used for intravenous induction. Opioids, such as fentanyl, are preferred for patients with advanced disease. Inhalational agents are usually used for maintenance of anaesthesia. Children may be satisfactorily induced with halothane inhalation. Potent inhalational agents depress cardiac output and decrease systemic vascular resistance and could potentially reverse a left-to-right shunt. However, this is unusual in the absence of marked pulmonary hypertension, when intravenous agents may be preferable.

The monitoring required does not differ from that appropriate for patients without atrial septal defects. Invasive monitoring is indicated for repair of the defect itself.

COMPLICATIONS

There is a constant hazard of air or particulate matter in all patients with atrial septal defects, including those with left-to-right shunting. Intravenous tubing and connectors must be rigorously checked for the presence of air. Bubbles tend to adhere to sites where there are changes in the diameter of the lumen of the tubing. Small bubbles can come out of solution over time and coalesce, making re-checking of apparatus important.

The prevention of infective endocarditis is guided by local microbiological protocols, which take into account differences in

Table 3.
A typical antibiotic prophylaxis regimen

Low-risk procedure	Amoxycillin 3 g p.o. 1 hour prior to procedure plus amoxycillin 3 g p.o. at 6 hours postoperatively or amoxycillin 1 g i.v. at induction plus 500 mg p.o. at 6 hours. *Penicillin allergic:* clindamycin 600 mg p.o. 1 hour prior to procedure.
High-risk procedure	Amoxycillin 1 g i.v. at induction plus gentamicin 120 mg i.v. plus amoxycillin 500 mg p.o. at 6 hours postoperatively. *Penicillin allergic:* vancomycin 1 g i.v. 2 hours prior to procedure, plus gentamicin 120 mg i.v. at induction.

bacterial prevalence and sensitivities. Isolated secundum defects are considered low risk, and many authorities do not consider that antibiotic prophylaxis is necessary. The risk of endocarditis is related to the velocity of blood flow, impact on cardiac structures, shear rate and likelihood of bacteraemia. Nasotracheal intubation is significantly more likely than orotracheal intubation to cause bacteraemia. A typical antibiotic prophylaxis regimen is outlined in Table 3.

BIBLIOGRAPHY

Baum V C, Perloff J K. Anaesthetic implications of adults with congenital heart disease. Anesthesia and Analgesia 1993; 76: 1342–58

Lake C L (ed). Pediatric cardiac anesthesia, 2nd edn. 1993, Appleton and Lange, Connecticut

Konstantinedes S, Geibel A, Olschewski M et al. A comparison of surgical and medical therapy for atrial septal defect in adults. New England Journal of Medicine 1995; 333:

CROSS REFERENCES

Adult congenital heart disease
Patient Conditions 4: 92
Pulmonary hypertension
Patient Conditions 4: 118

x "delta wave" describes the slurred upstroke of the QRS complex.

CARDIAC CONDUCTION DEFECTS

M. Wall and T. W. Feeley

WOLFF–PARKINSON–WHITE SYNDROME

Pathophysiology

Wolff–Parkinson–White (WPW) syndrome is one of the pre-excitation syndromes in which activation of accessory atrioventricular conduction pathways leads to early and rapid ventricular contractions. The ECG typically shows a short P–R interval (<0.12 s), a wide QRS (>0.12) and a delta wave.x The dysrhythmia commonly associated with WPW syndrome is paroxysmal supraventricular tachycardia.

Perioperative management

The patient's antidysrhythmic drugs should be continued. Monitoring should consist of at least continuous ECG and pulse oximetry. A defibrillator should be in the room and the ECG leads connected to the patient. Intraoperatively the goals are to avoid increases in heart rate and increases in sympathetic nervous system activation. Therefore, vagolytic drugs should be avoided, and adequate depth of anaesthesia needs to be obtained prior to laryngoscopy and during surgical stimulation.

Treatment of supraventricular tachycardia due to pre-excitation syndromes

- Avoid digoxin and calcium channel blockers, as in the acute setting these drugs may decrease the refractory period of the accessory pathways and, paradoxically, increase the ventricular response rate
- If haemodynamically unstable,

synchronous cardioversion with 25, 50, 100 J
- If haemodynamically stable:
  - Adenosine (6 mg followed by 12 mg i.v. push) which may convert the rhythm to sinus, *or*
  - Esmolol (250–500 μg kg^{-1} followed by an infusion of 50–300 μg kg^{-1} min^{-1}), *or*
  - Propranolol (0.025 mg kg^{-1}) to control rate, *then*
  - Procainamide (10 mg kg^{-1} load followed by 1–4 mg min^{-1}) to convert the rhythm to sinus.

PROLONGED QT INTERVAL

Congenital long QT interval syndrome

Pathophysiology

There are four types of congenital long QT interval syndrome (CLQTS) that are all characterized by a QT interval greater than 0.44 s. The congenital prolonged QT syndromes may or may not be associated with congenital neural deafness, epilepsy or a family history of sudden death. This syndrome is an important cause of sudden death in the young patient and has a mortality rate of up to 73% in untreated patients. The basic abnormality is still not fully understood, but the most accepted theory is that CLQTS results from an asymmetrical adrenergic stimulus to the heart. The result of this alteration in sympathetic tone is to delay repolarization of the ventricles (producing the prolonged QT interval) which then increases the susceptibility of the heart to dysrhythmias, most commonly ventricular tachycardia and fibrillation.

Treatment

Because of the high mortality, treatment is essential. Beta blockers shorten the QT interval in patients with CLQTS (beta blockers prolong the QT interval in normal patients) and decrease the mortality from 73% to 6%. Other drugs that may have a role include phenytoin, phenobarbitol, primidone, digoxin, verapamil and bretylium. Other treatment options include left stellate ganglion block or surgical ganglionectomy/sympathectomy if medical therapy has failed.

Preoperative management

The main anesthetic goal in the management of CLQTS is to avoid excessive sympathetic nervous system discharge during the entire pre-, intra- and post-operative periods. Patients who respond to beta blockade alone appear to have a low risk of developing malignant dysrhythmias. Patients who require more than beta blockers or who are unresponsive to beta blockade are at high risk of life-threatening dysrhythmias during surgery. These patients may benefit from preoperative left stellate ganglion blockade.

Premedication with a hypnotic agent on the night before surgery, and a narcotic and benzodiazepine on the morning of surgery is recommended. Antiarrhythmic drugs, a defibrillator, transcutaneous pacer and temporary transvenous pacemaker should be in the operating room and immediately available. There appears to be no difference between general and regional anaesthesia with respect to the development of arrhythmias. If local anaesthesia is used, adrenaline should be avoided.

Perioperative management

- *Induction:*
  - *Avoid* ketamine
  - Thiopental most commonly used.
- *Intubation:* the patient must be deeply anaesthetized.
- *Muscle relaxants*:
  - *Avoid* pancuronium, gallamine
  - Succinylcholine can be used with caution
  - Vecuronium probably safest.
- *Reversal of relaxants*: neostigmine plus atropine or glycopyrolate do not affect the QT interval.
- *Maintenance*:
  - *Avoid* halothane
  - Narcotics, nitrous oxide and isoflurane are safe.
- *Emergence*: Extubate deep, *or* prevent hypertension and tachycardia for awake extubation.
- *Postoperative care*:
  - Adequate analgesia is paramount
  - Resume preoperative medications
  - 24–48 h of monitoring on ITU.

Treatment of intraoperative arrhythmias

Ventricular dysrhythmias in patients who respond to beta blockers are usually responsive to further beta blockade. Primidone, bretylium or verapamil may be used in those who do not respond to beta blockade. In both groups, PVCs usually respond to lignocaine. Left stellate ganglion block may also be used. Standard advanced cardiac life support (ACLS) protocols (with the possible exception of using adrenaline last) should be followed for ventricular tachycardia or fibrillation.

Acquired long QT interval syndrome

Pathophysiology

Acquired long QT interval syndrome (ALQTS) is a separate syndrome, but is still associated with malignant dysrhythmias, especially torsade des points. It can be caused by:

- Cardiac disease
- Thermal and electrolyte abnormalities
- Drugs, especially antidysrhythmics
- Neurological disease
- Endocrine and metabolic disturbances.

Preoperative management

Correct the underlying cause. Remove or adjust drugs if ALQTS is drug induced.

Perioperative management

Avoid hypothermia, hypocalcaemia, hypokalaemia, and hypomagnesaemia. Thiopental and succinylcholine prolong the QT interval in normal patients and may increase it in ALQTS. Vagotomy and head and neck procedures can prolong the QT interval.

Treatment of intraoperative arrhythmias

Follow established ACLS guidelines initially. If the dysrhythmia does not respond, isoprenaline (which shortens the QT interval) may be useful. Temporary use of a pacemaker has also been described.

SICK SINUS SYNDROME

This is often caused by degenerative changes in the sinoatrial node that lead to inappropriate episodes of sinus bradycardia and supraventricular tachycardia. Patients with this disorder should have had a recent evaluation by a cardiologist to address the need for a transvenous pacemaker.

FIRST-DEGREE ATRIOVENTRICULAR HEART BLOCK

This is caused by a delay in conduction through the atrioventricular node which results in a P–R interval of greater than 0.2 s. This may be caused by ageing, ischaemia, myocarditis, cardiomyopathy, aortic regurgitation or any cause of increased vagal tone. This heart block is usually asymptomatic, and can easily be treated with atropine or glycopyrolate.

SECOND-DEGREE ATRIOVENTRICULAR HEART BLOCK

Mobitz type I (Wenckebach) is caused by a delay in conduction through the atrio-ventricular node and is characterized by progressive prolongation of the P–R interval until there is a dropped beat. This rhythm is usually asymptomatic and requires no specific therapy.

Mobitz type II, however, is caused by a block below the atrioventricular node (usually in the His–Perkinje fibres). The ECG shows sudden block of conduction without progressive elongation of the P–R interval. Because this may suddenly progress to complete heart block, a pacemaker is usually placed, even in patients without symptoms.

RIGHT BUNDLE BRANCH BLOCK

Right bundle branch block (RBBB), characterized by a QRS of >0.1 s and RSR complexes in V1–V3, is found in 1% of all hospitalized adults and does not always imply serious cardiac disease. The right bundle branch is usually supplied by a small septal branch of the LAD. There are no special anaesthetic concerns for patients with RBBB.

LEFT BUNDLE BRANCH BLOCK

The left bundle branch is made up by the smaller anterior fascicle with blood supply by the septal branches of the LAD and the larger posterior fascicle that usually has dual blood supply from the LAD and the RCA.

Left anterior hemiblock is block of the anterior fascicle which shows left axis deviation of more than −60° with minimal prolongation of the QRS complex. *Left posterior hemiblock* is a block of the posterior fascicle which on ECG shows right axis deviation greater than 120° with minimal prolongation of the QRS complex. The hemiblocks are associated with coronary artery disease so patients should have a thorough preoperative evaluation.

Complete left bundle branch block (*LBBB*) shows a QRS of >0.12 s, with notched R waves in all leads. *Incomplete LBBB* shows a similar pattern of wide R waves in all leads, but the QRS complex is 0.10–0.12 s. These two blocks are also associated with coronary artery disease.

Because placement of pulmonary artery catheters can cause RBBB, especially in patients with known coronary artery disease, this can lead to complete heart block in patients with prior hemiblocks or LBBB. Thus it is reasonable to have a transcutaneous pacemaker attached to the patient prior to the placement of the pulmonary artery catheter, or to use a pacing pulmonary artery catheter.

BIFASCICULAR HEART BLOCK

Bifasicular heart block is defined as a hemiblock and RBBB. This is also associated with coronary artery disease, and this block may over time progress to complete heart block. However, in the absence of symptoms there no evidence to support the placement of a prophylactic pacemaker prior to elective surgery with general or regional anaesthesia.

THIRD-DEGREE (COMPLETE OR TRIFASCICULAR) ATRIOVENTRICULAR HEART BLOCK

This is present when there is no conduction from the atria to the ventricles. If the block is above the atrioventricular node the rate is 45–55 beats min^{-1} and the QRS complex is normal. If the block is below the atrioventricular node the rate will be 30–40 beats min^{-1} and the QRS complex will be wide in all leads. This block should always be treated with a temporary or permanent pacemaker. Isoprenaline (1–4 $\mu g\ kg^{-1}\ min^{-1}$) may be used while the pacemaker is being placed.

ATRIOVENTRICULAR DISSOCIATION

Atrioventricular dissociation is not a diagnosis, but a symptom that is due to one of four causes:

- Slowing of the dominant pacemaker of the heart, which allows the escape of a latent pacemaker
- Acceleration of latent pacemaker that takes over control of the ventricles
- Block that prevents normal impulse conduction that allows the ventricles to beat under the control of a secondary pacemaker
- Any combination of the above three.

The treatment and anaesthetic management of atrioventricular dissociation will depend on the underlying cause of the rhythm and can range from:

- Atropine administration to patients with sinus bradycardia with ventricular escape beats
- Lignocaine administration for ventricular tachycardia
- Pacemaker insertion for patients with complete heart block.

BIBLIOGRAPHY

Galloway P A, Glass P S A. Anesthetic implications of prolonged QT interval syndromes. Anesthesia and Analgesia 1985; 64: 612–620

Hurst W J, Schlaut R C, Reekle C E et al (eds). Cardiac arrhythmias and conduction disturbances. In: The heart, 7th edn. McGraw-Hill, New York, 1990

Stoelting R K, Dierdorf S F, McCammon R L (eds). Abnormalities of cardiac conduction and rhythm. In: Anesthesia and co-existing disease, 2nd edn. Churchill Livingstone, New York, 1988

CROSS REFERENCES

Iatrogenic adrenocortical insufficiency
Patient Conditions 2: 54

Assessment of renal function 6: 155

CARDIOMYOPATHY

W. Aveling

The cardiomyopathies are a group of conditions characterized by progressive failure of ventricular function not caused by ischaemic, valvular or hypertensive heart disease. A variety of conditions (e.g. viral infection, alcohol toxicity, sarcoidosis) may be the cause, but many are idiopathic.

Classification

Classification by morphology and haemodynamic factors helps one understand the pathophysiology (Table 1).

PATHOPHYSIOLOGY

Dilated cardiomyopathy

This is characterized by progressive dilatation of both ventricles leading to intractable heart failure. The ejection fraction is low (<40%) and arrhythmias are a frequent problem. Death is either sudden, due to dysrhythmia, or a result of cardiac failure.

Restrictive and obliterative cardiomyopathies

These conditions are similar with markedly decreased ventricular compliance resulting in a picture like that of constrictive pericarditis or tamponade. Decreased diastolic filling and low cardiac output lead to congestive failure with dysrythmias again a problem.

Hypertrophic cardiomyopathy

This is frequently hereditary. Hypertrophic cardiomyopathy is very different from the other types. It is characterized by uneven myocardial hypertrophy which is usually greatest in the interventricular septum. This may cause left ventricular outflow obstruction (hypertrophic obstructive cardiomyopathy (HOCM)). The obstruction can mimic aortic stenosis but can be variable, which makes it such an intriguing anaesthetic problem.

Outflow obstruction is increased by:
- Increased myocardial contractility (beta stimulation, catecholamines, digoxin, tachycardia)
- Decreased preload (hypovolaemia, vasodilators, tachycardia)
- Decreased afterload (hypovolaemia, vasodilators, hypotension).

Outflow obstruction is decreased by:
- Decreased myocardial contractility (beta blockade, calcium antagonists, volatile anaesthetics)
- Increased preload (volume loading, bradycardia)
- Increased afterload (volume loading, alpha stimulation).

Table 1.
Classification of cardiomyopathies

	Dilated	Restrictive	Obliterative	Hypertrophic
Morphology	Biventricular dilatation	↓ Ventricular compliance	Thickened endocardium	Hypertrophy: Left ventricular ± septum
Ventricular volume	↑↑	→↑	↓	→↓
Ejection fraction	↓↓	→↓	→↓	↑↑
Ventricular compliance	→↓	↓↓	↓↓	↓↓
Ventricular filling pressure	↑↑	↑↑	↑	→↑
Stroke volume	↓↓	→↓	→↓	→↑

PREOPERATIVE ASSESSMENT

It is important to know which kind of cardiomyopathy one is dealing with because management of HOCM is so different from the others. Specialist cardiological opinion is needed here.

PERIOPERATIVE MANAGEMENT

Dilated, restrictive and obliterative cardiomyopathies

The aim should be to avoid drug-induced myocardial depression, maintain adequate filling pressures and reduce afterload. Full invasive monitoring including a pulmonary artery catheter may be required. High-dose opiates (e.g. fentanyl) are the mainstay of anaesthesia; the addition of nitrous oxide will be depressant, but isoflurane can be used to decrease afterload without depression. Inotropes may be needed to improve cardiac output.

Hypertrophic cardiomyopathy

In complete contrast to the above, efforts are directed at reducing outflow obstruction and avoiding factors that increase it (see Table 1). Premedication to reduce anxiety and sympathetic drive is valuable, and atropine should be avoided. Intravenous induction (not ketamine) followed by volatile agents producing mild cardiac depression (e.g. halothane) and filling to increase preload, will all help reduce obstruction. If systemic pressure falls this should be treated with α agonists (e.g. phenylephrine) *not* inotropes or β agonists.

BIBLIOGRAPHY

Stoelting R K, Dierdorf S F. Anesthesia and co-existing disease, 3rd edn. Churchill Livingstone, Edinburgh, 1993, p 97–102

CROSS REFERENCES

Preoperative assessment of pulmonary risk
Anaesthetic Factors 34: 697

CHILDREN WITH CONGENITAL HEART DISEASE – FOR NONCARDIAC SURGERY

R. Seal

Appropriate anaesthetic management of children with congenital heart disease undergoing noncardiac surgery requires an understanding of the pathophysiology of the child's anomalies and the changes imposed by the surgical procedure.

PATHOPHYSIOLOGY

Shunt lesions

With large defects, the direction and magnitude of shunting is determined by the ratio of pulmonary and systemic vascular resistances. As defects become smaller, shunting becomes largely independent of changes in vascular resistance and is primarily determined by defect size.

Right-to-left shunts:

- Cyanosis (decreased pulmonary blood flow, mixing)
- Increased cardiac work
- Decreased cardiac reserve
- Polycythaemia with increased risk of cerebral/renal thrombosis
- Increased blood volume and viscosity
- Coagulopathy with impaired platelet aggregation
- Alveolar hyperventilation
- Neovascularization.

Left-to-right shunts:

- Pulmonary overperfusion
- Volume overload
- May progress to pulmonary hypertension and congestive heart failure

- Increased risk of pulmonary hypertensive crisis
- Decreased cardiopulmonary reserve.

Obstructive lesions:
- Fixed cardiac output
- Cardiac hypertrophy
- Potential myocardial ischaemia (especially subendocardium)
- Inability to compensate for changes in vascular resistance
- Congestive heart failure
- Sudden serious arrhythmias
- Complete obstructive lesions are dependent upon patency of ductus arteriosus.

Complex shunt lesions:
- Outflow obstruction(s) plus central communication(s)
- Obstruction may be fixed or dynamic
- Resistance of obstruction is additive to that of corresponding side of circulation.

PREOPERATIVE ASSESSMENT

In addition to determining the nature of the cardiac anomaly, one must assess the patient's present status to determine the need for optimization or referral to a specialized facility. Patients may present with unrepaired, palliated, or repaired lesions. Repairs may be physiological, but not anatomical, and may be followed by residual problems (see below). In the history and physical examination, special attention should be directed toward cyanosis, dyspnoea, symptoms and signs of congestive heart failure (see list below), as well as exercise intolerance, repeated pulmonary infections, medications, and acute or chronic concurrent problems. Investigations should be directed by the history and physical findings and may include haematocrit, electrolytes, oximetry, electrocardiogram, cardiology consultation, echocardiography, and possible cardiac catheterization. Patient assessment also requires consideration of the physiological trespass imposed by anaesthesia and surgery. Children undergoing major procedures as well as those with congestive heart failure, pulmonary hypertension, or complex congenital heart disease are best managed in a specialized facility.

Residual problems following cardiac surgery:
- Arrhythmias (especially atrial repair of TGA)
- Conduction disturbance
- Ventricular dysfunction
- Residual shunts
- Valvular stenosis or regurgitation
- Pulmonary hypertension (especially Down's syndrome).

Signs and symptoms of congestive heart failure:
- Poor feeding
- Perspiring while feeding
- Failure to thrive
- Hepatomegaly
- Tachypnoea
- Peripheral oedema.

PERIOPERATIVE MANAGEMENT

Premedication

Suitable antibiotic prophylaxis should be used, except in children with an isolated atrial septal defect secundum, or an atrial septal defect secundum, ventricular septal defect, or PDA that has been repaired more than 6 months previously. The utility of sedative premedication should be assessed on an individual basis. While it may be beneficial in certain instances (e.g. tetralogy of Fallot), it may be hazardous in children with decreased cardiopulmonary reserve. Dehydration due to prolonged fasting should be avoided in children with polycythaemia (haematocrit >45%) to decrease the risk of thrombotic complications.

Induction

Induction should be smooth (minimal crying or struggling), with the choice of agents dictated by the patient's pathophysiology and the availability of vascular access. Thiopentone, ketamine, halothane, opioids, and combinations of these have all been used safely. A reduced dosage and careful titration of intravenous agents is required, especially in patients with decreased cardiac reserve or right-to-left shunts. Experience with propofol in this patient population is limited, and its use is not recommended in critically ill patients. Inhalation induction may be delayed in patients with right-to-left shunts. Non-depolarizing muscle relaxants have a slower onset of action with both left-to-right and right-to-left shunts. An increased dose of muscle relaxants may be required if the circulatory time is prolonged. Secure intravenous access should be established as soon as possible and care taken to avoid bubbles in the intravenous fluid (risk of systemic emboli is extremely high in patients with right-to-left shunts).

Maintenance

The method of maintaining anaesthesia should be based on both the patient's pathophysiology and the destabilizing effects of the procedure. Volatile anaesthetics are suitable in children with less severe disease. Ketamine or opioids may be used in children at risk of excessive myocardial depression with volatile anaesthesia. Careful fluid management is essential. Hypotension will lead to hypoxaemia in patients with pulmonary artery bands or those dependent upon shunts for pulmonary perfusion.

Intraoperative monitoring

Standard paediatric anaesthetic monitoring is used. In children with cyanotic congenital heart disease the $ETCO_2$ underestimates arterial carbon dioxide, and the difference between the two is not stable. Invasive monitoring is indicated for children with advanced disease or for major surgery.

Airway and ventilation

Ventilation should be adjusted to maintain an optimum pulmonary vascular resistance by control of lung volume, end-expiratory pressure, carbon dioxide and oxygen tensions. A 'pulmonary steal' phenomenon can occur in some left-to-right shunt lesions.

Emergence

Similar to induction, emergence should be smooth and well managed.

Treatment of 'tet spells'

In patients with tetralogy of Fallot, increased catecholamine levels secondary to stress or stimulation may cause right ventricular outflow tract spasm and right-to-left shunting. Treatment consists of:

- Deepening anaesthesia or sedation
- Hyperventilation with 100% oxygen
- Phenylephrine
- Aortic constriction
- Beta blockers.

POSTOPERATIVE MANAGEMENT

Monitoring and supplemental oxygen administration should be used until the child has fully recovered. The provision of adequate analgesia and careful fluid management are essential. Elective admission to a paediatric ITU should be considered for major procedures and for children with advanced cardiac disease or complex medical problems.

BIBLIOGRAPHY

Dajani A S, Bisno A L, Chung K J et al. Prevention of bacterial endocarditis. Recommendation of the American Heart Association. Journal of the American Medical Association 1990; 264: 2919

Ekert H, Sheers M. Preoperative and postoperative platelet function in cyanotic congenital heart disease. Journal of Thoracic and Cardiovascular Surgery 1974; 67: 184–190

Hickey P R. Anesthesia for children with heart disease. In: International Anesthesia Research Society Review Course Lectures. 1988; p 86–90

Laishley R S, Burrows F A, Lerman J, Roy W L. Effect of anesthetic induction regimens on oxygen saturation in cyanotic congenital heart disease. Anesthesiology 1986; 65: 673–677

Lazzell V A, Burrows F A. Stability of the intraoperative arterial to end-tidal carbon dioxide partial pressure difference in children with congenital heart disease. Canadian Journal of Anaesthesia 1991; 38: 859–865

Lebovic S, Reich D L, Steinberg L G, Vela F P, Silvay G. Comparison of propofol versus ketamine for anesthesia in pediatric patients undergoing cardiac catheterization. Anesthesia and Analgesia 1992; 4: 490–494

CROSS REFERENCES

Pulmonary hypertension
Patient Conditions 4: 118

The failing heart
Patient Conditions 4: 129

Polycythaemia
Patient Conditions 7: 186

CORONARY ARTERY DISEASE

W. Davies

The incidence of coronary artery disease is 3–4% of the population.

Approximately 10–15% of myocardial infarctions are silent. CAD and its consequences are the main cause of death in anaesthesia and surgery. Mortality following perioperative myocardial infarction is high (Table 1), although with aggressive monitoring and intervention it may be reduced. Prior, successful percutaneous balloon angioplasty (PTCA) and/or coronary artery bypass grafting (CABG) may lower the perioperative mortality associated with noncardiac surgery to 0–1.2%. Thoracic, upper abdominal, major aortic or other vascular surgery increase the risks two- to three-fold. Mortality following reinfarction is 50–70% (90% of deaths occurring within 48 h of reinfarction).

Table 1.
Incidence of perioperative myocardial infarction following noncardiac surgery

	%
Overall	0–0.7
With known CAD	0–1.1
With known triple-vessel disease (left anterior descending, circumflex and right coronary artery) (>70% stenosis)	6
History of previous myocardial infarction *	
>6 months ago	6
>3 but <6 months ago	10–15
<3 months ago	20–37

* more recent figures not as bad.

PATHOPHYSIOLOGY

Stable angina

Defined as angina with no change in precipitating factors, frequency or duration of pain for at least the previous 2 months, and generally relieved by glyceryl trinitrate.

Unstable angina

Defined as angina with a changing pattern indicative of impending infarction, e.g. more frequent, longer duration of pain, pain not relieved by glyceryl trinitrate, or pain at rest. Silent infarction does not evoke angina!

Coronary artery disease

CAD usually means >50% obstruction of the lumen of one or more coronary arteries by atheromatous plaque. Diameter reductions of 30%, 50%, 70% and 90% are equivalent to 50%, 75%, eccentricity of lesions are also important considerations. Ischaemia develops if myocardial oxygen demand exceeds supply. In stable disease, atheromatous plaque comprises a constant proportion of the arterial lumen. In unstable disease, intra-arterial thrombosis or acute plaque disruption is superimposed on plaque fissuring, causing total or subtotal obstruction. Sudden death is usually due to an ischaemic-induced arrythmia.

Risk factors for developing CAD:

- Increasing age, e.g. >40 years
- Male gender
- Cigarette smoking
- Genetic predisposition
- Hypertension
- Diabetes
- Obesity
- Hypercholesterolaemia (increased low density lipoproteins)
- Sedentary life-style.

Increased perioperative morbidity:

- Recent myocardial infarction (within the last 6 months)
- Congestive heart failure
- High-risk surgery, e.g. thoracic/upper abdominal surgery, or major vascular surgery on the aorta.

CLINICAL HISTORY

- Previous myocardial infarction.

4

- Angina (stable or unstable).
- Associated diseases:
  - Diabetes
  - CCF
  - Syncope
  - TIA/CVA
  - Peripheral vascular disease
  - Renal disease
  - Obstructive airways disease.
- Exercise tolerance: Can the patient climb two to three flights of stairs? Is it limited by chest pain, breathlessness or other factors?
- Orthopnoea/PND
- Drug history:
  - Nitrates
  - Beta blockers
  - Calcium channel blockers
  - Antiplatelet agents
  - Digoxin.

CLINICAL EXAMINATION

In particular, look for:

- Elevated JVP
- S_3 gallop
- Dyspnoea/basal crackles
- Pulsatile hepatomegaly
- Presence of peripheral pulses
- Resting BP and heart rate.

SPECIFIC INVESTIGATIONS

Chest X-ray:

- Cardiomegaly is associated with a decreased ejection fraction
- Venous engorgement.

ECG:

- Rate
- Rhythm
- Ischaemia (>1 mm S–T depression measured 60–80 ms after J point when slope of S–T segment is down going, or 1.5 mm when S–T segment is up going, suggests significant ischaemia)
- Infarction
- Dysrhythmias.

Exercise ECG

Standard or automated 24-h Holter ECG (with S–T segment analysis). Look for evidence of ischaemia, dysrythmia or hypotension.

Echocardiography:

- Predicts ejection fraction
- Wall-motion abnormalities (hypokinesia, dyskinesia, akinesia)

MUGA scan

Measures ejection fraction and detects wall-motion abnormalities.

Dipyridamole thallium scanning

Accurately highlights areas with poor or no perfusion.

Angiography

Used to assess left ventricular function and document extent of CAD. Mortality 0.01–0.1%.

Use the above data to assess ventricular function as shown in Table 2.

Table 2.
Ventricular function

	Good function	Poor function
Ejection fraction	>0.55	<0.4
LVEDP (mmHg)	<12	>18
CI (l min^{-1} m^{-2})	>2.5	<2
Dyskinesia	None	Ventricular

Ejection fraction

With an ejection fraction of <0.35, the incidence of perioperative myocardial infarction in high-risk surgery is 75–85%, whilst if the ejection fraction is >0.35 the perioperative risk is reduced to approximately 20%.

Risk of postoperative ischaemic event

In patients with known ischaemic heart disease, some useful predictors of developing a postoperative ischaemic event are:

- LVH on preoperative ECG
- History of hypertension
- Preoperative diabetes
- Confirmed CAD
- Preoperative digoxin therapy.

Risk of postoperative myocardial ischaemia in high-risk surgery increases progressively with the number of predictors present, e.g. 22% with none, 31% with one, 46% with two, 70% with three, 77% with four.

ANAESTHESIA AND CAD

Unstable disease:

- Postpone surgery if at all possible, and consider further assessment such as coronary angiography with a view to

improving current medical therapy and/or consider PTCA/CABG first!
- Exclude recent infarct by serial ECG/serial cardiac enzymes if possible.

Urgent surgery
Optimize medical therapy:

- Aspirin(?) (antiplatelet agents) – to reduce intravascular thrombosis.
- Consider transdermal patch with premedication) to:
  - Reduce LVEDP
  - Reduce preload
  - Improve collateral flow
  - Dilate stenotic areas
  - Decrease systemic BP.
- Beta blockers (atenolol 50 to 100 mg daily) – to reduce contractility and heart rate.
- Calcium channel blockers (diltiazem 60 mg t.d.s.) to:
  - Reduce SVR
  - Relieve coronary spasm.

CONDUCT OF ANAESTHESIA

Continue preoperative drug therapy (but consider stopping ACE inhibitors 24 h preoperatively, as they may potentiate 'induction' hypotension).

Premedication
Aim to provide adequate sedation and reduce apprehension, whilst continuing optimal medical therapy and oxygen therapy (benzodiazepine, scopolamine, opiate is satisfactory).

Preoperatively instigate invasive monitoring and attain large-bore venous access under local anaesthesia and/or sedation. (IBP, CVP, PAOP), depending on assessment of patient.

Attach appropriate noninvasive monitoring, e.g. ECG CM_5/V_5/lead II, oximetry, noninvasive BP.

Induction:
- Preoxygenation
- Moderate doses of potent opioids:
  - Fentanyl (25–50 μg kg^{-1})
  - Sufentanil (10–15 μg kg^{-1})
  - Alfentanil (50–100 μg kg^{-1}; infusion 0.5–1.0 g kg^{-1} min^{-1})
- Induction agent: etomidate > thiopentone > propofol, midazolam
- Choice of relaxant is dependent on desired haemodynamic effect and length of surgery, e.g. vecuronium, atracurium, pancuronium for short laryngoscopy.

Maintenance
IPPV with volatile agent/relaxant/further opioid. Consider isoflurane, enflurane and halothane; consider avoiding nitrous oxide. Combined general and regional anaesthesia is highly desirable, if appropriate.

Reversal:
- Edrophonium is preferable to neostigmine
- Glycopyrrolate is preferable to atropine.

Monitoring
The severity of disease and the magnitude of surgery will determine degree of monitoring:

- Invasive BP monitoring is mandatory for high-risk surgery
- ECG – lead II and V_5 (or CM_5), with continuous S–T analysis if available
- Oximetry
- Capnography
- Central venous pressure
- PAOP
- Core temperature
- Urethral catheter
- Transoesophageal echocardiography (TOE)
- Transoesophageal Doppler echocardiography.

Optimal myocardial oxygen supply–demand balance is achieved when the heart rate is *slow* (maximal diastolic time), *small* (reduced wall tension), and *well perfused* (adequate coronary perfusion pressure) (Table 3). A reduction in contractility may be beneficial to reduce demand, depending on left ventricular function.

The choice of agent or technique may have little or no influence on cardiac outcome. Avoid tachycardia, sympathetic stimulation, pain and hypoxaemia. Aim to keep cardiovascular parameters at or near to preoperative values (±20%). Use nitrates or calcium channel blockers as coronary vasodilators, inotropes to maintain ventricular performance, and beta blockers to control heart rate.

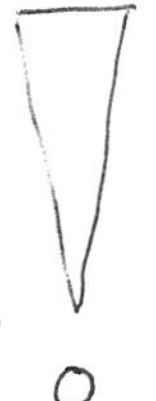

OUTCOME

Specific goals:
- Treat hypertension associated with tachycardia with labetalol, opioids or increased depth of anaesthesia
- Treat hypertension without tachycardia with increased depth of anaesthesia, opioids, hydrallazine, nicardipine or glyceryl trinitrate

Table 3.
Factors affecting myocardial oxygen delivery and demand

Factors increasing O_2 requirements	Factors decreasing O_2 delivery
• Sympathetic stimulation • Pain • Tachycardia • Systolic hypertension • Increased myocardial contractility • Increased afterload	• Decreased coronary perfusion pressure • Decreased CO_2 • Tachycardia • Diastolic hypotension • Coronary artery spasm • Decreased O_2 content: – Anaemia – Arterial hypoxaemia – Shift of O_2 dissociation curve to the left – Increased preload

4

- Treat hypotension with fluid, if hypovolaemic; vasoconstrictors (phenylephrine or ephedrine), if vasodilated; or positive inotropy (dopamine), if reduced contractility
- Actively treat metabolic acidosis by the use of inotropes, vasodilators and appropriate fluid replacement
- If persistent ischaemia develops despite the above measures, consider the use of a perioperative intra-aortic balloon pump.

Postoperative care:
- ITU/HDU stay for 48–72 h minimum
- Continue aggressive monitoring, intervention and oxygen therapy postoperatively for 48–72 h
- Adequate analgesia (ventilate if necessary!)
- Treat hypothermia, avoid shivering
- Actively and aggressively treat:
  - Hypotension
  - Hypertension
  - Acidosis
  - Hypercarbia
  - Hypocarbia
  - Hypoxaemia
  - Arrythmias
- Aim for a PCV of 33%
- Increase oxygen delivery, until oxygen consumption plateaus and is therefore no longer supply-dependent
- Aim to keep parameters within 20% of the preoperative baseline.

Overall morbidity and mortality may be reduced with appropriate invasive monitoring and aggressive treatment of adverse cardiovascular parameters, which should be continued into the postoperative period. Definitive treatment of unstable CAD should precede nonurgent noncardiac surgery.

BIBLIOGRAPHY

Anderson W G. Anaesthesia for patients with cardiac disease: postoperative management. British Journal of Hospital Medicine 1987; 411–418

Ballard P. Anaesthesia for patients with cardiac disease: intraoperative management. British Journal of Hospital Medicine 1987; 398–407

Fleisher L A, Barash P. Preoperative cardiac evaluation: a functional approach. Anaesthesia and Analgesia 1992; 74: 586–598

Masey S A, Burton G W. Anaesthesia for patients with cardiac disease: preoperative management. British Journal of Hospital Medicine 1987; 386–394

Thomas S J, Kramer J L. Manual of cardiac anaesthesia, 2nd edn. Churchill Livingstone, Edinburgh

Walter S N, Rowbotham D J, Smith G. In Reiz S, Mangano D T, Bennett S (eds) Anaesthesia, 2nd edn. Blackwell Scientific, Oxford, vol 2, p 1212–1263

West J N W, Gammage M D. Angina: strategies for management. Current Anaesthesia and Critical Care 1993; 4: 124–134

CROSS REFERENCES

Carotid endarterectomy
Surgical Procedures 22: 451

Coronary artery bypass grafting
Surgical Procedures 27: 511

HYPERTENSION

M. Aglan

Systemic hypertension is diagnosed by the physical finding of an elevation in the blood pressure. It is a silent killer. It afflicts nearly one-third of the adult population and half of the elderly. Nearly 30% of patients going for noncardiac surgery have a history of hypertension.

AETIOLOGY

- 95%: primary or essential hypertension
- 5%: secondary hypertension, e.g.
  - chronic renal failure
  - Endocrine (adrenocortical hyperfunction, pheochromocytoma).

MAJOR CONCERNS FOR THE ANAESTHETIST

- Hypertension affects end organs (heart, kidney and brain)
- Association with other atheromatous artery disease (cerebral, coronary and peripheral)
- Antihypertensive drug interactions, with each other and with anaesthetic agents
- Role of the anaesthetist as a screen for the patient.

PATHOPHYSIOLOGY

Sustained rise in blood pressure leads to adaptive muscular hypertrophy in both the arterioles and left ventricle and following the La Place law, this results in two major pathophysiological changes: high SVR and LVH (Figure 1).

SHOULD ELECTIVE SURGERY BE POSTPONED?

For rational *guidelines*, five important debatable questions need to be addressed.

1. Is the patient hypertensive?

- There is no physiological dividing line between normotension and hypertension.
- The WHO criterion is blood pressure >160/90 mmHg.
- A good definition is the level at which the benefits of action exceed the risks of inaction. Considering this, the 4th Joint National Committee on Detection, Evaluation and Treatment of High Blood Pressure classified hypertension thus:

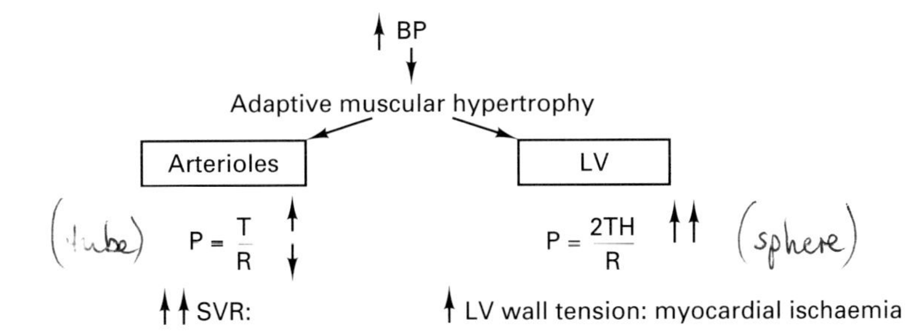

Figure 1
Physiological effects of hypertension.

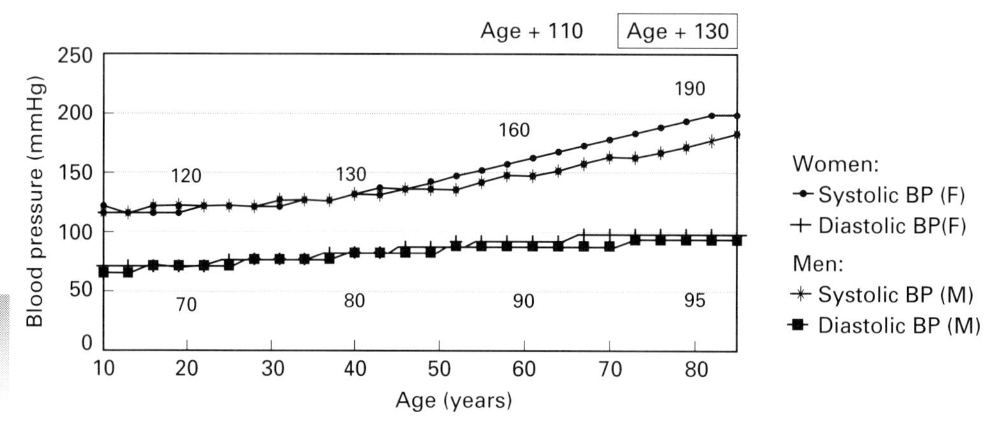

Figure 2
Age- and sex-adjusted blood pressure.

- Mild, diastolic BP 90–104 mmHg
- Moderate, diastolic BP 104–114 mmHg
- Severe, diastolic BP >115 mmHg

They also stressed the significance of systolic BP. However, systolic increases progressively with age (Figure 2). Good rules of thumb are:

Age + 110 = Upper limit of normal
Age + 130 = Significantly high systolic BP

2. Are hypertensives at higher risk?

- Dagnino & Prys-Roberts (1989), have shown that the incidence of postoperative myocardial infarction or reinfarction in hypertensive patients was almost consistently double that observed in normotensives.
- Systolic BP elevations are a better determinant of risk (strokes, myocardial infarction) than is diastolic BP.

3. Does treatment matter?

- *Severe* untreated hypertensive patients have greater variations in BP and a greater incidence of myocardial ischaemia and dysrhythmias.
- *Mild/moderate* untreated hypertension is more controversial. However, it seems that controlling treatment does matter and the presence of end organ involvement increases the risk.
- *Mild* untreated hypertension is associated with a high incidence of myocardial ischaemia during intubation and emergence from anaesthesia.

4. Is short-term 'cosmetic' therapy sufficient?

Acute treatment with vasodilatation reduces the numbers but does not alter the reactivity of blood vessels. Treatment should be given for several weeks to bring the regression of the curve back to normal (Figure 3).

5. Is local anaesthesia a safe alternative?

- Spinal/epidural: untreated hypertensives respond with a greater and unpredictable decrease in BP than do treated patients.

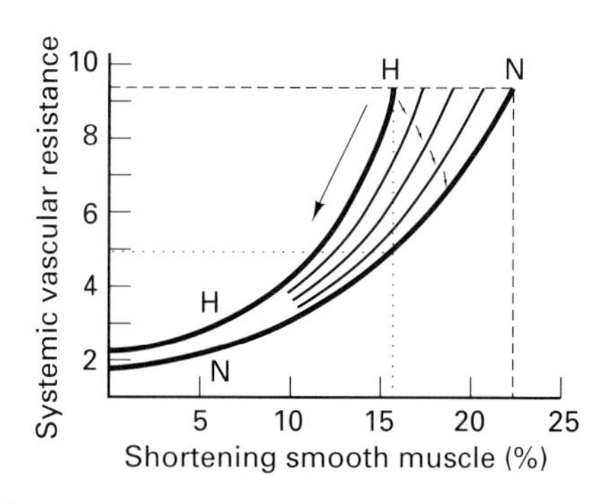

Figure 3
Is short-term therapy sufficient?

- Local infiltration/nerve block: this seems to be a simpler and safer technique; however, the possibility of inadequate block should be borne in mind.

PLAN OF ACTION

See Figure 4.

- Confirm that it is *sustained high BP* and not 'white coat syndrome':
  - In-patient: four BP measurements at 4-h intervals
  - Day-case: three BP measurements at 1-h intervals.
- Look for *evidence of end organ involvement*:
  - History of ischaemic heart disease, myocardial infarction, TIA or stroke.
  - Check ECG for left ventricular hypertrophy, and urea and electrolytes for renal involvement.
- Assess the *severity of SBP* (better determinant of risks).
- Assess the *severity of DBP*: For moderate uncontrolled group with *no* end organ involvement, the decision will depend on:
  - The experience of the anaesthetist,
  - The duration & type of surgery,
  - The patient's other medical conditions (obesity, diabetes mellitus, chronic obstructive airways disease).
- *Cancelled patient:*
  - Educate, the disease can be treated to improve their quality of life
  - Consult cardiologist to investigate and control BP.

MANAGEMENT

Aim

Optimize perfusion so that end organ ischaemia does not occur.

Preoperative:

- Continue antihypertensive medication, even during fasting period
- Adequate rehydration, as patients are relatively volume deficient.

Premedication:

- Anxiolytic
- Beta blocker or clonidine may protect against myocardial ischaemia.

Perioperative:

- Avoid stress response to laryngoscopy, intubation and extubation (intravenous opoid, lignocaine or esmolol)
- Control BP and heart rate within the range of adequate preoperative values

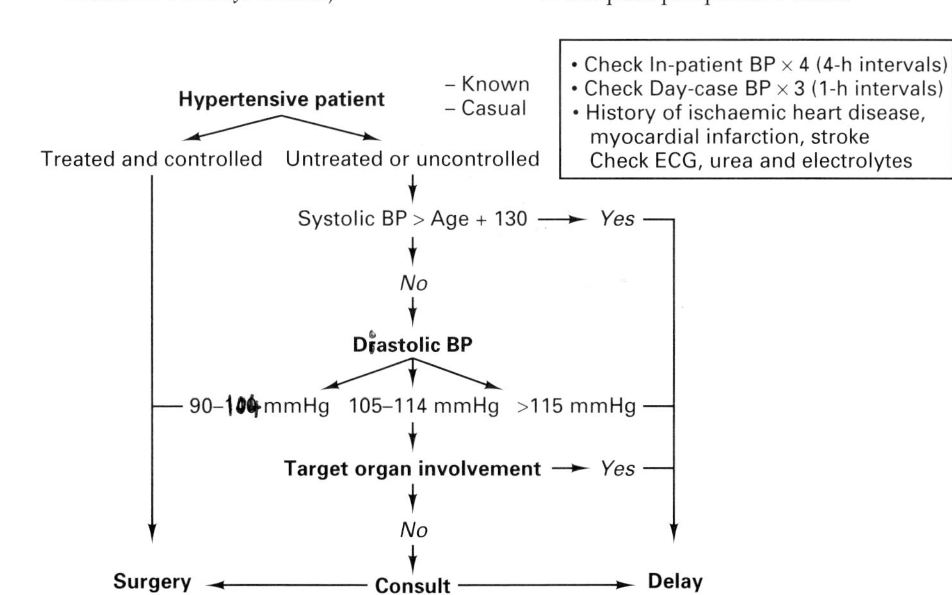

Figure 4

- Avoid hypoxaemia, hypercapnia, hypothermia and haemodynamic fluctuations.

Postoperative:
- Adequate analgesia
- Continue monitoring (on HDU) for severe uncontrolled hypertension
- Resume medication as soon as possible.

BIBLIOGRAPHY

Dagnino J, Prys-Roberts C. Strategy for patients with hypertensive heart disease. Baillière's Clinical Anaesthesiology 1989; 3: 261–289

Goldman L, Caldera D L. Risks of general anaesthesia and elective operation in hypertensive patients. Anesthesiology 1979; 50: 285–292

Hulyakar A R, Miller E D. Evaluation of the hypertensive patient. In: Rogers M C, Tinker J H, Covino B G, Longnecker D E (eds) Principles and practice of anesthesiology. Mosby-Year Book, St. Louis, 1993, p 155–167

Stone J G, Foex P, Sear J W et al. Myocardial ischaemia in untreated hypertensive patients: effect of a single small oral dose of a beta adrenergic blocking agent. Anesthesiology 1988; 68: 495–500

CROSS REFERENCES

Preoperative assessment of pulmonary risk
Anaesthetic Factors 34: 697

MITRAL VALVE DISEASE

M. Scallan

MITRAL STENOSIS

Pathophysiology

Due to the chronic underfilling of the left ventricle there is a decrease in both left ventricular end-diastolic pressure and left ventricular end-diastolic volume. In the early stages left ventricular function is preserved, but with time chronic underfilling leads to a decrease in contractility and the development of a cardiomyopathy.

When right heart failure occurs there may be a shift of the interventricular septum, which causes an additional impairment of left ventricular function.

The increase in the left atrial pressure causes atrial distension which in turn leads to a decrease in the left atrial contractility.

Later, sinus rhythm is lost and replaced by atrial fibrillation. Loss of atrial systole leads to an increase in the patient's symptoms, since atrial systole contributes approximately 30% to left ventricular filling in patients with mitral stenosis. A normal atrial contribution is 20%.

Atrial fibrillation causes a tachycardia. Because of the shorter diastolic time a greater gradient across the valve is necessary to maintain filling of the left ventricle. This increases further the left atrial pressure. The chronic increase in left atrial pressure may cause pulmonary vascular disease. Thrombi may form within the cavity of the atrium with a risk of systemic embolization.

Clinical features

Patients with mitral stenosis remain asymptomatic for 20 years. Thereafter their symptoms become rapidly progressive and they will have a severe disability at 7 years.

The main symptoms of mitral stenosis are dyspnoea, paroxysmal nocturnal dyspnoea, fatigue, pulmonary oedema and atrial fibrillation.

Anaesthesia

Avoid agents which impair ventricular contractility.

Maintain preload but avoid excess fluid as this may precipitate pulmonary oedema.

Tachycardias have a detrimental effect on left ventricular filling.

If pulmonary vascular disease is present hypercarbia, acidosis and hypoxia should be avoided at all times. Nitrous oxide should probably not be used because it increases pulmonary vascular resistance.

Pulmonary artery catheters are of value during the perioperative management of patients with mitral stenosis (Table 1).

Many patients will benefit from a period of postoperative IPPV.

Table 1.
Pulmonary artery catheters in mitral stenosis

- There is an increased risk of pulmonary artery rupture
- The catheter has a greater distance to travel which may make its insertion more difficult – the catheter may 'loop' within the enlarged right ventricle.
- Arrhythmias may occur during the insertion of catheters
- In the presence of pulmonary hypertension, the pulmonary artery diastolic pressure may not be a true reflection of the left atrial pressure
- The monitored waveforms may be distorted by left atrial pressure events – interpretation may be difficult

MITRAL REGURGITATION

Pathophysiology

In the early stages there is an increase in left ventricular end-diastolic volume and concentric hypertrophy of the myocardium.

The considerable increase in left ventricular stroke volume ensures that the forward flow to the aorta is maintained.

In the later stages forward flow is diminished and is associated with fatigue. There is a large increase in the volume of the left atrium.

The pressure in the left atrium is not increased in the early stages of the disease.

As in mitral stenosis, atrial fibrillation and pulmonary hypertension may occur.

Clinical features

Patients with chronic mitral regurgitation may remain asymptomatic for 20–40 years.

The symptoms associated with this disease are dyspnoea, orthopnoea, fatigue, pulmonary oedema and atrial fibrillation.

Anaesthesia

While the preload should be maintained, excess fluid should be avoided as this may cause further dilatation of the mitral valve ring.

Agents which impair ventricular contractility should be avoided.

Bradycardia should be avoided as this will increase regurgitation.

An increase in the systemic vascular resistance should be avoided as this will increase the regurgitant fraction.

If pulmonary vascular disease is present steps should be taken to avoid increases in the pulmonary vascular resistance. Postoperative mechanical ventilation may be required.

BIBLIOGRAPHY

Rappaport E. Natural history of aortic and mitral valve disease. Am J Cardiol 1975; 35: 221

CROSS REFERENCES

Marfan's syndrome
Patient Conditions 8: 199
Aortic valve surgery
Surgical Procedures 27: 517
Mitral valve surgery
Surgical Procedures 27: 520
Preoperative assessment of pulmonary risk
Anaesthetic Factors 34: 697

4

PATIENTS WITH PERMANENT PACEMAKERS IN SITU

N. Curzen

Permanent pacemakers (PPM) are fitted with increasing frequency to treat a variety of bradyarrhythmias as well as a few types of tachyarrhythmia. Modern systems are becoming more complex, but also safer.

PREOPERATIVE ASSESSMENT

Elective cases

Preoperative assessment should provide enough information to establish:

- The type of pacemaker present and its basic mode of operation
- Where it is sited (to minimize the chance of iatrogenic damage)
- Whether there is evidence that the unit is currently working
- Whether other factors are present that may influence the PPM function.

Pacemaker code

Produced by a combined Working Party of the North American Society of Pacing and Electrophysiology (NASBE) and the British Pacing and Electrophysiology Group (BPEG), the pacemaker code (Table 1) takes the form of a four-letter code to describe the PPM function in a systematic way.

Table 1.
Pacemaker code

First letter	*Paced* chamber	A atrium V ventricle D both
Second letter	*Sensed* chamber	A atrium V ventricle D both O none
Third letter	*Mode* of response to sensed events	I inhibited T triggered D inhibited and triggered O no response
Fourth letter	Rate responsiveness	R

Factors that can affect pacing function perioperatively

These factors can alter pacing threshold or make the myocardium more irritable (Table 2). For all but emergency cases it is important to know this information and, ideally, to have the unit fully checked by a PPM clinic, especially since a significant proportion of PPM units will be sensing most of the time, and there will be little evidence on the resting ECG as to whether they are functioning. In addition, it is not always possible to identify the specific program in which a unit is set (e.g. rate response) unless it is formally interrogated. There are some settings which would be better altered before general anaesthesia, but this decision is necessarily patient specific and should be made by an expert.

Table 2.
Factors that can affect pacing function perioperatively

Electrolytic	Hypokalaemia, hyperkalaemia
Acid–base	Acidosis, alkalosis
Myocardial	Ischaemia, acute infarction
Drugs	Digoxin toxicity, catecholamines, antiarrhythmic agents (e.g. lignocaine)
Metabolic	Hypothermia and thyroid disturbances

History:

- When and where was the unit fitted? Were there later box or lead changes?
- When was it last checked, and were the technicians happy, or did they ask for follow-up earlier than normal?
- Is the patient carrying a PPM card, which details unit and program?

- Any recent symptoms to suggest malfunction (e.g. syncope, dizzy spells)?

Examinations:
- Bradycardia; hypotension
- Where is the pacemaker generator (left, right, abdominal)?

Investigations:
- Electrolytes
- Chest X-ray:
  - Dual or single chamber?
  - Where is the generator?
- ECG:
  - What is the current rate and rhythm?
  - Is there evidence of satisfactory pacing?
  - If mode is known, is the PPM performing in that mode?
- Whenever possible, has there been a satisfactory pacing check before elective surgery?

EMERGENCY SURGERY

Even in these cases it will be possible to establish where the generator is and whether the patient is pacing or not. If there is doubt as to the functional integrity of the unit then:

- Place a magnet over the pacemaker generator (see Magnet Mode).
- If this fails to induce pacemaker activity, it may be advisable to request the placement of a temporary pacing wire.

MAGNET MODE

This should reprogram all commonly used units to the VOO, DOO or AOO mode (i.e. they pace the chamber(s) indicated at a fixed rate with no sensing of intrinsic activity) at rates that depend on the manufacturer and the unit, but are most often 70–90 beats min^{-1}. The magnet works in most modern PPM units by closing a reed switch and the PPM will remain in this setting until the magnet is removed, when it will revert to its previous mode. This property can therefore be useful:

- To confirm that the PPM is working, *or*
- To overcome sensing problems which may be causing pacing failure.

INTRAOPERATIVE MANAGEMENT

Monitoring

The ECG monitor will not identify malfunctions such as failure to capture. It is *essential* to have a system that monitors the BP or arterial waveform every beat (i.e. oximeter or arterial line) rather than just electrical activity, and this should ideally be accompanied by auditory output.

Diathermy

This is the equipment that interferes with PPM function most commonly. Most PPM will revert to asynchronous (nonsensing mode, e.g. VOO) when exposed to continuous electromagnetic interference (EMI). This may not occur with intermittent EMI, such as that generated by diathermy, and this can cause failure to pace. The major manufacturers recommend that diathermy is relatively contraindicated and that it is not used near to the generator.

- When unipolar electrocautery is used, keep the apparatus (especially the grounding plate) away from the generator and leads
- Use bipolar electrocautery if possible
- Use as little diathermy as possible
- The procedure should be followed by a formal PPM check.

Electrical cardioversion/defibrillation:
- Use the lowest possible energy level
- Paddles should be as far away from the generator as possible (not less than 10 cm)
- Paddles should be placed at right angles to the line between the generator and the lead tip
- The procedure should be followed by a formal PPM check.

Myopotential inhibition

This occurs when the PPM senses skeletal myopotentials which may be generated by:

- Mechanical ventilation
- Drug-induced myoclonic movements (e.g. propofol, ketamine, etomidate)
- Drug-induced fasciculation (e.g. depolarizing muscle relaxants).

It can present with pacing failure, in which case application of a magnet should restore fixed rate pacing (see Magnet Mode). It is more commonly a problem with unipolar systems.

Magnetic resonance imaging

This can affect PPM function in a number of ways, such as conversion to asynchronous mode, or even pacing failure. Because of this, MRI is contraindicated in pacing-dependent patients, and can damage the PPM of those who are not. It should only be performed if absolutely essential – and then only after planning by a pacing expert.

POSTOPERATIVE MANAGEMENT

It is advisable to have the function of any PPM checked after surgery; checking is *essential* following high-risk procedures including:

- Electrical cardioversion
- Diathermy.

Malfunction of the PPM in this period should be fully investigated. Possible contributory factors are included in Table 2.

BIBLIOGRAPHY

Atlee J. Cardiac pacing and electroversion. In: Kaplan J A (ed) Cardiac anaesthesia, 3rd edn. WB Saunders, Philadelphia

Bloomfield P, Bowler G M. Anaesthetic management of the patient with a permanent pacemaker. Anaesthesia 1989; 44: 42–46

Furman S, Hayes D L, Holmes D R. A practice of cardiac pacing, 2nd edn. Futura, New York, 1989

Hayes D L, Vlietstra R E. Pacemaker malfunction. Annals of Internal Medicine 1993; 119: 828–835

PULMONARY HYPERTENSION

B. Keogh

The definition of pulmonary hypertension is not clear. Generally accepted values include pulmonary artery pressure >35/15 mmHg or mean pulmonary artery pressure >20 mmHg. The condition may be primary or secondary, and in the latter case the primary condition may greatly influence both health and relevance to anaesthesia. Mild pulmonary hypertension is of little anaesthetic consequence, whereas pulmonary artery pressures approaching systemic levels represent a significant anaesthetic risk.

CLINICAL FINDINGS

Moderate pulmonary hypertension:

- Right ventricular heave
- Loud P2
- Exertional dyspnoea
- May be clubbed.

Advanced pulmonary hypertension:

- High JVP
- 'v' waves secondary to tricuspid regurgitation
- Central cyanosis (may occur early)
- Oedema
- Hepatomegaly and later ascites.

ECG:

- Right ventricular hypertrophy, usually right axis deviation
- P pulmonale (P >2 mm in lead 2).

Chest X-ray

Bilateral large pulmonary artery plus changes in primary cause.

Blood
Secondary polycythaemia.

AETIOLOGY

Primary
Pulmonary hypertension is rare and of unknown cause. It typically occurs in young females. The condition is advanced at presentation, and patients die from right ventricular failure within 2–5 years.

Secondary:
- Cardiac factors – mitral or aortic disease, left ventricular failure
- Congenital heart disease
- Chronic thromboembolic disease
- Pulmonary veno-occlusive disease
- Parenchymal pulmonary diseases
  - COPD, pulmonary fibrosis, granulomatous disease
  - Collagen and generalized vasculitic diseases
  - Secondary to kyphoscoliosis, or 'Pickwickian'.

COR PULMONALE

This is a confusing term. It is defined (WHO classification) as: right ventricular enlargement secondary to diseases of lung parenchyma or vasculature, excluding congenital and left-sided cardiac disease. Thromboembolic and veno-occlusive diseases are variously included or omitted from this group. Such patients have high right-sided pressures with low left atrial pressure and left ventricular end-diastolic pressure. By far the most common presenting group is COPD.

ANAESTHETIC IMPLICATIONS

The response of pulmonary hypertension patients to anaesthesia depends on the aetiology of the disease, disease progression and degree of decompensation. In many patients the underlying cause will bear greater relevance to anaesthesia than the pulmonary hypertension itself.

General principles:
- High F_{IO_2}; normocarbia, if possible.
- Maintain right ventricular preload; decrease right ventricular afterload.
- Orientation to cardiac output and oxygen delivery rather than P_{aO_2}.
- Vasodilators give disappointing results in established pulmonary hypertension. Options are:
  - Prostacyclin (2.5–20 ng kg^{-1} min^{-1} i.v.)
  - Prostacyclin (5–10 ng kg^{-1} min^{-1} nebulized)
  - Nitroglycerin (0.5–3 μg kg^{-1} min^{-1} i.v.)
  - Sodium nitroprusside (0.2–3 μg kg^{-1} min^{-1} i.v.)
  - Inhaled nitric oxide (NO) (2–50 ppm).
- All systemic vasodilators may decrease right ventricular preload.
- Right ventricular inotropy:
  - Phosphodiesterase inhibitors (e.g. milrinone 0.25–0.75 mg kg^{-1} min^{-1}) lower PVR
  - Dobutamine has a variable effect on PVR.
- Right ventricular lusitropy:
  - Phosphodiesterase inhibitors
  - May decrease tricuspid regurgitation.
- Switch oral anticoagulants to intravenous heparin.

N.B. Systemic vasoconstrictors may be required. An imbalance of oxygen supply–demand to the right ventricle can occur, resulting in right ventricular failure, when systemic pressure falls and right ventricular systolic and diastolic pressures remain elevated in the presence of fixed elevated PVR. Suggest noradrenaline (0.01–0.1 μg kg^{-1} min^{-1}) which has little effect on PVR in this context.

Pulmonary hypertension secondary to cardiac disease
Pulmonary hypertension secondary to left heart dysfunction mandates a high left-atrial pressure. Anaesthesia for left ventricular failure requires both preload and afterload reduction, e.g. by nitrate therapy or phosphodiesterase inhibitors. Specific therapy of valve lesions is discussed elsewhere. IPPV may have favourable effects on left ventricular function. In pulmonary hypertension, right ventricular preload must be maintained and may be difficult due to effects of tricuspid regurgitation. Direct arterial pressure monitoring and pulmonary artery catheters are indicated and right ventricular ejection-fraction catheters aid volume and pharmacology titration. A prudent anaesthetic approach to such patients includes induction with etomidate, fentanyl and vecuronium (a narcotic-based anaesthetic), followed by elective postoperative ventilation and full monitoring in the postsurgical and weaning

phase. Epidural-and-spinal anaesthesia has little to offer in such patients.

Cor pulmonale

Preoperative assessment

See COPD section (1:3:75)

- Pulmonary function tests mandatory
- Pulmonary circulation
  - Direct, by pulmonary artery catheter
  - Indirect, by Doppler echocardiography (assessment of right ventricular function, degree of tricuspid regurgitation and reasonable assessment of peak pulmonary artery pressure and pulmonary blood flow).

Choice of anaesthesia

Choice of anaesthesia will probably be dictated by the underlying aetiology.

- Primary pulmonary hypertension and chronic thromboembolic disease is probably best managed by 'cardiac'-type general anaesthesia (see elsewhere).
- In pulmonary parenchymal disease, regional techniques with judicious attention to right ventricular preload and SVR maintenance are likely to offer an advantage over general anaesthesia, especially if the right ventricle is coping.
- If there is clear evidence of right ventricular decompensation with gross peripheral oedema and ascites, the patient is at extremely high risk, whatever technique is applied. The author believes that general anaesthesia is the preferable option in this case.

Pharmacological manipulation

Vasodilators (as listed above) with attention to SVR maintenance, if necessary. The phosphodiesterase inhibitors have a particularly favourable pharmacological profile for use in pulmonary hypertension.

Facilities for prolonged ventilation

Patients are clearly at risk due to protracted recovery. The availability of postoperative ventilation facilities is mandatory and a low threshold for their use should be adopted.

Postoperative analgesia

A key factor in recovery. Epidural opiates are probably the analgesics of choice. The risks associated with epidural anaesthesia in some anticoagulated patients may need to be balanced against the perceived advantages.

BIBLIOGRAPHY

Power K J, Avery A F. Extradural analgesia in the intrapartum management of a patient with pulmonary hypertension. British Journal of Anaesthesia 1989; 63: 116–120

CROSS REFERENCES

Mitral valve disease
Patient Conditions 4: 114
Difficult airway
Anaesthetic Factors 30: 558
Preoperative assessment of pulmonary risk
Anaesthetic Factors 34: 697

SEVERE CHD IN ADULT LIFE

B. Keogh

Approximately 70% of congenital heart disease (CHD) patients reach adulthood, most of them after corrective or palliative surgery. Such patients are likely to present for noncardiac surgical procedures. Many have associated abnormalities as part of the syndrome complex. Mental retardation may be associated (40% of trisomy 21 patients have CHD).

PATHOPHYSIOLOGY

Enormous variability in anatomy and resultant dysfunction is observed, and this is compounded by varying success in surgical intervention. An understanding of the direction and quantity of blood flow is key to understanding individual physiology.

Adult CHD patient groups:

- Corrected patients:
  - Non cyanotic
  - Risk of valve and conduit dysfunction with degeneration
  - May have limited cardiac output.
- Palliated patients:
  - Commonly limited pulmonary blood flow
  - Often aortopulmonary shunts
  - Usually cyanotic; limited exercise tolerance with age
  - May progress to congestive cardiac failure.
- Untreated patients:
  - Balanced physiology
  - Usually moderately cyanotic.
- All-groups risk:
  - Arrhythmias, increasing with age
  - Infective endocarditis

MANIPULATION OF CARDIAC SHUNTS AND PULMONARY BLOOD FLOW

General principles:

SVR	PVR	Pulmonary blood flow	Shunt direction
↓		↓	R → L
↑		↑	L → R
	↓	↑	L → R
	↑	↓	R → L

Decrease PVR:

- $F_{I}O_2 = 1$
- Hyperventilate to $P_{a}CO_2 = 3.5$ kPa
- Short inspiratory time; no PEEP
- Prostacyclin (2–20 ng kg^{-1} min^{-1} i.v.; 3–10 ng kg^{-1} min^{-1} nebulized)
- Nitric oxide dose range uncertain (suggest 2–50 ppm).

Increase PVR:

- $F_{I}O_2 = 0.21–0.3$
- Hypoventilate to $P_{a}CO_2$ >7 kPa; add carbon dioxide to circuit (?)
- Long inspiratory time; PEEP rarely used clinically.

Increase SVR:

- Phenylephrine (0.25–0.5 μg kg^{-1})
- Metaraminol (0.5–1 μg kg^{-1})
- Noradrenaline (0.01–0.1 μg kg^{-1} min^{-1} infusion).

Decrease SVR:

- Sodium nitroprusside (infusion)
- Phentolamine (10 μg kg^{-1} bolus).

APPROACH TO ADULT CHD PATIENTS

- Identify basic congenital anatomy
- Consider functional effect of repair
- Consider associated medical conditions
- Always consider endocarditis
- Maintain antiarrhythmic therapy
- Potential for paradoxical emboli.

ANAESTHETIC MANAGEMENT

The majority of CHD patients who have stable cardiopulmonary physiology will tolerate anaesthesia without significant instability.

Due to extreme patient variability, it is difficult to construct a strict framework for anaesthetic management. In general it is advisable to maintain the pre-existing balance between SVR and PVR.

General principles:

- Avoid injection of air, clot, precipitates
- Adequate hydration; avoid prolonged fasting
- Isovolaemic venesection if haematocrit is >60%
- Switch anticoagulants to intravenous heparin
- Antithrombotic measures (TED stockings).

Antibiotic prophylaxis

Recommendations vary regionally and with the contemplated surgery. The regime should include anti-staphylococcal agents (e.g. flucloxacillin, teicoplanin or vancomycin) with broad-spectrum cover (e.g. gentamicin or second-generation cephalosporin).

Induction:

- Many options; CVS stability is the key
- Suggest etomidate, fentanyl or alfentanil, vecuronium
- Ketamine useful to maintain SVR
- Ketamine (i.m.) in retarded patients
- Inhalational anaesthesia is possible, but is unpredictable due to variable pulmonary blood flow.

Maintenance

Volatile or intravenous agents are equally acceptable. Marked decreases in SVR should be avoided. Tachycardia associated with isoflurane may be troublesome in some patients. In general, the balance between PVR and SVR is altered little by potent narcotics such as fentanyl, alfentanil and sufentanil. There is a theoretical risk of the use of nitrous oxide in patients with right-to-left shunts, in that the bubble size of inadvertently injected air will increase with nitrous oxide and, therefore, should probably be avoided in such patients.

Monitoring

Arm BP monitoring may underestimate the true systemic BP in patients who have had previous aortopulmonary shunts involving the subclavian artery. Peripheral Sa_{O_2} is mandatory, in addition to basic monitoring. Interpretation of ET_{CO_2} tracing is complex. ET_{CO_2} does not necessarily reflect $P_{a}CO_2$, but trends in ET_{CO_2} can indicate variations in pulmonary blood flow. A low threshold for arterial line and central venous pressure line placement is appropriate. Pulmonary artery catheterization is likely to yield valuable information in relatively few patients, and is anatomically impossible in a considerable number.

Haemodynamic support

This is a complex area and depends greatly on the anatomy. In addition to the manipulation of intracardiac shunt (see above), inotropic support of either ventricle may be required. The phosphodiesterase inhibitors milrinone (0.25–0.75 μg kg^{-1} min^{-1}) and enoximone (5–10 μg kg^{-1} min^{-1}) have proved useful in the cardiac sphere in view of associated pulmonary vasodilatation and positive lusitropy (ventricular relaxation), which can improve filling of often restrictive ventricles. Isoprenaline (0.02–0.05 μg kg^{-1} min^{-1}) is useful for rate support, but does decrease SVR. Adenosine (4–12 mg bolus) may successfully treat a troublesome tachycardia. In a desperate situation, adrenaline (0.01–0.2 μg kg^{-1} min^{-1} or even higher doses) tends to be the drug of choice.

Regional anaesthesia

Cardiac anaesthetists, regularly confronted with such patients, rarely consider epidural or spinal regional techniques. The decrease in SVR may be troublesome in some patients, but can be counteracted by vasoconstrictor infusions. Many patients are anticoagulated, representing a relative contraindication.

Day-case anaesthesia

The presence of CHD alone does not preclude day-case surgery. Patients with stable cardiopulmonary physiology undergoing limited surgical procedures may be considered suitable.

Cardiopulmonary resuscitation

This may be difficult due to anatomy. External cardiac compression is ineffective in some patients, e.g. those with a right ventricle to pulmonary artery conduit which lies behind the sternum and is blocked by compression. Systemic vasoconstrictors are useful in many circulations and in a deteriorating situation may improve pulmonary blood flow and avoid need for cardiopulmonary resuscitation.

General comments
Polycythaemic patients with decreased plasma volume have an increased bleeding tendency and require extra haematological support. Patients with relatively simple lesions, e.g. ASD, who have not had access to medical therapy are at risk of acute decompensation. Discussion with the congenital cardiothoracic centre staff is advisable before undertaking anaesthesia, especially if the cardiopulmonary connections are difficult to understand.

SURGERY IN HEART TRANSPLANT RECIPIENTS

M. Wall and T. Feeley

BACKGROUND

The most common reason an anesthesiologist will manage a heart-transplant recipient is that the patient is requiring surgery for some other procedure. In the past 10 years there has been tremendous growth in the number of procedures performed yearly (IHLTS 1993) (Figure 1). Continually improving survival (Figure 2) has meant that many heart-transplant patients are receiving surgical treatment at hospitals which are not transplant centres. Surgical procedures performed on these patients are usually due to the complications of the transplant surgery or chronic immunosuppression. Surgery may be needed for mediastinal bleeding, late infection such as an abscess, or joint replacement for aseptic necrosis. Two recent reviews of surgery in heart-transplant patients found that cholecystectomy was the commonest general surgical procedure and may be related to altered bile metabolism caused by cyclosporin (Yee et al 1990, Melendez et al 1991).

PATHOPHYSIOLOGY

The two main concerns for the anesthesiologist are:

- The denervated heart
- The consequences of chronic immunosuppressive therapy (Kanter & Samuels 1977, Shaw et al 1991).

The denervated heart responds to stress by

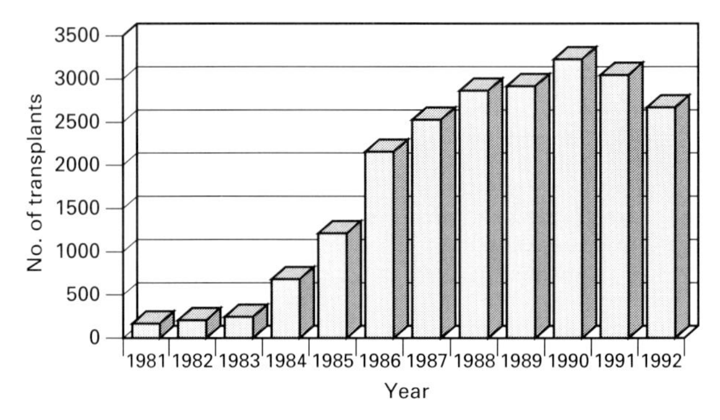

Figure 1
Number of heart transplants performed world-wide between 1981 and 1992. Over 2500 transplants have been performed yearly since 1987, and 87% of all transplants performed have occurred since 1984. From the registry of the International Heart and Lung Transplantation Society (IHLTS 1993).

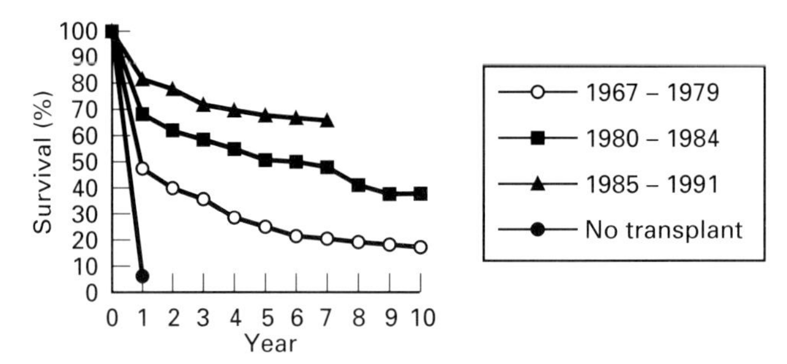

Figure 2
Survival following heart transplantation in patients transplanted during three periods. Patients in the no transplant group were selected for transplantation but no suitable donor could be found. Most recent data reflect improved survival associated with the introduction of cyclosporin and the growth of the numbers of centres performing transplantation.

increasing cardiac output from increased preload and later by direct effects of circulating catecholamines. Changes in heart rate are late and occur from the direct effects of catecholamines. The denervated heart is preload dependent, making regional anesthesia potentially problematic, and making the heart rate an unreliable guide to the patient's volume status and the adequacy of anaesthesia. Vasodilators can be hazardous, since they may cause a fall in cardiac output without an increase in heart rate. Myocardial depressants should also be used with care since the denervated heart typically increases cardiac output by increasing stroke volume rather than rate. When treating bradycardia and hypotension in these patients direct acting drugs such as isoproterenol are more efficacious than indirect agents such as atropine or drugs with mixed effects such as ephedrine. The transplanted heart typically has a high resting heart rate since it is denervated from its vagal tone. It also has a higher density of α and β receptors due to denervation up-regulation. Despite this experimental finding, there is no clinical evidence of hypersensitivity to catecholamines. Dysrhythmias are not common in transplanted hearts; however, they are more common in the first 6 months and are associated with episodes of rejection. Hypertension is not uncommon in heart transplant recipients. Cyclosporin is nephrotoxic and many patients have mild renal insufficiency

Table 1.
The effect of various drugs on the normal and transplanted heart

	Action	Heart rate		Pressure	
		Normal	Transplant	Normal	Transplant
Atropine	Indirect	Increase	None	None	None
Neostigmine	Indirect	Decrease	None	None	None
Ephedrine	Both	Increase	Small increase	Increase	Small increase
Epinephrine	Direct	Increase	Increase	Increase	Increase
Phenylephrine	Direct	Decrease	None	Increase	Increase

and hypertension and are often on vasodilating agents. Myocardial ischaemia will probably be painless, and transplanted hearts are prone to atherosclerosis. Ventricular function is generally good, unless there is rejection.

THE EFFECT OF DRUGS

Drugs which have direct actions on the heart are not affected by the presence of a transplanted heart. Drugs which have indirect actions (mediated by the autonomic nervous system) will not have their ordinary effects on the transplanted heart. Drugs with mixed actions (both direct and indirect) will have their full effects attenuated by the absence of innervation. Phenlyephrine has no direct cardiac effects; however, it has a direct effect on the peripheral vessels. In the normal circulation, vagal innervation slows the heart when the pressure increases due to vasoconstriction. In the transplant patient, phenylephrine results in increased BP, but no reflex decrease in heart rate.

PREOPERATIVE ASSESSMENT

The heart-transplant patient should be carefully evaluated for evidence of rejection, especially before elective surgical procedures. Most transplant patients undergo frequent evaluations of the function of their heart, and often present with extensive information. Endomyocardial biopsies are performed regularly, and most centres perform yearly coronary angiography to look for new coronary disease. Both liver and renal function should be evaluated prior to surgery, in addition to routine blood tests, chest X-ray and ECG.

PERIOPERATIVE MANAGEMENT

Strict sterile technique needs to be observed at all times. Virtually all anaesthetic techniques have been used with success in heart-transplant recipients. Despite concerns about the preload dependence of the denervated heart, conduction anaesthesia has been used successfully in conjunction with administering a moderate amount of intravenous fluids prior to the block (Melendez et al 1991, Shaw et al 1991). Thiopental and propofol are not contraindicated, but the dose should be reduced. Isoflurane has been advocated for maintenance of anaesthesia due to its absence of significant myocardial depression. However, halothane and enflurane have also been used successfully.

Fluids are used to maintain preload. Most patients are haemodynamically stable during surgery, as long as they are not undergoing acute rejection. The major haemodynamic differences which can be observed are the absence of immediate haemodynamic response to tracheal intubation and surgical incision, as well as a slowly progressive increase in heart rate during surgery, which is probably secondary to increasing levels of circulating catecholamines (Melendez et al 1991). Invasive monitoring is therefore not needed due to the presence of a transplanted heart per se, but is dictated by the procedure being performed.

Several studies have suggested that cyclosporin may have effects both on sedative drugs as well as neuromuscular blocking agents. However, clinical observations of delayed awakening from anaesthesia have not been described, despite this experimental concern. Care must be taken, however, in the use of muscle relaxants, since the preservative in cyclosporin potentates the block and may make reversal difficult if normal doses are given. Reduced doses and careful monitoring are used. If careful monitoring is used, this complication can also be avoided (Melendez et al, 1991). The chronic use of steroids mean that prophylactic stress doses of steroids are necessary. OKT-3 has no known interactions with anaesthetic agents. Azothioprine may cause resistance to muscle relaxants; however, the effects of cyclosporin are more relevant and overdose is more commonly seen than resistance to neuromuscular blocking agents. Common anaesthetic problems must be watched for in these patients. Ventilation and oxygenation must be maintained, and cannot be lost sight of while worrying about the transplanted heart.

4

POSTOPERATIVE PERIOD

- Prompt extubation of trachea.
- Resume immunosuppression (Shaw et al 1991):
  - Oral, if possible, at preoperative doses
  - Intravenous if NBM
    Azothioprine – same as oral dose
    Cyclosporin – 25% of oral dose twice daily over 6 h
    Methylprednisolone – 0.8 of oral dose of prednisolone.

Cyclosporin blood levels should be carefully monitored, aiming for blood levels of 150–250 mg ml^{-1}.

BIBLIOGRAPHY

IHLTS. The registry of the International Society for Heart and Lung Transplantation: tenth official report – 1993. Journal of Heart and Lung Transplantation 1993; 12: 541–548

Kanter S F, Samuels S I. Anesthesia for major operations on patients who have transplanted hearts. A review of 29 cases. Anesthesiology 1977; 46: 65–68

Melendez J A, Delphin E, Lamb J, Rose E. Noncardiac surgery in heart transplant recipients in the cyclosporin era. Journal of Cardiothoracic and Vascular Anesthesia 1991; 5: 218–220

Shaw I H, Kirk A J B, Conacher I D. Anaesthesia for patients with transplanted hearts and lungs undergoing non-cardiac surgery. British Journal of Anaesthesia 1991; 67: 772–778

Yee J, Petsikas D, Ricci M A, Guerraty A. General surgical procedures after heart transplantation. Canadian Journal of Surgery 1990; 33: 185–188

TETRALOGY OF FALLOT

B. Keogh

Tetralogy of Fallot (TOF) accounts for 10% of congenital heart disease. Both early surgical correction (<6 months) and palliative aortopulmonary shunt followed by later definitive correction are widely practised. Only 5% of untreated patients survive beyond age 25 years.

ANATOMY

- Ventricular septal defect
- Pulmonary stenosis
- Right ventricular hypertrophy
- Aorta overriding ventricular septal defect (VSD).

CLINICOPATHOPHYSIOLOGICAL FEATURES

- Right-to-left shunt
- Cyanosis and clubbing
- Polycythaemia
- Dyspnoea on exertion.

HYPERCYANOTIC SPELLS

These intermittent cyanotic episodes are characteristic of children with TOF. Right ventricular infundibular (subpulmonary but supra-VSD) muscle spasm increases right-to-left shunt, resulting in profound hypoxaemia. Children squat in response to this phenomenon, resulting in increased SVR and decreased venous return, both of which decrease the right-to-left shunt. Propranolol therapy is indicated to control spells.

COMPLICATIONS AND SEQUELAE

- Increasing dyspnoea with age
- Arrhythmia
- Infective endocarditis
- Paradoxical emboli
  - Cerebral thrombosis
  - Cerebral abscess
- Ischaemic cardiomyopathy.

INVESTIGATIONS

Chest X-ray

'Boot shaped' heart and oligaemic lung fields.

ECG

Right ventricular hypertrophy and right axis deviation.

Blood

Polycythaemia (haematocrit >50%) and thrombocytopenia (uncommon).

Sao_2

Range 70–90%.

ANAESTHETIC MANAGEMENT

Anaesthesia for TOF correction lies within the province of the cardiothoracic anaesthetist. Palliated or uncorrected TOF patients may present at any age for noncardiac or, particularly, emergency surgery. Relevant issues are discussed below.

PREOPERATIVE ISSUES

- Sedative premedicants are indicated in younger patients
- Avoid prolonged NBM period; consider intravenous hydration
- Continue beta blockers and antiarrhythmics perioperatively
- Antibiotic prophylaxis is mandatory
- Switch anticoagulation to intravenous heparin
- General antithrombotic measures (TED stockings)
- Reduced plasma volume (may need coagulation support)
- Venesect if haematocrit is >60%; replace with albumin in children.

Induction

Inhalational induction is commonly used in children, but may precipitate a hypercyanotic spell. Inhalational induction may be slower in

TOF due to limited pulmonary blood flow, especially during a spell. Both halothane and isoflurane are advocated. There is no indication to alter the preferred inhalational agent.

Intravenous induction (after EMLA cream) allows induction to be achieved with little patient awareness, potentially decreasing the risk of a spell. Ketamine (intramuscular or intravenous) maintains SVR with little increase in PVR in TOF, thus decreasing the right-to-left shunt, but is popular in few centres. Increased right-to-left shunt with routine induction agents due to decreased SVR may be antagonized by vasoconstrictors (e.g. phenylephrine 0.5 μg kg^{-1} i.v. or metaraminol 1 μg kg^{-1} i.v.). In practice, vasoconstrictors are rarely required.

Monitoring

Besides ECG, monitoring of peripheral Sa_{O_2} is mandatory in monitoring a right-to-left shunt and ET_{CO_2} trends can reflect variations in pulmonary blood flow. A low threshold for direct intravascular monitoring of arterial pressure and central venous pressure is appropriate. Pulmonary artery catheterization is unhelpful, technically difficult, and in fact contraindicated.

Maintenance

Volatile or intravenous techniques are equally appropriate as long as marked falls in SVR are avoided. Low-dose noradrenaline infusion (typically 0.01–0.05 μg kg^{-1} min^{-1}) can control SVR changes. Potent narcotics (e.g. alfentanil) may ablate undesired cardiovascular responses. Spontaneous respiration may be employed for minor cases. Adequate fluid replacement is vital.

Management of a hypercyanotic spell under anaesthesia

The drug of choice is intravenous propranolol; a dose of 0.05–0.1 mg kg^{-1} decreases infundibular spasm. Resistant spells require vasoconstrictors by bolus and by infusion (see doses above). In addition, extra sedatives (e.g. opiates), aggressive hyperventilation and correction of the cause of metabolic acidosis are indicated. The use of sodium bicarbonate is, as always, controversial.

Other special considerations

There is a substantial risk of paradoxical embolus through the VSD. Injection of air, drug precipitates or clots in lines must be avoided.

Regional anaesthesia

Reduced SVR due to spinal and epidural anaesthesia is likely to increase right-to-left shunt. Fluid resuscitation will exacerbate this effect. If regional techniques are considered truly preferable to general anaesthesia, manipulation of SVR with a vasoconstrictor infusion is integral to the safety of an unpredictable technique.

POSTOPERATIVE FACTORS

The same general principles apply, but in addition avoid the oxygen demands of excessive shivering. Treatment of spells is as described above. Arrhythmias are common, and amiodarone is useful in these patients.

UNCORRECTED, PALLIATED AND CORRECTED PATIENTS

Uncorrected patients are severely at risk of complications and adverse haemodynamic sequelae. Palliated patients, while at risk of paradoxical emboli and consequences of polycythaemia, do not spell as pulmonary blood flow is maintained by the aorto-pulmonary shunt. The presence of residual intracardiac shunts should be determined by echocardiography in patients who have had correction of TOF. Antibiotic prophylaxis is indicated. The vast majority of TOF patients who have undergone successful repair can be expected to exhibit normal cardiopulmonary interactions.

THE FAILING HEART

W. Aveling

The presence of a failing heart in a patient presenting for noncardiac surgery is known to increase mortality and morbidity. Patients will fall into two categories:

- Treated, not likely to improve further
- Untreated or undertreated.

As always, the problem in untreated or undertreated patients is to balance the risk of delaying surgery against the benefit of medical improvment.

PATHOPHYSIOLOGY

The factors affecting ventricular performance are described below.

Preload

The Frank–Starling relationship (Figure 1) describes how stroke volume increases as end-diastolic volume (i.e. cardiac muscle fibre length) increases within limits. End-diastolic pressure is easier to measure and can be substituted for volume. Preload can easily be manipulated to produce maximum cardiac output by judicious filling of the circulation.

Afterload

The tension that the left ventricle must develop to move blood forward depends on the state of the aortic valve (fixed), and the systemic vascular resistance. Reducing resistance by vasodilation can increase output in the failing heart.

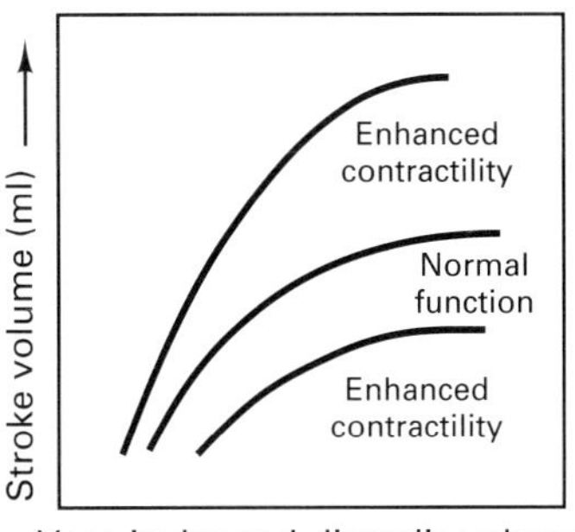

Figure 1

Inotropic state

The force of contraction for a given fibre length can be increased by sympathetic stimulation (intrinsic) or β sympathomimetic drugs. In heart failure there is a depletion of catecholamines and a decreased density of β receptors, resulting in decreased response to β stimulation.

Rate

As

$$\text{Cardiac output} = \text{Stroke volume} \times \text{Rate}$$

one might expect increase in rate to increase cardiac output. However, at high rates, diastole is reduced, and with it coronary perfusion. Manipulation of rate by chronotropes is only helpful in bradycardia.

PREOPERATIVE ASSESSMENT

- History – exercise tolerance and dypsnoea.
- Right ventricular function – raised JVP and oedema are early signs.
- Left ventricular function – tachycardia, basal creps and a third heart sound.
- Chest X-ray – upper lobe diversion (early), bat's-wing shadowing (late).
- Many cardiological investigations:
  - Ejection fraction is a simple and useful guide (<50% impaired; <30% poor; <10% very poor)
  - A pulmonary artery catheter can be used to measure cardiac output
  - Wedge pressure reflects left atrial pressure
  - Full cardiac catheterization gives most information (left ventricular end-diastolic pressure increases to >12 mm in left ventricular failure).
- Renal and liver function aren often impaired.

PREOPERATIVE TREATMENT

Where time permits, cardiac function should be optimized.

- *Vasodilation* to offload the ventricle. ACE inhibitors are now the first-line treatment, but they have to be given orally (captopril 25–75 mg). If time presses, intravenous infusion of nitroprusside (0.5–5 μg kg^{-1} min^{-1}; venous and arteriolar) or nitroprusside (0.5–5 μg kg^{-1} min^{-1}; mainly arteriolar) or isosorbide (2–40 mg kg^{-1} min^{-1}; venous and arteriolar). Dosage is limited by hypotension.
- *Adjustment of filling pressures* requires at least central venous pressure monitoring. It is better to use a pulmonary artery catheter so that cardiac output and pressures can be measured in response to aliquots of 200 ml colloid.
- *Inotropes.* Digoxin is still useful, but even when given intravenously takes 30 min. Dobutamine (5–20 μg kg^{-1} min^{-1}) can be used for an immediate effect.
- *Phosphodiesterase inhibitors* increase cyclic AMP. Known as 'inodilators', they can be of benefit in intractable failure. Milrinone (50 μg kg^{-1} bolus then 0.4–0.75 μg kg^{-1} min^{-1} infusion).
- *Intra-aortic balloon* counterpulsation can be inserted percutaneously preoperatively in severe cases.

ANAESTHESIA

The haemodynamic consequences of extensive regional blockade make this a hazardous choice. General anaesthesia with minimum cardiovascular disturbance is preferred.

Monitoring:
- Arterial and central venous lines
- Urine output
- Consider placing a pulmonary artery catheter.

Premedication
Premedication is either minimal or not required.

Induction
Ketamine, etomidate or midazolam plus an opiate (i.v.).

Maintenance
Opiates are the mainstay of maintenance. Use fentanyl (10–20 μg kg^{-1}) or alfentanil (50 μg kg^{-1} bolus, then 50 μg kg^{-1} min^{-1} infusion). Note that nitrous oxide depresses myocardial function in the presence of opiates.

POSTOPERATIVE MANAGEMENT

Continue monitoring on the ITU.

BIBLIOGRAPHY

Stoelting R K, Dierdorf S E. Congestive heart failure. In: Anaesthesia and co-existing disease, 3rd edn Churchill Livingstone, Edinburgh, 1993, ch 6

CROSS REFERENCES

Preoperative assessment of pulmonary risk
Anaesthetic Factors 34: 697

5

GI TRACT

T. Peachey

CARCINOID SYNDROME

M. Brunner

Carcinoid syndrome is caused by peptides, particularly serotonin (5-hydroxytryptamine (5-HT) and bradykinin, which reach the systemic circulation in abnormally high concentrations after release by carcinoid tumours. It occurs in approximately 8/100 000 people.

PATHOPHYSIOLOGY

Carcinoid tumours are derived from argentaffin cells and occur in several locations, e.g. bronchus and pancreas, although 75% are found in the gastro-intestinal tract, most commonly in the appendix. Appendicial tumours are usually benign and nonsecreting. The amines and peptides responsible for the symptoms of carcinoid syndrome are produced by malignant tumours. Up to 20 peptides and amines have been isolated, e.g. serotonin, bradykinin which is derived from kallikrein, histamine, somatostatin, vasoactive peptide and substance P. However, only 7% of people with carcinoid tumours exhibit carcinoid syndrome, as only 25% of malignant tumours produce peptides and these are normally cleared from the portal circulation by the liver. Carcinoid syndrome is usually associated with ileal tumours with liver secondaries which secrete peptides directly into the hepatic veins. Bronchial tumours release peptides which bypass the portal circulation, resulting in symptoms at an earlier stage.

PREOPERATIVE EVALUATION

Patients may have symptoms caused by:

- The primary tumour:
  - Intestinal obstruction
  - Haemoptysis.
- Right heart valve lesions.
- The systemic effects of peptides released by the tumour, most commonly serotonin, bradykinin and histamine.

Serotonin:

- Watery diarrhoea (75% of patients) associated with cramps may be severe, resulting in dehydration, hyponatraemia, hypokalaemia and hypochloraemia. Malabsorbtion with steatorrhoea and hypoproteinaemia is less common.
- Pallor.
- Hypertension, as 5-HT stimulates the release and inhibits the uptake of nor-adrenaline and potentiates the response of $\alpha_1$adrenoreceptors to catecholamines.
- Tachycardia, as 5-HT is a positive chronotrope.
- Hyperglycaemia.
- Right heart failure (33% of patients) due to pulmonary stenosis and tricuspid regurgitation resulting from subendocardial fibrosis.
- Raised urinary 5-hydroxyindoleacetic acid (5-HIAA) levels, which are diagnostic of carcinoid syndrome.

Bradykinin:

- Flushing (90% of patients) of the face and upper body increases in duration as the disease progresses
- Hypotension
- Bronchospasm (20% of patients), especially in previous asthmatics and in the presence of cardiac disease.

Histamine

Particularly in some patients with gastric carcinoid.

- Flushing
- Hypotension
- Bronchospasm.

Preoperative drug therapy

Preoperative drug therapy is aimed at antagonizing the mediators of carcinoid syndrome or preventing their release from carcinoid tumours.

Serotonin antagonists:
- Cyproheptadine and methysergide are effective against gastrointestinal manifestations.
- Ketanserin blocks the effects of serotonin mediated by the 5-HT_2 receptor, i.e. vasoconstriction, bronchoconstriction and platelet aggregation. It also has adrenergic antagonist activity and reduces central sympathetic outflow, and is therefore used to treat hypertension in patients with carcinoid.

Bradykinin antagonists:
- Aprotinin inhibits the kallikrein cascade. By infusion it is used to control flushing and treat hypotension.
- Steroids, e.g. methylprednisolone, reduce the synthesis of prostaglandins which mediate the action of bradykinin.

Histamine antagonists

H_2 antagonists or combination antihistamines are more effective than H_1 blockers on their own.

Inhibitors of mediator release by tumours:
- Somatostatin inhibits the release of mediators from carcinoid tumours. It has a short half-life and must be given by infusion.
- Octreotide, a long-acting synthetic octapeptide somatostatin analogue, has been used as a sole agent to treat diarrhoea, hypertension, hypotension and bronchospasm in patients with carcinoid syndrome. It reduces the plasma levels of mediators by inhibiting their release from carcinoid tumours.

ANAESTHETIC CONSIDERATIONS

- Hypovolaemia and electrolyte abnormalities may be significant in patients with severe diarrhoea.
- Prevent the release of mediators, i.e. somatostatin and somatostatin analogues
- Avoid factors which trigger carcinoid crisis by causing the release of mediators, e.g.
  - Catecholamines, which mediate the release of peptides from carcinoid tumours
  - Anxiety, hypercapnia, hypothermia and hypotension which release catecholamines
  - Drugs which release histamine, e.g. morphine, atracurium, suxamethonium
  - Hypertension, which causes the release of bradykinin.
- Prepare for carcinoid crisis, i.e. resistant bronchospasm and sudden variations in arterial pressure, particularly at induction of anaesthesia and when the tumour is handled.

PREOPERATIVE MANAGEMENT

- Correct fluid and electrolyte abnormalities secondary to severe diarrhoea, and consider nutritional support if malabsorption is severe.
- Octreotide, 100 μg subcutaneously two or three times a day for 2 weeks prior to surgery followed by 100 μg intravenously at induction of anaesthesia and a slow postoperative wean over a few days (Roy et al 1987), reduces mediator release.
- Continue antagonists of serotonin, bradykinin and histamine to minimize symptoms and maintain haemodynamic stability.
- All antimediator drugs, e.g. ketanserin, cyproheptadine, somatostatin, antihistamines and aprotinin, should be available for immediate administration if required perioperatively.
- Premedication should include an anxiolytic drug and a sedative antihistamine, e.g. benzodiazepine and promethazine.

PERIOPERATIVE MANAGEMENT

Monitoring starts prior to induction and should include:

- Intra-arterial BP
- ECG
- Central venous pressure (CVP)
- Blood gases
- Blood sugar
- Airway pressure
- In patients with right-sided heart lesions, pulmonary hypertension must be avoided and pulmonary artery catheterization should be considered.

Regional anaesthesia is relatively contra-indicated, as hypotension may occur. General anaesthesia should be induced with drugs which maintain haemodynamic stability, obtund the hypertensive response to laryngoscopy and tracheal intubation, and do not release histamine. Suxamethonium should be avoided. Volatile agents may delay recovery and cause myocardial depression.

Therefore a technique including high-dose narcotics may be indicated for maintenance. A flow-generating ventilator may be required to overcome bronchospasm.

Hypotension should be treated with fluid guided by the CVP or with an infusion of aprotinin. Angiotensin and vasopressin have also been used. Catecholamines should not be given as they cause the release of peptides. Hypertension is controlled with intravenous ketanserin and cyproheptadine. Adrenergic receptor antagonists and clonidine have also been used, but can precipitate hypotension. Somatostatin and its analogues prevent pre- and peri-operative episodes of hypertension (Hughes & Hodkinson 1989), hypotension (Marsh et al 1987) and bronchospasm which may be resistant to other forms of drug therapy.

POSTOPERATIVE MANAGEMENT

As recovery from anaesthesia in this group of patients may be delayed and close monitoring should continue, the patient should be sent to either a HDU or ITU in the immediate postoperative period. If octreotide has been used preoperatively it should be reduced slowly over the first postoperative week (Roy et al 1987).

CONCLUSION

In patients with carcinoid syndrome, the severity of symptoms does not predict the severity of perioperative complications, so that patients with minor preoperative symptoms may have significant intraoperative complications. Perioperative preparation and vigilance is of great importance in the anaesthetic management of these patients. The introduction of somatostatin and its analogues has shifted the emphasis of treating perioperative carcinoid crises from antagonizing mediators which have been released to inhibiting their release from carcinoid tumours altogether.

BIBLIOGRAPHY

Hughes E W, Hodkinson B P. Carcinoid syndrome: the combined use of ketanserin and octreotide in the management of an acute crisis during anaesthesia. Anaesthesia and Intensive Care 1989; 17: 367–370

Marsh H M, Martin Jr J K, Kvols L K et al. Carcinoid crisis during anesthesia: succesful treatment with somatostatin analogue. Anesthesiology 1987; 66: 89–91

Roy R C, Carter R F, Wright P D. Somatostatin, anaesthesia and the carcinoid syndrome. Anaesthesia 1987; 42: 627–632

CROSS REFERENCES

Pulmonary hypertension
Patient Conditions 4: 118
Obstruction or perforation
Surgical Procedures 18: 372
Intraoperative bronchospasm
Anaesthetic Factors 33: 632
Intraoperative hypertension
Anaesthetic Factors 33: 636

CHRONIC LIVER DISEASE

R. J. Alcock

There are numerous causes of chronic hepatic dysfunction, but cirrhosis is the most common and its incidence is increasing. These patients present an extreme risk for surgery.

PATHOPHYSIOLOGY

Gastrointestinal tract:

- Portal hypertension and associated oesophageal varices
- Ascites, causing increased intra-abdominal pressure
- Delayed gastric emptying and hyperacidity
- Poor hepatocellular function with decreased drug clearance and increased free drug concentration.

Cardiovascular system:

- Vascular shunts – arteriovenous, intrapulmonary, pleural, portosystemic
- Hyperdynamic circulation with decreased peripheral vascular resistance and increased cardiac output
- Increased circulating volume
- Low incidence of coronary artery disease.

Respiratory

Patients with cirrhosis, particularly end-stage disease, have arterial hypoxaemia, due to:

- Intrapulmonary shunts (not corrected with supplementary oxygen)
- Ventilation perfusion mismatch (correctable with supplementary oxygen)
- Restrictive defects due to pleural effusions and ascites
- Smokers (COAD).

Nervous system

Encephalopathy, aggravated by sedatives and diuretics.

Renal and metabolic:

- Increased sodium and water retention
- Metabolic alkalosis with obligatory kalluresis
- Susceptible to renal failure; acute tubular necrosis and hepatorenal failure.

Bleeding and clotting

There are numerous causes of coagulopathy in patients with end-stage liver disease:

- Decreased production of vitamin-K-dependent factors
- Decreased production of non-vitamin-K-dependent factors
- Thrombocytopenia
- Abnormal platelet function
- Hyperfibrinolysis.

PREOPERATIVE ASSESSMENT

History and examination

- Associated disease (cardiomyopathy, COAD)
- Degree of ascites
- Degree of encephalopathy (caution with sedatives)
- Bleeding varices and Sengstaken tube
- Neomycin (may prolong neuromuscular blockade)
- Cimetidine (may prolong action of drugs, e.g. fentanyl)
- Peripheral oedema
- Nutrition status.

Investigations:

- ECG.
- ABGs:
  - P_aO_2 (if low, see if corrected with oxygen)
  - Acid–base status.
- Renal function: urea, creatinine, creatinine clearance.
- Full blood count:
  - Hb
  - White cell count; look for infection
  - Platelet count.
- Chest X-ray: pleural effusions, heart size.
- Lung function: restrictive or obstructive defects.
- Electrolytes: dilutional hyponatraemia, low potassium.
- Coagulopathy:
  - PT
  - PTT
  - Bleeding time.
- Assess infection risk: hepatitis B, C antigens.

PREOPERATIVE PREPARATION

- Ascites should be controlled in consultation with a hepatologist.
- Improve poor nutritional status and optimize coexisting disease.
- Have adequate blood cross-matched, especially for abdominal surgery. The need for fresh frozen plasma (FFP) and cryoprecipitate should be anticipated.
- Give vitamin K several days prior to surgery.
- Start an intravenous infusion from point of starvation.

PREMEDICATION

Opioids are not well tolerated. Avoid intramuscular premedication if there is a coagulopathy, and avoid drugs relying on phase I liver metabolism. Oral lorazepam is an effective anxiolytic. Anticholinergic drugs can be prescribed if necessary. Acid aspiration prophylaxis should be given.

PERIOPERATIVE MANAGEMENT

Monitoring

Routine:
- ECG
- Pulse oximeter
- Temperature
- Urinary catheter (hourly urine output)
- BP – noninvasive/direct
- Capnography
- Neuromuscular monitoring.

All but minor surgery:
- Arterial line:
  - Hourly ABGs
  - Hb
  - Sodium and potassium
  - Glucose
  - Calcium
  - Clotting studies.
- Central venous pressure/pulmonary artery catheter.

Induction

Appropriate prophylactic antibiotics should be given before surgery. Thiopentone, etomidate or propofol are all quite satisfactory for induction.

The action of suxamethonium may be prolonged in severe disease, but avoidance must be weighed against the increased risk of aspiration in these patients.

Maintenance

Intubation and controlled ventilation for all but minor procedures, avoiding hypocapnia. Use technique based around volatile agent; isoflurane, enflurane satisfactory. Supplement cautiously with fentanyl, unless postoperative ventilation is contemplated. Nitrous oxide is best avoided during abdominal surgery as bowel distension can make surgery more difficult. Atracurium is the ideal muscle relaxant, though no muscle relaxants are contraindicated.

Urine output

Maintenance of urine output is of paramount importance:

- Aim to maintain output at above 50 ml h^{-1} in adults.
- Crystalloid infusion during surgery (dextrose 5~). Avoid excessive volumes of saline solutions.
- 100-ml boluses of 20% mannitol.
- Dopamine infusion at 3–5 μg kg^{-1} min^{-1} throughout the perioperative period.
- Loop diuretics should be used with caution.

Coagulopathy

During major surgery with marked blood loss, regular assessment of clotting should guide replacement therapy. Laboratory tests such as PT, PTT and platelet count may be used, but thromboelastography has also been found to be a reliable and effective guide to blood product requirements.

Blood product usage can be reduced by the use of intraoperative aprotinin, which decreases the hyperfibrinolysis seen in these patients. Aprotinin is given as a loading dose of 2 million units i.v. followed by an infusion of 500 000 units per hour.

Temperature

Avoid hypothermia. Wrap patient in reflective blanketing. The use of a warming mattress and the warming of all fluids is vital.

POSTOPERATIVE MANAGEMENT

- Analgesia: opiates are best administered intravenously either by infusion or via a patent-controlled system. Regional analgesia is worth considering, provided

Table 1.
Pugh's modification of Child's classification of risks for cirrhotic patients undergoing surgery: low risk < 6 points, moderate risk 7–9 points, high risk >10 points

Clinical and biochemical measurements	Points scored for increasing abnormality		
	1	2	3
Encephalopathy (grade)	None	1 or 2	3 or 4
Ascites	Absent	Controlled	Not controlled
Albumin ($g\ l^{-1}$)	>35	28–35	<28
Prothrombin time (seconds prolonged)	1–4	4–6	>6
Bilirubin ($\mu mol\ l^{-1}$)	<40	40–50	>50

there is no coagulopathy. Nonsteroidal analgesics are not recommended.
- Elective ventilation should be considered for:
  - Prolonged surgery
  - Severe blood loss
  - Continuing haemorrhage
  - Hypothermia.

Careful monitoring of urine output, coagulation, and the administration of analgesia and supplementary oxygen is best carried out in a HDU.

OUTCOME

The leading causes of death in the surgical patient are:

- Infection
- Liver failure
- Renal failure
- Haemorrhage.

There have been few studies on survival not involving surgery for portosystemic shunts or bleeding oesophageal varices. The Pugh score divides patients into three groups, classifying them as good, moderate and poor surgical risks (Table 1).

Other factors associated with high mortality include:

- Respiratory failure
- Cardiac failure
- Infection, particularly intra-abdominal
- Emergency surgery.

BIBLIOGRAPHY

Mallett S, Cox D. Thromboelastography. British Journal of Anaesthesia 1992; 69: 307–313

Pugh R N H, Murray-Lyon I M, Dawson J L, Pietroni M C, Williams R. Transection of the oesophagus for bleeding oesophageal varices. British Journal of Surgery 1973; 60: 646–649

CROSS REFERENCES

The full stomach
Patient Conditions 5: 139

DISORDERS OF THE OESOPHAGUS AND OF SWALLOWING

T. Peachey

5

Disorders of the oesophagus and the swallowing mechanism present hazards to the patient undergoing anaesthesia because mechanisms to clear the pharynx of foreign material and keep it clear may be compromised.

PATHOPHYSIOLOGY

Anatomical:

- *Hiatus hernia* results in compromise to the functional integrity of the lower oesophageal sphincter.
- *Pharyngeal pouch and other diverticulae* in the oesophagus may contain solid food particles or fluid for many hours after ingestion. They may also contain partially putrefied food. Discharge of the contents of the pouch may occur with changes in posture, or unexpectedly, and present an aspiration risk.
- *Tracheooesophageal fistula*, a direct communication between the trachea and oesophagus.
- *Tumours of the oesophagus* usually present with dysphagia which may be partial or complete at the time of surgery. Residual food particles may remain in the oesophagus as may liquid in the case of complete aphagia. Where obstruction is complete the patient will not be able to clear saliva.
- *Achalasia of the cardia* is a hypertrophy of the muscular layer at the lower end of the oesophagus resulting in increasing obstruction to the passage of material into the stomach. Whilst the risk of regurgitation is very low in these patients, the oesophagus may be greatly dilated above the obstruction and may contain significant volumes of swallowed material. This is demonstrated on a preoperative barium swallow. The dilated oesophagus does not contain stomach acid.

Physiological:

- *Oesophageal motility* is reduced in scleroderma. The lower oesophageal sphincter is functionally incompetent in these patients and this may result in reflux of gastric contents into the oesophagus. A history of heartburn can often be elicited, but is absent in patients taking omeprazole.
- *Neurogenic cerebrovascular accident.*

PREOPERATIVE ASSESSMENT

The history should determine whether or not obstruction of the oesophagus is present and whether the patient can swallow liquid without regurgitation. A history of regurgitation of solid material hours after food suggests the presence of either a diverticulum or a dilatation above an obstruction. In the case of a pharyngeal pouch the patient may be able to prevent filling of the pouch or empty it by pressure on the neck. Prolonged avoidance of solid food allowing free fluids may help to clear solid material. A nasogastric tube placed in the oesophagus may be useful in achalasia of the cardia.

PREMEDICATION

- Antacids are of no value in oesophageal obstruction. However, where surgery relieves an obstruction, reflux of stomach acid may occur postoperatively.
- Drying agents are beneficial if the patient is unable to swallow saliva.

ANAESTHETIC MANAGEMENT

- Rapid sequence induction of anaesthesia is required where the oesophagus may not be empty at the time of induction.
- In the case of pharyngeal pouches the source of the risk is above the cricoid cartilage and cricoid pressure is of no value. Induction of anaesthesia in the lateral position should be considered with the pouch dependent.

- Intubation of the trachea with a cuffed tube is required for protection of the airway. For oesophageal tumour resections a double-lumen tube may be required.
- If the patient is unable to swallow saliva, induction in the lateral position should be considered.

POSTOPERATIVE MANAGEMENT

- Extubate the trachea with the patient awake and in the lateral position, since the risk to the airway may persist into the postoperative period.
- After intubation of an oesophageal tumour, reflux of stomach acid may occur through the tube.
- Surgery for achalasia of the cardia may render the lower oesophageal sphincter incompetent and be followed by acid reflux in the postoperative period.
- Full competence of the protective laryngeal reflexes may take several hours to return.

THE FULL STOMACH

T. Peachey

The avoidance of aspiration of gastric contents into the airway is of paramount importance during the administration of anaesthesia. Aspiration of solid material may cause obstruction of the airway, leading to asphyxia, lobar pneumonia or lung abcess formation. Irritation of the vocal cords during light anaesthesia by regurgitated material may cause laryngeal spasm, whilst aspiration of as little as 25 ml of liquid of pH less than 2.5 may cause bronchospasm, pneumonitis, bronchopneumonia and adult respiratory distress syndrome.

PATHOPHYSIOLOGY

Both the active process of vomiting and the passive process of regurgitation of gastric contents present a hazard in a patient with a full stomach. Vomiting is a hazard at induction, during recovery, and if anaesthesia is light. Regurgitation is a hazard immediately following induction and throughout maintenance, and may occur silently. Regurgitation is predisposed to by a full stomach any reduction in the functional integrity of the lower oesophageal sphincter (LOS).

Failure of preparation

The rate of emptying of the stomach after oral intake is variable. No patient can be assumed to have a completely empty stomach. In general, for a normal healthy patient stomach emptying is complete within 6 h after food, 4 h after liquid and 3 h after water.

Delayed gastric emptying:
- Obstruction of the gastrointestinal tract:
  - Pyloric stenosis
  - Tumours.
- Ileus:
  - Postoperative
  - Metabolic.
- Peritonitis of any cause.
- Pain.
- Fear/anxiety.
- Pregnancy (third trimester).
- Drugs
  - Opiates
  - Alcohol.

Reflux of material from the bowel
In prolonged intestinal obstruction, faeculent material may enter the stomach retrogradely.

The lower oesophageal sphincter:
- Increased pressure zone (not anatomically distinct)
- Pinch-cock action of the diaphragm
- Mucosal one-way valve.

PREOPERATIVE ASSESSMENT

History:
- Last oral intake of food/drink, especially alcohol
- Possibility of swallowed blood
- Factors known to delay gastric emptying
- History of reflux, heartburn or hiatus hernia
- Drugs known to reduce LOS tone:
  - Alcohol, opiates
  - Anticholinergics
  - Tricyclics
  - Dopamine
  - Beta agonists.

Preparation
Delay surgery where possible to allow time for the stomach to empty. Induction of vomiting is not normally practical, and residual emetic tendency at the time of induction is dangerous. Passing a nasogastric tube and aspirating gastric contents may not be fully effective, but in the case of liquid contents will reduce intragastric pressure and thus the tendency to regurgitation. At the time of induction the presence of the tube may compromise the function of the LOS. Administration of a nonparticulate acid neutralizing drug (sodium citrate) offers protection from the effects of acid aspiration, but does not protect against regurgitation. Administrations of H_2 blocking drugs or omeprazole (not currently licensed for this purpose) only offer protection if the acid in the stomach has already been neutralized. Administration of prokinetic drugs such as metoclopramide may increase the rate of gastric emptying. Metoclopramide also increases the LOS tone. Anticholinergic drugs do not reliably increase gastric pH.

PERIOPERATIVE MANAGEMENT

Premedication
Avoid opiates and anticholinergics – both reduce LOS tone and delay gastric emptying.

Anaesthetic management
Management of the induction of anaesthesia depends on the cause of the full stomach and clinical circumstances. Intubation of the trachea with a cuffed tube in order to both secure and protect the airway is required.

In most cases, a rapid sequence induction with full preoxygenation and cricoid pressure is preferred. In the case of blood in the stomach where bleeding into the airway is responsible (e.g. post-tonsillectomy bleeding) an inhalation induction with the patient in the lateral position and tilted head-down is safest. (N.B. Although suxamethonium increases intragastric pressure it also increases LOS tone.) Head-up tilt may reduce the incidence of regurgitation, but predisposes to aspiration of any material in the pharynx into the lungs. Emptying of the stomach during anaesthesia with a gastric tube should be considered. Emergence from anaesthesia carries the same potential hazards as induction, and the patient should be placed in the lateral position before anaesthesia is terminated. The trachea should be extubated only on return of protective airway reflexes.

POSTOPERATIVE MANAGEMENT

- Risk continues until larynx is competent
- Delayed gastric emptying due to pain/ opiates
- Maintain lateral position
- Avoid sedative agents.

HIATUS HERNIA

I. J. Crabb

Hiatus hernia is a condition caused by migration of a portion of the stomach through the oesophageal hiatus in the diaphragm; it is common, particularly in later life.

Two forms are usually described, the sliding type (85% of cases) where the gastro-oesophageal junction passes into the thorax, and the rolling type where the stomach itself migrates into the thorax, the gastro-oesophageal junction remaining in the abdomen.

A higher incidence of hiatus hernia is associated with the following:

- Increasing age
- Obesity
- Pregnancy.

Although often associated with symptoms of reflux oesophagitis, a hiatus hernia may be symptomless; equally, reflux oesophagitis may occur in the absence of hiatus hernia. Reflux is associated with decreased pressure in the lower oesophageal sphincter (LOS).

THE LOWER OESOPHAGEAL SPHINCTER

An anatomically indistinct area of the oesophagus found around the diaphragmatic hiatus, 3–5 cm long, detectable as a high-pressure zone by manometry. It is usually closed at rest. The important variable is not LOS tone, but barrier pressure (LOS pressure – Gastric pressure). Reflux is unlikely to occur if barrier pressure is greater than 13 cmH_2O, although there is wide variation between individuals.

The normal response to an increase in gastric pressure is an increase in LOS pressure, but this adaptation is lost in those who develop reflux. The response is decreased by atropine, vagotomy, and in symptomatic pregnant women at term. Drugs affecting LOS pressure are shown in Table 1.

Table 1.
Drugs affecting lower oesophageal pressure

Increase LOS pressure	Decrease LOS pressure
Antiemetics:	Anticholinergics:
Metoclopramide	Atropine
Prochlorperazine	Glycopyrrolate
Domperidone	Thiopentone
Anticholinesterases:	Opioids
Neostigmine	Alcohol
Edrophonium	Nicotine
α-Receptor agonists	Dopamine
Histamine	α-Receptor antagonists
Suxamethonium	β-Receptor agonists
	Tricyclic antidepressants
	Ganglion blockers

Of more anaesthetic relevance is evidence of gastric reflux rather than the presence of a hiatus hernia per se.

PREOPERATIVE ASSESSMENT

History:

- Epigastric or retrosternal pain and heartburn, promoted by bending or lying down, pregnancy or obesity, relieved by antacids (sliding type)
- Discomfort or 'crushing' chest pain due to distension of the stomach with food (rolling type – symptoms of reflux are unusual)
- Waterbrash and reflux of bitter fluid into the pharynx and mouth
- Dysphagia – rare, and usually denotes oesophageal stenosis; may prevent further regurgitation and, therefore, produce a reduction in symptoms
- Nocturnal cough – suggesting regurgitation and aspiration; may lead to aspiration pneumonitis.

Investigations:

- Full blood count – chronic blood loss is common, resulting in iron-deficiency anaemia.
- Chest X-ray – to exclude aspiration pneumonia.
- Recent barium study.

PERIOPERATIVE MANAGEMENT

Premedication

Consideration should be given to the preoperative use of antacids or H_2 receptor antagonists, if not already prescribed. If the patient is symptomatic, opioids should be used with caution. Since anticholinergic drugs cause a reduction in LOS pressure, which may make regurgitation more likely, careful consideration must be given to their use as part of premedication. Metoclopramide (or domperidone) will increase LOS pressure, and negate the effects of anticholinergic drugs.

Airway
If the patient is asymptomatic, there are no factors present likely to increase the risk of regurgitation, and the surgery itself is short and does not require tracheal intubation, then spontaneous ventilation using a laryngeal mask following antacid premedication may be considered.

However, if there is any doubt about the patient's safety, then full precautions to prevent regurgitation and aspiration of stomach contents must be employed, i.e. preoxygenation, rapid sequence induction with cricoid pressure, and tracheal intubation. This is mandatory if the hiatus hernia is symptomatic.

Emergence
Ensure emergence/extubation with the patient in the lateral position.

POSTOPERATIVE MANAGEMENT

Semirecumbent or sitting position, when practical.

BIBLIOGRAPHY

Cotton B, Smith G. The lower oesophageal sphincter. In: Kaufman L (ed) Anaesthesia review. Churchill Livingstone, London, 1982, vol 1

Stoelting R K, Dierdof S F, McCammon R L. Anaesthesia and co-existing disease. Churchill Livingstone, New York, 1988

Vickers M D, Jones R M. Medicine for anaesthetists. Blackwell, Oxford, 1989

CROSS REFERENCES

Obesity
Patient Conditions 5: 148
Antacid prophylaxis
Surgical Procedures 20: 400

THE JAUNDICED PATIENT

J. Appleby

In the jaundiced patient presenting for surgery, liver disease may be divided into:

- Hepatocellular
- Cholestatic (obstructive).

Causes of hepatocellular jaundice include toxins, viruses and drugs. Surgery in this group carries a poor prognosis and must be avoided; emergency procedures only.

Cholestasis may be extrahepatic; obstruction commonly caused by calculus, stricture and cancer, or intrahepatic. Viral hepatitis may mimic intrahepatic obstruction (hence the importance of serology). Drugs may cause a hypersensitivity hepatitis (e.g. chlorpromazine, carbemazepine, erythromycin, imipramine, azathiaprine) or present a pure intrahepatic cholestatic picture (e.g. synthetic oestrogens). Presentation for surgery is not uncommon. Aetiology is difficult to ascertain clinically.

Complications of surgery increase with:

- Haematocrit <30% on presentation
- Plasma bilirubin >200 mmol l^{-1}
- Presence of malignancy
- Duration of jaundice (secondary biliary cirrhosis develops).

ASSOCIATED PROBLEMS

Acute oliguric renal failure
Occurs in 9% of all jaundiced patients undergoing surgery, with a mortality of 50%; 75% will have a fall in glomerular filtration rate postoperatively. Factors implicated include:

- Hypovolaemia and hypotension
- The presence of bile salts
- Bilirubin
- Endotoxin.

Glomerular and peritubular fibrin deposition has been demonstrated in affected kidneys. Hepatorenal syndrome may occur associated with deterioration of hepatic function.

Coagulopathy
Vitamin K deficiency reduces clotting factors 2, 7, 9 and 10 (exacerbated by cholestyramine) prolongs prothrombin time (>4 s of control is abnormal), but hepatocellular coagulopathy is refractory to vitamin K administration. Disseminated intravascular coagulation is associated with secondary biliary tract infection (and possibly endotoxaemia), and increases mortality.

Altered drug handling
Drugs excreted via the biliary system have prolonged elimination half-life in cholestasis. Increased volume of distribution and reduced clearance produces initial pancuronium resistance. Repeated dosing is associated with prolongation of action. Atracurium is the drug of choice for paralysis. Narcotics may produce spasm in the sphincter of Oddi (colic, and difficulty with cholangiography).

Pseudocholinesterase has a very long half-life, and suxamethonium apnoea is not a feature, even in fulminant liver failure.

Gastrointestinal tract
Stress ulceration occurs, with gastrointestinal haemorrhage demonstrated in 16% of cases.

Wound healing
This is significantly reduced, and correlates closely with degree of malnutrition, and the presence of sepsis and malignancy.

PREOPERATIVE ASSESSMENT

History and clinical examination
Look for malnutrition, malignancy, anaemia, dehydration, deep jaundice, pyrexia, signs of drug abuse, concomitant diseases.

Investigations:
- Haemoglobin – at presentation and current
- White cell count – cholangitis, isolates and sensitivities
- Platelet count – reduced with severe infection and DIC
- Clotting screen – note effect of vitamin K administration
- Urea, electrolytes, creatinine, glucose – creatinine clearance if poor or deteriorating renal function
- Serum bilirubin (N.B. >200 mmol l^{-1})
- Serum albumin, calcium and magnesium
- Serum transaminases – raised in hepatocellular dysfunction
- Blood gases – respiratory alkalosis and hypoxaemia
- Serology – consider risks to staff
- Biopsy – pattern and degree of damage.

PREOPERATIVE PREPARATION

Depends on severity of disease. Commonly required preparation involves:

- Rehydration
- Appropriate cross-match and preoperative transfusion
- Perioperative antibiotic administration
- Administer vitamin K
- If PT remains abnormal, arrange clotting factors
- H_2 antagonism
- Catheterize early
- Optimization of concurrent disease
- Percutaneous drainage (symptoms improve, prognosis unaltered).

Administration of taurocholate and selective gut decontamination is controversial.

Premedication:
- Anxiolysis; with coagulopathy avoid intramuscular route
- With hepatocellular disease consider duration of action of drugs
- Avoid sedatives in encephalopathy
- Continue H_2 antagonism and vitamin K.

PERIOPERATIVE MANAGEMENT

Poor prognosis may relate to reduction in hepatic blood flow associated with general anaesthetics, and total hepatic necrosis can occur. Renal insult must be avoided. Therefore stable anaesthesia avoiding hypotension is essential. Preserve cardiac output with fluid loading. Adequate circulating volume and haematocrit are essential. Isoflurane does not have major deleterious effect in animal models of hepatic circulation. Hypercarbia produces sympathetic activation, IPPV to P_aCO_2 35–40 mmHg would be advisable. Altered drug metabolism dependent upon high and low extraction ratio and, therefore, difficult to predict. Acid–base disturbance may occur; alterations in electrolytes may contribute to encephalopathy and should be monitored.

Preservation of urine output with mannitol (0.5 g kg^{-1}) and diuretics has been advocated. This should not be at the expense of circulating volume. Replace massive diuresis. Aggressive replacement of blood loss is essential. Hypoglycaemia may occur (with severe injury); monitor and treat.

In all cases a low threshold for invasive monitoring is to be recommended. In the presence of hepatocellular disease it is essential. If resuscitation is required, a Swan–Ganz catheter sited preoperatively is advisable. Dopamine may be beneficial in preservation of renal function perioperatively.

Hypothermia worsens coagulopathy. Therefore warm fiuids, use humidification and reduce body surface heat losses.

POSTOPERATIVE MANAGEMENT

Consider intensive care. Hypoxaemia is common. Drain losses should be aggressively replaced; hepatocellular disease may require additional clotting factors. Monitoring with thromboelastography is helpful. Replace urine losses appropriately. Continue dopamine until cardiovascularly stable. Catacholamines may reduce hepatic and renal blood flow. Epidural analgesia can be considered in the absence of coagulopathy. Intramuscular opiate administration is inappropriate in all but minor cases.

OUTCOME

Relates to severity of disease. Minor worsening of liver function tests is not uncommon; morphological change is. The following may worsen jaundice postoperatively:

- Blood transfusion.
- Haemolysis.
- Hepatocellular damage:
  - Postoperative cholestasis
  - Circulatory failure
  - Drug induced
  - Exacerbated chronic disease.
- Extrahepatic obstruction:
  - Duct stone
  - Bile duct injury
  - Postoperative pancreatitis.

Laparotomy in presence of hepatocellular disease has been associated with perioperative mortality of 9.5% and morbidity of 12%. Approximately 25% of jaundiced patients undergoing surgery for relief of biliary obstruction have subsequently been demonstrated to have hepatocellular disease. A combination of anaemia at presentation, serum bilirubin >200 mmol l^{-1} and presence of malignancy carries a mortality of 60%.

BIBLIOGRAPHY

Dixon J M, Armstrong C P, Duffy S W, Davies G C. Factors affecting morbidity and mortality after surgery for obstructive jaundice a review of 373 patients. Gut 1983; 24: 845–852

Haville D D, Dummerskill W H J. Surgery in acute hepatitis. Causes and effects. Journal of the American Medical Association 1963; 184: 257

Wilkinson S P, Moodie H, Stamatakis J D et al. Endotoxaemia and renal failure in cirrhosis and obstructive jaundice. British Medical Journal 1976; 2: 1415

CROSS REFERENCES

Acute renal failure
Patient Conditions 6: 154
Open cholecystectomy
Surgical Procedures 18: 375

MALNUTRITION

M. Brunner

Malnutrition occurs when protein/calorie supplies are inadequate to meet requirements and is found in approximately 50% of surgical patients, resulting in an increased incidence of postoperative complications.

Malnutrition is defined as:
- Moderate: 15% loss of ideal body weight
- Severe: 30% loss of ideal body weight

Calculation of ideal body weight (IBW) (Broca's index):
- For men: IBW (kg) = Height (cm) – 100
- For women: IBW (kg) = Height (cm) – 105

PATHOPHYSIOLOGY

General effects

These include: rapid weight loss; muscle wasting and fatigue; delayed ambulation following surgery, with an increased incidence of postoperative respiratory complications; bed sores and wound infections.

Pulmonary function:

- Diaphragmatic muscle mass falls in a linear fashion with body weight. There is a fall in vital capacity and maximal ventilatory volume, an increased incidence of postoperative respiratory failure and difficulty in weaning from mechanical ventilation.
- Decreased surfactant production and emphysematous changes in the lung causes alveolar atelectasis.
- Increased incidence of chest infection results from a depressed immune response, alveolar atelectasis and an ineffective cough.
- The ventilatory response to hypoxia is markedly depressed.
- The work of breathing is increased.

Visceral protein deficiency:

- Depletion of serum proteins, enzymes, immunoglobulins and vital organs
- Reduced cardiac output, stroke volume, contractility and reserve
- Hypoalbuminaemia results in interstitial and pulmonary oedema and reduced binding of metabolites, drugs and toxins
- Anaemia (folate or iron deficiency or mixed)
- Low serum transferrin
- Low T-lymphocyte count and function
- Impaired antibody response
- Low serum IgA
- Pseudocholinesterase deficiency in severe malnutrition (serum albumin $<2\ g\ dl^{-1}$).

PREOPERATIVE ASSESSMENT

Nutritional assessment

Many of the indices of malnutrition (Table 1) lack specificity and are poor predictors of perioperative morbidity and mortality. Immunological changes and loss of hand grip power, however, do predict those patients likely to have an increased risk of perioperative problems. Patients who demonstrate anergy at 48 h to the intradermal injection of several antigens (*Candida*, mumps, trychophyton), have a marked increase in postoperative morbidity and mortality and may benefit from preoperative nutritional support.

Clinical assessment:

- Evidence of fat and muscle wasting, e.g. weight loss, fatigue, hypothermia
- Symptoms of vitamin deficiency, e.g. anaemia (vitamin E), bleeding tendency (vitamin K)
- Reduced pulmonary function, e.g. shortness of breath
- Heart failure, e.g. peripheral oedema, orthopnoea
- Arrythmias
- Increased frequency of infection.

Table 1.
Nutritional evaluation

Value measured	Normal value	Degree of malnutrition: Mild	Moderate	Severe	Causes of error
Weight (%)	100	80–90	70–79	<70	
Weight loss (%)	0	<10	10–20	>20	Dehydration
Fat reserves					
Triceps skin fold (%)	100	80–90	60–79	<60	Oedema
Somatic protein					
Arm muscle circumference (%)	100	80–90	60–79	<40	Oedema
Weight (% of ideal)	100	80–90	70–79	<70	Dehydration
Weight (% of usual)	100	90–95	80–89	<80	Dehydration
Creatine/height index (%)	100	60–80	40–59	<40	Renal disease
Visceral protein					
Serum albumin (g dl^{-1})	3.5–5.0	2.8–3.4	2.1–2.7	<2.1	Liver disease
Serum transferrin (mg dl^{-1})	175–300	150–175	100–150	<100	Trauma, surgery
Retinol-binding protein (mg dl^{-1})	3–6	2.7–3.0	2.4–2.7	<2.4	State of hydration
Prealbumin (mg dl^{-1})	15.7–29.6	10–15	5–9.9	<5	Increased protein loss or demand, e.g. trauma
Total lymphocytes (mm^{-3})	1500–5000	1200–1500	800–1200	<800	Abnormal white cell count
Cell-mediated immunity		Reactive	Relative anergy	Non reactive	Steroids, immune deficiency

Investigations

Investigation	Result
ECG	AV block, prolonged Q–T
Echocardiogram	Reduced contractility
Pulmonary function tests	FVC <50 ml kg^{-1} in the absence of obvious lung disease; reduced maximal ventilatory volume

PREOPERATIVE MANAGEMENT

Preoperative nutrition should be discussed with surgeons and dieticians. Enteral and total parenteral nutrition (TPN) are equally beneficial.

Examine patient for the complications associated with TPN (Table 2) and correct serum electrolytes and blood glucose abnormalities. TPN must not be stopped suddenly, as rebound hypoglycaemia may occur. It should be either:

- Continued at the same rate, controlling hyperglycaemia perioperatively as in the diabetic patient

Table 2.
Complications of TPN

Catheter related
Improper central line placement
Infection

Fluid overload
Especially in the elderly and patients with heart failure

Metabolic
Hyperglycaemia
Hypercarbia
Hypokalaemia
Hypomagnesaemia
Hypophosphataemia

- Weaned to half the maintenance rate over 12 h preoperatively
- Replaced by 10% glucose infused at the same rate (in unstable patients).

Blood transfusion for anaemia and correction of clotting abnormalities may be required. The impact of a low plasma albumin and its correction with albumin solutions on post-operative outcome in the malnourished patient has yet to be shown. Endogenous albumin production should be encouraged with nutritional support. Exogenous albumin actually reduces the amount of albumin production by the liver. The effect of preoperative albumin infusions to increase plasma oncotic pressure is ill defined, although they may play an important role as a result of increasing the binding of metabolites, drugs and toxins.

PERIOPERATIVE MANAGEMENT

Monitoring includes measurement of:

- Central venous pressure (CVP)
- Blood sugar
- $ETco_2$.

Careful positioning of the patient and aseptic line placement reduces the incidence of sepsis and injury.

Mechanical ventilation is indicated by preoperative pulmonary function tests. Ability to sustain head raise, FVC greater than 15 ml kg^{-1} and maximum inspiratory force greater than –25 cmH_2O indicate adequate muscle strength prior to extubation. The malnourished heart functions at the peak of the Starling curve, and so cardiac output may fall with increased diastolic filling, precipitating cardiac failure. Judicious fluid management with CVP monitoring may be required.

There is an increased sensitivity to:

- Intravenous induction agents
- Suxamethonium in severe malnutrition (albumin <2.0 g dl^{-1}), since pseudocholinesterase deficiency may exist
- Nondepolarizing neuromuscular blockers in the presence of hypocalcaemia, hypophosphataemia and hypomagnesaemia
- Drugs bound to albumin, e.g. diazepam
- Drugs bound to sekeletal muscle, e.g. digoxin.

POSTOPERATIVE MANAGEMENT

- ITU/HDU in patients with severely reduced cardiorespiratory reserve
- Mechanical ventilation in the case of
  - Fatigue
  - Increased CO_2 production due to glucose feed
  - Impaired response to hypoxaemia
- Supplemental oxygen on the ward
- Physiotherapy
- Analgesia to allow an effective cough
- Restart nutritional support slowly over 12–24 h postoperatively
- Monitor blood glucose and serum potassium and avoid hypophosphataemia.

OUTCOME

Several studies have shown an increased incidence of postoperative complications in the malnourished patient, e.g. respiratory complications, wound infections and bed sores. The role of pre- and post-operative nutritional support in the malnourished patient are poorly defined. Both reduce postoperative complications and improve pulmonary function in patients with fistulae, short bowel syndrome, burns and acute renal failure, and may have a place in patients who have lost more than 20% of their usual body weight. For the maximum nutritional benefit, feeding (whether enteral or parenteral) should be started 1 week to 10 days preoperatively.

BIBLIOGRAPHY

Hill G L, Pickford I, Young G A et al. Malnutrition in surgical patients: an unrecognised problem. Lancet 1977; i: 689–692

Meakins J L, Pietsch J B, Bubenick D et al. Delayed hypersensitivity: Indicator of aquired failure to host defences in sepsis and trauma. Annals of Surgery 1977; 186: 241–250

Meguid M M, Campos A C, Hammond W G. Nutritional support in surgical practice. The American Journal of Surgery 1990; 159: 345–358

Rochester D F, Arora N S. Respiratory muscle failure. Medical Clinics of North America 1983; 67: 573–597

5

OBESITY

J. C. Goldstone

Obesity is a chronic nutritional disorder characterized by hypertension, cardiovascular and respiratory disease, diabetes, cirrhosis and hiatus hernia. Although medical morbidity is corrected with weight, few prospective studies have been performed relating obesity and anaesthetic outcome (Figure 1).

Obesity may be defined as:
- Simple: Weight greater than 30% of ideal
- Morbid: Weight greater than 100% of ideal *or* Weight 45 kg in excess of ideal

Calculation of ideal body weight (IBW) (Broca's index)
- For men: IBW (kg) = Height (cm) – 100
- For women: IBW (kg) = Height (cm) – 105

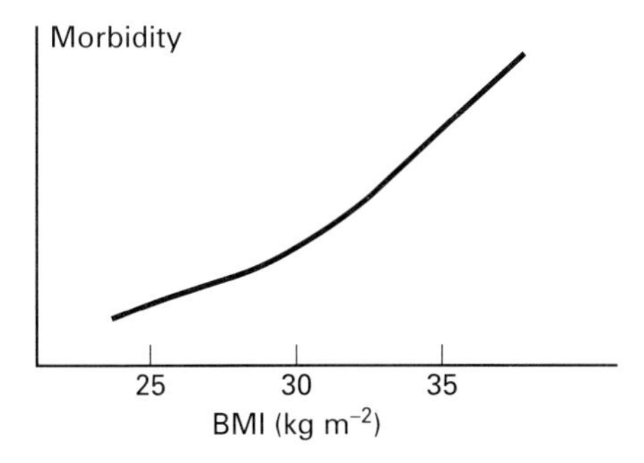

Figure 1
Relationship between body mass index and morbidity.

PATHOPHYSIOLOGY

Cardiovascular system
In the absence of ischaemic heart disease, obesity raises end-diastolic ventricular volume, increases stroke volume, and thereby increases cardiac output. Left ventricular work rises, in part due to the increased systemic vascular resistance, and is compensated for by biventricular hypertrophy. Filling pressure and cardiac output rise promptly with exercise, which includes moving body position in the morbidly obese.

Respiratory system
Obesity acts to impose a load on the chest wall, such that the work of breathing is raised, although lung compliance, in the absence of coexisting disease, is normal. Lung volume is reduced, and falls further with recumbency. In the morbidly obese, tidal breathing falls within the closing volume range. Arterial hypoxaemia is common, and increases pulmonary vascular resistance. In some morbidly obese patients (8%) the response to carbon dioxide is diminished, termed the *obesity hypoventilation syndrome* (OHS).

Gut
Both gastric acid and fasting gastric volume are raised in the obese. Abdominal pressure increases linearly with weight gain, and the incidence of hiatus hernia is high.

Endocrine system
Glucose tolerance in the obese is impaired and frank diabetes is common.

Coagulation
Laboratory evidence of hypercoagulability is slight, although some clinical reports suggest that the incidence of deep venous thrombosis (DVT) is raised.

PREOPERATIVE ASSESSMENT

Morphological:
- Assessment of veins/arteries
- Airway – mouth/jaw/dentition/neck
- Posture for epidural, if appropriate
- Transportation to theatre.

History:
- Systematic review of associated cardiovascular and respiratory disease
- OHS:
  - *Day time* somnolence, poor concentration

– *Night time* respiratory obstruction, nightmares and restlessness.
- Right ventricular failure
- Smoking history.

Investigations

See Table 1.

Table 1.
Investigations

Investigation	Result
ECG	Ventricular hypertrophy Ischaemia Evidence of pulmonary hypertension
Echocardiography	Right or left chamber enlargement
Spirometry (standing/supine)	Flow limitation VC FRC
Blood gas analysis (standing/supine)	Hypoxaemia when standing; falls when supine

PERIOPERATIVE MANAGEMENT

Premedication

Respiratory depressant drugs should be used with caution, and morbidly obese patients at risk of OHS should be monitored (Sao_2) and receive face-mask oxygen after premedication. Acid aspiration prophylaxis should be given. Anticholinergic agents should be given when intubation is anticipated as being difficult.

Monitoring

This should commence in the anaesthetic room:

- ECG (CM_5)
- Arterial cannula
- Sao_2

Airway

Spontaneous respiration is contraindicated. Obese patients deoxygenate 3–5 times quicker than non-obese controls. Both face-mask ventilation and intubation may be impossible.

When weight exceeds 75% of ideal, a suggested plan is to perform direct laryngoscopy under topical anaesthesia in the anaesthetic room prior to theatre. If the larynx cannot be seen, awake fibre-optic intubation is the safest approach.

When intubation is possible, a rapid sequence intubation should be performed. A range of intubating equipment should be available, including the polio blade. Obese patients have increased plasma pseudocholinesterase, and may require increased doses of suxamethonium.

Mechanical ventilation

- May be required with a volume preset constant flow generator
- Oxygenation may be impaired despite high inspired oxygen tensions and PEEP
- Head-up tilt.

Metabolism of inhaled agents is increased, and isoflurane is therefore theoretically advantageous. The usefulness of nitrous oxide may be limited by the need for high inspired oxygen tensions.

Cardiovascular depression is likely during general anaesthesia, leading to rises in filling pressure and declining cardiac output. Aortocaval compression may occur in the supine posture, increasing systemic vascular resistance and decreasing venous return. Left ventricular function has been shown to continue to decline in the postoperative phase as compared with the non-obese.

Physical positioning and lifting may be impossible in the morbidly obese, requiring modifications to the theatre to accommodate heavy lifting equipment. Severe cases may require a dry-run to ensure that facilities are adequate.

Regional anaesthesia

Although this may be technically difficult if the bony landmarks are obscured, subarachnoid and epidural anaesthesia have been advocated in the morbidly obese. Dose requirements are generally reduced compared to those in the non-obese (75–80%). Cardiovascular decompensation has been reported in cases where the sympathetic block was variably higher than the somatic blockade. Motor blockade of the respiratory muscles limits the height of blockade to T7.

POSTOPERATIVE CARE

- Semirecumbant/sitting position
- Continuous oxygen therapy
- Humidification
- Physiotherapy/early mobilization
- Analgesia

5

- Deep venous thrombosis therapy
- ITU/HDU for the morbidly obese and those with cardiorespiratory disease.

OUTCOME

Although epidemiological studies have shown obesity to correlate with mortality, this is not the case with anaesthetic mortality. From the limited literature available, similar mortality has been recorded for hysterectomy (1%) and gastric bypass (1.2%) when these results have been matched to non-obese controls. This is attributable to improvements in anaesthetic technique.

BIBLIOGRAPHY

Ashbaugh D G, Bigelow D B, Petty T L, Levine B E. Acute respiratory distress in adults. Lancet 1967; ii: 319–323

CROSS REFERENCES

Diabetes mellitus (IDDM)
Patient Conditions 2: 42
Hypertension
Patient Conditions 4: 111
Preoperative assessment of pulmonary risk
Anaesthetic Factors 34: 697

PREVIOUS LIVER TRANSPLANT

S. Mallett

The first human orthotopic liver transplant (OLT) was performed in 1963. This was recognized as a therapeutic procedure for end-stage liver disease in 1983. Improvements in organ preservation, surgical and anaesthetic techniques and immunosuppression (cyclosporin) led to an exponential increase in centres and number of cases performed over the next decade. In 1993 over 3500 OLTs were performed in the USA and 700 in the UK. Today, there are many thousands of patients alive who have had a successful OLT. One-year survival is 75–85% and the 5-year survival approaches 65%.

PATIENT CHARACTERISTICS

- Age: from infants to 70 years and over; majority are 30–60 years old.
- Medical status is generally good:
  - Reversal of cardiovascular and pulmonary effects of chronic liver disease (hyperdynamic circulation and shunting) reported within 3 months of OLT
  - Increased incidence of renal insufficiency in OLT patients (pre- and intra-operative factors and cyclosporin)
  - High incidence of hypertension reported after OLT.
- Normal liver function unless there is rejection, sepsis or recurrence of original disease.
- Immunosuppression increases susceptibility to infection.

SPECIFIC COMPLICATIONS OF OLT

- *Early*: vascular occlusion, bleeding and primary nonfunctional graft
- *Late*: biliary leak and duct stenosis requiring reconstruction.

These will usually be dealt with at a primary transplant centre and are not further considered here.

PREOPERATIVE ASSESSMENT AND INVESTIGATIONS

- Full systemic review for intercurrent or chronic problems and any evidence of infection
- Formal clinical and biochemical assessment of liver function (chronic rejection, recurrent disease, biliary obstruction)
- Arrange conversion of immunosuppression from oral to intravenous administration
- Steroid cover intraoperatively
- Liaise with transplant centre if any queries.

Investigations:
- FBC: Hb, white blood cells (may be low with azothioprin)
- Liver function tests
- Chest X-ray
- Urea and electrolytes, creatinine and creatinine clearance
- Coagulation: PT, PTTK platelets ± bleeding time
- ECG.

PERIOPERATIVE MANAGEMENT: LAPAROTOMY

The aim is to avoid any deterioration or compromise in:

- *Liver function*, by optimizing hepatic oxygenation and blood flow. Maintain $P_{a}O_2$ above 15 kPa, normal $P_{a}CO_2$ and pH and normovolaemia at all times. Central venous pressure (CVP) and direct arterial monitoring is therefore desirable.
- *Renal function*, by optimizing volume status and using low-dose dopamine (1–3 μg kg^{-1} min^{-1}) and, if patient jaundiced, mannitol infusion.
- Be aware of *increased infection risk*. All invasive monitoring must be inserted with 'no touch' aseptic technique.

Anaesthesia:
- Isoflurane is the agent of choice: minimal metabolism (<0.2%) and best preservation of hepatic arterial and mesenteric flow
- Avoid halothane
- Atracurium for neuromuscular relaxation
- Maintain normocapnia and normal acid–base status to minimize effects on liver blood flow
- Analgesia: epidural ideal for postoperative analgesia (N.B. check coagulation). If liver function deranged, fentanyl is the safest choice intraoperatively.

Bleeding risk
May be increased because:

- Previous surgery with possibility of vascular adhesions
- Abnormal liver function:
  - Deranged coagulation
  - Obstructive jaundice (vitamin-K-dependent factors)
  - Decreased synthesis of clotting proteins.

Management:
- Correct prolonged PT with fresh frozen plasma prior to surgery and invasive procedures
- If platelet count <80 000, have platelets available for surgery
- Drugs such as DDAVP and aprotinin (Trasylol) are useful in reducing blood loss resulting from platelet dysfunction and fibrinolysis; Trasylol also decreases 'ooze' from vascular adhesions.
- Coagulation monitoring: thrombelastography and/or serial clotting screens.

POSTOPERATIVE MANAGEMENT

For major procedures these patients will require HDU care for a minimum of 24 h.

- Post operative analgesia:
  - Epidural opiates/low-dose bupivicaine infusion
  - Intravenous opiate infusion/patient-controlled analgesia pumps
- Continue to ensure good oxygenation and optimize haemodynamics and volume status
- Renal-dose dopamine for 24 h postoperatively
- Antibiotic prophylaxis
- Continue immunosuppression and steroid cover.

OUTCOME

Increasing numbers of patients have successful liver transplants and may present months to years later with unrelated surgical problems. Careful preoperative assessment is essential, especially in relation to liver and kidney function. Perioperative management is directed to avoiding any factors that might compromise hepatic and renal function and minimizing the infection risk with antibiotic prophylaxis and careful aseptic techniques.

BIBLIOGRAPHY

Hawker F. Liver transplantation. In: Park G (ed) The liver. W B Saunders, Philadelphia, 1993, ch 5, p 196–249

Mallett S V, Cox D J A. The monitoring and treatment of coagulopathy during major surgery. British Journal of Anaesthesia 1992; 69: 307–313

Stock P G, Payne W D. Liver transplantation. Critical care of the transplant patient. Critical Care Clinics 1990; 6: 911–926

CROSS REFERENCES

Liver transplantation
Surgical Procedures 23: 464

6

GU TRACT

J. C. Goldstone

ACUTE RENAL FAILURE

P. Saunders and K. Pearce

This condition can be defined as an acute decline in renal function sufficient to result in the retention of nitrogenous end-products of metabolism, which is not reversible by manipulation of extrarenal factors. Patients are not necessarily oliguric.

Causes:

- *Pre-renal* – inadequate perfusion
- *Renal* – intrinsic renal disease
- *Postrenal* – obstructive uropathy.

The most common situation is the development of 'acute tubular necrosis', due to ischaemia, or occasionally, renal toxins.

ACUTE TUBULAR NECROSIS (ATN)

Causes:

- *Hypoperfusion*, i.e. decreased intravascular volume, sepsis, cardiogenic shock, cardiac tamponade.
- *Embolic occlusion* of the renal arteries.
- *Severe hypoxia* will also contribute to ischaemic damage.
- *Drugs*:
  - Aminoglycosides
  - Amphotericin B
  - Radiocontrast agents
  - Nonsteroidal analgesics
  - Frusemide
- *Endogenous toxins*:
  - Haemoglobin after a transfusion reaction
  - Myoglobin from rhabdomyolysis of massive trauma
  - Abnormal reaction to succinylcholine
  - Myeloma renal damage.

Prevention of pre-renal causes of ANT

Preoperative assessment

This must begin before surgery, i.e. may require an intravenous infusion the night before surgery.

Assessment of high-risk states

- Preoperative renal disease
- Preoperative 'shock' states
- Cirrhosis
- Biliary obstruction
- Sepsis
- Multiple system trauma
- Multiple organ system failure
- Cardiac failure
- Extracellular fluid volume deficit
- Elderly patients
- Aortorenal vascular disease

Peri- and post-operative management

Prevention of the development of renal failure in the perioperative period involves avoiding those manoevres that lead to a reduction in renal blood flow and pharmacological means to support renal function:

- Maintain oxygenation
- Maintain normocarbia
- Maintain renal perfusion pressure (>80 mmHg)
- Optimize intravascular volume and cardiac output
- Drug therapy.

Frusemide is controversial, if patients respond they are certainly easier to treat.

Dopamine increases renal blood flow.

Mannitol administered before an ischaemic insult will reduce renal damage, probably by its action as a free-radical scavenger.

If acute renal failure occurs in the perioperative period, the mortality is very high (60–75%), which probably reflects the severity of the insult. Although mortality is high, few patients die as a result of the renal disease.

An abnormal urine output does not preclude the presence of renal failure. Beware the blocked urinary catheter. Acute tubular necrosis may recover and be followed by a period of polyuria, usually after 1–2 weeks.

ACUTE RENAL FAILURE – ESTABLISHED

Anaesthetic assessment

A full history is taken, with particular attention to previous renal disease, infection, stones or prostatism. Examination includes the state of fluid balance, i.e. evidence of postural hypotension, reduced skin turgor, poor circulation, weight and thirst. Patient must have a urinary catheter and central venous pressure monitor.

Investigations:

- Serum urea, creatinine and electrolytes
- Ratio of urine/blood osmolality if over 1.5:1 suggests hypovolaemia
- Urine.

The specific gravity is >1015, and the urea concentration is >2 g/100 ml, when oliguria is due solely to hypovolaemia. Intrinsic renal failure leads to a fixed specific gravity of 1010 and a urea concentration of <600 mg ml^{-1}.

Perioperative and postoperative management:

- Avoid drugs that require renal function for elimination
- Maintain renal perfusion pressure
- Monitor any urine output.

BIBLIOGRAPHY

Byrick R J, Rose D K. Pathophysiology and prevention of acute renal failure: the role of the anaesthetist. Canadian Journal of Anaesthesia 1990; 37: 457–467

Gokhale Y A, Marathe P, Patil R D et al. Rhabdomyolysis and acute renal failure following a single dose of succinylcholine. Journal of the Association of Physicians India 1991; 39: 968–970

CROSS REFERENCES

The jaundiced patient
Patient Conditions 5: 142

ASSESSMENT OF RENAL FUNCTION

P. Saunders and K. Pearce

An assessment of renal function aids in an overall estimate of the degree of physiological derangement and reserve of the individual.

Factors affecting renal function tests:
Intrinsic renal disease
Intra- and extra-vascular fluid status
Cardiovascular function
Neuroendocrine factors

Perioperative acute renal failure accounts for 50% of all patients requiring dialysis and carries a high mortality rate. Preoperatively it is important to try to identify those patients at risk, and take measures to protect them from developing renal complications following surgery. There is no single comprehensive test of renal function; all results should be viewed together with any significant history and examination.

Basic functions of the kidney:

- Glomerular
- Tubular
- Endocrine.

The glomeruli are responsible for filtration and subsequent excretion of nitrogenous wastes. Tubular function involves the movement of water, sodium and the maintenance of fluid balance, along with the excretion/reabsorption of hydrogen ions in acid–base homeostasis. The endocrine activity involves the metabolism of vitamin D, prostaglandins and erythropoietin.

Normal variables:

Cardiac output	5000 ml min^{-1}
Renal blood flow	1250 ml min^{-1}
Renal plasma flow	750 ml min^{-1}
Glomerular filtration rate	125 ml min^{-1}
Urine flow	2 ml min^{-1}

HISTORY AND EXAMINATION

Symptoms:
- Polyuria
- Polydypsia
- Fatigue
- Dysuria
- Oedema

Signs:
- Long-standing hypertension
- Hypovolaemic signs if overdialysed.

Medication:
- Diuretics
- Potassium supplements
- Immunosuppressive agents
- Antihypertensive therapy
- Dialysis schedule.

INVESTIGATIONS

Plasma:

Sodium	140 mmol l^{-1}
Potassium	3.5–5.0 mmol l^{-1}
Chloride	95–105 mmol l^{-1}
Osmolality	280–295 mOsm kg^{-1}
Urea (blood urea nitrogen (BUN))	2.5–7.0 mmol l^{-1}
Creatinine	40–120 mmol l^{-1}
Bicarbonate (HCO_3^-)	21–25 mmol l^{-1}
Calcium	2.1–2.8 mmol l^{-1}
Magnesium	0.7–1.0 mmol l^{-1}

Urine:

Sodium	50–200 mmol/24 h
Potassium	30–100 mmol/24 h
Chloride	100–300 mmol/24 h
Osmolality	300–1000 mOsm kg^{-1}
Specific gravity (SG)	1003–1030
Creatinine	9.0–18 mmol l^{-1}
Creatinine clearance	110–130 ml min^{-1}
Urea clearance	60–95 ml min^{-1}
H^+	60 mEq/24 h

URINALYSIS

As a sole investigation, urinalysis is sufficient screening in patients with no history of renal or systemic disease.

Appearance
- *Gross*: bleeding, infection.
- *Microscopic*: casts, bacteria, cell forms.

pH
Normally urine is acidic. Therefore acidification is a measure of function.

Specific gravity
SG refers to the concentration of solutes in urine; the ability to concentrate is a measure of tubular function. This is, however, nonspecific.

Substances/conditions affecting SG:
- Protein
- Glucose
- Mannitol
- Dextran
- Diuretics
- Age extremes
- Antibiotics (carbenicillin)
- Temperature
- Hormonal inbalance (pituitary, adrenal and thyroid disease).

Osmolality
Osmolality = No. osmotically active particles/ Unit solvent

Osmolality is more specific than SG, and is helpful at extreme values:

- Oliguria + Osmolality >500 suggests pre-renal azotaemia (PRA)
- Oliguria + Osmolality <350 likely to be ATN

Oliguria itself also affects the osmolality value. Osmolality is only useful in low urine output states, coupled with a low SG. An osmolality of <350 mOsm kg^{-1} suggests an inability to concentrate urine and excrete electrolytes.

Protein:
- *<150 mg/24 h*: excretion in health (exercise and standing can increase this).
- *>750 mg/24 h*: specific indicator of renal parenchymal disease.
- *Massive*: glomerular damage.

Glucose
Freely filtered and reabsorbed. Glycosuria occurs when an abnormally heavy load is presented to the tubules (e.g. diabetes mellitus, intravenous glucose.).

BUN and creatinine
Indicators of general function, urea being filtered at the glomerulus and 33% reabsorbed when the urine flow <2 ml min^{-1}. There is a steady production of creatinine (proportional to body mass) which is never reabsorbed. BUN and creatinine values vary widely, and do not increase despite a fall in glomerular and tubular function by as much as 50%.

Creatinine > 180 mmol l^{-1} indicates renal failure.

Nonrenal variables affecting BUN and creatinine levels:
Increased nitrogen absorption
Increased nitrogen waste production
Diet
Body mass
Activity
Hepatic disease
DKA
Large haematoma
Gastrointestinal bleeding
Drugs (steroids)

Creatinine clearance
Measures the glomerular filtration of creatinine (Cr) which approximates to glomerular filtration rate.

$$\text{Cr clearance} = \frac{\text{Urine Cr} \times \text{UV}}{\text{Plasma Cr}}$$

where UV is the urine volume.

Creatinine clearance of <25 ml min^{-1} indicates severe renal failure, 50–80 ml min^{-1} indicates mild renal dysfunction.

$$\text{Cr clearance} = \frac{140 - \text{Age} \times \text{Weight (kg)}}{72 \times \text{Plasma Cr}}$$

This approximation overestimates values in females by 15%, and is invalid in gross renal failure.

Plasma electrolytes
Sodium, potassium, chloride and bicarbonate remain normal until advanced disease, when one sees a hyperkalaemic, hyperchloraemic acidosis. These changes will exacerbate dysrhythmias and compromise resuscitation. Frank renal failure results in hypocalcaemia, hyperphosphataemia and hypermagnesaemia.

Haematology
- End-stage renal failure (ESRF): Hb = 3–9 g dl^{-1}.
- White cell count and platelets are deranged if the patient is immunosuppressed or has a coagulopathy.

Chest X-ray
It is important to look for signs of hypertensive cardiovascular disease, pericardial-pleural effusions and, rarely, uraemic pneumonitis.

ECG
Toxic effects of:

- Hyperkalaemia:
  - Tall peaked T-waves
  - ST depression
  - QRS widening
  - Ventricular dysrhythmias.
- Hypocalcaemia.
- Signs of hypertension.
- Signs of ischaemic heart disease.

Echocardiography
In the presence of symptoms and signs of heart failure, left ventricular dysfunction should be evaluated. If present, the patient is at increased risk of developing renal failure following major surgery.

CONCLUSION

At present, the measurement of creatinine clearance is the most sensitive test of renal function. However, it is time consuming, has an inherent delay factor, and does not offer the anaesthetist a simple, single-shot assessment of renal reserve. One relies on electrolytes, BUN and creatinine levels, which are not reliable indices of glomerular or tubular function.

BIBLIOGRAPHY

Katz, Benumof, Kadis (eds). Renal diseases. In: Anesthesia and uncommon diseases, 3rd edn. W B Saunders, Philadelphia, 1990

Kellen M, Aronson S, Roizen M F, Barnard J, Thisted R A. Predictive and diagnostic tests of renal function: a review. Anesthesia and Analgesia 1994; 78: 134–142

Prough D S, Foreman A S. Anesthesia and the renal system. In: Barash, Cullen, Stoelting (eds) Clinical anesthesia. J B Lippincott, Philadelphia, 1989, ch 39, p 1079–1109

Strunin L, Pettingale K W. Renal disease. ch 4

Thompson F D. Modern tests of renal function and drugs affecting the kidney. In: Kaufman L (ed) Anaesthesia review. Churchill Livingstone, Edinburgh, 1990, vol 7, ch 4

6

CHRONIC RENAL FAILURE

P. Saunders and K. Pearce

Chronic renal failure results from a reduction in renal function by a chronic disease process, which causes a retention of nitrogenous waste products and inability of the kidneys to maintain fluid, electrolyte and acid–base homeostasis in the face of normal variations of fluid and dietary intake and of physical activity. It is characterized by uraemia.

Anaesthesia in this condition is complicated by a number of factors. Each patient may have a widely varying cardiovascular status, blood volume and biochemical profile. Consideration needs to be given to other associated medical conditions, such as diabetes, to their often multiple medications, and to their treatment requirements (i.e. peritoneal or haemodialysis).

Aetiology:
- Chronic pyelonephritis
- Chronic glomerulonephritis
- Essential (primary) malignant hypertension
- Polycystic disease
- Systemic lupus erythematosus
- Diabetes mellitus
- Amyloidosis
- Gout
- Analgesic nephropathy
- Nephrocalcinosis.

PATHOPHYSIOLOGY

Biochemical:
- Uraemia
- High serum creatinine (>180 mmol l^{-1})
- Hyperkalaemia
- Hyponatraemia
- Metabolic acidosis.

Cardiovascular:
- Hypertension
- Fluid overload (unless dialysed)
- Cardiac failure (secondary to hypertension and increased cardiac output)
- Pericarditis ± pericardial effusion.

Haematological:
- Anaemia (3–9 g dl^{-1})
- Bleeding tendency (abnormal platelet function).

Immunological:
- Tendency to acquire infections.

Neurological:
- Drowsiness, convulsions and coma (uraemia)
- Peripheral and autonomic neuropathies, especially if diabetic.

Gastrointestinal:
- Autonomic neuropathy may lead to delayed gastric emptying and risk of aspiration.

Skeletal:
- Bone disease leading to pathological fractures.

PREOPERATIVE ASSESSMENT

History:
- Drug history:
  - Immunosuppression
  - Antihypertensives
  - Hypoglycaemics.
- Systematic review of cardiovascular disease.
- Method and time of last dialysis.

Examination:
- Signs of fluid overload
- Weight (in relation to dialysis record)
- Location of any arteriovenous fistula sites.

Investigations:
- Full blood count (normochromic, normocytic anaemia)
- Clotting studies (including bleeding time)
- Full biochemical screen
- ECG
- Chest X-ray.

Premedication

Premedication with sedative drugs and opioids is unpredictable and potentially dangerous. The decreased tolerance to these drugs is due to abnormal levels of plasma proteins and the effect of altered blood pH on their pharmacokinetics.

PERIOPERATIVE MANAGEMENT

Patients should be preoxygenated and monitored prior to induction. Avoid using intravenous access that may compromise the use of veins for future arteriovenous fistulae formation.

Central venous access should be established for monitoring fluid balance.

Induction

Use barbiturates with caution and in lower dosage because of the patient's requirement of a high cardiac output to maintain oxygen delivery, in the face of chronic anaemia and the low levels of plasma proteins, leading to an increased percentage of free drug during the initial bolus effect.

Avoid suxamethonium if the serum potassium level exceeds 5 mmol l^{-1} or if there is peripheral neuropathy.

For neuromuscular blockade, atracurium and mivacurium are preferred due to their rapid elimination and independence of renal metabolism and excretion. Neuromuscular blockade with vecuronium has a longer duration of action, and is best used as a single dose, not by infusion.

Maintenance

- Maintain blood volume and blood pressure whilst monitoring filling pressures to prevent overload.
- Monitor urine output, if indicated.
- Regional techniques, such as brachial plexus blocks for fistulae formation may be employed, but watch for bleeding tendencies. Bupivacaine and lignocaine may be safely used and have been shown not to accumulate.
- Isoflurane and desflurane are ideal inhalational agents, with minimal metabolism and good muscle relaxation. Enflurane may be used, but its use is controversial due to the potential accumulation of fluoride ions, usually <15 μmol l^{-1}. Nephrotoxicity is seen when levels are in excess of 50 μmol l^{-1}.

Analgesia

Use morphine and pethidine with caution, as their metabolites (morphine-6-glucuronide, norpethidine) tend to accumulate.

POSTOPERATIVE MANAGEMENT

- Watch fluid balance closely, whilst monitoring filling pressures and urine output, if any
- Oxygen therapy to maximize carrying capacity
- Monitor electrolytes
- Avoid transfusion, unless excessive blood loss.

The later postoperative period:

- Bleeding may occur
- Patients may require many further anaesthetics, usually for vascular access surgery for dialysis, or for transplantation.

6

BIBLIOGRAPHY

Chauvin M, Sandouk P, Scherrmann J M, Farinotti R, Strumza P, Duvaldestin P. Morphine pharmacokinetics in renal failure. Anesthesiology 1987; 66: 327–331

Dyson D. Anesthesia for patients with stable end-stage renal disease. Veterinary Clinics of North America, Small Animal Practice 1992; 22: 469–471

Grejda S, Ellis K, Arino P. Paraplegia following spinal anaesthesia in a patient with chronic renal failure. Regional Anesthesia 1989; 14: 155–157

McEllistrem R F, Schell J, O'Malley K, O'Toole D, Cunningham A J. Interscalene brachial plexus blockade with lidocaine in chronic renal failure – a pharmacokinetic study. Canadian Journal of Anaesthesia 1989; 36: 59–63

Rice A S, Pither C E, Tucker G T. Plasma concentrations of bupivacaine after supraclavicular brachial plexus blockade in patients with chronic renal failure. Anaesthesia 1991; 46: 354–357

CROSS REFERENCES

Hypertension
Patient Conditions 4: 111
Anaemia
Patient Conditions 7: 168

GOODPASTURE'S SYNDROME

P. Saunders and K. Pearce

6

Although originally described in an 18-year-old male, who developed haemoptysis and died, following an influenza-type illness, it was not until later that the term 'Goodpasture's syndrome' was used to describe the entity of *pulmonary haemorrhage* and *glomerulonephritis*.

The pathogenetic mechanism appears to involve the development of antibodies to pulmonary and glomerular basement membranes, with an ensuing autoimmune process accounting for the renal lesions (crescentic glomerulonephritis), and pulmonary alveolitis resulting in haemoptysis.

Antiglomerular basement membrane antibodies (anti-GBM) and antineutrophil cytoplasmic autoantibodies (ANCA) can be assayed by immunofluorescence, allowing for a more rapid and accurate diagnosis than was possible in the past. It must be stressed that the term 'Goodpasture's syndrome' refers to the clinical situation of glomerulonephritis with pulmonary haemorrhage, and therefore includes those diseases which are also antibody negative, such as:

- Polyarteritis nodosa
- Wegener's syndrome
- Primary crescentic glomerulonephritis
- Following treatment with penicillamine
- Systemic lupus erythematosus.

PATHOPHYSIOLOGY

History:

- Male preponderance 2:1
- Caucasians
- HLA/DRA association (inherited?).

Presenting features:

- *Pulmonary features*, appear early:
  - Dyspnoea
  - Haemoptysis (rusty sputum to massive bleed).
- *Renal*:
  - Haematuria
  - Nephrotic picture
  - Oliguria/anuria
  - Hypertension.

Clinical course and outcome

Once respiratory symptoms develop, oliguria and anuria usually follow rapidly. Those with early oligoanuria or requiring haemodialysis seldom recover renal function. Treatment involves renal support, plasmapheresis, steroids and immunosuppression with cytotoxic drugs (azathiaprine). Pulmonary signs and symptoms are improved by reducing anti-GBM titres with plasmapheresis and immunosuppression.

Clinical lapses during treatment are characterized by fever and reduced pulmonary and renal function.

Mortality is usually due to overwhelming sepsis or pulmonary haemorrhage.

PREOPERATIVE MANAGEMENT

Elective surgery should be carried out during quiescent periods (low DLco). Preoperative blood transfusion and dialysis may be necessary to optimize fluid, electrolyte and haemodynamic status.

Investigations:

- Full blood count – microcytic hypochromic anaemia
- Clotting – usually normal
- Urea and electrolytes – derangement reflects degree of renal impairment
- Chest X-ray – small discrete shadowing; confluent densities; bilateral alveolar infiltrates
- Pulmonary function – restrictive picture; DLco elevated
- ECG – electrolyte abnormalities; systemic hypertension; pulmonary hypertension.

ANAESTHESIA

Premedication:
- Avoid respiratory depression
- Steroid cover.

Monitoring:
- Routine (defined by needs of surgery)
- Airway pressures and compliance.

Specific problems:
- If employing IPPV, smaller tidal volumes and increased frequency are necessary to minimize risk of alveolar capillary membrane rupture.
- Pulmonary haemorrhage leads to airways/ endotracheal tube obstruction. Therefore frequent endotracheal suctioning is recommended.
- Avoid renal excreted NMBs.
- Aseptic techniques for immunosuppressed patients.

POSTOPERATIVE MANAGEMENT

- Physiotherapy
- Monitor renal function
- Increased steroid dosage.

BIBLIOGRAPHY

Katz, Benumof, Kadis (eds). Respiratory diseases. In: Anaesthesia and uncommon diseases, 3rd edn. W B Saunders, London, 1990

Katz, Benumof, Kadis (eds). Renal diseases. In: Anesthesia and uncommon diseases, 3rd edn. W B Saunders, London, 1990

Prough D S, Foreman A S. Anaesthesia and the renal system. In: Barash, Cullen, Stoelting (eds) Clinical anaesthesia. Lippincott, Philadelphia, 1989, ch 38, p 1079–1104

Stoelting R K, Dierdorf S F (eds). Renal disease in anesthesia and coexisting disease, 3rd edn. Churchill Livingstone, Edinburgh, 1993

CROSS REFERENCES

Restrictive lung disease
Patient Conditions 3: 80

HAEMOLYTIC URAEMIC SYNDROME

P. Saunders and K. Pearce

The haemolytic uraemic syndrome is the most important cause of renal failure in infancy and childhood. Following a prodromal illness, usually gastroenteritis, the patient may rapidly develop the typical triad of *renal failure, haemolytic anaemia* and *thrombocytopenia.* Many viral agents have been implicated, and bacteria such as *Shigella* and *Salmonella* have been recovered from these patients.

Most patients present for anaesthesia for the creation of arteriovenous fistulae and shunts.

PATHOPHYSIOLOGY

It is a multisystem disease involving not only the kidneys, erythrocytes and platelets, but also the gastrointestinal tract, liver, heart and CNS.

Cardiovascular system
Myocarditis, congestive heart failure and severe systemic hypertension.

Respiratory system
Severe respiratory insufficiency may occur, unrelated to volume overload, pulmonary oedema or congestive heart failure.

CNS
Drowsiness, seizures, hemiparesis and coma.

Biochemical:
- Evidence of acute renal failure, including acid–base and electrolyte disturbances
- Abnormal liver function tests associated with hepatitis.

Haematological:
- Haemolysis rapidly appears; haemoglobin falls to as low as $4\ g\ l^{-1}$
- Thrombocytopenia (lasting 7–14 days)
- Hepatosplenomegaly.

Renal system
Proteinuria, haematuria and oliguria, leading to anuria.

Gastrointestinal tract
Haemorrhagic gastritis.

Immunological
Severe infections are common, e.g. peritonitis, meningitis and osteomyelitis.

PREOPERATIVE ASSESSMENT

Examination:
- Full neurological and cardiovascular examination
- Evidence of hepatic dysfunction
- Evidence of clotting disorders.

Investigations:
- Full blood count
- Urea and electrolytes, and creatinine
- Liver function tests
- Glucose
- Clotting studies
- Arterial blood gases
- Chest X-ray
- ECG.

PREOPERATIVE MANAGEMENT

Premedication is unnecessary as patients in the acute phase tend to be lethargic and drowsy. Correction of acid–base status, electrolyte and coagulation disorders should be arranged prior to surgery. Preoperative transfusion may be necessary, and any anticonvulsant therapy should be continued perioperatively.

PERIOPERATIVE MANAGEMENT

General anaesthesia is preferred due to presence of coagulation disorders in an uncooperative and severely ill child. A reduction in the dose of thiopentone (less protein binding in hepatic disease) is usual. Rapid sequence induction should be performed. Isoflurane and atracurium are the ideal agents for maintenance, although the newer agents desflurane and mivacuronium would be attractive alternatives. In most surgery, continual monitoring of acid–base and electrolyte status, temperature and urine output will be required.

POSTOPERATIVE MANAGEMENT

Postoperative ventilation may be required in patients with severe cerebral involvement. Sepsis is a common postoperative complication.

The later postoperative period
Repeated procedures are common. Haemolytic crisis may last more than 2 weeks, but the anaemia continues for months. Renal function may recover completely, or the child may require permanent haemodialysis.

BIBLIOGRAPHY

Johnson G D, Rosales J K. The haemolytic uraemic syndrome and anaesthesia. Canadian Journal of Anaesthesia 1987; 34: 196–199

NEPHROTIC SYNDROME

P. Saunders and K. Pearce

Although of multifactorial aetiology, 80% of cases are due to glomerulonephritis.

Presenting features
- Proteinuria (>3 g/24 h)
- Hypoalbuminaemia
- Hypercholesterolaemia
- Thromboembolic episodes.

Hypoalbinaemia leads to a fall in plasma oncotic pressure, retention of sodium and water with the build up of peripheral oedema, ascites, pleural effusions and a hypovolaemic patient. This physiologically deranged state puts the individual at risk of thromboembolic episodes, commonly venous (deep venous thrombosis, renal vein thrombosis), but also arterial.

Diagnosis
Renal biopsy.

Nephrotic syndrome		
50% Hypovolaemic		50% Normal or increased Blood volume
	RBF	Normal/low renin
Aldosterone		but still retain water/sodium
	GFR	
Renin		
Sodium/water retention		? Primary renal mechanism causes salt retention
Oedema		

Treatment:
- Prednisolone
- Cyclophosphamide
- Chlorambucil
- Cyclosporine.

Without treatment most cases spontaneously remit. Renal failure is rare.

Hypertension

PREOPERATIVE MANAGEMENT

- Drug history: diuretics, steroids, antihypertensives
- Clinical signs of oedema
- Assess circulation, with central venous pressure monitoring if necessary

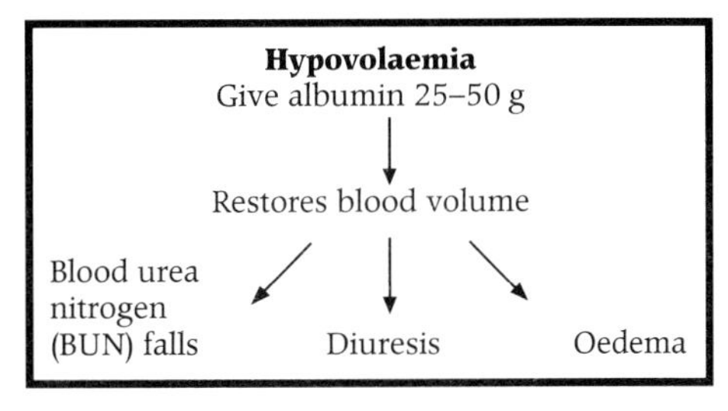

- Assess renal function to determine the degree of the renal lesion
- Potassium supplementation may be required; any deficiency may be due to the disease itself, or induced by diuretics/ steroids.

ANAESTHETIC CONSIDERATIONS

- Precautions and care, as for any patient with renal impairment/failure.
- Remember: low protein levels make drugs more active. Therefore, reduce dose of induction agents, especially STP. Monitor neuromuscular blockade.

POSTOPERATIVE MANAGEMENT

Thromboembolic prophylaxis.

POLYCYSTIC DISEASE

Autosomal dominant inheritance. The disease progresses slowly leading to end-stage renal failure in middle age.

Pathophysiology:
- Hypertension
- Proteinuria
- Reduction in urine concentrating ability early in the disease.

Associated cysts:
- Liver
- CNS (intracranial aneurysms).

Treatment:
- Dialysis
- Renal transplantation.

Anaesthetic considerations

As for end-stage renal failure, if present.

PATIENT WITH A TRANSPLANT

P. Saunders and
K. Pearce

In the UK, more than 2000 cadaveric renal transplants (RT) are performed each year. The perioperative mortality is <1.0%, and 80% are functioning at 1 year. These recipients may present for any surgery, and it is imperative that no damage occurs to the organ. Most elective procedures are well tolerated and the renal handling of drugs is good, although renal function is rarely normal.

Reasons for RT:
- Diabetes mellitus
- Glomerulonephritis
- Polycystic disease
- Hypertension.

Problems commonly seen following RT:
- Opportunistic infection
- Hepatitis B (<5% due to vaccine)
- Cancer risk (increased 30–100 times)
- Associated medical conditions
- Large cell lymphoma (Epstein–Barr virus infection).

PREOPERATIVE PREPARATION

Discuss the patient with the renal physician. A formal assessment of renal function, coupled with a careful history and examination of any associated medical conditions should be undertaken. Take note of any drug therapy, e.g. immunosuppressives, antihypertensives.

Specific cardiovascular changes

- Hypertension:
  - Essential
  - Secondary to end-stage renal failure

- Left ventricular failure:
  - Secondary to hypertension
  - Secondary to a chronic increase in cardiac output (shunts, atrioventricular fistulae and anaemia).
- Ischaemic heart disease: accelerated atherosclerosis
- Peripheral vascular disease
- Autonomic neuropathy: postural hypotension

MAIN ANAESTHETIC CONSIDERATIONS

- Continue immunosuppressive regime peri-operatively (cyclosporin A reduces RBF and glomerular filtration rate by preglomerular afferent arteriolar vasoconstriction, but produces less bone marrow depression (? reduced infection risk)).
- Risk of aspiration.
- Infection risk.
- Avoid damage to arteries, veins and fistulae.
- Gastrointestinal bleeding:
  - Steroid therapy
  - Stress of surgery/anaesthesia.
- Osteoporosis (care in moving and handling of patients).
- Potential for altered renal handling of drugs.

Premedication:

- Prophylactic antibiotics
- Steroid cover
- H_2 blockers/metoclopramide
- Benzodiazepines (avoid diazepam due to its long half-life)
- Atropine/glycopyrulate (20–50% renal excretion)
- Opioids are not contraindicated
- Continue immunosuppression.

Anaesthetic technique

Local, general and regional techniques are well tolerated, any general anaesthetic will reduce RBF, but avoid hyperventilation, hypercapnia and high concentrations of volatile agents. Enflurane and sevoflurane are metabolized to produce fluoride ions (usually $<15\ \mu mol\ l^{-1}$; nephrotoxicity at $>50\ \mu mol\ l^{-1}$). Isoflurane and desflurane require minimal metabolism and give good muscle relaxation, and are therefore recommended.

If the graft is functioning, all relaxants and anticholinesterases are easily dealt with, but atracurium and mivacuronium are the ones of choice.

Likewise with opioids, but beware of the possible build up of morphine-6-glucuronide and norpethidine (convulsant potential).

If one is considering a regional technique, and there is a degree of doubt concerning graft function, or the patient is on dialysis, then coagulation studies, including bleeding time, are mandatory.

POSTOPERATIVE MANAGEMENT

Most surgery is performed without any specific complications. However, one should monitor renal function closely, especially if undertaking major procedures. Immunosuppression should be continued, with antibiotics if indicated, and any infection appropriately dealt with.

If there is any doubt concerning graft function, opioid infusions are best avoided.

Causes of death in transplant recipients:
- Sepsis
- Cardiovascular disease
- Suicide
- Gastrointestinal perforation

BIBLIOGRAPHY

Castaneda M A, Garvin P J. General surgical procedures in renal allograft recipients. American Journal of Surgery 1986; 152: 717–721

Katz, Benumof, Kadis (eds). Renal diseases. In: Anesthesia and uncommon diseases. W B Saunders, Philadelphia, 1990, p 537–559

Kaufmann (ed). Anaesthesia for renal transplantation. In: Kaufmann L (ed). Anaesthesia review. Churchill Livingstone, Edinburgh, 1991, vol 8, ch 8

Miller (ed). Anesthesia and the renal and genitourinary systems. In: Miller R D. Anesthesia. Churchill Livingstone, Edinburgh, 1990, ch 55

Stoelting R K, Dierdorf S F (eds). Anesthesia and coexisting disease. Churchill Livingstone, Edinburgh, 1993, ch 20

CROSS REFERENCES

Diabetes mellitus (IDDM)
Patient Conditions 2: 42

Iatrogenic adrenocortical insufficiency
Patient Conditions 2: 54

Hypertension
Patient Conditions 4: 111

Fluid and electrolyte balance
Anaesthetic Factors 33: 626

7

THE BLOOD

W. Harrop–Griffiths

ANAEMIA

J. Jones

7

Anaemia
- A common condition which rarely puts fit patients at increased risk
- There is no universally accepted minimum haemoglobin concentration
- The management of anaemia must depend on the cause, the patient's overall medical status and the surgery being contemplated

Definition

The World Health Organization defines anaemia as a haemoglobin (Hb) concentration of less than:

- 13 g dl^{-1} in adult men
- 12 g dl^{-1} in adult women
- 11 g dl^{-1} in children aged from 6 months to 6 years
- 12 g dl^{-1} in children aged between 6 and 14 years.

Causes

The causes of anaemia may be divided into three categories:

- Defective red cell production
- Haemolysis
- Haemorrhage.

PATHOPHYSIOLOGY

The essential feature of all forms of anaemia is a reduction in the Hb content of the blood. Since

Arterial oxygen content $\propto$ Arterial oxygen saturation $\times$ Hb concentration
and

Oxygen delivery = Arterial oxygen content $\times$ Cardiac output

it follows that a fall in Hb concentration will, in the absence of compensatory mechanisms, be followed by a fall in oxygen supply to the tissues.

COMPENSATORY MECHANISMS

In acute normovolaemic anaemia in otherwise healthy individuals, two mechanisms compensate for the fall in oxygen-carrying capacity:

- An increase in cardiac output
- A reduction in blood viscosity.

In chronic anaemia a third mechanism comes into play:

- Increased 2,3-diphosphoglycerate (2,3-DPG) concentration in the red cells which shifts the oxygen dissociation curve to the right and promotes the release of oxygen to the tissues.

CLINICAL FEATURES

The symptoms and signs of anaemia include dyspnoea on exertion, tachycardia, palpitations, angina, increased arterial pulse pressure and capillary pulsation. However, in mild chronic anaemia which is well compensated, there may be no symptoms or signs. Anaemia is poorly tolerated by patients with coronary artery disease or pre-existing myocardial dysfunction. Such patients, who are often elderly, may present with cardiac failure.

PREOPERATIVE ASSESSMENT

In some surgical patients anaemia is to be anticipated as a feature of the disease for which operation is indicated. In other surgical patients anaemia is an unexpected and unrelated finding revealed only by routine preoperative haematological testing.

Routine blood count and blood film examination will disclose:

- The severity of the anaemia
- The type of anaemia, thus suggesting its cause (see Table 1).

FURTHER INVESTIGATIONS

It is always desirable to know the exact cause of any patient's anaemia. If surgery cannot be postponed, blood should be taken preoperatively so that investigations may be performed on a specimen which is undiluted by transfused blood.

Table 1.
Classification of causes of anaemia according to red cell morphology

Type	Cause
Hypochromic microcytic (reduced MCV, MCH, MCHC)	Iron deficiency; thalassaemia
Normochromic macrocytic (increased MCV)	Vitamin B_{12} or folate deficiency; alcohol
Polychromatic macrocytic (increased MCV)	Haemolysis
Normocytic normochromic (normal indices)	Chronic disease; renal failure; haemorrhage; hypothyroidism; hypopituitarism; marrow aplasia or infiltration
Leukoerythroblastic	Marrow infiltration

Renal failure is a common and often unsuspected cause of anaemia. The blood urea or plasma creatinine should always be checked.

CORRECTION OF ANAEMIA

What preoperative Hb level is acceptable?

There is no Hb concentration which must be met by all patients in all circumstances. Although the figure of 10 g dl^{-1} was generally accepted for many years, clinical experience, for example with patients in renal failure, suggests that in patients who are otherwise fit surgery may safely be carried out with Hb concentrations as low as 6 g dl^{-1}. The degree of anaemia which is acceptable depends on the cardiac reserves of the patient. A frail old patient with severe coronary artery disease may develop cardiac failure even at a Hb concentration of 10 g dl^{-1}.

How may the patient's Hb level be raised?

By treating the cause of anaemia

Obviously the ideal solution, but most cases of anaemia are not amenable to treatment or the treatment is surgery.

By giving specific haematinics

Appropriate in specific deficiency states (iron, vitamin B_{12} or folic acid) only. Blind, blunderbuss haematinic treatment is useless and expensive.

By red cell transfusion

Transfusion has only a limited place because:

- A moderate degree of anaemia is well tolerated in otherwise fit patients (see above)
- Transfusion has many hazards; in particular, it is easy to overload the circulation of a normovolaemic anaemic patient.

The only patients in whom preoperative transfusion is certainly indicated are some patients with sickle cell anaemia and severely anaemic patients with cardiac decompensation in whom surgery is urgent. To minimize the risks of circulatory overload, red cell concentrates should be transfused and a diuretic administered at the same time.

PERI- AND POST-OPERATIVE MANAGEMENT

The anaesthetist's aim is to maintain oxygen delivery. To this end:

- An adequate supply of blood must be crossmatched, and blood which is lost at operation should be promptly replaced
- Particular care should be taken to ensure that:
  - Hypoxaemia never develops
  - The cardiac output is not depressed.

Within this framework there is a wide choice of anaesthetic techniques at the anaesthetist's disposal. There is virtually no evidence to suggest that anaemia is associated with an increased morbidity or mortality at elective surgery.

BIBLIOGRAPHY

Consensus conference: perioperative red blood cell transfusion. Journal of the American Medical Association 1988; 260: 2700–2703

Messmer K, Lewis D H, Sunder-Plassman L, Klovekorn W P, Mendler N, Holper K. Acute normovolaemic haemodilution. European Surgery Research 1972; 4: 55

Nunn J F, Freeman J. Problems of oxygenation and oxygen transport during anaesthesia. Anaesthesia 1964; 19: 206

Stehling L. Perioperative morbidity in anaemic patients. Transfusion 1989; 29: 375

CROSS REFERENCES

Intraoperative bronchospasm
Anaesthetic Factors 33: 632

Intraoperative hypotension
Anaesthetic Factors 33: 638

DISSEMINATED INTRAVASCULAR COAGULATION (DIC)

N. Watson

7

Disseminated intravascular coagulation (DIC):
- Often associated with life-threatening conditions
- Usually manifests as uncontrolled bleeding but can also cause thrombotic complications
- Treatment is by eliminating cause, if possible, and with blood components

Table 1.
Conditions associated with DIC

Tissue damage	Trauma Surgery – especially cardiac, vascular, neurosurgery, prostate Burns Dissecting aortic aneurysm Hypoxia, particularly with hypotension
Infection	Bacterial – especially Gram-negative organisms Viral Fungal Parasitic
Obstetric causes	Eclampsia Abruptio placentae Amniotic fluid embolism Retained fetal products
Neoplastic	Promyelocyte leukaemia Adenocarcinoma – lung, pancreas, prostate
Other causes	Fat embolism Drug reactions Severe liver disease Anaphylactic or haemorrhagic shock Transfusion reaction Cavernous haemangioma Snake venom

Definition
Disseminated intravascular coagulation (DIC) involves widespread activation of those haemostatic mechanisms which normally operate locally to halt bleeding from injured vessels. The diagnosis of DIC requires the identification of a bleeding disorder with evidence of fibrinolysis and consumption of platelets and clotting factors. Microvascular thrombosis occurs and may be associated with multiple organ failure.

PATHOPHYSIOLOGY

DIC may be triggered by a variety of conditions (see Table 1) and in a variety of ways, all of which act through a procoagulant stimulus to the production of thrombin. Irrespective of the triggering mechanism, the result is widespread intravascular fibrin deposition and haemorrhage associated with depletion of clotting factors and consumption of platelets.

Coagulopathy
In acute DIC, depletion of clotting factors and platelets may result in clinically significant bleeding. When the process is subacute or chronic, hepatic synthesis of clotting factors may keep pace with consumption, and only minor abnormalities may be detected.

Activation of the fibrinolytic system occurs as a secondary phenomenon, fibrin and fibrinogen being broken down by plasmin to fibrin degradation products (FDPs), which are themselves anticoagulant.

Thrombosis
Microvascular thrombosis may cause tissue ischaemia and necrosis, resulting in organ dysfunction which typically affects the kidneys, lungs and liver.

The thrombotic tendency is exacerbated by depletion of the natural anticoagulant antithrombin III which acts by forming complexes with activated clotting factors and which is also consumed by the process of DIC.

PREOPERATIVE ASSESSMENT

Surgery which is related to the cause of the DIC, e.g. evacuation of the retained products of conception (ERPC), should be delayed no longer than is necessary to correct coagulopathy to an acceptable level and ensure cardiorespiratory stability.

History and examination

- The underlying disease is often of greater clinical significance than the DIC
- Coagulopathy may cause purpura or bruising, oozing from vascular access sites and surgical incisions and bleeding from gastrointestinal, genitourinary or respiratory tracts
- Thrombosis may cause renal or respiratory failure, hepatic dysfunction, skin infarcts and multiple organ failure.

Investigations for a patient with DIC are given in Table 2.

PREOPERATIVE PREPARATION

- Treat the underlying cause if possible, e.g. give antibiotics for infections.
- Correct hypotension, hypoxia, acidosis, electrolyte imbalance (using haemodialysis if necessary) and anaemia.
- Attempt to correct coagulation abnormalities using fresh frozen plasma and platelet concentrates. An adequate supply of blood components should be available before surgery is commenced.
- The use of heparin to prevent thrombosis and consumption coagulopathy is controversial and may result in increased bleeding. Its main use is in those subjects in whom the procoagulant stimulus cannot be halted or in fulminant DIC in which replacement therapy cannot keep up with blood loss. The value of antithrombin III therapy is as yet unproven.
- Premedication is usually unnecessary or inadvisable in the critically ill patient. Avoid intramuscular injections.

PERIOPERATIVE MANAGEMENT

Coagulopathy contraindicates most loco-regional anaesthetic techniques, and therefore general anaesthesia is usually employed.

Monitoring

This should be tailored to the patient's clinical condition and the surgery planned, and will often include invasive cardiovascular monitoring.

Induction and maintenance

If, as is likely, cardiovascular instability is present or probable, anaesthetic agents should be chosen which will minimize cardiovascular depression. Large-bore intravenous lines are necessary to allow the rapid transfusion of blood and blood products. Methods to achieve warming of intravenous fluids should be available. Controlled ventilation is recommended. Nasal intubation should be avoided if coagulopathy is significant.

Haematological management

Blood loss should be measured and promptly replaced. During prolonged procedures, blood

Table 2.
Investigations suggested for a patient with DIC

Investigation	Possible abnormalities in DIC
Full blood count	Thrombocytopenia, microangiopathic anaemia
Coagulation screen	Prolonged thrombin time, increased FDPs and decreased fibrinogen. APTT may be short or slightly prolonged, PT may be normal
Urea and electrolytes	May be deranged due to critical illness and renal failure
Liver function	Abnormalities due to hepatic dysfunction
Arterial gases	Hypoxaemia, hypercarbia, acidosis
Chest X-ray	Adult respiratory distress syndrome, pneumonia, trauma
ECG	Should be performed to exclude significant arrhythmia or ischaemia
Other, e.g. blood culture	

should be taken regularly for haemoglobin concentration, platelet count, thrombin time, partial thromboplastin time and XDP estimations (an estimate of breakdown products now more commonly performed than FDP measurement). Note that the prothrombin time may not be significantly abnormal in quite severe DIC. Platelet concentrates and fresh frozen plasma should be given as indicated.

Postoperative management

Patients with clinically significant DIC are best managed on an ITU and often require mechanical ventilation for actual or anticipated respiratory failure. Intensive monitoring of the cardiovascular, respiratory and renal systems should continue, as should frequent haematological surveillance.

Surgery, particularly in obstetric practice, may remove the cause of DIC, resulting in rapid resolution. However, coagulopathy, thrombosis and the results of thrombosis may persist for a considerable time.

Mortality from severe acute DIC may be as high as 86%, probably reflecting the severity of underlying disease.

BIBLIOGRAPHY

Giles A R. Disseminated intravascular coagulation. In: Bloom A L et al. (eds) Haemostasis and thrombosis. Churchill Livingstone, Edinburgh, 1994

Mant J, King E. Severe acute disseminated intravascular coagulation. The American Journal of Medicine 1979; 67: 557–563

Preston F E. Disseminated intravascular coagulation. British Journal of Hospital Medicine 1982: 129–137

Thijs L G, de Boer J P, de Groot M C M, Hack C E. Coagulation disorders in septic shock. Intensive Care Medicine 1993; 19: S8–S15

Weinberg S, Phillips L, Twersky R, Cottrell J E, Braunstein K M. Hypercoagulability in a patient with a brain tumor. Anesthesiology 1984; 61: 200–202

GLUCOSE-6-PHOSPHATE DEHYDROGENASE DEFICIENCY

N. Denny

Glucose-6-phosphate dehydrogenase deficiency:

- An inherited condition
- Haemolysis, which may be severe, can be triggered by certain agents
- Few triggering agents are in routine anaesthetic usage

Glucose-6-phosphate dehydrogenase (G6PD) deficiency is the most common inherited metabolic disorder of red blood cells (RBCs), affecting over 100 million people world-wide with varying degrees of severity. G6PD governs the rate at which RBCs consume, utilize and detoxify oxygen. Its deficiency makes RBCs vulnerable to haemolysis. G6PD deficiency will not usually result in complications during or after anaesthesia, provided oxidant agents known to trigger haemolysis are avoided.

PATHOPHYSIOLOGY

Low levels of G6PD result in failure to generate NADPH which is needed to maintain red cell glutathione in a reduced state. Low levels of reduced glutathione render red cell proteins susceptible to oxygenation, resulting in the formation of masses of denatured globin (Heinz bodies) which are attached to the red cell membrane. Heinz bodies are pitted out of the red cells by macrophages during passage through the spleen. The inclusion-free red cells have damaged

Table 1.
Some oxidant drugs capable of triggering haemolysis in patients with G6PD deficiency

Analgesics	Aspirin in high dose Phenacetin Acetanilide
Sulphonamides	
Antibiotics	Ciprofloxacin Chloramphenicol
Antimalarials	Primaquine Chloroquine Quinine
Miscellaneous drugs	Methylene blue Vitamin K Nalidixic acid Naphthalene Quinidine Probenecid Phenylhydrazine Nitrates Nitrofurantoin Ascorbic acid in high dose

membranes and are haemolysed. Table 1 lists oxidant drugs which may cause haemolysis in patients with G6PD deficiency, though the response is somewhat idiosyncratic.

CLINICAL MANIFESTATIONS

The structural gene for G6PD resides on the X chromosome and is therefore inherited as a sex-linked characteristic. G6PD deficiency is most common in hemizygous males but is also seen in homozygous females. Heterozygous females may occasionally have clinical manifestations. There are more than 200 variants of G6PD and the clinical manifestations range from negligible to severe, depending upon the activity of the abnormal G6PD and whether the patient is a heterozygote or a homozygote/hemizygote. Two distinct clinical syndromes may result:

- In the African variant (the gene in this variant is termed A^-) the patient is asymptomatic until exposed to oxidant drugs or a severe infection. 11% of black Americans have the A^- gene.
- In the Mediterranean and Oriental groups of variants the G6PD deficiency is generally more severe and may be a cause of neonatal jaundice. Nevertheless, the patient is usually asymptomatic until a drug or infection precipitates haemolysis. Some individuals can also develop a fulminant haemolytic anaemia after exposure to the fava bean (favism).

ANAESTHETIC MANAGEMENT

Elective surgery should not be carried out during a haemolytic crisis. The classical features of such a crisis include abdominal pain, jaundice, a decrease in haemoglobin concentration, a rising reticulocyte and the presence of Heinz bodies in the peripheral blood film.

When providing anaesthetic care for patients with G6PD deficiency it is important to avoid oxidant agents associated with the triggering of haemolysis. These are listed in Table 1. In addition to these it has been recommended that nitroprusside be avoided along with prilocaine in large amounts.

BIBLIOGRAPHY

Handl J. Heinz body hemolytic anemias. In: 'Blood'. Textbook of hematology, 1st edn. Little, Brown & Co, Boston, 1987, p 338–341

Smith C L, Snowdon S L. Anaesthesia and glucose-6-phosphate dehydrogenase deficiency. Anaesthesia 1987; 42: 281–288

Vickers M D, Jones R M. Blood disorders. In: Medicine for anaesthetists, 3rd edn. Blackwell Scientific, Oxford, ch 11, p 384–386

HIV AND AIDS

P. Ward

7

HIV and AIDS:
- Can adversely affect all major body systems
- Patients may be infectious without having AIDS or being HIV positive

Definitions

HIV positive A state in which a person has produced an antibody response as a result of having been exposed to and infected by the human immunodeficiency virus (HIV).

AIDS Acquired immunodeficiency syndrome – a clinical diagnosis by which a patient has presented with one or more of the 23 definitive or more than two of the presumptive conditions listed in Table 1.

AIDS can be divided into three categories according to the 1993 Classification (see below).

UK data as of October 1993

Number of patients known to be HIV positive or suffering from AIDS:

- HIV positive 20 590 (of which 2673 are female)
- AIDS 8115 (of which 619 are female)

63% of reported AIDS cases have died.

PATHOPHYSIOLOGY

Most organ systems can be affected by HIV and AIDS.

Respiratory system

There are numerous effects on the airway, ranging from oral candidiasis, ulcers and herpes simplex to serious haemorrhagic lesions of Kaposi's sarcoma which can be distributed throughout the airway. Of greatest concern are those conditions listed in Table 1 which can affect gas exchange, e.g. *Pneumocystis carinii* pneumonia (PCP), histoplasmosis, tuberculosis (TB), cytomegalovirus (CMV) and bacterial infections.

Cardiovascular system

HIV can cause autonomic neuropathy, cardiomyopathy, viral pericarditis and lymphomatous infiltration of the myocardium. Kaposi's sarcoma in the gut or respiratory tract can cause cardiovascular collapse due to haemorrhage.

Central nervous system

Infection with herpes simplex and CMV can cause malaise, headache, confusion, pyrexia and focal or generalized epileptiform attacks. Invasive conditions such as non-Hodgkin's lymphoma can give rise to limb weakness and visual loss, while degenerative disease can cause poor cerebration and progressive dementia.

Gastrointestinal system

The whole of the gut is at risk from HIV-related infections. Chronic diarrhoea is common and leads to pain, debility and

CATEGORY A	Acute (primary) HIV infection or asymptomatic infection or persistent generalized lymphadenopathy
CATEGORY B	Symptomatic with conditions other than those included in categories A or C attributed to HIV infection or which are indicative of a defect of cell mediated immunity, e.g. bacillary angiomatosis
CATEGORY C	Clinical condition listed in the AIDS surveillance case definition definitively or presumptively (as given in Table 1)

Table 1.
AIDS indicator diseases

(The ticks and crosses indicate whether a definitive or presumptive diagnosis can (√) or cannot (×) be used towards a diagnosis of AIDS)

	Definitive	Presumptive
Bacterial infection (multiple in a child aged less than 13 years)	√	√
Candidiasis: trachea, bronchi or lungs	√	√
Candidiasis: oesophageal	√	√
Cervical carcinoma, invasive	√	√
Coccidiomycosis: extrapulmonary	√	√
Cryptococcosis: extrapulmonary	√	×
Cryptosporidosis: with diarrhoea for over 1 month	√	×
Cytomegalovirus (CMV) retinitis	√	√
CMV disease not in liver, spleen or nodes	√	√
Encephalopathy (dementia) due to HIV	√	√
Herpes simplex: ulcers for over 1 month or bronchitis, pneumonitis, oesophagitis	√	×
Histoplasmosis: disseminated or extrapulmonary	√	√
Isosporiasis: with diarrhoea for over 1 month	√	√
Kaposi's sarcoma	√	√
Lymphoid interstitial pneumonia or pulmonary lymphoid hyperplasia in child <13 years	√	√
Lymphoma, Burkitt's, or equivalent	√	√
Lymphoma, immunoblastic or equivalent	√	√
Lymphoma, primary in brain	√	×
Mycobacterium avium: extrapulmonary	√	√
M. tuberculosis: pulmonary	√	√
M. tuberculosis: extrapulmonary	√	√
Mycobacterium of other or unidentified species, disseminated	√	√
Pneumocystis carinii pneumonia	√	√
Pneumonia: recurrent within a 12-month period	√	√
Progressive multifocal leukoencephalopathy	√	√
Salmonella septicaemia, recurrent	√	√
Toxoplasmosis of brain	√	√
Wasting due to HIV	√	×

weight loss and may cause significant fluid and blood loss. Colonic perforation may be associated with CMV colitis. Malignant involvement with Kaposi's sarcoma, or non-Hodgkin's lymphoma may result in bleeding and bowel obstruction.

Genitourinary tract

Urinary tract infections are common and may lead to pyelonephritis. Malignant involvement of the kidneys is rare. The external genitalia are prone to herpes and papilloma infections.

Haematology

As a result of chronic infection, malaise, anorexia, diarrhoea and bone marrow suppression (TB), patients are often anaemic. Anaemia is commonly compounded by drug therapy such as AZT. The possibility of sudden marked blood loss is always present.

Systemic

A wide variety of other systemic effects such as depressed liver function, adrenal failure and widespread skin changes and infections are well recognized.

ANAESTHETIC MANAGEMENT

Preoperative

Assessment is guided by the clinical presentation and knowledge of the potential complications. Careful cardiovascular, hepatorenal and respiratory evaluation should be conducted and optimization pursued. In the wholly asymptomatic patient, preoperative management is as for any healthy patient.

Perioperative

Management must be responsive to disease processes identified in the preoperative assessment. Great care is required in protecting staff and other patients during surgical procedures from infection, either from the HIV virus itself or from the possibility of resistant infections.

Postoperative

Continuing careful management of infection and major systems complications must continue into the postoperative period.

STAFF/PATIENT PROTECTION

It is well recognized that blood-borne viruses can be transmitted to health-care workers via broken skin and 'sharps injuries'. The risk of hepatitis B infection through a penetrating injury is of the order of 30%, that of hepatitis C is around 3%. It is thought that the risk of the transmission of HIV is 0.4% or less from a single injury. The risk of HIV transmission by contamination of mucous membranes is thought to be extremely small. There are two approaches to occupational exposure limitation:

- Identify all infected or potentially infected patients and take extra care. This approach requires compulsory testing of all patients. Although at present the ethical correctness of this approach to HIV infection is under discussion, it is likely that compulsory testing will gain increasing support. It must be borne in mind that the tests available are not infallible (HIV seroconversion may take some months).
- Adopt a high level of care with all patients – assume that every patient poses a threat to health-care workers from blood-borne infection.

IDIOPATHIC THROMBOCYTOPENIC PURPURA (ITP)

T. Ainley

Idiopathic thrombocytopenic purpura (ITP):
- Thrombocytopenia can lead to severe haemorrhage
- Platelet count should be raised to above $100 \times 10^9\ l^{-1}$, if possible
- Patients may be taking drugs, e.g. steroids, with significant side-effects
- Platelet transfusions may raise the platelet count for no more than 1 h

PATHOPHYSIOLOGY

ITP is a destructive thrombocytopenia caused by the presence of an antibody (usually IgG) against platelet membrane glycoproteins IIb/IIIa. The binding of antibody to platelets leads to their phagocytosis by cells of the reticulo-endothelial system (mainly in the spleen, but also in the liver) and, therefore, to a shortened platelet life-span.

ITP may be acute or chronic. The acute form occurs most commonly in children (of both sexes). It is usually preceded by a viral infection and leads to spontaneous remission in the vast majority of patients. The chronic form of the disease affects mainly young women and is a relatively common haematological disorder.

CLINICAL FEATURES

- Petechial haemorrhage
- Easy bruising
- Skin purpura

- Menorrhagia
- Mucosal bleeding
- Rarely, intracranial haemorrhage.

DIAGNOSIS

- Reduced platelet count (usually $10–50 \times 10^9\ l^{-1}$)
- Increased megakaryocytes in an otherwise normal marrow
- Splenomegaly is unusual and suggests another diagnosis
- Increased platelet-associated IgG (PAIgG) in most patients (this test is not widely available and its significance is being ascertained).

TREATMENT

High-dose corticosteroids can lead to a rapid rise in platelet numbers and long-term remission, but continued low-dose therapy is often required to produce adequate platelet counts. As the side-effects of long-term steroid therapy are not inconsiderable, the aim of therapy should be to provide adequate platelet numbers for haemostasis rather than to achieve a normal platelet count.

Splenectomy is often recommended if steroid therapy fails. The operation carries a low mortality in experienced hands and the response, if it occurs, is usually rapid with normalization of platelet count within 2 weeks. Unfortunately, relapse is common. Prophylaxis against pneumococcal infection must be given to patients who have undergone splenectomy.

Around 70–85% of patients achieve remission with steroid therapy and/or splenectomy. For patients refractory to these treatments the options are many, but even if therapy is successful, relapse is common. The treatment options include vinca alkaloids, cyclophosphamide, azathiaprine, danazol, colchicine and intravenous gammaglobulins.

ITP IN PREGNANCY

ITP may occur de novo in a pregnant patient or pregnancy may occur in a patient with pre-existing ITP. Intra- and post-partum haemorrhage may prove life-threatening to the mother. As PAIgG can cross the placenta, the fetus may become thrombocytopaenic and is at risk of haemorrhage, particularly in the CNS. There is therefore debate on whether vaginal delivery or Caesarean section is the safer option for the baby. In the neonate, the platelet count may be low and continue to fall in the first week of life.

The mother with ITP does not need therapy if the platelet count is over $100 \times 10^9\ l^{-1}$. If the platelet count falls below this level, low-dose steroid therapy or immunoglobulin may be given. The neonate may also receive steroids and immunoglobulin if necessary.

ANAESTHETIC MANAGEMENT

Advice should be sought from a haematologist. If the procedure is elective, steroid and immunoglobulin administration may increase platelet count sufficiently for surgery to be undertaken safely. A platelet count of $100 \times 10^9\ l^{-1}$ or more is an acceptable target. Platelet transfusion is rarely indicated, as platelet survival is usually less than 1 h; however, it may be the only option in acute life-threatening haemorrhage.

Regional anaesthetic techniques should normally be avoided if the platelet count is less than $100 \times 10^9\ l^{-1}$.

The side-effects of drug therapy should be looked for and managed appropriately if present. For steroids these include hyperglycaemia, hypokalaemia and hypertension.

BIBLIOGRAPHY

Andersen J C. Response of resistant idiopathic thrombocytopenic purpura to pulse high dose dexamethasone therapy. New England Journal of Medicine 1994; 330: 1560–1564

McVerry B A. Management of ITP in adults. British Journal of Haematology 1985; 59: 203–208

INHERITED COAGULOPATHIES

M. Price

7

Inherited coagulopathies:
- Rare
- Most patients presenting for anaesthesia are already aware of their disease
- Specific concentrates are available for all the commoner types

Inherited coagulopathies are rare, but the anaesthetist may encounter the following more common conditions:

- Factor VIII deficiency (haemophilia A or classical haemophilia)
- Factor IX deficiency (haemophilia B or Christmas disease)
- Von Willebrand's disease
- Factor XI deficiency
- Factor VII deficiency.

HAEMOPHILIA

There are about 5500 patients with haemophilia A in the UK, of whom 34% are HIV positive. There are about 1100 patients with haemophilia B in the UK, of whom 5% are HIV positive.

The genes for factor VIII and factor IX production are carried on the X chromosome, and consequently haemophiliacs are usually male. The severity of haemophilia A is determined by the level of functional factor VIII (see Table 1).

Table 1. Relationship between plasma factor VIIIc levels and severity of bleeding in classical haemophilia*

Factor VIIIc level (units/100 ml)	Bleeding symptoms
50	None
25–50	Excess bleeding after major surgery or accident
5–25	Excess bleeding after minor surgery
1–5	Severe bleeding after minor surgery and some spontaneous haemorrhage
<1	Spontaneous haemorrhage

*Adapted from Rizza (1977).

Clinical manifestations

The mild form (factor VIII levels 25–50 units/100 ml) is asymptomatic, and the diagnosis may not be made until the patient has surgery. Any family history of abnormal bleeding, however vague, should be taken seriously and the patient's haemostatic mechanisms thoroughly investigated. In the severe form, spontaneous bleeding into joints, muscles and other organs occurs and can give rise to long-term dysfunction of the sites of bleeding. The clinical manifestations of haemophilia B are similar and depend on the level of factor IX.

The activated partial thromboplastin time (aPTT) is prolonged in haemophilia and can be corrected by the addition of normal plasma. Quantitative assays of factor VIII or IX will identify the type and severity of the disease.

Management

A haematological opinion should be sought if possible. For minor surgery, factor VIII or IX levels should be 50% of normal or more. For major surgery the levels should be as near normal as possible preoperatively and should be maintained above 50% of normal for several days postoperatively.

Cryoprecipitate and fresh frozen plasma should only be given to patients with haemophilia in extreme emergencies, as the possibility of viral transmission has given rise to medico-legal concern. Most hospitals now have adequate supplies of factor VIII and factor IX concentrates, all of which have been subject to some form of virucidal treatment. Hospitals which do not stock these concentrates can usually obtain supplies within 24 h.

Older patients who received factor concentrates before 1985 when heat treatment was introduced may be infected with some or all of the following viruses:

- Hepatitis B
- Hepatitis C
- Human immunodeficiency virus (HIV)

VON WILLEBRAND'S DISEASE

Von Willebrand's disease (vWD) is an autosomal dominant disease and is therefore seen in both sexes. Severe forms of the disease are probably about as common as factor IX deficiency. It is caused by a deficiency of Von Willebrand's factor (vWF), which has a complex molecular biology. It can be associated with gene deletion, point mutations or intragenic replications. Although the frequency of abnormal genes may be as high as 1 in 2000 in the UK population, relatively few affected people have a haemostatic abnormality.

vWF is a multifunctional plasma glycoprotein which is secreted by endothelial cells and binds to factor VIII, collagen, heparin and to platelet membrane glycoproteins. In severe vWD, platelets do not adhere to endothelium, and the factor VIII level is low due to lack of carrier protein.

Clinical manifestations

The severity of the disease depends upon the vWF levels. Problems range from frequent nose bleeds, heavy periods and marked bleeding after dental extraction to more serious problems such as mucosal bleeds and haemarthroses. Diagnosis is by the demonstration of a prolonged bleeding time, the ristocetin induced platelet agglutination test and by a quantitative vWF radioimmunoassay.

Management

DDAVP treatment can raise vWF levels for a few days, but does so at the expense of body stores. For severe forms of the disease, replacement therapy can be given using intermediate-purity factor VIII concentrate which contains some vWF (high-purity factor VIII concentrate is unsuitable as it contains no vWF).

FACTOR XI DEFICIENCY

There are about 250 patients with factor XI deficiency in the UK, of whom around half are Ashkenazi Jews. It is an autosomally inherited condition. A heat-treated factor XI concentrate is available on a named-patient basis from Blood Product Laboratories (BPL).

FACTOR VII DEFICIENCY

Factor VII deficiency is very rare and, in the UK, is usually seen in Muslims of Indian origin, probably as a result of consanguinity. It is autosomally inherited. BPL make a specific heat-treated concentrate for treatment of Factor VII deficiency; it is released on a named-patient basis.

BIBLIOGRAPHY

Rizza C R. Clinical management of haemophilia. British Medical Bulletin 1977; 33: 225

7

MASSIVE TRANSFUSION, MICROVASCULAR HAEMORRHAGE AND THROMBOCYTOPENIA

H. Dodsworth

Massive transfusion:
- Unlikely to result in coagulopathy until at least one blood volume transfused
- Thrombocytopenia clinically more significant than lack of clotting factors
- Give platelets when count less than 80×10^9
- Give fresh frozen plasma when prothrombin time or activated partial thromboplastin times are greater than 1.5 times normal range

Definition

Massive transfusion can be defined as the transfusion of a volume of donor blood equivalent to the patient's total blood volume within a 24 h period. This is approximately equal to the administration of between 15 and 18 units of blood to a 70 kg adult (Table 1).

Table 1.
Contents of donor units

Red cells in additive
• SAGM unit = 350 ± 70 ml
• Buffy-coat poor unit (e.g. Optipress or Compamat) = 280 ± 60 ml
Platelet concentrates
• Single unit = 50 ± 10 ml fresh plasma containing >55 × 10^9 platelets
• Pooled platelet pack = 320 ± 26 ml plasma containing >250 × 10^9 platelets
Fresh frozen plasma
• Single unit = 150 ml (factor VIIIc >0.7 iu ml^{-1})

Massive transfusion is frequently associated with microvascular haemorrhage and, in the absence of inherited disorders of haemostasis, the main causes are dilutional thrombocytopenia and disseminated intravascular coagulation (DIC).

PATHOPHYSIOLOGY

In the absence of DIC the platelet count falls steadily with the transfusion of each successive unit (see Figure 1). During surgery, excessive haemorrhage due to thrombocytopenia is unlikely to occur until the platelet count falls below $80 \times 10^9\ l^{-1}$, unless platelet function is abnormal. Extracorporeal circulatory techniques used in cardiac surgery, the administration of aspirin and the

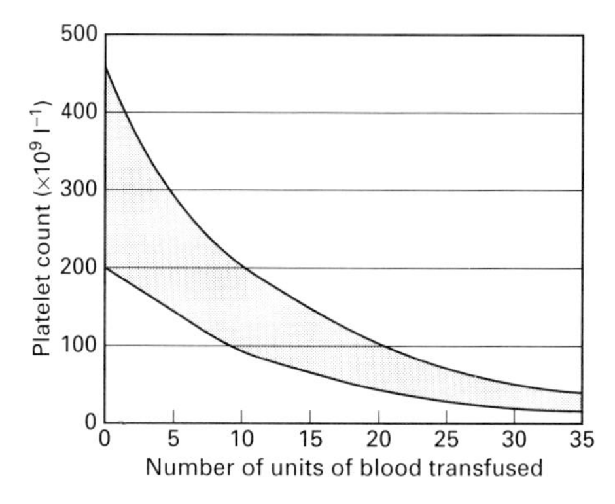

Figure 1
The likely progressive decrease in platelet count during massive transfusion over a range of initial platelet counts.

intake of large amounts of alcohol will affect platelet function, causing prolongation of the bleeding time and decreased platelet aggregation in response to ADP or collagen. This may result in bleeding with a platelet count in excess of 80×10^9 l^{-1}.

Moderate deficiency of coagulation factors is common in massively transfused patients, but does not contribute to microvascular haemorrhage until levels fall below 20% of normal. These levels are reliably reflected by prolongation of the prothrombin and activated partial thromboplastin times (PT and aPTT) to values of more than 1.5 times the control value. Synthesis and release of factor VIII and fibrinogen are stimulated by stress, and deficiency of these factors is not a problem in massively transfused subjects unless the situation is complicated by DIC.

MANAGEMENT

If massive blood loss is inevitable during an operation, e.g. thoracoabdominal aneurysm repair or liver transplantation, then it is reasonable to request a bag of pooled platelets when ordering blood before the operation.

The primary responsibility of the anaesthetist during periods of heavy blood loss is the maintenance of an adequate circulating volume. Crystalloids and synthetic colloids may be used initially and should then be followed by the administration of blood if bleeding continues. Whole blood is difficult to obtain, but the use of red cells suspended in saline, adenine, glucose and mannitol (SAGM) is appropriate. There is no evidence that plasma replacement per se is necessary.

Correctly identified samples of blood should be taken for blood grouping and cross-matching, for coagulation studies and for biochemical tests. Accurate identification of transfusion specimens and of designated units of blood, platelets and fresh frozen plasma (FFP) is particularly important in patients undergoing massive transfusion. It is important to remember that the majority of incompatible transfusions, i.e. the transfusion of blood designated for another person, occur in emergency situations and many patients receiving massive transfusions fall into this category.

Formula replacement therapy (i.e. the automatic administration of a unit of FFP and/or platelets for each set number of units of blood transfused) has been shown not to be effective in preventing microvascular haemorrhage (see Table 2). The results of regular haemostatic tests should be monitored and transfusions of platelets and FFP should be given when appropriate. If the platelet count is 80×10^9 l^{-1} or less, one bag of pooled platelets should be given, checking the platelet count post-transfusion to ensure an adequate incremental rise. If the PT and aPTT are more than 1.5 times the midpoint of the normal ranges, 4 units of FFP should be given. Transfusion of FFP rarely normalizes the results of coagulation tests completely. Minor abnormalities of coagulation unassociated with thrombocytopenia do not give rise to abnormal bleeding and are not an indication for treatment with FFP.

Table 2.
Failure of formula replacements, with FFP and platelets, to correct significant abnormalities in platelet count and coagulation studies in massively transfused patients*

No. of patients	Transfusion regime	Mean No. units	Abnormal (%)				
			Platelets	PT	aPTT	TT	FDP
64	1	12	75	54	31	23	30
66	2	11.5	88	65	48	36	47
42	3	11	90	57	24	31	48

Tranfusion regimes:
1. Blood alone
2. 1 unit of FFP after every 3 units of blood
3. 2 units of FFP and 3 units of platelets after every 10 units of blood

* Modified from Manucci et al (1982).

Haematological monitoring should be continued postoperatively. The platelet count should be maintained above $80 \times 10^9\ l^{-1}$ for 3 days after operation. Following cardiopulmonary bypass, thrombocytopenia may persist for up to 3 days.

BIBLIOGRAPHY

BCSH Blood Transfusion Task Force. Guidelines for transfusion for massive blood loss. Clinical and Laboratory Haematology 1988; 10: 265–273

Counts R B, Haisch C, Simon T L, Maxwell N G, Heimbach D M, Carrico C J. Haemostasis in massively transfused trauma patients. Annals of Surgery 1979; 190: 91–99

Manucci P M, Federici A B, Sirchia G. Haemostasis testing during massive blood replacement. A study of 172 cases. Vox Sanguinis 1982; 42: 113–123

Miller R D, Thomas O R, Tong M J, Barton S L. Coagulation defects associated with massive blood transfusion. Annals of Surgery 1971; 174: 794–801

Woodman R C, Harker L A. Bleeding complications associated with cardiopulmonary bypass. A review article. Blood 1990; 76: 1680–1697

7

MASTOCYTOSIS

K. Merrett

Mastocytosis:
- Rare but dangerous
- Premedicate with antihistamines and cromoglycate
- Avoid histamine-releasing agents
- Expect cardiovascular instability

Definition

Mastocytosis is a rare clinical disorder characterized by an abnormal proliferation and infiltration of mast cells in the skin (either localized or generalized) and/or in body organs (particularly those of the reticulo-endothelial system: gut, bone marrow, liver and spleen). It is usually regarded as a malignancy. Symptoms are related to the release of chemical mediators from within the mast cell. These include histamine, prostaglandins (particularly PGD_2), heparin, proteolytic enzymes, lipid-derived proinflammatory products, cytokines, leukotrienes and chemotactic factors. Histamine and PGD_2 are the most important clinically.

PATHOPHYSIOLOGY

The aetiology of the initial mast cell proliferation is not understood, although there is speculation that interleukin-3 and perhaps one or more of the colony stimulating factors may have a role.

The histamine release from the mast cells results in:

- Small blood vessel dilation with a localized

or generalized increase in skin blood flow leading to local erythema or widespread flushing. There may be a decrease in systemic vascular resistance and a fall in arterial blood pressure.
- Relaxation of tight junctions with transudation of fluid and the development of tissue oedema.
- Smooth muscle contraction causing bronchoconstriction, gut hypermotility and, if severe, uterine contraction.
- Exocrine secretion from the upper airway, lung and gut.
- Pruritus.

PGD_2 release produces:

- Flushing and systemic hypotension.

Although mast cells can be found in the bone marrow, the skin is the most frequently identified site of infiltration. The lesions are most commonly the red-brown or yellow macules, papules and plaques of urticaria pigmentosa.

SYMPTOMS

Symptoms exist in varying combinations with a paroxysmal nature and marked interpatient variability in both the severity and duration of 'attacks'.

Symptoms resulting from mast cell degranulation most commonly include flushing, headache, abdominal pain (with or without diarrhoea), vascular collapse or hypotension, palpitations, pruritus, urticaria, rhinitis, wheezing and syncope. Less commonly reported symptoms include dyspnoea, dizziness, chest pain, chronic fatigue, lethargy, nausea and vomiting, vertigo and CNS disturbances. Rarely, chronic diarrhoea, malabsorption, paraesthesiae, focal neurological symptoms and haemorrhage occur. Symptoms resulting from organ infiltration may include anaemia, thrombocytopenia, hepatosplenomegaly, bleeding diathesis, pathological fractures and osteoporosis.

PRECIPITATING FACTORS

Mast cell degranulation in patients with mastocytosis primarily results from non-immune IgE mediated mechanisms
- *Nonpharmacological factors*: physical exertion, anxiety, extremes of temperature, mechanical irritation and trauma to the skin.
- *Pharmacological factors*: opioids, neuromuscular blocking agents, dextrans, NSAIDs (including aspirin), preservatives (including sodium metabisulphite and parabens), β antagonists, α agonists, cholinergic agents, radiological dyes, alcohol, etc.

PREOPERATIVE ASSESSMENT

Review the results of investigations relevant to mastocytosis which may include: full blood count, coagulation studies, lung function tests, plasma histamine levels and a 24 h collection for raised levels of tryptase and PGD_2 metabolites. Unfortunately, the urinary levels of the above substances are not consistent indicators of the severity of the disease. To assess the systemic involvement of the disease further tests may include a marrow, lymph node or liver biopsy, bone scan, gastrointestinal tract evaluation, and perhaps an electroencephalogram.

PREOPERATIVE PREPARATION

Preoperative pharmacological treatment with H_1 and H_2 antagonists, cyclo-oxygenase inhibitors to prevent PGD_2 synthesis, and mast cell stabilization with sodium cromoglycate is recommended. Oral steroids have not been shown to be of value.

Aspirin has been advocated due to its action as an inhibitor of PGD_2 synthesis. However, its use is controversial as it has been implicated as a triggering agent and has effects on platelet function.

Intradermal skin testing of drugs to be used in the perioperative period is of limited value unless there is systemic disease with high levels of circulating mast cells.

PERIOPERATIVE MANAGEMENT

Premedication

An adequate dose of benzodiazepine provides both anxiolysis and sedation without affecting mast cells.

Monitoring

Haemodynamic instability should be anticipated and, therefore, invasive BP monitoring should be used in addition to standard monitoring. Core temperature should be measured.

Induction and maintenance

A large-bore intravenous line should be in place before induction. Avoid agents with histamine-releasing potential. Suitable agents might include etomidate, fentanyl, volatile anaesthetics, vecuronium, glycopyrrolate, benzodiazepines and preservative-free amide local anaesthetics. Suxamethonium should perhaps be avoided unless specifically indicated. Locoregional anaesthesia is acceptable if clotting studies are normal.

Environment

A calm, quiet, warm environment should be provided. Active measures should be taken to prevent hypothermia. Particular care should be taken in handling and positioning the patient to avoid skin irritation and trauma. Adrenaline should be readily available along with antihistamines, bronchodilators and intravenous fluids.

POSTOPERATIVE MANAGEMENT

Temperature monitoring and action to achieve and maintain normothermia should be continued into the postoperative period. The availability of adrenaline and other resuscitative drugs should be ensured.

BIBLIOGRAPHY

Duffy T P. In: Hoffman R (ed) Systemic mastocytosis in hematology: basic principles and practice. Churchill Livingstone, London, 1991, ch 82, p 1058–1061

Greenblatt E P, Chen L. Urticaria pigmentosa: an anesthetic challenge. Journal of Clinical Anesthesia 1990; 2: 108–115

Marney S R. Mast cell disease. Allergy Proceedings 1992; 13: 303–310

MULTIPLE MYELOMA

C. Gomersall

Myeloma
Can cause:

- Severe bone pain and spontaneous fractures
- Renal failure
- Hypercalcaemia

Definition

Multiple myeloma is a diffuse proliferation of B lymphocytes and plasma cells largely confined to bone marrow. It is characterized by the production of a paraprotein and the occurrence of osteolytic bone lesions. The diagnosis is made by the coexistence of at least two of the following:

- Excess plasma cells in the marrow
- Paraprotein concentration of greater than 1 g dl^{-1} (IgG or IgA) or excess light chains in the urine
- X-ray evidence of lytic lesions

It is a disease of the elderly, with a mean age at diagnosis of 60 years.

PATHOPHYSIOLOGY

Bone lesions

Lytic lesions, through which pathological fractures occur, result from the secretion of an osteoclast-stimulating cytokine by the abnormal plasma cells. Bones fracture either spontaneously or following trivial injuries; vertebral collapse is particularly common. Patients often suffer from severe bone pain.

Hypercalcaemia
In general this occurs only in those patients with extensive osteolysis. It is exacerbated by dehydration secondary to vomiting and the inability to retain salt and water due to renal involvement. It may also be precipitated by bed rest and infection. Hypercalcaemia can cause vomiting, constipation, anorexia, depression, confusion, drowsiness and even coma.

Renal impairment
Renal impairment is due to a combination of dehydration, hypercalcaemia, pyelonephritis, deposition of myeloma protein in the kidney, and in some cases renal amyloidosis. In acute renal failure secondary to myeloma the most important measure is correction of dehydration and treatment of any precipitating renal infection.

Haematological abnormalities
Normochromic, normocytic anaemia is common and may be severe due to marrow failure or renal failure. Haemostatic abnormalities may be due to interference with clotting and platelet function by paraprotein, hyperviscosity, renal failure or, rarely, thrombocytopenia as a result of marrow infiltration or chemotherapy.

Hyperviscosity
This is a rare complication associated with high plasma levels of paraprotein. It is more likely to occur in IgA myelomatosis where there is polymerization of paraprotein molecules. It can cause a variety of neurological, ocular, haematological and cardiac problems, including cardiac failure. It may also result in spurious hyponatraemia and predispose to venous thrombosis.

Immune system
Synthesis of all immunoglobulins apart from the paraprotein is depressed, leading to increased susceptibility to infection, especially by staphylococci and Gram-negative organisms.

Nervous system
The most important neurological manifestations are peripheral neuropathy, paraplegia secondary to an epidural plasmacytoma, and spinal root compression due to paravertebral masses or collapsed vertebrae.

ANAESTHETIC MANAGEMENT

There has been little research into the anaesthetic management of patients with multiple myeloma; no papers have been published in the English literature on this subject in the last 10 years and, therefore, all recommendations have to be based purely on an understanding of the abnormalities associated with the disease.

Preoperative
Management should be directed towards the detection and correction of abnormalities associated with myeloma, with particular attention to fluid balance, hypercalcaemia, haemostatic abnormalities and renal impairment. Patients with symptomatic hyperviscosity should be treated with plasmapheresis preoperatively.

Intraoperative

Regional anaesthesia
This may be absolutely contraindicated for medical reasons (haemostatic abnormalities) or relatively contraindicated for medico-legal reasons (active neurological disease).

General anaesthesia
Attention to the positioning of the patient is essential in view of the increased susceptibility to fractures. Strict asepsis is important in view of the impairment of immune function which may be further impaired by general anaesthesia. In theory, adjustment of doses of intravenous agents may be necessary in view of changes in plasma proteins.

Postoperative
Duration of immobility should be minimized to decrease the risk of precipitating hypercalcaemia and of developing venous thromboses.

BIBLIOGRAPHY

Dewhirst W E, Glass D D. Haematological diseases. In: Katz J, Benumof J L, Kadis L B (eds) Anaesthesia and uncommon diseases. W B Saunders, Philadelphia, 1990, p 406–408

CROSS REFERENCES

Chronic renal failure
Patient Conditions 6: 158
Water and electrolyte disturbances
Patient Conditions 10: 246

POLYCYTHAEMIA

W. Harrop-Griffiths

7

Polycythaemia:
- Is often secondary to clinically significant conditions
- Can give rise to abnormal bleeding during and after surgery
- Postoperative thromboembolic events are common
- Poses a greater risk to the patient than anaemia

Definition

Polycythaemia may be defined as an increase in red blood cell mass such that haemoglobin (Hb) concentration and haematocrit exceed the following values:

	Male	Female
Haemoglobin (g dl^{-1})	17.5	15.0
Haematocrit	0.52	0.48

It is possible to exceed these values with a normal red cell mass if plasma volume is substantially reduced. This can occur in a number of clinical situations such as plasma loss in burns and severe fluid loss suffered as a result of gross dehydration or prolonged bowel obstruction.

Causes:
- Polycythaemia rubra vera (PRV)
- Polycythaemia secondary to an increase in erythropoietin secretion
- 'Spurious' polcythaemia – due to a slight increase in red cell mass and a slight decrease in plasma volume.

POLYCYTHAEMIA RUBRA VERA

This is a stem cell disease of clonal origin and gives rise to an increase in granulocyte and platelet count in addition to an increase in red cell mass. Hb can exceed 20 g dl^{-1}, platelet count is often in the range 450–800 × 10^9 and can exceed 1000 × 10^9. It is a disease of older adults, with a mean age of onset of 60 years. Less than 5% of cases present before the age of 40 years. Splenomegaly and hepatomegaly are common. High blood viscosity resulting from the high haematocrit can lead to episodes of thrombosis with resulting ischaemic damage. Although thrombosis is more common in subjects with a high platelet count, it can occur with normal platelet numbers. Paradoxically, patients with PRV can also suffer from abnormal bleeding as platelet function is sometimes abnormal. Rarely, patients with PRV may present with anaemia as a result of chronic gastrointestinal haemorrhage. Without treatment the median survival of patients with PRV is about 2 years after diagnosis. Treatment is with repeated phlebotomy, chemotherapy and/or phosphorus-32.

SECONDARY POLYCYTHAEMIA

Erythropoietin secretion is stimulated by hypoxaemia and, therefore, any cause of chronic hypoxaemia can cause polycythaemia. Common causes include chronic obstructive airways disease and right-to-left cardiac shunts.

Abnormal excess secretion of erythropoietin may occur in hypernephroma, hepatoma, cerebellar haemangioblastoma and phaeochromocytoma.

Polycystic and transplanted kidneys can secrete inappropriately large amounts of erythropoietin.

ANAESTHESIA AND POLYCYTHAEMIA

Polycythaemia probably presents a much greater risk to the patient undergoing surgery than anaemia. It is not surprising that controlled randomized studies of patients who have undergone surgery with or without treatment of their polycythaemia are not available. A retrospective, uncontrolled and nonrandomized study reported over 30 years ago (Wasserman & Gilbert 1964) suggests some important points about the anaesthetic and surgical management of patients with PRV:

- Patients with untreated PRV experience substantially greater morbidity and mortality after surgery than those with adequately treated PRV
- Patients with adequately treated PRV may have a similar morbidity and mortality to unaffected patients
- The commonest complications in patients with untreated PRV are haemorrhage and thrombosis
- The reduction in postoperative morbidity and mortality seen in patients whose PRV has been treated is proportional to the duration of effective haematological control.

Preoperative management

Polycythaemia most often comes to light during the investigation of some other disorder or at routine preoperative testing. It should be considered if small vessel occlusive disease is the indication for surgery, or if the patient has plethoric facies, a history of ischaemic heart disease or abnormal bleeding.

If a high Hb concentration or haematocrit is identified preoperatively, acute plasma volume reduction as a cause can usually be excluded on history and clinical grounds. If true polycythaemia is identified, hypoxaemia as a cause can be readily excluded by performing arterial blood gas measurement. If the surgical procedure is elective, the patient should then be referred to a haematologist for investigation and treatment. It has been suggested that the peripheral blood count and the blood volume should be normalized before surgery.

If surgery is urgent and blood volume is clinically normal, isovolaemic haemodilution can be performed by venesecting the patient and replacing the withdrawn volume with colloid. It is logical to retain the withdrawn blood for administration to the patient should surgical blood loss be excessive. Subcutaneous heparin administration should be considered.

Peroperative management

If the polycythaemia is secondary then steps must be taken to account for the primary disease process, e.g. chronic obstructive airways disease, right-to-left cardiac shunts.

Venous stasis and hypotension, both of which can cause thrombosis, should be avoided. Regional anaesthesia offers advantages to the polycythaemic patient in that the incidence of postoperative thromboembolic events may be reduced. The anaesthetist should take care to ensure that the results of clotting and platelet function tests are normal before embarking on neuraxial blocks.

Cyanosis occurs when the concentration of reduced (deoxygenated) haemoglobin exceeds a value of about 5 g dl^{-1}. This will occur at higher oxygen saturations in patients with a high Hb concentration. If the Hb concentration exceeds 20 g dl^{-1} cyanosis may occur at saturations equal to the normal mixed venous oxygen saturation, i.e. 75%. Figure 1 shows the oxygen saturation at which cyanosis may occur for a range of Hb concentrations.

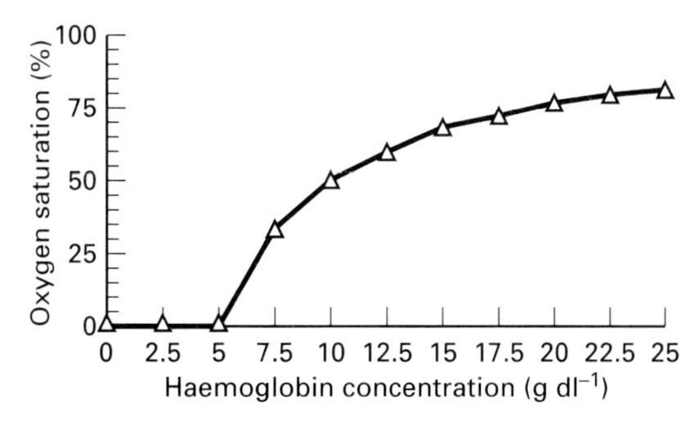

Figure 1
Oxygen saturation at which cyanosis may occur over a range of haemoglobin concentrations.

BIBLIOGRAPHY

Wasserman L R, Gilbert H S. Surgical bleeding in polycythaemic patients. Annals of the New York Academy of Science 1964; 115: 122–138

CROSS REFERENCES

COPD and anaesthesia
Patient Conditions 3: 75
Patients with a transplant
Patient Conditions 6: 164
Phaeochromocytoma
Surgical Procedures 25: 488

SICKLE CELL SYNDROME

I. Munday

Sickle cell syndromes:
- Include HbSS, HbSC and HbSThal
- Sickle crises, which can be life-threatening, occur
- Finding compatible blood can be difficult as a result of red blood cell antibodies

Definition

Sickle cell syndromes are inherited haemoglobinopathies in which the dominant haemoglobin (Hb) is the unstable haemoglobin S. They include sickle cell anaemia (HbSS) and the double heterozygote conditions sickle C (HbSC) and sickle thalassaemia (HbSThal).

PATHOPHYSIOLOGY

The sickle gene causes a single amino-acid substitution on the β chain of the Hb molecule. There is some evidence that haemoglobin S confers a limited resistance to infection with malaria, a fact that may explain the greater incidence of the sickle gene in equatorial Africa.

When haemoglobin S is deoxygenated, the molecules polymerize into long chains called 'tactoids' and become insoluble. This results in deformation of the red cell membrane into the characteristic sickle shape. Although the process is often reversible with oxygenation, haemolysis will occur if the cell membrane is damaged. During prolonged periods of deoxygenation irreversible sickling may occur. In this situation the cells aggregate and occlude small blood vessels, which leads to tissue infarction and further hypoxia. Hypoxia is aggravated by lung infarction which is a common cause of death. The major features of sickle cell disease are therefore a chronic anaemia and the occurrence of sickle cell 'crises' when multiple episodes of tissue infarction occur.

Sickling occurs in individuals who are homozygous for the sickle gene (HbSS) and also in those in whom the sickle gene is inherited along with another variant such as HbC or β thalassaemia. Tactoid formation is enhanced in the presence of HbC compared with the normal HbA. Patients with HbSC may have a Hb concentration towards the lower end of the normal range but are liable to sickle and have a high incidence of venous thrombosis. Inheritance of the β thalassaemia gene results in greatly reduced β chain synthesis.

Individuals with sickle cell trait (HbAS) are usually asymptomatic, although sickling may occur under conditions of severe hypoxaemia. Patients with sickle cell trait are not at increased risk during a properly conducted anaesthetic, although the use of a tourniquet may be hazardous.

PREOPERATIVE ASSESSMENT

Patients from susceptible populations should be screened for haemoglobin S with a quick haemoglobin solubility test (e.g. Sickledex), although this in itself does not distinguish between HbAS and the more dangerous phenotypes. If time allows, haemoglobin electrophoresis can be performed to determine the proportions of normal and abnormal haemoglobin.

In general, patients with sickle cell anaemia have a haemoglobin concentration in the range 6.5–10.5 g dl^{-1}. Therefore, if the Sickledex test is positive and the patient has a haemoglobin greater than 10.5 g dl^{-1} it is safe to assume that the patient does not have HbSS.

The optimum haemoglobin concentration for patients who are HbSS is debatable, and the question of preoperative blood transfusion should be discussed with a haematologist. Patients who have required multiple transfusions in the past may have red blood cell antibodies which can make the finding of compatible blood exceedingly difficult. A reduction in HbS concentration by transfusion or exchange transfusion is often recommended when the risk of haemoglobin desaturation due to hypoxia is greater than usual. Situations where this is likely to occur include major abdominal and thoracic surgery, orthopaedic operations in which the use of a tourniquet is felt to be essential, and in patients with coexisting respiratory disease.

Adequate hydration must be ensured during a preoperative starvation period and intravenous fluid administration is often recommended. Elective preoperative alkalinization with sodium bicarbonate solutions is no longer considered necessary.

See also Table 1.

PERIOPERATIVE MANAGEMENT

No specific anaesthetic technique is recommended although the use of

Table 1.
Points to note in preoperative assessment of patients with Sickle cell disease

Cardiovascular system	Cardiomegaly Raised cardiac output at rest Blood pressure typically low
Respiratory system	Pulmonary infarctions common Consider measuring arterial blood gases
Blood	Oxyhaemoglobin dissociation curve shifted to left Low arterial oxygen saturation Increased blood viscosity
Abdomen	Abdominal crises may mimic a surgical emergency
Renal	Impaired concentration ability causes polyuria Chronic renal failure common
Neurological	Cerebral infarction may result in focal deficits Proliferative sickle retinopathy

locoregional anaesthesia, where appropriate, is thought to be advantageous. If general anaesthesia is used, preoxygenation with 100% oxygen is sensible and the continuous administration of oxygen-enriched breathing mixtures (i.e. an F_IO_2 of at least 0.5) is recommended. Continuous monitoring of arterial oxygen saturation by pulse oximetry is particularly useful.

Adequate intravenous fluid replacement to maintain circulating volume is essential. If blood replacement is necessary, excessive transfusion must be avoided to reduce the risk of increased blood viscosity. Steps should be taken to maintain body temperature. Tourniquets should not normally be used. However, if the use of a tourniquet is thought to be necessary it should be applied as distally as possible (to minimize the volume of stagnant blood), the limb must be thoroughly exsanguinated, and the ischaemic time should be minimized.

A reduction in arterial oxygen saturation is common in all patients after major surgery and poses an additional threat to those with sickle cell syndromes. Therefore the high standard of care and monitoring in the operating theatre must be continued into the postoperative period. Admission to an ITU or HDU is advisable. Supplementary oxygen administration and monitoring of oxygen saturation for some time postoperatively is important. Management of postoperative pain relief and fluid balance should not be delegated to the most inexperienced member of the surgical team.

BIBLIOGRAPHY

Banarjee A K, Layton D M, Rennie J A, Bellingham A J. Safe surgery in sickle cell disease. British Journal of Surgery 1991; 78: 516–517

Esseltine D G, Baxter M R, Bevan J C. Sickle cell states and the anaesthetist. Canadian Journal of Anaesthesia 1988; 35: 385–503

THALASSAEMIA

M. Weisz

Thalassaemia:

- β Thalassaemia major, a transfusion-dependent anaemia, is the form most likely to present problems
- The major problems are:
  - Cardiomyopathy and liver disease as a result of haemosiderosis
  - Difficult airway management
  - Difficulty in finding compatible blood

Definition

The thalassaemias are an inherited group of haematological disorders in which there is deficient synthesis of globin chains. They are most frequently found in peoples originating in the Mediterranean area, Central Africa, China and South East Asia.

In healthy individuals the majority of haemoglobin is HbA which has two α and two β chains. There are four genes controlling α-chain production (two on each chromosome 16) and two genes controlling β-chain production (one on each chromosome 11). The type and severity of the disease depends upon the number and type of these genes which are deleted.

α THALASSAEMIA

Deletion of one of the four genes which controls α-chain production has no discernible adverse effects.

In the thalassaemia trait two genes are deleted and the resulting anaemia is mild and of no anaesthetic or clinical consequence.

α Thalassaemia intermedia results from the deletion of three genes. The anaemia causes persistent stimulation of erythropoietin production, and as a result large amounts of excess β chain are made. Insoluble tetramers

(HbH) form from the excess β chains. The resulting anaemia is moderately severe and is associated with haemolysis as a result of red cell deformation by HbH. The haemolysis is increased by oxidant drugs.

α Thalassaemia major results from the inability to produce any α chains, and is incompatible with life.

β THALASSAEMIA

Heterozygotes have β thalassaemia minor which is associated with mild iron-resistant hypochromic anaemia, but little or no other disability.

Homozygotes have β thalassaemia major and are unable to produce normal β chains. Production of fetal haemoglobin ($\alpha 2\gamma 2$) leads to a total Hb concentration of the order of 30–50% of normal adult levels. The condition is associated with severe, chronic transfusion-dependent anaemia. Transfusion is necessary from the first year of life, and patients almost invariably develop alloantibodies to both white and red cell antigens. Compatible blood may prove extremely difficult to find.

β Thalassaemia may coexist with a sickle gene and will produce sickle thalassaemia, one of the sickle syndromes (see p. 1.7.188). These patients only rarely have a transfusion-dependent anaemia.

CLINICAL FEATURES OF THALASSAEMIA

Clinically significant thalassaemia is associated with bone marrow hyperplasia as a result of excessive erythropoietin secretion. This can cause head bossing, prominent maxillae, a sunken nose and a variety of other skeletal abnormalities. Difficult intubation has been associated with thalassaemia. Hepatosplenomegaly may be gross and there may be hypersplenism.

Treatment of the anaemia is by repeated transfusion which invariably results in iron overload. Desferrioxamine, an iron-chelating agent, is given to limit the extent of haemosiderosis. Bone marrow transplantation has proved an effective treatment, but availability is limited.

Haemosiderosis may result in cardiomyopathy, left ventricular dysfunction and clinically significant heart failure. Haemosiderosis can also lead to hepatic failure, diabetes, hypothyroidism, hypoparathyroidism and adrenal insufficiency.

PREOPERATIVE ASSESSMENT

The patient's airway should be carefully assessed. Ease of venous access should be assessed, as repeated transfusions may have damaged peripheral veins. Skeletal abnormalities should be noted. Symptoms and signs of cardiac, hepatic or endocrine disorders should be sought.

Investigations should include a full blood count, liver function tests, blood glucose estimation, an ECG and further cardiovascular testing if cardiomyopathy is suspected.

PERIOPERATIVE MANAGEMENT

Appropriate steps should be taken to account for associated abnormalities identified. Transfusion to normal levels of haemoglobin is not normally justified unless protracted and bloody surgery is contemplated or in order to optimize the patient's cardiorespiratory status.

If cardiomyopathy is present as a result of haemosiderosis, intensive chelation treatment may improve cardiac function.

Individuals who have had a splenectomy for hypersplenism should have been immunized with pneumococcal vaccine and may receive antibiotic prophylaxis.

BIBLIOGRAPHY

Aldouri M A, Wonke B, Hoffbrand A U et al. High incidence of cardiomyopathy in β thalassaemia patients receiving regular transfusion and iron chelation. Acta Haematologica 1990; 84: 113–117

Modell B, Letskey E A, Flynn D M. Survival and desferrioxamine in thalassaemia major. British Medical Journal 1986; 284: 2031–2039

Orr B. Difficult intubation: a hazard in thalassaemia. British Journal of Anaesthesia 1967; 39: 585

Zurlo M G, de Stefans P, Borgna-Pignatti C et al. Survival and causes of death in thalassaemia major. Lancet 1989; ii: 27–30

CROSS REFERENCES

Cardiomyopathy
Patient Conditions 4: 103
The difficult airway
Anaesthetic Factors 30: 558

8

BONES AND JOINTS

J. C. Goldstone

ANKYLOSING SPONDYLITIS

C. Hamilton-Davies

Ankylosing spondylitis is an inflammatory arthropathy affecting or likely to affect 1.6% of the population, although most cases are likely to be relatively mild. Despite primarily affecting the joints it is a systemic disorder and 50% will experience extraspinal involvement at some time. There is a known association between the development of the disease and presence of the genetic marker HLA-B27 (96% of patients with ankylosing spondylitis compared with 4% of controls and 51% of first-degree relatives of patients with the disease).

PATHOPHYSIOLOGY

Musculoskeletal disease

The disease usually starts in the sacroiliac joints and then spreads up to involve the spine and the costovertebral joints. Decreased movement of the lumbar spine results with a proportion progressing to ankylosis and complete rigidity with a classical X-ray picture of 'bamboo spine'.

Cervical spine disease ranges from mild limitation of flexion/extension to complete ankylosis. These patients also have an increased incidence of cervical fracture (often undiagnosed) and may have associated neurological deficit.

Thoracic spinal disease may lead to restrictive lung disease due to reduced rib-cage movement. Involvement of the lumbar spine leads to calcification of the intraspinous ligaments of the vertebral column.

Incidence of temporomandibular joint involvement varies between 10–40%. Cricoarytenoid disease may present as dyspnoea or hoarseness.

Respiratory system

Upper lobe pulmonary fibrosis is a recognized complication of long-standing ankylosing spondylitis. Along with the costovertebral involvement this may significantly impair the respiratory reserve of the patient.

Cardiovascular system

Disease of the connective tissue of the aorta and aortic valve cusps may give rise to aortitis and aortic incompetence. As in rheumatoid disease the conduction tissue of the heart may lead to conduction defects. Cardiovascular involvement occurs in up to 10% of patients with severe spondylitis. Long-term disease is associated with a greatly increased cardiovascular mortality.

Neurological system

In long-standing spondylitis, one study found that 22% had neurological symptoms and signs. Spinal cord compression, cauda equina syndrome and vertebrobasilar insufficiency have all been described. As mentioned previously, there is a higher than normal incidence of vertebral fractures which may lead to neurological symptoms.

Other

Uveitis is found in up to 40% of sufferers and, rarely, there may be evidence of renal impairment secondary to an IgA nephropathy.

NSAIDs and phenylbutazone are often used for pain relief, with the usual associated gastrointestinal morbidity. One study demonstrated death from peptic ulcer to be four times greater in spondylitics than controls. Phenylbutazone may rarely cause severe blood dyscrasias, and monitoring is essential. Steroid therapy is reserved for eye involvement.

PREOPERATIVE ASSESSMENT

Morphological:

- Neck movement/mouth opening/dentition
- Suitability for regional techniques
- Joint limitations.

History:

- Previous anaesthetic problems

- Complete respiratory and cardiovascular history
- Drug history.

Investigations
See Table 1.

Table 1.
Investigations and results

Investigation	Result
Full blood count	Anaemia (? iatrogenic gastrointestinal bleed) Pancytopenia (? iatrogenic – NSAIDs)
Urea and electrolytes	Abnormal Iatrogenic NSAIDs
ECG	Left ventricular hypertrophy Valvular disease
Chest X-ray	Upper lobe fibrosis
Spirometry	Restrictive flow pattern

PERIOPERATIVE MANAGEMENT

Regional techniques are frequently not possible in these patients due to ankylosis of the intervertebral joints, or are ill-advised due to neurological complications of the disease. Careful airway management of the patient with this condition is paramount.

Premedication
If fibre-optic intubation is to be performed or difficulty with intubation is anticipated then an antisialogogue should be prescribed with or without an antacid.

Airway
In this group of patients it is prudent to ensure a secure airway before embarking on a surgical procedure where there is a risk of having to convert to an emergency intubation due to either loss of airway control or failure of regional technique. In severe spondylitics early consideration should be given to awake fibre-optic intubation methods. Excessive force to overcome a fixed flexion cervical spine deformity whilst trying to intubate under general anaesthesia may result in vertebral fractures.

The 'intubate at all costs' approach is not appropriate for elective surgery, and if maintaining the airway is reasonably easy a laryngeal mask is useful. If airway maintenance is extremely difficult or impossible, then allowing the patient to wake up and postponing the surgery is prudent.

In the emergency situation there may be insufficient skill/equipment available to perform fibre-optic intubation and emergency tracheostomy/cricothyrotomy may be necessary.

Respiratory system
Preoperative assessment should indicate whether any degree of respiratory compromise exists and if consideration should be given to postoperative ventilation.

Cardiovascular system
Aortic or mitral incompetence should be treated as in primary cardiac disease, with caution over the use of vasodilating drugs. Antibiotic cover may be appropriate and preoperative pacing may be necessary.

Conduct of anaesthesia
There are no specific contraindications to the use of any anaesthetic agent. Care should be taken with regard to patient positioning for the surgery in order to avoid vertebral or neurological damage and minimize backache postoperatively.

Ensuring that the patient has full control of the airway prior to extubation is essential, as reintubation may prove impossible.

POSTOPERATIVE MANAGEMENT

Analgesia often proves to be difficult in these patients, as regional techniques will rarely be available even for the most major procedures and high doses of opioids must be balanced against the risk of oversedation and compromising the airway. Patient-controlled analgesia (PCA) may be very useful in these circumstances.

Re-establishment of regular NSAID therapy will help to relieve pain due to ankylosing spondylitis, which may be greater than the surgical pain.

LONG-TERM MANAGEMENT

Patients with ankylosing spondylitis may present for any type of surgery, but as the duration of the disease lengthens so does the likelihood of the surgery relating to the disease or complications of its treatment.

Previous anaesthetic notes are essential, with particular reference to intubation/airway difficulties.

BIBLIOGRAPHY

Calin A. Seronegative spondarthritides. Medicine International 1984; 22: 146–149

Sinclair J R, Mason R A. Ankylosing spondylitis – the case for awake intubation. Anaesthesia 1984; 39: 3–11

CROSS REFERENCES

Restrictive lung disease
Patient Conditions 3: 80

Aortic valve disease
Patient Conditions 4: 95

Conduction defects
Patient Conditions 4: 99

Mitral valve disease
Patient Conditions 4: 114

DWARFISM

A. T. Lovell

People with short stature conventionally are divided into two categories: those with proportionate growth and those with disproportionate growth, and it is the latter group that are classified as dwarfs. Patients with dwarfism are often considered as having a single disease entity, but this is an over-simplification. There are over 100 different types of dwarfism, many of which pose specific anaesthetic problems.

INCIDENCE

Although each particular type of dwarfism is relatively rare, the large number of types means that any practising anaesthetist is likely to meet dwarfs. Achondroplasia, the commonest cause of dwarfism, has an incidence of 150 per million births.

ANAESTHETIC PROBLEMS

It is only through an understanding of the multiple abnormalities that are present in dwarfs that anaesthesia can be safely delivered.

Monitoring and anaesthetic techniques need to be considered in relation to both the underlying diagnosis as well as the planned surgical procedure.

Traditionally, general anaesthesia has been the technique of choice. This is despite the risks of airway obstruction with some syndromes. This is in part due to the problems that may be encountered in performance of spinal and epidural blockade due to a variety of spinal deformities. Nevertheless, there are numerous reports of successful spinal and epidural anaesthesia for Caesarean section.

PREOPERATIVE ASSESSMENT

Respiratory system:
- Clinical assessment of airway
- Obstructive airway lesions, especially in patient with mucopolysaccharidoses
- Previous problems with airway maintenance or intubation
- Restrictive defects secondary to rib hypoplasia and kyphoscoliosis
- Sleep apnoea.

Cardiovascular system
- Pulmonary hypertension
- Congenital heart disease
- Coronary artery disease
- Valvular heart disease
- Cardiomyopathy.

Neurological system
- Macrocephaly and hydrocephaly
- Cervical spine instability
- Spinal cord compression
- Nerve root compression
- Temperature regulation problems.

Other
- Endocrinopathy
- Bleeding problems.

PREMEDICATION

Anticholinergic agents are used widely in patients with marked secretions, and those in whom problems with the airway or intubation are anticipated. Sedatives are avoided in patients with potential upper airway obstruction.

VENOUS ACCESS

Peripheral and central access are often difficult. These patients are frequently obese and, in addition, may possess subcutaneous infiltrates. Cervical abnormalities, including very short necks and, frequently, stabilization devices, may make access to the jugular vein extremely difficult. In these circumstances there may be no option but to use either a femoral or subclavian approach.

INDUCTION

Awake intubation or an inhalational induction with the maintenance of spontaneous respiration are thought to be relatively safe techniques in patients in whom difficulties with airway maintenance or intubation are predicted. Restrictive lung disease, if present, will prolong an inhalational induction. It is vital that muscle relaxants are avoided until it is certain that the patient can be ventilated by mask.

INTUBATION

This can prove to be extremely difficult and exposure of the larynx may prove impossible with a conventional laryngoscope in some dwarfs with very short necks. In these circumstances a short-handled laryngoscope may enable visualization of the glottis, but if this fails then fibre-optic guided intubation either awake or under general anaesthesia will be required. In patients with foramen magnum stenosis or atlantoaxial instability it is important to avoid neck movements during attempts at intubation, and under these circumstances fibre-optic control of the airway may be preferable.

There is some controversy as to the selection of correct size of tracheal tube. For achondroplastics the formula

$$\frac{\text{Age}}{4} + 4$$

usually correctly predicts the internal diameter correctly. In extreme circumstances a tracheostomy may be necessary, but in patients with mucopolysaccharidoses this may not completely relieve the tracheal obstruction due to distal tracheal distortion.

RESPIRATORY SUPPORT

The low FRC and high closing volume frequently found in dwarfs with respiratory involvement predisposes these patients to atelectasis and V/Q mismatching. This may cause severe problems with oxygenation and renders the use of pulse oximetry and capnography mandatory. For all but the shortest and simplest surgical procedures, arterial canulation for intra- and post-operative blood gas estimation is strongly recommended for any dwarf with respiratory dysfunction. Postoperative ventilation, which can be prolonged, may be required, especially in patients with thoracic dystrophy.

CARDIOVASCULAR PROBLEMS

The assistance of a cardiologist is frequently required to delineate the extent of cardiac compromise. Pulmonary hypertension is the most frequent cardiovascular complication seen in dwarfs and requires careful consideration. Clinical suspicion may be raised by the presence of a parasternal heave, a loud widely split second heart sound and a pulmonary systolic ejection murmur. Right ventricular enlargement can be confirmed either by electrocardiography or echocardiography. In patients with pulmonary hypertension the anaesthetic has to be planned to avoid pulmonary arterial vasoconstriction whilst still maintaining an adequate cardiac output. Care must be taken to avoid respiratory or metabolic acidosis which can cause profound rises in pulmonary artery pressures. In mildly affected individuals oxygen and halothane or isoflurane anaesthetics are often used. In patients with right ventricular failure, high-dose narcotic techniques are preferred. In children, ketamine has been safely used, even in cases with right ventricular failure, although this is not recommended in adults. In patients with congenital heart lesions, or corrected lesions, endocarditis prophylaxis is mandatory.

NEUROLOGICAL PROBLEMS

Most of these problems revolve around the stability of the cervical spine, especially at the atlantoaxial and craniocervical junctions, and problems with raised intracranial pressure (ICP). In patients with spinal cord compression an autonomic hyperreflexic state may develop.

The problems of anaesthetizing a dwarf with raised ICP are formidable: an inhalational induction can be associated with hypercapnia and a rise in ICP, whilst an intravenous induction can be associated with apnoea in a patient who cannot be intubated or ventilated. These patients thus require consideration on a case-by-case basis.

Rarely, hyperthermia, usually without the clinical features of malignant hyperthermia (MH), develops. Therapy consists of simple cooling measures alone. A few cases that are clinically indistinguishable from MH have been observed in patients with osteogenesis imperfecta. It was only by muscle biopsy that the diagnosis was able to be refuted. Thus potential trigger agents do not need to be avoided unless MH is clinically suspected.

BLEEDING PROBLEMS

Osteogenesis imperfecta is the only chondrodystrophy associated with a coagulopathy. These patients require formal evaluation with a bleeding time preoperatively. Platelets and fresh frozen plasma should be available.

BIBLIOGRAPHY

Berkowitz I D, Raja S N, Bender K S, Kopits S E. Dwarfs: pathophysiology and anesthetic implications. Anesthesiology 1990; 73: 739–759

Borland L M. Anesthesia for children with Jeunne's syndrome (asphyxiating thoracic dystrophy). Anesthesiology 1987; 66: 86–88

Walts L F, Finerman G, Wyatt G M. Anaesthesia for dwarfs and other patients of small stature. Canadian Journal of Anaesthesia 1975; 22: 703–709

CROSS REFERENCES

Pulmonary hypertension
Patient Conditions 4: 118
Cardiomyopathy
Patient Conditions 4: 103
Adult congenital heart disease
Patient Conditions 4: 92
Monitoring
Anaesthetic Factors 31: 583
Difficult airway – overview
Anaesthetic Factors 30: 558

MARFAN'S SYNDROME

V. Taylor

Marfan's syndrome is a generalized connective tissue disorder. It is inherited as an autosomal dominant trait, with variable expression. Its incidence is 1–6 per 100 000 births. The mean age of death is early in the fourth decade, often from cardiovascular causes.

PATHOPHYSIOLOGY

Cardiovascular manifestations

There is degeneration of the media of the pulmonary artery, aorta and distal arteries, leading to 'cystic medial necrosis' and weakness. This causes aneurysm formation, especially in the aortic root and the ascending aorta. The dilatation of the aortic root leads to aortic regurgitation, ventricular hypertrophy, dilatation, mitral valve regurgitation, heart failure and angina. There may be mitral regurgitation due to stretching of the chordae tendineae, and dilatation of the pulmonary artery. Conduction abnormalities are seen (especially bundle branch block).

Dissection of an aneurysm may cause aortic regurgitation or it may extend into the pericardium with cardiac tamponade. Intimal tears with dissection may occur in the absence of an aneurysm.

Skeletal manifestations

There is disproportionate growth of long bones, leading to arachnodactyly with hyperextensible joints, which are prone to dislocation. Patients have high arched palates. Kyphoscoliosis and pectus excavatum may be present.

Respiratory manifestations

Patients with Marfan's syndrome are prone to develop emphysema, accentuating the lung defect secondary to kyphoscoliosis. Spontaneous pneumothorax may occur.

Ocular manifestations

These include lens dislocation, myopia, retinal detachment and cataracts.

PREOPERATIVE ASSESSMENT

Particular attention should be paid to cardiopulmonary investigations. These should include chest X-ray, ECG, echocardiography, lung function tests and arterial blood gas estimation.

Vital capacity and FEV_1 may appear to be lower than expected when compared with predicted values, due to greater height or arm span.

PERIOPERATIVE MANAGEMENT

Prophylactic antibiotics must be given due to the high risk of bacterial endocarditis.

Careful handling and positioning are essential to avoid joint trauma and dislocation.

Intubation may be difficult, and the temporomandibular joint may sublux.

Surges of blood pressure should be avoided, e.g. on laryngoscopy or in response to surgical stimulation. Beta blockade will reduce aortic wall tension. Blood pressure should be maintained with the diastolic pressure high enough to ensure good coronary flow, but not too high so as to risk dissection. There may be little cardiac reserve, and volatile agents may be very depressant.

Spontaneous pneumothorax may become a tension pneumothorax in a patient on positive pressure ventilation.

The risk of malignant hyperthermia may be increased.

Monitoring:

- ECG
- Pulse oximetry
- Capnography
- Airway pressures

- Arterial cannulation (but increased risk of morbidity because of weak arterial wall)
- Temperature.

CHOICE OF ANAESTHETIC

The choice of anaesthetic technique is broad and no one agent or technique is suggested. Following careful induction with thiopentone, propofol or etomidate while monitoring blood pressure, anaesthesia may be maintained with nitrous oxide/oxygen/narcotic/muscle relaxant/volatile agent. Blood pressure may be further controlled by beta blockade, if needed. Care must be taken to maintain intravascular volumes and filling pressure.

BIBLIOGRAPHY

Katz J, Benumof J L, Kadis L B (eds). Anaesthesia and uncommon diseases, 3rd edn. W B Saunders, Philadelphia, 1990; p 144–145, 294–295

Steolting R K, Dierdors S F, McCammon R L (eds). Anaesthesia and co-existing disease, 2nd edn. Churchill Livingstone, Edinburgh, 1988; p 640–641

CROSS REFERENCES

Restrictive lung disease 3: 80
Aortic valve disease
Patient Conditions 4: 95
Cardiac conduction defects
Patient Conditions 4: 99
Mitral valve disease
Patient Conditions 4: 114
Cataract surgery
Surgical Procedures 13: 288
Abdominal aortic reconstruction – elective
Surgical Procedures 22: 446

METABOLIC AND DEGENERATIVE BONE DISEASE

A. T. Lovell

OSTEOMALACIA

Osteomalacia is a metabolic disease of bone in which normal bone is replaced by unmineralized osteoid. When this condition occurs in children the disease is called rickets. Clinically it can be extremely difficult to differentiate osteomalacia and osteoporosis. The finding of a low serum phosphate suggests osteomalacia, but the only certain diagnostic method is to take a bone biopsy.

Osteomalacia is caused by an inadequate level of 1,25-dihydrocholecalciferol (1,25-DHCC); this is an active metabolite of vitamin D. The commonest cause for osteomalacia is deficiency of vitamin D due to diet or inadequate exposure to sunlight. Rarely, malabsorption can interfere with absorption of vitamin D leading to osteomalacia. Severe renal disease is a potent cause of osteomalacia because 25-hydroxycholecalciferol is only converted to the active 1,25-DHCC in the kidney. Osteomalacia may develop in patients on long-term therapy with drugs that induce the hepatic mixed function oxidase, because this interferes with vitamin D metabolism.

Treatment is based on replacement of vitamin D. This may be administered either as calciferol or the active metabolite 1-α-cholecalciferol. Any replacement therapy must be closely monitored since there is a risk of hypercalcaemia developing. Calcium supplements are only used if the patient is hypocalcaemic.

Anaesthetic problems of osteomalacia:
- Abnormal drug metabolism of mixed function oxidase induced
- Potential for hypercalcaemia if on therapy with vitamin D supplements
- Great care with positioning (fractures can easily occur)
- Deformity, if occurs before epiphyseal fusion.

OSTEOPOROSIS

In osteoporosis the overall quantity of bone is reduced, whilst its shape, composition and morphology remain normal. It generally occurs in elderly Europeans, especially women. The commonest precipitating factor is the menopausal withdrawal of oestrogens. However, endocrinopathies, long-term corticosteroid therapy and immobilization can also result in osteoporosis. The net effect appears to be a relative overactivity of the osteoclasts, leading to bone loss. Because of the bone loss, fractures occur far more readily, frequently after minimal trauma.

Common sites of fractures in osteoporosis:
- Vertebrae (usually crush or wedge fractures)
- Neck of femur
- Distal radius
- Proximal humerus
- Pelvis.

Multiple vertebral fractures leading to a kyphosis are not uncommon. This may be associated with marked respiratory impairment. Despite their frequency it is unusual for vertebral fractures to be associated with serious neurological sequelae, although sciatica is common.

Treatment is unsatisfactorily since no long-term study has shown an increase in bone density. Patients may require surgical stabilization, but any immobilization tends to worsen the conditions. Current attempts are directed at prevention by increasing the bone mass before the menopause with the aid of calcium supplementation, and to reducing the rate of bone resorption by using hormone replacement therapy.

PAGET'S DISEASE

Paget's disease is a metabolic disease of unknown aetiology. It is characterized by excessively rapid remodelling of bone. The new bone formed is architecturally distorted and its mineralization is defective. The affected bones and bone marrow are initially very vascular. Eventually, the bone may become dense and hard with a reduced vascularity. It is these sclerotic areas that are weak and lead to the common complication of fractures.

The incidence of Paget's disease is 2–8% of over 55 year olds and tends to run in families. The most frequently affected sites are the pelvis, femur, tibia, skull and the spine. Because of the involvement of the skull and spine, spinal cord compression, atlantoaxial instability and brainstem compression may develop.

Patients may be asymptomatic, but commonly bone pain or fractures are the presenting feature. Occasionally, patients present in high output cardiac failure due to the increased bone vascularity. The mechanism of the high output failure is uncertain.

Specific treatment is indicated for patients with symptoms or complications of the disease. Calcitonin, which acts primarily as an inhibitor of bone resorption, has been used in patients with bone pain and before orthopaedic procedures to reduce the vascularity of the bone. Increasingly, the diphosphonates are being used to control bone pain, their effect often far outlasting the duration of treatment. Mithramycin has been used for the rapid control of bone pain and in the presence of spinal cord compression.

Anaesthetic management of Paget's disease:
- Careful evaluation for atlantoaxial and craniocervical instability.
- Assess lung function in patients with a kyphosis.
- Cardiac failure, if present, must be treated.
- Careful moving and positioning of the patient (fractures occur very easily).
- General or regional techniques may be used. Spinal and epidural placement can be difficult. Most dental cases are performed under general anaesthesia because extractions are difficult and the risk of postoperative bleeding is increased.
- Corticosteroid treatment may be required, depending upon previous treatment.
- Consideration should be given to the use of calcitonin before major orthopaedic procedures.

OSTEOARTHRITIS

Osteoarthritis is the commonest degenerative

disease articular cartilage. Unlike rheumatoid arthritis there is minimal inflammatory reaction. The aetiology is unclear, but may be related to joint trauma. The incidence rises with increasing age. There are changes in the surrounding joint capsule and bone with an increase in bone vascularity.

Patients usually complain of pain on motion, and of stiffness that improves with use. Characteristically, the hip and knee joints are involved, but there may be involvement of the distal interphalangeal joints and degeneration of the spine. The middle and lower cervical spinal and lower lumbar spine are the areas most likely to be involved. Spinal cord compression or nerve root compression can occur due to degenerative disks. Spinal fusion is rare. Frequently, asymptomatic changes are found on radiographs.

Treatment of osteoarthritis is symptomatic, using physiotherapy and NSAIDs. Corticosteroids are not used since they are associated with a worsening of the degenerative process. Reconstructive joint surgery has much to offer these patients, but can be associated with considerable blood loss and carries a high risk of thromboembolic phenomena. The use of regional anaesthesia for these procedures, either alone or in combination with general anaesthesia, has been shown to reduce the blood loss and to decrease the incidence of deep venous thrombosis from 33% to 9%. Many centres additionally use graduated compression stockings and heparin prophylaxis in an attempt to further reduce the incidence of thromboembolism.

CROSS REFERENCES

Repair of fractured neck of femur
Surgical Procedures 24: 479
Epidural and spinal anaesthesia
Anaesthetic Factors 32: 594

RHEUMATOID DISEASE

C. Hamilton-Davies

Rheumatoid disease is a systemic chronic inflammatory disease affecting up to 3% of women and 1% of men in the UK. It may involve every organ system in the body, but of particular relevance to the anaesthetist are the disorders of the musculoskeletal system and the respiratory system. These patients present for surgery commonly due to the degenerative nature of the condition.

PATHOPHYSIOLOGY

Musculoskeletal

The destructive synovitis associated with rheumatoid disease attacks the small joints of the hands, ankles, knees, temporomandibular joints, wrists, elbows and joints of the spinal column. The disease is believed to have an autoimmune component and progresses until the inflammation eventually moves into a fibrotic phase, leaving characteristic fixed deformities in the joints of the hands. The cervical spine is involved in the disease process in up to 80% of affected individuals, with 30% showing clinical signs of cervical spine instability. Involvement of the temporomandibular and cricoarytenoid joints are also commonly seen.

Respiratory

Pleural disease occurs in 3–12.5% of patients, with rheumatoid disease being more common in men. Rib-cage stiffness and interstitial lung fibrosis combine to produce a restrictive picture of lung disease. Other pulmonary manifestations include the presence of rheumatoid nodules in the lungs that may rupture or cavitate and become sites of infection. Pulmonary vasculitis should be considered as a potential cause of pulmonary hypertension. Iatrogenic pulmonary disease occurs in up to 5% of patients treated with methotrexate, and appears as a progressive interstitial fibrosis. Sulphasalazine, a drug whose use has become more commonplace in the management of rheumatoid arthritis over the past decade, may lead to the development of eosinophilic pneumonitis.

Cardiovascular

The prevalence of cardiovascular disorders has been estimated to be up to 35%, with pericardial disease being the most common. Of rheumatoid patients, 1%–5% have mitral valve disease, with other valves being less commonly involved. Direct myocardial involvement rarely causes symptoms, although involvement of the conduction pathways may lead to heart block. Systemic vasculitis is rare but is more common in patients with high titres of rheumatoid factor. Symptoms of mononeuritis multiplex indicate neurovascular involvement and indicate extensive, severe, vasculitic disease.

Haemopoietic

A mild normocytic anaemia is common in rheumatoid patients and tends to correlate with disease activity. It is important that other causes of anaemia are excluded, in particular bleeding from the gastrointestinal tract secondary to either steroid or NSAID therapy. The normal responses to infection may not be present due to concomitant immuno-suppressive therapy. Methotrexate therapy may induce bone marrow suppression.

Other

Gastrointestinal symptoms are generally secondary to drug therapy, NSAIDs and steroids causing ulceration, azathioprine leading to nausea and vomiting and possibly even pancreatitis, and oral gold therapy causing irritation of the gut.

Renal impairment may occur secondary to gold or NSAIDs. Recently, the use of cyclosporin in rheumatoid disease has been considered, but renal toxicity will probably limit its use.

Methotrexate therapy alters the hepatic metabolism of coumarin anticoagulants, thereby potentiating their effects, and causes gastrointestinal disturbances in a large proportion of patients.

PREOPERATIVE ASSESSMENT

Morphological:

- Neck movement/mouth opening/dentition
- Veins/arteries/bruising
- Presence of painful joints and limitations
- Suitability for regional technique.

History:

- Complete neurological, respiratory and cardiovascular history
- Drug history
- Previous anaesthetic problems.

Investigations

See Table 1.

Table 1.
Investigations and results

Investigations	Result
Full blood count	Anaemia normochromic, normocytic (severe, hypochromic – ? gastrointestinal bleed)
Urea and electrolytes	Abnormal (iatrogenic – gold, cyclosporin)
ECG	Heart block Ischaemic (arteritis) Left ventricular hypertrophy – (valvular heart disease)
Chest X-ray	Rheumatoid nodules
Cervical spine X-ray (? lateral and odontoid views)	Atlantoaxial subluxation; subatlanto axial subluxation
Spirometry	Restrictive flow pattern
Indirect laryngoscopy	Degree of cricoarytenoid involvement

PERIOPERATIVE MANAGEMENT

Consideration should be given to performing the procedure under local or regional blockade if feasible, as this will avoid the need for airway manipulation. However, the involvement of the spine may make epidural or spinal anaesthesia difficult if not impossible. Maintenance of awkward positions for surgery may not be feasible in the rheumatoid patient, due to discomfort.

If general anaesthesia is to be used then the cervical spine and airway are the areas likely to cause most concern.

Premedication

If fibre-optic intubation is to be performed or difficulty with intubation is anticipated, then an antisialogogue should be prescribed.

Cervical spine

On induction of anaesthesia the cervical spine will lose any protective spasm around the unstable neck, and thus it is important to determine the range of comfortable neck movement before induction and limit it to this with the use of sandbags, etc. If tracheal intubation is necessary it may be that with severe cervical spine involvement early consideration should be given to awake fibre-optic intubation.

Where intubation is not required, then oropharyngeal or nasopharyngeal airways may reduce the amount of cervical manipulation required. The laryngeal mask is useful in longer procedures, although the larynx may be displaced in cervical spine disease, making placement difficult.

Airway

Temporomandibular joint involvement may lead to difficulty in mouth opening and forward jaw protrusion, thus leading to difficulty in inserting a laryngoscope as well as viewing the larynx. Anticipated problems or previous difficulty should lead to early consideration of the fibre-optic laryngoscope.

Conduct of anaesthesia

There are no restrictions on anaesthetic agents used in rheumatoid disease, although iatrogenic, hepatic or renal disease may alter the amount of free drug available and increments should be administered with care.

Great care should be taken to protect the joints during anaesthesia, with careful handing and positioning of the patient and protection of pressure points.

Mechanical ventilation may be necessary in those patients with severe pulmonary disease.

POSTOPERATIVE MANAGEMENT

Analgesia is the main problem in the postoperative period, as these patients tend to be more sensitive to opioids. Patient-controlled analgesia (PCA) may be difficult for the rheumatoid patient due to hand deformities. Regional blockade may provide the optimal form of analgesia in this group of patients, if appropriate.

Early physiotherapy is indicated, both to prevent chest infections in a patient that has a restrictive lung defect, and thus a propensity to develop atelectasis, and for a patient who is more difficult to mobilize due to musculoskeletal dysfunction.

Steroid cover should be continued where indicated, and there should be close monitoring of renal function, especially if preoperative dysfunction was present.

LONG-TERM MANAGEMENT

These patients tend to require multiple surgical procedures due to the relentless progression of their disease. Careful attention should be paid to previous anaesthetic notes and any problems with intubation, analgesia, etc., noted.

BIBLIOGRAPHY

Helmers R, Galvin J, Hunninghake G W. Pulmonary manifestations associated with rheumatoid arthritis. Chest 100: 235–238

Macarthur A, Kleiman S. Rheumatoid cervical joint disease – a challenge to the anaesthetist. Canadian Journal of Anaesthesia 1993; 40: 154–159

Skues M A, Welchew E A. Anaesthesia and rheumatoid arthritis. Anaesthesia 1993; 48: 989–997

CROSS REFERENCES

Mitral valve disease
Patient Conditions 4: 114
Anaemia
Patient Conditions 7: 168
Iatrogenic adrenocortical insufficiency
Patient Conditions 2: 54
Athroscopy
Surgical Procedures 24: 476
Difficult and failed intubation
Surgical Procedures 20: 408

SCOLIOSIS

W. E. Edge

Scoliosis is a complex deformity of growth of the vertebral column resulting in lateral curvature and rotation of the vertebrae. The spinous processes rotate toward the concavity of the curve. In the thoracic spine, scoliosis results in abnormal development of the thoracic cage and, consequently, abnormalities of respiratory and cardiovascular function.

AETIOLOGY

Scoliosis is a sign, not a disease. It may arise from several different causes; although presentation, complications and management may be similar, the prognosis may differ greatly for different aetiologies. The anaesthetic relevance of identifying the aetiology lies in the recognition of problems associated with the underlying cause.

CLASSIFICATION OF SCOLIOSIS

Functional scoliosis

Secondary to discordant leg length, etc. Curve disappears when patient lies down.

Structural scoliosis

There are three main groups:

- *Congenital* – associated with vertebral anomalies. May have abnormalities of the heart and genitourinary tract.
- *Idiopathic* – accounts for 60–80% of cases and has the best prognosis of all aetiologies. This is a diagnosis of exclusion.
- *Neuromuscular* – scoliosis occurring secondary to a neuropathy (upper or lower motor neurone or other neuropathy) e.g. cerebral palsey, poliomyelitis, etc., or myopathy, e.g. Duchenne's muscular dystrophy. This group includes many of the syndromes associated with scoliosis, e.g. Prader–Willi syndrome.

In addition:

- *Mesenchymal* – abnormalities of the tissues, e.g. Marfan's syndrome, Ehlers–Danlos syndrome.
- *Trauma.*
- *Tumours* – intraspinal or skeletal.
- *Metabolic* – this category includes several miscellaneous causes, e.g. rickets, hyperphosphatasia.

The severity of scoliosis can be defined by the Cobb angle (Figure 1) which is measured from an anteroposterior radiograph of the spine. The first line is taken from the most tilted vertebral body above the scoliosis and extended laterally. The second line is taken from the most tilted vertebra below the scoliosis. The measured angle is at the intersection of these two lines. Although occasional patients may have a scoliosis which is largely in the lumbar region, it is more often the case that the thoracic vertebrae are involved. In these circumstances, the larger the angle, the more severe is the scoliosis and the greater the likelihood of compromised respiratory and cardiovascular function.

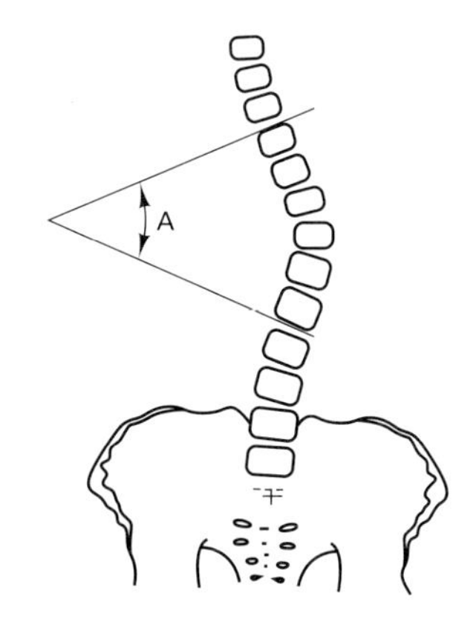

Figure 1
The Cobb angle (A).

PATHOPHYSIOLOGY

Respiratory system

Respiratory impairment usually shows a restrictive pattern, with lung volumes being related inversely to the angle of curvature. Vital capacity is the most severely affected, but total lung capacity and functional residual capacity are also reduced. The abnormalities of rib-cage development cause abnormal development of the underlying lung, with alveolar volume being compressed to, or below, FRC. Rib abnormalities result in mechanical disadvantage of muscles of respiration and reduced chest wall compliance. This results is alveolar hypoventilation. The commonest arterial blood gas abnormality is a reduced $P_{a}O_2$.

Associated with the compressed alveoli is restricted development of the pulmonary vascular bed and diversion of blood into high-resistance extra-alveolar vessels. The resulting ventilation/perfusion mismatch causes an increased alveolar to arterial oxygen gradient and exacerbates the alveolar hypoventilation. An increase in $P_{a}CO_2$ occurs late and is a poor prognostic indicator. In addition, patients with scoliosis have a decreased respiratory sensitivity to elevated $P_{a}CO_2$.

Cardiovascular system

Thoracic scoliosis of any aetiology may result in right-sided cardiac problems. The ventilation/perfusion mismatch causes an increased pulmonary vascular resistance.

Low lung volumes, chronic hypoxia and abnormal development of the pulmonary vascular bed all contribute to these changes. Right atrial dilatation and right ventricular hypertrophy are late in appearance. ECG changes are rare and occur late.

PREOPERATIVE ASSESSMENT

Assessment involves determining the aetiology of the scoliosis and associated problems.

Assessment of respiratory function:

- Exercise tolerance.
- Chest expansion and ability to cough.
- Formal lung function tests – if the scoliosis is <65° or lung function tests are greater than 30% of the predicted value, ventilation problems are rare. If VC <30% the patient is more likely to need postoperative mechanical ventilation.
- Arterial blood gas measurements – if the patient is unable to perform lung function tests or has scoliosis >65°.

Assessment of cardiac function:

- Clinical examination – right ventricular enlargement, loud pulmonic second sound, murmur of pulmonary insufficiency.
- ECG – P wave >2.5 mm and R<S in V_1 and V_2. These changes are rare and occur late.
- Echocardiography – a more sensitive detector of cardiac abnormalities secondary to pulmonary hypertension.

PERIOPERATIVE MANAGEMENT

Premedication

Narcotics should be avoided if there is significant respiratory impairment (curve >60 or lung function <30% predicted). Consider an anticholinergic if cough is inadequate or there are problems clearing secretions.

Monitoring

Monitoring should be started in the anaesthetic room.

- ECG
- SaO_2
- BP – arterial cannulation is useful both for measuring blood pressure and for postoperative measuring of arterial blood gasses.
- Core temperature – there is a higher incidence of malignant hyperthermia in patients with scoliosis.
- Nasogastric tube – decompression of the stomach assists ventilation, and distraction of the spine may be associated with the development of paralytic ileus.
- Consider: central venous pressure and urine output monitoring, particularly for surgery associated with high blood loss.

Anaesthesia

- Hyperkalaemia may occur following the use of suxamethonium in patients with neuromuscular problems.
- Rhabdomyolysis and myoglobinuria may occur following the use of suxamethonium and halothane in patients with myopathies.

SURGERY – GENERAL

Evidence of pulmonary hypertension or right ventricular hypertrophy carry a poor prognosis. Right ventricular failure must be treated before surgery.

There is no specific contraindication to local or regional anaesthesia.

SURGERY – FOR SCOLIOSIS

Aims:
- Correction of curve
- Prevention of progression of curve
- Relief or prevention of back pain
- Cosmetic.

Patients usually present for corrective surgery before the onset of pulmonary hypertension. Surgery may be via an anterior approach, posterior approach, or both (carried out as two separate procedures several days apart or during a single session). The anterior approach requires access to the vertebrae on the convex side of the curve. This is achieved via thoracotomy and costectomy and usually precedes posterior fusion. The posterior approach requires the patient to be placed prone with all its attendant problems.

Anaesthetic – specific considerations

- Blood loss may be considerable and rapid. Hypotensive techniques have been associated with spinal cord ischaemia and paresis.
- Postoperative pain, hypoventilation and atelectasis are severe following thoracotomy. Thoracic epidural analgesia provides good operating conditions and excellent pain relief and may be continued for several days postoperatively.
- Anaesthesia must facilitate spinal cord monitoring ('wake-up' test, sensory or motor evoked potentials). Total intravenous anaesthesia using an infusion of propofol is a suitable technique.

POSTOPERATIVE CARE

- ITU or HDU following corrective scoliosis surgery, major general surgery and minor surgery under general anaesthesia if there is significant respiratory or cardiovascular compromise
- Postoperative IPPV may be required
- Continuous oxygen therapy
- Regular physiotherapy
- Analgesia.

BIBLIOGRAPHY

Kafer E R. Respiratory and cardiovascular functions in scoliosis and the principles of anaesthetic management. Anesthiology 1980; 52: 339–351

Sharrad W J W. Congenital and developmental abnormalities of the spine. In: Paediatric orthopaedics and fractures, 3rd edn. Blackwell Scientific, Oxford, 1993, vol 1, p 556–659

CROSS REFERENCES

Muscular dystrophies
Patient Conditions 2: 60
Restrictive lung disease
Patient Conditions 3: 80
Marfan's syndrome
Patient Conditions 8: 199

9

CONNECTIVE TISSUES

G. B. Smith

BULLOUS AND VESICULAR SKIN DISORDERS OTHER THAN EPIDERMOLYSIS BULLOSA

J. Powell

Pemphigus and *pemphigoid* are rare autoimmune conditions characterized by a bullous eruption of the skin and mucous membranes. There are several variants of each disease. In pemphigus, blisters form intra-dermally; in pemphigoid, lesions occur at the dermal–epidermal junction.

Erythema multiforme (EM) is more common and is an acute, self-limiting eruption of the skin and mucous membranes. Stevens–Johnson syndrome is a more severe form of EM, with involvement of mucosal surfaces and viscera in association with marked constitutional symptoms.

PATHOPHYSIOLOGY

Pemphigus vulgaris is the most common form of pemphigus and occurs predominantly in patients of Mediterranean or Jewish origin, with a peak incidence between 30 and 50 years of age. It was uniformly fatal before the advent of steroid therapy. There is a familial tendency and an increased incidence of HLA-13 amongst affected individuals. There may be an association with other autoimmune diseases such as thymoma, myasthenia gravis and systemic lupus erythematosus. The large (>1 cm), superficial, flaccid blisters may occur spontaneously or in response to trauma and are found in the groins, axillae and over the trunk. Oral lesions may predate the cutaneous bullae by several months. Pressure with torsion may result in blister formation in normal looking skin (Nikolsky's sign). The bullae are fragile, rupturing easily with coincident loss of large areas of skin; healing occurs without scarring. Lesions may occur on the lips and in the mouth, nose, pharynx and larynx causing difficulty in eating and hoarseness. *Pemphigus vegetans* has a course similar to pemphigus vulgaris.

In some variants of pemphigus, e.g. *pemphigus erythematosus* and *pemphigus foliaceous*, bullous formation occurs more superficially within the epidermis. These forms tend to be less severe.

There are two forms of pemphigoid – *bullous pemphigoid* and *cicatricial pemphigoid*. Bullous pemphigoid is clinically similar to pemphigus, but occurs predominantly in patients over 50 years of age. Untreated, it follows a chronic relapsing course and the mortality is low. It tends to be self-limiting and the patient's health remains good. The characteristic feature of the condition is large, tense bullae, often occurring on the inner aspects of the thighs, on the flexor surfaces of the forearms, axillae and groins and over the lower abdomen. The oral cavity may be affected but, unlike pemphigus, is rarely the initial manifestation. Blister formation is thought to result from the activation of complement in association with neutrophil and eosinophil migration. *Cicatricial pemphigoid* is rare and primarily affects the mucous membranes. Skin is involved in 10–30% of cases, but rarely in the absence of mucosal lesions. It is a chronic condition and the lesions usually heal with scarring. This may lead to nasal obstruction, dysphagia and laryngeal stenosis. Blindness may complicate ocular involvement.

Treatment in both pemphigus and pemphigoid is with steroids and, occasionally, other immunosuppressant drugs, e.g. methotrexate, azathioprine or cyclophosphamide. Lower doses of corticosteroids are used in pemphigoid. Gold injections and plasmapheresis may also be used in pemphigus.

Erythema multiforme is characterized by the distinctive target or iris lesions. Of cases of EM, 50% have no identifiable cause but, for the rest, a wide variety of triggers, including infective agents, drugs and neoplasms, has been described. Those of particular importance to the anaesthetist include barbiturates, antibiotics, anticonvulsants, antipyretics and cimetidine. The pathogenesis of EM is not fully understood, but there is evidence that it may be a hypersensitivity reaction. It may present in various forms (hence its name), ranging from a mild, self-limited, skin eruption through to the Stevens–Johnson syndrome (SJS) with its systemic involvement and high mortality (5–15%) if untreated. EM may present as symmetrical target lesions (dull red macules up to 2 cm in diameter with a clear centre) on the extensor surfaces of the extremities, as a series of urticarial plaques or with vesicle or bullae formation.

The SJS has a prodrome lasting up to 14 days consisting of fever, malaise, myalgia, arthralgia, respiratory and gastrointestinal symptoms. It is followed by the explosive eruption of bullous lesions of the mouth, lips and conjunctivae, and variable skin involvement. In severe cases the oesophagus and respiratory tree are involved. Pneumonitis, pleural effusions and bullae of the visceral pleura are seen, the latter occasionally leading to pneumothorax or even bronchopleural fistula. Myocarditis, atrial fibrillation and renal failure are recognized complications. There may also be anaemia and fluid and electrolyte imbalance. Treatment in SJS is supportive, although steroids have also been used for SJS and in severe cases of EM.

PREOPERATIVE ASSESSMENT

History and examination:

- Fully assess the disease together with its extent and the duration of the illness. In particular, assess the distribution and severity of lesions, especially those involving the airway.
- Assess nutritional state.
- Note drug therapy and dose, especially systemic corticosteroids and immunosuppressants.
- Consider the effects of plasmapheresis on cholinesterase levels in pemphigus.

Investigations:

- Full blood count
  - Anaemia may occur in SJS
  - Leucopenia and thrombocytopenia may result from immunosuppressant therapy.
- Urea and electrolytes – abnormalities may exist in SJS or as a result of steroid therapy.
- Assess renal function, especially in SJS.
- Blood glucose – may be raised due to steroid therapy.
- Flow-volume loops may be of use where upper respiratory tract stenosis is suspected.
- Consider cholinesterase activity following plasmapheresis.

Premedication:

- Ensure that premedication is sufficient to prevent struggling during induction. Struggling may risk new bullous formation.
- The intramuscular route might appear unsuitable for fear of inducing new lesions; however, when intramuscular premedication has been used in pemphigus and SJS, new bullae formation has not been reported.

PERIOPERATIVE MANAGEMENT

Induction:

- Intramuscular ketamine has been used successfully in pemphigus and SJS.
- Suture intravenous cannulae in place or secure with vaseline gauze and ties.
- Avoid barbiturates in EM or SJS.
- For children, encourage the presence of parents in the anaesthetic room in order to reduce the chances of struggling and restlessness on induction, thereby reducing chances of blister formation.

Airway considerations

A major concern in all the blistering diseases must be the potential to cause new bullae during airway manipulation or intubation. Insufficient data exist to assess the true risks, and consequently manoeuvres to avoid unnecessary airway manipulation are advised.

- Use face-masks with a soft air cushion.
- Pad face-masks with vaseline gauze.
- Place vaseline gauze under chin to protect skin from anaesthetist's fingers.
- If possible, avoid the use of airway adjuncts, such as Guedel airways.
- An inhalational induction may be required where laryngeal stenosis is present. Helium/oxygen mixtures may help.
- Consider the use of an 'anaesthetic hood' for inhalational induction.
- Protect front of neck with vaseline gauze if cricoid pressure must be employed.
- Laryngoscopy and oral intubation may be difficult in all of the blistering diseases due to pre-existing airway bullae.
- Laryngeal stenosis has been reported in SJS and cicatricial pemphigoid. The use of small uncuffed endotracheal tubes may be necessary.

- The use of nasotracheal tubes has not been reported in pemphigus, pemphigoid, EM or SJS.
- Secure endotracheal tubes with simple ties rather than with adhesive tape.

Maintenance:
- IPPV may be hazardous in SJS because of the risk of pneumothoraces/bronchopleural fistulae
- Drug disposition will be affected by hypoalbuminaemia and renal disease in SJS
- Intravenous ketamine and diazepam infusions, in the absence of intubation, have proven useful in SJS.

Regional techniques:
- Intrathecal and epidural anaesthetic techniques appear safe in pemphigus and pemphigoid. No new lesions have occurred at the sites of spinal needle insertion.
- Modifications should be made to the skin cleansing routine, e.g.:
  - Soak skin using betadine swabs or pour betadine over skin
  - Avoid skin scrubbing
  - Avoid subcutaneous injections of local anaesthetic solutions.
- Use EMLA cream for skin anaesthesia.

Monitoring:
- Well-padded noninvasive BP cuffs do not appear to cause bullae, probably because direct pressure is less harmful in EB than frictional or shearing forces
- Pulse oximeters can be attached to the patient using simple clips rather than adhesive or tape
- Use ECG pads without adhesive; needle ECG electrodes may be an alternative
- A weighted untaped precordial stethoscope may be useful
- Arterial lines may be of considerable use; secure with sutures.

Positioning:
- Keep sheets and other linen free from creases
- Pad heals, elbows and bony prominences using foam
- Allow patients to move themselves onto trolleys or the operating table in order to minimize skin trauma
- Inform operating-room staff of the need for special care during patient positioning
- Take care with the positioning of a diathermy pad.

Emergence and recovery:
- Use protective vaseline gauze under oxygen masks
- For children, encourage the presence of parents in the recovery room in order to reduce the chances of struggling and restlessness on emergence
- Regional techniques may allow the provision of high-quality continuous postoperative analgesia.

POSTOPERATIVE MANAGEMENT

- New skin lesions are a common complication
- Continue steroid supplements.

BIBLIOGRAPHY

Cucchiara R F, Dawson B. Anesthesia in Stevens–Johnson syndrome: report of a case. Anesthesiology 1971; 35: 537–539

Drenger B, Zidenbaum M, Reifen E, Leitersdorf. Severe upper airway obstruction and difficult intubation in cicatricial pemphigoid. Anaesthesia 1986; 41: 1029–1031

Prasad K K, Chen L. Anesthetic management of a patient with bullous pemphigoid. Anesthesia and Analgesia 1989; 69: 537–540

Vatashsky E, Aronson H B. Pemphigus vulgaris: anaesthesia in the traumatised patient. Anaesthesia 1982; 37: 1195–1197

CROSS REFERENCES

Iatrogenic adrenocortical insufficiency
Patient Conditions 2: 54
Assessment of renal function
Patient Conditions 6: 155
Anaemia
Patient Conditions 7: 168

DISORDERS OF EPIDERMAL CELL KINETICS AND DIFFERENTIATION

G. B. Smith

Several skin disorders affect the epidermal layer of the skin causing combinations of erythema, scaling and dryness. *Psoriasis* is a skin disorder associated with an increased rate of epidermal protein synthesis which results in rapid epidermal cell growth. *Ichthyosis* is a disorder of keratinization characterized by clinically dry and scaly skin. *Erythroderma* describes a generalized inflammatory disorder in which there is widespread scaling and erythema of skin, occasionally in association with marked systemic effects.

PATHOPHYSIOLOGY

Psoriasis

Psoriasis is a chronic skin disorder, characterized by an accelerated epidermal turnover and epidermal hyperplasia. These are caused by a shortened epidermal cell cycle and an increase in the proliferative cell population. The exact aetiology of psoriasis is unknown, although both genetic and environmental factors are thought to play a part. The lesions, which tend to involve the extensor surfaces (elbows, knees), sacral area and scalp, consist of loosely adherent, thickened, noncoherent, silver skin scales which have an increased vascularity. Mechanical trauma leading to removal of skin causes small blood droplets to appear on the skin (Auspitz's sign). Psoriatic lesions often follow trauma of the skin (Koebner's phenomenon). Psoriatic arthropathy occurs in 5–10% of patients and resembles seronegative rheumatoid arthritis. Psoriasis is also associated with ulcerative colitis and Crohn's disease. Psoriatic lesions have a tendency to increased colonization by bacteria, especially *Staphylococcus aureus*, compared with normal skin. Severe psoriasis may be associated with hyperuricaemia, anaemia (chronic illness, folate or vitamin B_{12} deficiency), negative nitrogen balance, iron loss and hypoalbuminaemia.

Two forms of psoriasis produce marked systemic effects on the body: psoriatic erythroderma (see below) and generalized pustular psoriasis. The latter is characterized by waves of sterile pustules over the skin of the trunk and extremities, together with fever up to 40°C lasting for several days. There may be associated weight loss, muscle weakness, congestive cardiac failure and hypocalcaemia.

The treatment of psoriasis involves the use of topical steroids, coal tar or dithranol, ultraviolet light (with or without a psoralen), retinoids (vitamin A derivatives), cytotoxic agents (e.g. methotrexate, azathioprine) and, recently, cyclosporin A.

Erythroderma

Eyrthroderma (or exfoliative dermatitis) describes a generalized inflammatory disorder in which there is widespread scaling and erythema of the skin. The skin is hot and oedematous, and the disorder is associated with systemic effects, including disturbances of the cardiovascular, thermoregulatory and metabolic systems. In the acute stages of the disorder there may be marked hypothermia, pyrexia-related hypovolaemia and heart failure. The more common causes are psoriasis, eczema, drug reactions and the reticuloses. Normally, total skin blood flow is approximately 1 l min^{-1} at 37°C; however, in erythroderma, this may increase to 5 l min^{-1}, reaching as much as 10 l min^{-1} in the presence of pyrexia. As a result, high output cardiac failure is a risk and may be exacerbated by hypovoalbuminaemia, hypercatabolism and an iron- or folate-deficiency anaemia. Treatment of erythroderma relies on treating the cause of the disorder.

Ichthyosis

Ichthyosis describes a group of conditions which are characterized by the accumulation of large amounts of dry scales on the skin. The most common form is ichthyosis vulgaris, an autosomal dominant disease. Other common forms include X-linked ichthyosis, lamellar ichthyosis (autosomal recessive) and epidermolytic hyperkeratosis (autosomal dominant). Ichthyosis is also seen in association with neoplasia such as lymphoma, multiple myeloma and carcinomas of the lung and breast. Treatment of ichthyosis is directed at increasing the water content of the skin (urea-containing creams), causing separation of the cells using keralytic agents (salicylic acid ointment), or by affecting epidermal metabolism (lactic acid ointment). Occasionally, methotrexate and the retinoids are used.

PREOPERATIVE ASSESSMENT

History and examination:

- Fully assess the disease together with its extent and the duration of the illness. In particular, assess the distribution and severity of lesions.
- Assess nutritional state.
- Assess any cardiovascular dysfunction, e.g. congestive cardiac failure in erythroderma or generalized pustular psoriasis.
- Exclude hypovolaemia (due to increased transepidermal water loss or pyrexia) in erythroderma.
- Check core temperature in eythroderma and pustular psoriasis.
- Note drug therapy and dose, especially immunosuppressants.

Investigations:

- Full blood count:
  - Anaemia may be due to chronic illness or deficiencies of iron, vitamin B_{12} or folate
  - Leucopenia and thrombocytopenia may result from immunosuppressant therapy.
- Urea and electrolytes:
  - Abnormalities may exist in erythroderma
  - Measure calcium levels if hypoalbuminaemia exists.
- Assess renal function in erythroderma.
- ECG and chest X-ray if there is clinical evidence of heart failure.
- Cross-match blood in erythroderma (risk of blood loss).

Premedication

Do not inject intramuscular premedication into areas of psoriasis (risk of Auspitz's phenomenon and infection due to skin colonization).

PERIOPERATIVE MANAGEMENT

Induction:

- Avoid using psoriatic sites for intravenous access (risk of Auspitz's phenomenon and infection due to skin colonization).
- Suture intravenous cannulae in place or secure with vaseline gauze and ties. Adhesive tape is likely to denude skin (ichthyosis or psoriasis), cause bleeding (psoriasis) or the Koebner phenomenon (psoriasis).
- The hyperdynamic circulation in erythroderma may alter the speed of onset of intravenous and inhalational anaesthetic agents.
- Hypervolaemia, hypovolaemia, congestive cardiac failure, hypoalbuminaemia and a reduction in renal blood flow may affect the kinetics of drug distribution and excretion.

Maintenance:

- Hypervolaemia, hypovolaemia, congestive cardiac failure, hypoalbuminaemia and a reduction in renal blood flow may affect the kinetics of drug distribution and excretion.
- The increased skin blood flow and high cardiac output in erythroderma may lead to excessive bleeding during surgery.
- Use space or warming blankets with care in erythroderma because of the risk of hyperthermia. These patients cannot regulate body temperature, have an increased metabolic rate and may not be able to sweat.

Regional techniques:

- Avoid using psoriatic sites for regional techniques (risk of Auspitz's phenomenon and infection due to skin colonization).
- Modifications should be made to the skin-cleansing routine, e.g.:
  - Soak skin using swabs soaked in an aqueous solution of antiseptic or pour solution over skin in ichthyosis (alcohol-based solutions may cause intense pain)
  - Avoid skin scrubbing.
- Secure extradural catheters using bandage, as adhesive tape may cause skin loss.

Monitoring:

- Central venous pressure monitoring will be of use in erythroderma where fluid replacement must be undertaken with care
- Use ECG pads without adhesive in ichthyosis/erythroderma

- A weighted untaped precordial stethoscope may be useful in ichthyosis/erythroderma
- Monitor core temperature in erythroderma
- BP cuffs may cause the Koebner phenomenon.

BIBLIOGRAPHY

Love J B, Wright C A, Hooke D H et al. Exfoliative dermatitis as a risk factor for epidemic spread of methicillin resistant *Staphylococcus aureus*. Intensive Care Medicine 1992; 18: 189

Smart G, Bradshaw E G. Extradural analgesia and ichthyosis. Anaesthesia 1984; 39: 161–162

CROSS REFERENCES

Assessment of renal function
Patient Conditions 6: 155
Anaemia
Patient Conditions 7: 168

EHLERS–DANLOS SYNDROME

G. Krishnakumar

Ehlers–Danlos syndrome (EDS) consists of a group of hereditary disorders of connective tissue characterized by hypermobile joints, extensibility and fragility of skin, and easy bruising. The syndrome is divided into nine distinct types (I to IX) depending on biochemical studies, the severity of joint and skin manifestations and the degree of involvement of other tissues and organs.

PATHOPHYSIOLOGY

In most forms of EDS, the condition is inherited as an autosomal trait. Specific mutations of some of the 20 collagen genes have been described in most of the different types of EDS. Variations in the specific types of collagen involved and their distribution in different tissues result in diverse clinical manifestations (Table 1). Type-IV EDS (ecchymotic form), due to abnormalities in type-III collagen, is the most severe form.

Other features of EDS include cardiac conduction defects, mitral valve prolapse, pes planus, scoliosis, herniae, bladder diverticuli, pulmonary emphysema, spontaneous pneumothorax, periodontitis and loose teeth. Clotting is usually normal, but severe bruising, due to friable vessels, is common.

PREOPERATIVE ASSESSMENT

History and examination:

- Determine the exact form of EDS and its severity

Table 1.
Clinical manifestations of different forms of EDS

Form	Effects
I, III, V, VI, VII, X	Hyperextensible joints resulting in recurrent dislocations
IV	Thin skin with prominent veins Spontaneous rupture of: major vessels, uterus, bowel Aneurysmal dilatation
VI	Blue sclera Rupture of eye
Most types	Laxity of skin
I, IV, VIII	Easily torn skin that heals with 'cigarette paper' scars
V	Mitral/tricuspid valve prolapse

- Assess pre-existing cardiovascular and arterial disease with emphasis on valvular abnormalities, aneurysms and arrhythmias
- Assess jaw opening
- Assess cervical spine mobility
- Check for loose teeth and periodontitis.

Investigations:
- Coagulation studies, especially bleeding time
- Cross-match blood (large volumes may be required)
- ECG to exclude dysrhythmias and conduction defects.

PERIOPERATIVE MANAGEMENT

Premedication:
- The patient should be warned of the risks of specific modes of anaesthesia
- Avoid intramuscular premedication (risk of haematoma formation)
- Ensure prophylaxis for subacute bacterial endocarditis if mitral valve disease is present
- Consider cardiac pacing in the presence of conduction defects.

Induction:
Cannulation of vessels may be difficult:

- Lax mobile skin makes vessel fixation difficult
- There may be loss of the normal sensation when a vessel wall is pierced
- Vessels may be fragile
- Risk of haematoma formation with all vessel punctures, especially of arteries and central veins
- Securing cannulae may be difficult due to mobile skin
- Subcutaneous extravasation may be marked and undetected due to skin laxity.

Maintenance:
- Care with insertion of nasogastric tubes (risk of haemorrhage)
- Avoid systemic hypertension (risk of haemorrhage and aneurysmal rupture).

Airway considerations
Avoid tracheal intubation if possible:

- Tracheal intubation may cause local haemorrhage
- Modify the hypertensive response to intubation as it may risk aneurysmal rupture
- Special care should be taken during intubation (risk of cervical spine damage)
- Use oral route in preference to nasal.

Avoid IPPV if possible as there is a risk of pneumothorax if high inflation pressures are required.

Regional techniques
Regional techniques are said to be inadvisable in patients with easy bruising because of risk of haematoma formation. However, intradural and epidural (caudal and lumbar) extradural techniques have been employed without complication.

Positioning
Lax and fragile skin demands that extra care be taken when positioning the patient for surgery.

Other considerations
- During surgery meticulous attention should be paid to haemostasis
- Risk of major blood loss
- Ligaments and skin may not hold sutures – risk of wound dehiscence.

Postoperative care
- Intramuscular injections are best avoided in case of haematoma formation
- Intravenous opiate infusions or continuous regional techniques would appear to be most suitable.

BIBLIOGRAPHY

Abouleish E. Obstetric anaesthesia and Ehlers–Danlos syndrome. British Journal of Anaesthesia 1980; 62: 1283–1286

Brighouse D, Guard B. Anaesthesia for Caesarian section in a patient with Ehlers–Danlos syndrome type IV. British Journal of Anaesthesia 1992; 69: 517–519

Dolan P, Sisko F, Riley E. Anaesthetic considerations for Ehlers–Danlos syndrome. Anesthesiology 1980; 52: 266–269

Prockop D J. Heritable disorders of connective tissue. In: Harrison's principles of internal medicine, 12th edn. McGraw-Hill, New York, 1991, p 1866–1867

CROSS REFERENCES

Abdominal aortic reconstruction – elective
Surgical Procedures 22: 446

Blood transfusion
Anaesthetic Factors 33: 616

EPIDERMOLYSIS BULLOSA

G. B. Smith

9

Epidermolysis bullosa (EB) encompasses a group of diseases characterized by blistering of skin, either spontaneously or following minimal mechanical trauma (direct pressure to the skin seems less likely to damage the skin than frictional or shearing forces). Over 20 different subtypes of EB exist, but they can be classified into three major groups – dystrophic (EBD), junctional (EBJ) and simplex (EBS) – depending on the level of blistering within the skin. EBD is the form of greatest anaesthetic significance.

PATHOPHYSIOLOGY

Dystrophic epidermolysis bullosa

EBD may be transmitted as either an autosomal dominant or recessive disorder with an incidence ranging from 1 in 50 000 to 1 in 300 000 births. An abnormality of type-VII collagen, possibly due to excessive collagenase activity, is implicated in some forms. Blister formation occurs beneath the lamina densa of the epidermal basement membrane. The disease may start at birth or in early infancy, and is characterized by extensive skin bullae, scarring and dystrophic nail lesions. The bullae are large, flaccid and may become infected or haemorrhagic. In the hand, scar formation eventually results in digital fusion with the formation of 'mitten-like' hands. Flexural contractures also occur. Involvement of the mucous membranes of the mouth, pharynx and oesophagus may lead to feeding difficulties, fixation of the tongue to the floor of the mouth, and oesophageal stricture. Anaemia is common and poor nutrition leads to growth retardation in severe cases. The skin lesions of EB have often been confused with those of porphyria cutanea tarda (PCT) and have led to the suggestion that there is a strong association between EBD and porphyria. However, these two diseases can now be distinguished on the basis of histopathologic, immunofluorescence and porphyrin studies. Equally, PCT does not hold the same significance for the anaesthetist as do the hepatic porphyrias.

Junctional epidermolysis bullosa
EBJ describes a group of autosomal recessive conditions leading to blister formation immediately above the basal membrane in the lamina lucida. Death usually occurs in the first 2 years of life. Patients who survive infancy often develop many of the complications of EBD.

Simplex epidermolysis bullosa
EBS may be generalized or localized. Some forms are inherited as autosomal dominant disorders, others as autosomal recessives. EBS is the least disabling form of EB.

TREATMENT

EB has been treated using systemic corticosteroids or drugs with collagenase activity, e.g. phenytoin and monocycline. Patients with EB often require repeated surgery for repair of syndactyly, oesophageal dilatation, skin grafting, dental surgery, removal of skin cancer or change of dressings.

PREOPERATIVE ASSESSMENT

History and examination:
- Fully assess the form of EB, together with the extent and duration of the illness
- Note drug therapy, especially systemic corticosteroids and phenytoin
- Assess venous access.

Investigations:
- Full blood count – anaemia and thrombocytosis are both common; anaemia may be due to iron or folate deficiency
- Urea and electrolytes – abnormalities may exist in severe EB; assess renal function
- Serum iron, folate and vitamin B_{12} levels.
- Liver function tests
- Albumen level – hypoalbuminaemia is common
- Phenytoin levels (to exclude toxicity).

Premedication:
- Ensure that premedication is sufficient to prevent struggling during induction (struggling may risk new EB lesions)
- Traditionally, the intramuscular route has been avoided for fear of inducing new EB lesions; however, it now seems unlikely that intramuscular injections cause such problems
- Prophylaxis against gastric aspiration (ranitidine, metoclopramide, sodium citrate) may be required if oesophageal complications exist.

PERIOPERATIVE MANAGEMENT

Induction:
- Venous access may be difficult and cut-down or central vein cannulation may be necessary
- An inhalation induction may be needed if venous access is difficult
- Intramuscular ketamine has proven extremely useful
- Suture intravenous cannulae in place or secure with vaseline gauze and ties
- Suxamethonium appears safe in EB:
  - There have been no new EB lesions reported after muscle fasciculations
  - Hyperkalaemia response is not seen, despite obvious muscle atrophy
- Thiopentone appears to be safe, despite fears of associated porphyria
- For children, encourage the presence of parents in the anaesthetic room in order to reduce the chances of struggling and restlessness on induction.

Airway considerations
Concern has been expressed over the possibility of causing new EB lesions during airway manipulation or intubation. Although pharyngeal lesions do occur, the hazards of intubation appear to have been overstated, since there are no reports of laryngeal or tracheal lesions following endotracheal intubation or tracheostomy. However, spontaneous EB lesions are possible in all of these sites.

- Use face-masks with a soft air cushion
- Pad face-masks with vaseline gauze
- Place vaseline gauze under chin to protect skin from anaesthetist's fingers

- If possible, avoid the use of airway adjuncts, such as Guedel airways
- On theoretical grounds, the laryngeal mask airway (LMA) would seem inappropriate because of the risk of producing pharyngeal lesions; however, studies to date suggest that the use of well-lubricated and carefully placed LMAs may be safe
- Consider the use of an 'anaesthetic hood' (a bag or a box) for inhalational induction
- Use a rapid sequence induction when there are oesophageal symptoms (regurgitation is a risk)
- Protect front of neck with vaseline gauze when applying cricoid pressure
- New head and neck lesions are often associated with difficult or failed intubation
- Laryngoscopy and oral intubation may be difficult:
  - Poor dentition
  - Limited mouth opening
  - Adhesion of tongue to floor of mouth
  - Consider fibre-optic intubation
- There are no reports of nasal lesions following nasotracheal intubation
- Use small uncuffed endotracheal tubes if possible, always taking into account the surgical field and the need to prevent airway soiling
- Secure endotracheal tubes with simple ties rather than with adhesive tape
- Treat haemorrhage from mucous membrane lesions using sponges soaked in adrenaline (1:200 000)
- Avoid nasogastric tube if possible (risk of oesophageal lesions).

Maintenance

Drug disposition will be affected by decreased muscle bulk, hypoalbuminaemia and any renal disease.

Regional techniques

- Although regional anaesthesia has traditionally been avoided, the following blocks have been used without complication:
  - Brachial plexus blocks (use the supraclavicular approach if there are axillary contractures)
  - Subarachnoid blocks
  - Epidural anaesthesia (lumbar and caudal)
  - Femoral nerve block
  - Digital block
  - Wrist block
  - Lateral cutaneous nerve of thigh blocks.
- Modifications should be made to the skin cleansing routine, e.g.:
  - Soak skin using betadine swabs or pour betadine over skin
  - Avoid skin scrubbing
  - Avoid subcutaneous injections of local anaesthetic solutions
  - Use EMLA cream for surface anaesthesia.
- Landmarks are usually easy to locate.
- Tourniquets do not appear to be hazardous if the skin is protected by sufficient padding; however, intravenous regional anaesthesia remains an unreported option.

Monitoring:

- Well-padded non-invasive BP cuffs do not appear to cause bullae, probably because direct pressure is less harmful in EB than frictional or shearing forces
- Pulse oximeters are of benefit as they can be attached to the patient using simple clips rather than adhesive or tape
- Use ECG pads without adhesive; needle ECG electrodes may be an alternative
- A weighted untaped precordial stethoscope may be useful
- Arterial lines may be of considerable use; secure with sutures.

Positioning:

- Protect the eyes using bland ointment and vaseline gauze pads (bullae may lead to corneal ulceration and globe perforation)
- Keep sheets and other linen free from creases
- Pad heals, elbows and bony prominences using foam
- Allow patients to move themselves onto trolleys or the operating table to minimize skin trauma
- Inform operating-room staff of the need for special care during patient positioning
- Take care with the positioning of a diathermy pad.

Emergence and recovery:

- Use protective vaseline gauze under oxygen masks
- For children, encourage the presence of parents in the recovery room in order to reduce the chances of struggling and restlessness on emergence.

POSTOPERATIVE CARE

- Common problems/complications:
  - New skin lesions
  - Regurgitation during anaesthetic induction may lead to aspiration pneumonia.

- Other medical therapy – continue steroid supplements.

BIBLIOGRAPHY

Boughton R, Crawford M R, Vonwiller J B. Epidermolysis bullosa – a review of 15 years' experience, including experience with combined general and regional anaesthetic techniques. Anaesthesia and Intensive Care 1988; 16: 260–264

Fine J, Bauer E A, Briggaman R A et al. Revised clinical and laboratory criteria for subtypes of inherited epidermolysis bullosa. Journal of the American Academy of Dematology 1991; 24: 119–135

Griffin R P, Mayou B J. The anaesthetic management of patients with dystrophic epidermolysis bullosa. A review of 44 patients over a 10 year period. Anaesthesia 1993; 48: 810–815

James I, Wark H. Airway management during anaesthesia in patients with epidermolysis bullosa dystrophica. Anesthesiology 1982; 56. 323–326

CROSS REFERENCES

Assessment of renal function
Patient Conditions 6: 155
Peripheral limb surgery
Surgical Procedures 16: 337
Paediatric plastic surgery
Surgical Procedures 16: 340
Rigid bronchoscopy
Surgical Procedures 17: 360
Difficult airway – difficult direct laryngoscopy
Surgical Procedures 30: 560

MUCOPOLY-SACCHARIDOSES

B. L. Taylor

A group of rare familial disorders caused by deficiencies of enzymes required to metabolize the mucopolysaccharide (MPS) constituents of connective tissue. MPS accumulates in skin, bone, blood vessels, brain, heart, liver, spleen, cornea and the tracheobronchial tree, causing anatomical and biochemical malfunction. All sufferers exhibit progressive joint, skeletal, and craniofacial abnormalities. Survival beyond the second decade is rare, the majority of childhood deaths being attributable to recurrent pneumonia or cardiac disease. In later years, death occurs from cardiac failure or related complications.

PATHOPHYSIOLOGY

MPS enzyme deficiencies are recessively inherited. All variants are autosomal, with the exception of the Hunter syndrome which is X linked. Urinary excretion of connective tissue substrates assists diagnosis, but skin biopsy and biochemical enzyme analysis may also be required. Anaesthesia may be required for surgical correction of anatomical abnormalities, relief of distressing symptoms, diagnostic investigation or coincidental disease. The MPSs present a wide range of potential anaesthetic problems (Table 1).

Cardiovascular system

The mitral and aortic valves are distorted and thickened, causing incompetence, or stenosis. Myocardial and coronary vessel involvement leads to hypertrophic cardiomyopathy,

Table 1.
Anaesthetic problems associated with various syndromes

Syndrome (type)	Major anaesthetic considerations
Hurler (I)	Macroglossia, kyphoscoliosis, odontoid hypoplasia, mitral incompetence, cardiomegaly
Scheie (I)	Macroglossia, prognathia, short neck, aortic incompetence
Hurler–Scheie (I)	Macroglossia, micrognathia, short neck, mitral and aortic incompetence
Hunter (II)	Hydrocephaly, short neck, ischaemic cardiomyopathy
San Filippo (III)	Macroglossia, vertebral abnormalities
Morquio (IV)	Kyphoscoliosis, odontoid hypoplasia, short neck, C1/C2 instability, aortic regurgitation
Maroteaux–Lamy (VI)	Macroglossia, kyphoscoliosis, odontoid hypoplasia, mitral and aortic valve lesions
Sly (VII)	Contractures, thoracic gibbus, odontoid hypoplasia, mitral and aortic valve lesions, aortic dissection

congestive cardiac failure, myocardial ischaemia and infarction. Arryhthmias and conduction block may occur. Chronic respiratory disease and airway obstruction may produce cor pulmonale.

Respiratory system

Airway obstruction may occur due to an enlarged tongue, orofacial abnormalities, adenotonsillar hypertrophy, laryngomalacia, tracheomalacia, and mucosal deposition of MPS throughout the respiratory tree. Excessive secretions may cause further compromise. Age-related anterocephalad displacement of the larynx occurs in some types. Kyphoscoliosis and obstructive lung disease increase susceptibility to pulmonary sepsis. Mitral valve disease, pulmonary hypertension and chronic right ventricular failure may further affect respiratory function.

Central nervous system

Mental function ranges from normal intellect to severe retardation. Intellectual deterioration may arise from the disease process or be secondary to hydrocephalus and raised intracranial pressure (ICP). Visual and hearing impairment may complicate assessment.

Gastrointestinal tract

Hepatosplenomegaly is routinely present, but liver and splenic function are usually unaffected. Umbilical and inguinal herniae are common owing to abdominal wall weakness.

Skeletal

Macrocephaly, hypertelorism, and abnormalities of the oropharynx and temporomandibular joints occur frequently. Abnormalities of the neck and cervical spine are common, including 'silent' atlanto-occipital subluxation and delayed vertebral ossification. Joint deformities may be aggravated by muscle contractures.

PREOPERATIVE ASSESSMENT

History:

- Previous operations and anaesthetic problems
- Physical and mental disability
- Respiratory or cardiovascular history
- Symptoms of obstructive sleep apnoea.

Examination

General

- Skeletal abnormalities (craniofacial, contractures, etc.)
- Skin and peripheral veins.

Respiratory

- Upper airway and orofacial abnormalities
- Axial anomalies (cervical spine, kyphoscoliosis, etc.)
- Proximal and distal airways obstruction
- Evidence of chronic lung disease
- Secretion and sputum production
- Active pulmonary infection.

Cardiovascular

- Cardiac valve incompetence or stenosis
- Cardiomegaly, left ventricular hypertrophy
- Cor pulmonale
- Univentricular and biventricular failure
- Arrhythmias.

Central nervous system

- Raised intracranial pressure, papilloedema
- Visual and hearing impairment.

Investigations

See Table 2.

Table 2.

Investigation	Result
Spirometry	Decreased vital capacity, FRC, TLC
Arterial blood gases	Hypoxaemia, hypercapnia
Chest radiograph	Pneumonia, atelectasis, subglottic narrowing
Electrocardiogram	LVH, RVH, arrhythmias, conduction block
Echocardiogram	Decreased ejection fraction, valve lesions, dyskinesia
Cardiac catheterization	Valve pressure gradients, coronary artery occlusion
CAT scan of brain	Hydrocephaly, increased ICP
Cervical spine X-rays	Decreased ossification, atlanto-occipital instability
Haematology profile	Increased white cell count, anaemia
Urea and electrolytes	Diuretic and digoxin effects
Liver function tests	Liver dysfunction

PREOPERATIVE PREPARATION

- Treatment of active respiratory infection
- Chest physiotherapy
- Treatment of cardiac failure and arrhythmias
- Full discussion with parents, and consideration of parental accompaniment to anaesthetic room.

Premedication

- Increased sensitivity to narcotic analgesics
- Risk of respiratory depression/sleep apnoea
- Antisialogogue advisable (use glyco-pyrrolate if tachydysrhythmias are predicted)
- Benzodiazepines effective, but unpredictable
- Ketamine useful if difficult airway anticipated
- Consider the need for SBE prophylaxis
- Use of EMLA cream helps maintain cooperation of child.

PERIOPERATIVE MANAGEMENT

Induction:

- Arrange a full range of airway adjuncts
- Endotracheal tube size not predictable from age/weight; therefore a full range of sizes must be available
- Oral abnormalities and temporomandibular stiffness may reduce airway access
- Fibre-optic laryngoscopy may be necessary
- Nasal intubation may cause epistaxis; adenoidal tissue may obstruct nasal tube
- Laryngeal mask airway is useful, but may cause excessive secretions or laryngospasm
- Inhalational induction with oxygen/halothane is useful if difficult airway is likely
- Small titrated doses of intravenous anaesthetic drug maintaining spontaneous ventilation may be used until the airway is secured
- Ketamine is often used; avoid if ICP is raised
- Intravenous induction agents should be used cautiously, as they may precipitate apnoea
- Avoid neuromuscular blockade until trachea intubated or ventilation can be assured.

Regional techniques

These are seldom appropriate for surgery alone due to mental retardation of many patients.

Airway considerations:

- Always consider cervical spine involvement
- Oral airways may cause obstruction by pushing epiglottis backwards; nasal airways less so
- Difficult intubation is common, and becomes progressively more so with increasing age
- Cartilaginous softening/airway distortion may make tracheostomy/cricothyrotomy difficult.

Maintenance:

- Nitrous oxide/volatile agent mix appropriate
- Use caution with narcotic analgesics because of increased sensitivity
- Spontaneous breathing techniques are generally inadvisable unless the procedure is of short duration or intubation proves impossible.

Positioning
This may be difficult due to kyphoscoliosis.

Emergence and recovery:
- Delayed awakening is a recognized problem
- Extubate when awake to avoid airway obstruction; consider nasopharyngeal airway.

Analgesia:
- Titrate narcotic analgesics in reduced dosage
- Local or regional techniques beneficial.

POSTOPERATIVE CARE

- Consider ITU admission for close monitoring
- Chest physiotherapy and antibiotics.

Common problems include:

- Restlessness or aggressive behaviour
- Arrhythmias
- Respiratory obstruction/depression
- Obstructive sleep apnoea
- Pulmonary infection
- Reduced cough and secretion clearance.

OUTCOME

With appropriate management, the perioperative morbidity and mortality of patients with mucopolysaccharidoses is low.

BIBLIOGRAPHY

Diaz J H, Belani K G. Perioperative management of children with mucopolysaccharidoses. Anesthesia and Analgesia 1993; 77: 1261–1270

CROSS REFERENCES

Aortic valve disease
Patient Conditions 4: 95
Cardiomyopathy
Patient Conditions 4: 103
Mitral valve disease
Patient Conditions 4: 114
Difficult airway – overview
Anaesthetic Factors 30: 558
Raised ICP/CBF control
Anaesthetic Factors 33: 662

POLYARTERITIS NODOSA

G. B. Smith

Polyarteritis nodosa (PAN) is a rare systemic disease in which a necrotizing arteritis affects the medium and small arteries. The consequence of this vasculitis depends on the site and number of vessels involved and may range from localized lesions with clinically insignificant effects to life-threatening organ failure. Typically, there is aneurysm formation in the medium-sized arteries, and both haemorrhage and infarction in major organs. Prognosis in PAN is significantly influenced by the size of vessel affected and by the presence of renal involvement. Up to 40% of patients with PAN die within a year of diagnosis.

PATHOPHYSIOLOGY

The histology of *classical polyarteritis nodosa* is a fibrinoid necrosis of the media of affected arteries associated with infiltration of the intima and media by polymorphs. The male/female ratio of incidence is approximately 2:1, with a peak incidence in the 40–50 year age group. Presenting symptoms often include malaise, fever and weight loss. Approximately 60% have arthralgia, 50% a rash (erythematous, purpuric or vasculitic) and 40% a peripheral neuropathy. The gastrointestinal system is involved in about 45% of cases; gut or gallbladder infarction, gastrointestinal haemorrhage and pancreatitis being the common presentations. Approximately 25% have renal impairment. Myalgia may also be a presenting symptom. Classical PAN is treated with immunosuppressive drugs (e.g. cyclophosphamide) and systemic corticosteroids.

In some patients with polyarteritis there is little evidence of major organ involvement, with the exception of severe renal disease (necrotizing glomerulonephritis). This disorder, which has a mean age of onset of 50 years and a male predominance, is often termed *microscopic polyarteritis*. Although all of the features of classical PAN can occur in microscopic polyarteritis, they are less frequent. The patient often presents with haematuria (microscopic or macroscopic), proteinuria or oliguria. Haemoptysis, frank pulmonary haemorrhage (occasionally requiring mechanical ventilation), pleurisy and asthma may also be the initial symptoms. In microscopic polyarteritis histological examination reveals a focal segmental necrotizing glomerulonephritis with fibrinoid necrosis and thrombosis of the glomerular tufts. Treatment of microscopic polyarteritis is as for PAN; azathioprine is occasionally added. Plasmapheresis may be used where cytotoxics and steroids appear to have no benefit.

PREOPERATIVE ASSESSMENT

History and examination:

- Assess the extent and duration of the illness. Discover whether the patient has an acute arteritis or is in remission, as this will affect perioperative risk and outcome.
- Assess systemic involvement:
  - Cardiovascular (angina, heart failure, cardiomegaly, pericarditis)
  - Resiratory (asthma, pneumonia, haemoptysis, pleurisy)
  - Renal (renal failure, hypertension)
  - CNS (peripheral neuropathy, CVA)
  - Airway (acute pharyngeal oedema).
- Check drug history:
  - Systemic corticosteroids
  - Other immunosuppressant drugs
  - Cardiac drugs.

Investigations

ECG:

- Cardiac ischaemia, myocardial infarction
- Dysrhythmias
- Pericarditis.

Echocardiography

Assess cardiac contractility, pericardial effusions.

Chest X-ray

- Pulmonary infection, haemorrhage
- Pulmonary infiltrates (pulmonary eosinophilia)
- Pulmonary fibrosis
- Cardiac failure.

Arterial blood gases

- Look for hypoxaemia
- The critically ill patient is likely to have a metabolic acidosis.

Urea and electrolytes

- Usually normal until disease is very severe
- Baseline test of renal function (creatinine and potassium).

Full blood count

- Anaemia is common
- Leucocytosis is a frequent finding
- Leucopenia may result from immunosuppressant drug therapy.

Liver function tests

- Albumin; clotting factors as indicators of liver function
- Approximately 30% of patients with PAN carry the hepatitis B surface antigen.

Lung function tests

- Request if there is clinical evidence of lung disease
- Pulmonary fibrosis will cause a restrictive defect.

Coagulation studies

May be abnormal due to hepatic involvement.

HBsAg

Approximately 30% of patients carry the hepatitis B surface antigen.

Urinalysis

PAN may cause the nephrotic syndrome.

Plasma cholinesterase levels

- Reduced by plasmapheresis
- Action inhibited by cyclophosphamide.

PREOPERATIVE PREPARATION

- Preoperative optimization of cardiovascular and respiratory systems:
  - Chest-physiotherapy
  - Antibiotics
  - Control of hypertension
  - Treatment of angina (e.g. nitrates).

- Patients with severe cardiovascular disease may require perioperative invasive haemodynamic monitoring (e.g. central venous catheter, pulmonary artery catheter).
- If surgery is required urgently for patients with acute complications of PAN, e.g. gut ischaemia, the following may be required perioperatively:
  - Invasive haemodynamic monitoring
  - Mechanical ventilation
  - Inotropic/vasopressor agents
  - Renal replacement therapy.
- Perioperative steroid cover will be needed for the patient receiving systemic steroids.

PERIOPERATIVE MANAGEMENT

Throughout the perioperative phase there should be scrupulous anti-infection measures because of the high risk of sepsis in PAN.

Premedication:
- Use an anxiolytic to reduce the risk of tachycardia and hypertension from catecholamines
- Avoid anticholinergic premedication (risk of tachycardia).

Induction:
- Avoid drugs and techniques likely to cause tachycardia, hypertension, hypotension or reduced myocardial contractility (e.g. ketamine, thiopentone)
- Use a 'cardiac' anaesthetic (e.g. opiate induction ± intravenous lignocaine) to limit the hypertensive response to laryngoscopy
- Preoxygenate prior to induction
- Administer high concentrations of oxygen when there is a history of cardiac or respiratory disease
- Maintain good tissue blood and oxygen supply.

Airway considerations
Pharyngeal oedema, although rare, has been reported in PAN.

Maintenance:
- Avoid drugs and techniques likely to cause tachycardia, hypertension, hypotension or reduced myocardial contractility
- Administer high concentrations of oxygen when there is a history of cardiac or respiratory disease
- Maintain good tissue blood and oxygen supply
- Avoid hypotension and maintain fluid balance, especially in patient with renal involvement
- Drug metabolism is altered in renal disease. Avoid drugs which are primarily metabolized/excreted by the kidneys
- Hypoalbuminaemia will affect drug distribution
- Avoid vasoconstrictor drugs, if possible, because of the risk of vascular occlusion
- When plasmapheresis has been recent, remember that the action of ester drugs (e.g. suxamethonium) will be prolonged
- The action of suxamethonium may be prolonged by cyclophosphamide.

Regional techniques:
- Avoid use of adrenaline-containing local anaesthetic solutions because of the risk of vascular occlusion
- Document existing sensorimotor neuropathies prior to use of regional techniques.

Monitoring:
- CM_5 ECG useful to detect myocardial ischaemia and arrhythmias
- Radial artery cannulation may be inadvisable in the presence of aneurysmal disease because of the risk of vascular occlusion
- BP measurement essential
- Transoesophageal echocardiography may be helpful intraoperatively if there is severe cardiac disease; it has been used during surgery in infant PAN.

POSTOPERATIVE MANAGEMENT

Common problems/complications are:

- Deterioration in cardiovascular function
- Respiratory failure may result from pneumonia
- Risk of systemic sepsis.

Continue systemic steroid supplements.

CROSS REFERENCES

Chronic renal failure
Patient Conditions 6: 158
Obstruction or perforation
Surgical Procedures 18: 372

9

POLYMYOSITIS AND DERMATOMYOSITIS

G. B. Smith

Dermatomyositis (DM) and polymyositis (PM) are members of an uncommon group of connective tissue disorders known as idiopathic inflammatory myopathies (IIM) (Table 1). Their cause is unknown but genetic factors, toxins, drugs and infectious agents probably all play a part; the incidence of malignancy is increased in patients with IIM. Both DM and PM present with muscle weakness, usually involving proximal muscle groups, and are associated with other multisystem connective tissue diseases such as systemic lupus erythematosus, rheumatoid arthritis, Hashimoto's thyroiditis and systemic sclerosis. In DM there are characteristic violaceous skin lesions, often involving the upper eyelid.

Table 1.
Idiopathic inflammatory myopathies

Polymyositis
Dermatomyositis
Cancer-associated myositis
Connective-tissue-disease-associated myositis
Childhood dermatomyositis
Inclusion body myositis
Eosinophilic myositis
Other rare forms

PATHOPHYSIOLOGY

Muscle

Chronic inflammation leads to weakness, muscle tenderness, myalgia and, eventually, both atrophy and fibrosis of skeletal muscle. Characteristically there is a rise in serum enzymes derived from muscle, e.g. creatine phosphokinase (CPK), and their levels usually parallel disease activity. Myoglobin may be released from muscle, leading to myoglobinaemia and myoglobinuria. The risk of malignant hyperthermia in patients with IIM is unknown, but recent in vitro studies have shown that muscle from some patients produces significant contracture to caffeine or halothane, but not both (i.e. malignant hyperthermia equivocal).

Respiratory

Of the patients with IIM, 5–10% have associated interstitial pulmonary disease, predominantly fibrosis. Pulmonary compromise can also occur because of intercostal and diaphragmatic weakness or aspiration pneumonia. Patients with myositis who have no pulmonary symptoms and a normal chest radiograph may exhibit abnormal pulmonary function tests. Vocal cord dysfunction may exist.

Cardiac

Cardiac disease is a major cause of death in IIM. The prime cardiac manifestations are dysrhythmias, conduction defects, myocarditis, cardiomyopathy, and cor pulmonale. Steroid-induced hypertension may occur.

Gastrointestinal

Poor coordination of swallowing, nasal regurgitation and pooling of secretions in the vallecula and cricopharyngeal spaces may predispose to pulmonary aspiration. There may also be oesophageal reflux, delayed gastric emptying and decreased intestinal motility.

Treatment

First-line therapy in IIM involves oral steroids. In some cases, other immunosuppressive drugs such as azathioprine, cyclophosphamide, methotrexate or cyclosporin are added. Patients may present with side-effects of therapy. Plasmapheresis has also been employed in IIM and may lower plasma cholinesterase levels.

PREOPERATIVE ASSESSMENT

From data available from the limited number of case reports of anaesthesia for patients with

IMM, the potential problems associated with these diseases do not seem to hold major implications for the anaesthetist.

History and examination:
- Systematic review of associated cardiovascular, respiratory and gastrointestinal disease
- Systemic assessment for other associated autoimmune disorders
- Review of drug therapy and its possible complications.

Investigations
See Table 2.

Table 2.

Investigation	Possible findings
ECG	Tachyarrhythmias Conduction abnormalities Ventricular hypertrophy Cor pulmonale
Chest X-ray	Pulmonary fibrosis Ventricular dilatation
Spirometry	Decreased vital capacity Decreased FRC Decreased tidal volume
Blood gas analysis	Hypoxaemia Hypercapnia
Full blood count	Anaemia Leucopenia

Preoperative preparation
Treat any chest infection.

Premedication:
- Continue systemic steroid cover
- Avoid intramuscular injections.

PERIOPERATIVE MANAGEMENT

Induction/maintenance:
- Avoid malignant hyperthermia trigger agents
- Controlled-ventilation should be used in presence of preoperative ventilatory compromise.

Muscle relaxants
Conflicting evidence exists regarding the use of neuromuscular blocking agents in IIM. Suxamethonium has produced an abnormal muscle contraction prior to relaxation in a child with DM. The use of suxamethonium has been avoided by other workers because of the potential, yet unproven, risk of malignant hyperthermia and hyperkalaemia.

The use of nondepolarizing neuromuscular blocking agents (NDNMBs) has also resulted in conflicting evidence. Several workers have noted no problem with NDNMBs, yet there are reports of prolonged neuromuscular paralysis following the use of both vecuronium in PM and atracurium in eosinophilic myositis. A myasthenic-like response to NDNMBs has been reported, but this may be related more to associated malignancy than to myositis.

- Use small doses of short-acting neuromuscular blocking agents, preferably after a test dose (remember reduced muscle mass)
- Avoid suxamethonium if possible (because of the potential risk of malignant hyperthermia or, in acute myositis, hyperkalaemia).

Airway considerations:
- The use of an endotracheal tube is strongly recommended, especially if there is risk of aspiration
- Rapid sequence induction should be used if pharyngeal, oesophageal or gastric symptoms are present.

Intraoperative monitoring:
- Neuromuscular monitoring is essential
- Extubation and termination of assisted ventilation should follow measurement of lung volumes (e.g. tidal volume, vital capacity).

POSTOPERATIVE CARE

Posture
Extubate awake or in the lateral position, because of the risk of aspiration.

Common problems/complications
Immediate postoperative recovery appears to be normal in most patients with IIM, yet the following complications might be expected from knowledge of the disease:

- Prolonged recovery from neuromuscular blockade, requiring IPPV
- Lung atelectasis
- Postoperative pneumonia
- Postoperative respiratory failure
- Aspiration if pharyngeal muscles are weak.

Other medical therapy:

- Continue systemic steroid supplementation postoperatively
- Avoid intramuscular analgesics; titrate small intravenous doses of opiates to avoid respiratory depression
- Postoperative physiotherapy, where necessary.

OUTCOME

Morbidity and mortality in patients with IIM undergoing anaesthesia seems to be low. When it occurs it is usually because of respiratory disease.

BIBLIOGRAPHY

Flusche G, Unger-Sargon J, Lambert D H. Prolonged neuromuscular paralysis with vecuronium in a patient with polymyositis. Anesthesia and Analgesia 1987; 66: 188–190

Gabta R, Campbell I T, Mostafa S M. Anaesthesia and acute dermatomyositis/polymyositis. British Journal of Anaesthesia 1988, 60: 854–858

Heytens L, Martin J J, Van de Kleft E, Bossaert L L. In vitro contracture test in patients with various neuromuscular diseases. British Journal of Anaesthesia 1992; 68: 72–75

Johns R A, Finholt D A, Stirt J A. Anaesthetic management of a child with dermatomyositis. Canadian Anaesthetists Society Journal 1986; 33: 71–74

Plotz P H, Dalakas M, Leff R L, Love L A, Miller F W, Cronin M E. Current concepts in the idiopathic inflammatory myopathies: polymyositis, dermatomyositis, and other related disorders. Annals of Internal Medicine 1989; 111: 143–157

CROSS REFERENCES

Rheumatoid disease
Patient Conditions 8: 202

Systemic lupus erythematosus
Patient Conditions 9: 234

PSEUDOXANTHOMA ELASTICUM

B. L. Taylor

Pseudoxanthoma elasticum (PXE) is an inherited disorder of elastic and collagen tissue in which there is progressive calcification and degeneration of elastin fibres and the supportive collagen matrix in skin and mucous membranes of affected areas. Similar processes may affect the media of the arterial system, leading to arterial occlusion and ischaemia. Ocular and myocardial involvement may also occur.

PATHOPHYSIOLOGY

The underlying biochemical lesion in PXE, also known as Groenblad–Strandberg disease, is unknown, but the condition is inherited as either an autosomal dominant or recessive disorder. Diagnosis is usually confirmed by skin biopsy. It is unclear why the areas of the body most rich in elastic tissue (e.g. aorta, lungs, palms, soles) are spared, and the pattern follows more closely the distribution of collagen. The prevalence of PXE is estimated to be between 1 in 50 000 and 1 in 200 000 adults, with females being more commonly affected. Acceleration of symptoms may occur during pregnancy, supporting the theory that some aspects of the disease may be hormonally influenced. The disease occurs at any age and, although average life expectancy is normal, premature death in childhood is a recognized risk.

Skin

There is a variable tendency to loosening of the skin, particularly in the neck, face, axillae, abdomen and groin (including the genitalia). Most affected individuals show evidence of these changes by their second decade, but some may have minimal involvement even in later life. The loose skin becomes thickened and 'pebbled', sometimes being described as '*peu d'orange*'. A characteristic skin deposition of yellowish lesions, mainly in the antecubital fossae, gives a xanthoma-like appearance and the disorder its name. Similar deposition and calcification may occur in mucous membranes, commonly the lower lip, rectum and vagina.

Airway and respiratory system:
- Laryngeal involvement with PXE has been reported. This may cause loss of elasticity of the layrngeal structures leading to difficult tracheal intubation.
- Respiratory complications may occur secondary to cardiac involvement.

Vascular system:
- Arterial involvement may lead to a reduction or absence of peripheral pulses, often with associated medial calcification. Distal ischaemic problems are uncommon, presumably because the slow process allows time for collateral circulation to develop.
- Renovascular arterial occlusion may cause severe hypertension, even in young patients.
- Vascular aneuryms also occur in PXE.

Heart:
- Calcification within the endocardium may affect conduction, and predisposes to arrhythmias.
- Mitral valve thickening and incompetence have been reported.
- Coronary arterial lesions may result in severe angina, even in the young; myocardial ischaemia and infarction may result. Coronary artery bypass grafting has been necessary in teenage sufferers and a fatal myocardial infarction has been reported in a 6-week-old infant.

Eye

PXE produces well-recognized ocular manifestations in the form of retinal streaks extending radially from the optic disc over the fundus. The 'angioid streaks' are the result of reduced elasticity of Bruch's membrane, and may lead to scarring and retinal or vitreous haemorrhage.

Gastrointestinal system

Acute gastrointestinal haemorrhage is common, often presenting in children and young adults. The cause appears to be vascular involvement which prevents normal healing responses to minor abrasions of the mucosa. Peptic ulceration and oesophagitis also occur.

Central nervous system

Psychiatric disturbances are commonly associated with the condition. Cerebral ischaemia and haemorrhage are also recognized complications of PXE.

PREOPERATIVE ASSESSMENT

Patients with PXE may require surgery for the ocular, cardiovascular or gastrointestinal complications of the disease. Increasingly, patients present for the surgical treatment of disfiguring cutaneous manifestations.

History and examination:
- Assess the extent of the disease, taking note of the degree of involvement of the cardiovascular and respiratory systems:
  - Angina, myocardial infarction
  - Dyspnoea
  - Syncopal attacks (dysrhythmias)
  - Arterial pulses
  - Blood pressure
  - Heart murmurs.
- Assess venous access, both peripheral and central.

Investigations:
- ECG
- Chest X-ray
- Urea and electrolytes as a baseline test of renal function.

Preoperative preparation

Temporary cardiac pacing may be indicated in selected patients with conduction defects.

PERIOPERATIVE MANAGEMENT

Induction:
- Venous access may be difficult due to the loose and thickened skin
- The antecubital fossae are often unsuitable for intravenous access
- Neck involvement may prevent use of the internal jugular veins
- Groin involvement may prevent use of the femoral veins
- Venous cut-down may be necessary
- An inhalation induction may be necessary.

Anaesthetic technique
There appear to be no specific contraindications to the use of any particular anaesthetic drug during induction of anaesthesia in PXE. However, in planning the anaesthetic technique, the following points should be borne in mind:

- Risks of undiagnosed cardiac ischaemia and dysrhythmias
- Risk of major haemorrhage
- Risks of hypertension, e.g. subendocardial ischaemia, intracranial haemorrhage.

Airway considerations:
- Endotracheal intubation may be difficult because involvement of the laryngeal ligaments and cartilages may cause laryngeal rigidity
- Rigid bronchoscopy has been necessary to assist with endotracheal intubation in PXE.

Maintenance
See induction (above).

Care should be taken to avoid upper gastro-intestinal trauma from the use of a nasogastric tube.

Regional techniques
Thickened loose skin may make regional techniques difficult.

Monitoring:
- BP monitoring, although essential, may be difficult:
  - Noninvasive oscillotonometric methods are likely to be unreliable in the presence of occlusive arterial disease
  - Invasive BP monitoring may be difficult because of arterial occlusion or vessel calcification.
- Central venous access for central venous pressure monitoring may be difficult (see above).
- Care should be taken to avoid upper gastrointestinal trauma from the use of an oesophageal stethoscope or oesophageal temperature probe.

OUTCOME

The majority of patients with PXE who undergo anaesthesia and surgery have an uncomplicated course and outcome. Those with severe cardiovascular involvement are at greater risk, as are those suffering complications such as gastrointestinal haemorrhage, requiring emergency surgery.

BIBLIOGRAPHY

Levitt M W D, Collison J M. Difficult endotracheal intubation in a patient with pseudoxanthoma elasticum. Anaesthesia and Intensive Care 1982; 10: 62–64

Wilson Krechel S L, Ramirez-Inawat R C, Fabian L W. Anesthetic considerations in pseudo-xanthoma elasticum. Anesthesia and Analgesia 1981; 60: 344–347

CROSS REFERENCES

Cardiac conduction defects
Patient Conditions 4: 99
Hypertension
Patient Conditions 4: 11
Coronary artery bypass grafting
Surgical Procedures 27: 511

SCLERODERMA

G. Krishnakumar

Scleroderma, or progressive systemic sclerosis, is a chronic multisystem disorder of unknown cause characterized by fibrosis of skin, blood vessels and viscera, including the gastrointestinal tract, lungs, heart and kidneys.

PATHOPHYSIOLOGY

Scleroderma results from an excessive deposition of collagen and extracellular matrix in affected tissues. Sufferers often possess certain common HLA antigens and there is evidence that both disordered cell-mediated immunity and abnormal endothelial cell function play a part in the development of the disease. Additionally, some chemicals (e.g. silica) induce scleroderma-like syndromes. Most cases of scleroderma fall into one of two subsets: diffuse cutaneous systemic sclerosis (DSSC) or limited cutaneous systemic sclerosis (LSSC) (Table 1).

- The skin is shiny, waxen and taut. There is loss of skin folds. Perioral contractures may limit mouth opening.
- Oesophageal involvement occurs in about 80% of cases resulting in dysphagia and stricture formation.
- The heart is involved in approximately 50% of patients leading to cardiac arrhythmias, conduction defects, cardiomyopathy, pericarditis and pericardial effusions.
- Lung involvement causes pulmonary fibrosis and pulmonary hypertension.
- Weakness of the intercostal muscles and diaphragm have been reported. Skin of the chest wall may be involved.
- Renal disease may lead to hypertension.
- Gut involvement may cause malabsorption.
- Other findings in scleroderma include peripheral neuropathies, Sjogren's syndrome and diminished sweating.

The *crest syndrome*, a variant of scleroderma,

Table 1.
Clinical features and natural history of scleroderma subtypes*

Diffuse cutaneous systemic sclerosis		
	Early (<5 years after onset)	*Late (>5 years after onset)*
Early onset of Raynaud's (<1 year) Truncal and acral skin involved Early systemic disease (interstitial lung fibrosis, renal failure, gastrointestinal and myocardial involvement) Antitopoisomerase antibody in 30%	Rapid progression of skin thickening Increased risk of renal, cardiac pulmonary, articular, vascular complications and digital ulcers	Skin involvement stable or regresses Progression of existing visceral disease, but reduced risk of new visceral involvement
Limited cutaneous systemic sclerosis		
	Early (<10 years after onset)	*Late (>10 years after onset)*
Raynaud's phenomenon for years Face, hands, feet and forearm skin affected Late incidence of pulmonary hypertension, trigeminal neuralgia, skin calcification and telangiectasia Anticentromere antibody in 70–80%	No progression of skin lesions Raynaud's phenomenon, digital tip ulceration, oesophageal symptoms are common	No progression of skin lesions Raynaud's phenomenon, digital ulceration and calcification, oesophageal stricture, malabsorption and pulmonary hypertension

*Modified from LeRay (1988) and Steen & Medsger (1990).

is the combination of calcinosis, Raynaud's phenomenon, oesophageal involvement, sclerodactyly and multiple telangiectasia of the skin, lips, oral mucosa and gut.

PREOPERATIVE ASSESSMENT

History and examination:

- Assess the extent and duration of the illness
- Assess venous access
- Assess oral aperture
- Assess state of dentition (often poor)
- Look for mucosal telangiectasia in mouth
- Assess neck mobility
- Assess degree of cardiac and respiratory symptoms (e.g. exertional dyspnoea or the dry cough of pulmonary fibrosis); examine for cardiac dysrhythmias, a pericardial effusion and signs of pulmonary hypertension
- Check preoperative blood pressure
- Exclude dysphagia and oesophageal reflux
- Ask about symptoms of Raynaud's phenomonen
- Check for evidence of chronic renal failure
- Examine for peripheral neuropathies
- Check drug history:
  - Systemic corticosteroids
  - Other immunosuppressant drugs.

Investigations

ECG

24-h ECG recording (conduction defects): the presence of a normal resting ECG does not exclude involvement of the heart in scleroderma. Up to 40% of such patients may have abnormalities on 24-h rhythm analysis.

Chest X-ray:

- Look for signs of pulmonary fibrosis
- Exclude preoperative inhalation of gastric contents.

Cervical spine radiograph

Assess associated spinal disease.

Arterial blood gases

Look for hypoxaemia.

Urea and electrolytes

Baseline test of renal function.

Full blood count

Look for anaemia or leucocytosis due to treatment.

Lung function tests:

- Determine if illness is of a long duration or there is clinical evidence of lung disease
- Pulmonary fibrosis may lead to decreased lung compliance and reduced TLC or vital capacity
- Impaired gas transfer may occur (DLCO is abnormal in 70% of cases of DSSC)
- Most lung function tests are poor indicators of pulmonary hypertension in scleroderma.

Coagulation studies

These may be abnormal due to malabsorption.

Thyroid function tests

Hypothyroidism may occur in scleroderma.

Preoperative preparation:

- Preoperative pulmonary artery catheterization may help to diagnose pulmonary hypertension
- Xerostomia and poor dental hygiene may be helped by frequent preoperative mouthwashes
- Steroid cover will be needed for the patient receiving systemic corticosteriods
- Use prophylactic H_2 blockers and prokinetic drugs, such as metoclopramide, when oesophageal disease is present
- Vitamin K may be required where malabsorption has led to a bleeding tendency
- Temporary cardiac pacing may be indicated in selected patients with conduction defects.

PERIOPERATIVE MANAGEMENT

Induction:

- Venous access may be difficult due to vasoconstriction; cut-down or central vein cannulation may be necessary
- An inhalation induction may be necessary
- Intravenous injection of methohexitone in scleroderma has induced severe pain and cyanosis (? due to Raynaud's-like phenomenon).

Airway considerations:

- A rapid sequence induction may not be practicable if intubation difficulties are anticipated
- Cricoid pressure may be ineffective if the oesophagus is fibrosed
- Consider induction of anaesthesia in the head-up position
- Consider awake fibre-optic intubation

- Intubation should be performed very gently to avoid injury to the mouth
- Use oral intubation in preference to the nasal route as telangiectasia may lead to bleeding
- In very severe cases, consider tracheostomy.

Maintenance:
- Maintain patient's temperature at 37°C (risk of Raynaud's phenomenon)
- Warm all intravenous fluids
- Reduced lung and chest-wall compliance may make ventilation difficult
- Dry eyes (Sjogren's syndrome) make eye care especially important: eyelids should be taped shut; use bland ointments or artificial tears
- Use heat and moisture exchanger in Sjogren's syndrome
- Avoid hypotension and maintain fluid balance, especially in patient with renal involvement
- Drug metabolism is altered in renal failure
- Avoid vasoconstrictor drugs, if possible
- Increased concentrations of oxygen may be required.

Regional techniques:
- Ischaemic effects of tourniquets make the use of intravenous regional anaesthesia unwise
- Nerve blocks, including brachial plexus and sciatic nerve, have been used successfully, but may be associated with prolonged neural blockade (this may be beneficial)
- Raynaud's phenomenon may follow wrist blocks
- Avoid use of adrenaline-containing local anaesthetic solutions
- Unilateral local anaesthetic stellate ganglion blocks have worsened Raynaud's phenomenon on the contralateral side.

Monitoring:
- Limb contractures may make blood pressure measurement difficult
- Radial artery cannulation may cause reflex spasm and should be avoided if possible
- ECG monitoring to detect arrhythmias and conduction defects.

Positioning

Consider the risks of pressure effects on fibrotic skin during prolonged operations.

Emergence and recovery:
- The maintenance of a head-down position is advisable until patient is fully conscious
- Patients should be nursed upright once awake, in order to prevent regurgitation
- Increased oxygen requirements may result from a diffusion block in cases of lung fibrosis.

POSTOPERATIVE MANAGEMENT

Common problems/complications are:

- Postoperative chest infection
- Respiratory failure may result from respiratory muscle weakness or pneumonia
- Postoperative analgesic requirements may be increased (possibly due to increased numbers of sensory nerve fibres in skin).

Continue systemic steroid supplements.

BIBLIOGRAPHY

Black C M, Stephens C. Systemic sclerosis (scleroderma) and related disorders. In: Maddison P J et al (eds) Oxford textbook of rheumatology. Oxford, 1993, p 771–794

Leroy E C, Black S, Eleischmajor R, et al. Scleroderma (systemic sclerosis): classification, subsets and pathogenesis. Journal of Rheumatology 1988; 15: 202–205

Neill R S. Progressive systemic sclerosis. Prolonged sensory blockade following regional anaesthesia in association with a reduced response to systemic analgesics. British Journal of Anaesthesia 1980; 52: 623–625

Omote K, Kawamata M, Namiki A. Adverse effects of stellate ganglion block on Raynaud's phenomenon associated with progressive systemic sclerosis. Anesthesia and Analgesia 1993; 77: 1057–1060

Smoak L R. Anesthesia considerations for the patient with progressive systemic sclerosis (scleroderma). Journal of the American Association of Nurse Anesthetists 1982; 50: 548–554

Steen V D, Medsger T A. Epidemiology and natural history of systemic sclerosis. Rheumatic Diseases Clinic of North America 1990; 16: 1–10

Younker D, Harrison B. Scleroderma and pregnancy. Anaesthetic considerations. British Journal of Anaesthesia 1985; 57: 1136–1139

CROSS REFERENCES

Disorders of the oesophagus and of swallowing
Patient Conditions 5: 138

Difficult airway – difficult mask anaesthesia/ventilation
Anaesthetic Factors 30: 565

SYSTEMIC LUPUS ERYTHEMATOSUS (SLE)

G. B. Smith

9

Systemic lupus erythematosus (SLE) is an inflammatory disease affecting most body systems and characterized by abnormal immune function. Increased numbers of hyperactive B lymphocytes, together with impaired T-cell regulation, lead to the production of IgG antibodies which are specific for exogenous and endogenous antigens. The serum in SLE contains a variety of autoantibodies directed against nuclear material (e.g. anti-DNA antibodies), and histological examination of affected tissue shows evidence of immune complex deposition. The origin of SLE appears to be multifactorial – diet, drugs, toxins, infection, environment, hormones, genetics, etc., all seem to play a part. Drug-induced SLE occurs with isoniazid, hydralazine, anticonvulsants, procainamide and chlorpromazine.

SLE is more common in females than males (9:1), and the usual onset is in the third and fourth decades. It is an episodic disease with periods of prolonged remission punctuated by life-threatening exacerbations. Usually the onset involves arthralgia, fever, weight loss, rash and leucopenia; involvement of other organs produces a wide clinical spectrum of disease (Table 1).

Table 1.
Clinical features of SLE

Bones/joints
Flitting arthralgia
Polyarthritis (wrists, elbows, knees)
Aseptic necrosis of large joints
Skin
'Butterfly' rash in malar region
Photosensitivity
Raynaud's phenomenon
Cardiovascular system
Pericarditis/pericardial effusion
Myocarditis
Endocarditis
Leg ulcers
Limb gangrene
Necrotic finger pulp lesions
Respiratory system
Pleurisy/pleural effusions
Pulmonary infiltration
Diffusion block
Renal system
Proteinuria
Nephrotic syndrome
Hypertension
Acute and chronic renal failure
Muscular system
Myalgia
Myositis
Wasting/weakness
Nervous system
Seizures
Psychosis
Peripheral sensorimotor neuropathy
Hemiplegia
Cranial nerve palsies
Gastrointestinal system
Peritonitis
Gastrointestinal haemorrhage
Vasculitic ischaemia
Haematological system
Anaemia
Leucopenia
Thrombocytopaenia
Bleeding diathesis (circulating anticoagulants)

Of particular note to the anaesthetist is involvement of the cardiovascular, respiratory and renal systems by SLE. Myocarditis occurs in approximately 15% of cases, pericarditis in up to 60% and valvular lesions (Libman–Sach's endocarditis) in almost 25%. Pleuritic pain is found in about 50% of cases of SLE, pleural effusions in 25% and interstitial fibrosis, pulmonary vasculitis and interstitial pneumonitis in 20%. Renal disease is the most common cause of death in SLE. Of patients with renal disease, 50% have hypertension.

Up to 30% of patients with SLE have a circulating anticoagulant (lupus anticoagulant), which may prolong the activated partial thromboplastin time but also risks the formation of arterial and venous thromboses and predisposes to recurrent abortions. The presence of the anticardiolipin antibody is also associated with these problems.

Treatment of SLE is with a combination of NSAIDs, antimalarial agents, corticosteroids and immunosuppressant drugs (e.g. cyclophosphamide, azathioprine, etc.). Some centres use plasmapheresis for patients who are resistant to conventional therapy.

PREOPERATIVE ASSESSMENT

History and examination

- Assess the extent and duration of the illness. Discover whether the patient has acute disease or is in remission, as this will affect perioperative risk and outcome.
- Assess systemic involvement:
  - Cardiovascular (tachycardia, heart failure, cardiomegaly, pericardial effusion, valve lesions)
  - Respiratory (pleurisy, dyspnoea)
  - Renal (renal failure, hypertension)
  - CNS (peripheral neuropathy, CVA)
  - Raynaud's phenomenon.
- Check drug history:
  - NSAIDs
  - Antimalarials
  - Systemic corticosteroids
  - Other immunosuppressant drugs
  - Cardiac drugs
  - Use of plasmapheresis.

Investigations

ECG

- Myocarditis
- Dysrhythmias
- Pericarditis.

Echocardiography

Assess cardiac contractility, pericardial effusions.

Chest X-ray

- Pulmonary effusion
- Pulmonary fibrosis
- Pericardial effusion
- Cardiac failure.

Arterial blood gases

Look for hypoxaemia, usually with a normal or low $P_{a}CO_2$.

Urea and electrolytes

Baseline test of renal function (creatinine and potassium).

Full blood count:

- Anaemia is common
- Leucopenia may result from immunosuppressant drug therapy or from SLE itself
- Thrombocytopaenia may occasionally occur.

Lung function tests:

- Clinical signs, symptoms and chest radiograph do not reflect degree of pulmonary involvement
- Pulmonary fibrosis will cause a restrictive defect
- Diffusing capacity may be reduced.

Coagulation studies

- Look for anticardiolipin antibody and lupus anticoagulant. Their presence may be associated with a prolonged APTT or KCCT. However, PT may be normal.
- Clotting factor assays.

Urinalysis

SLE may cause the nephrotic syndrome.

Plasma cholinesterase levels:

- Reduced by plasmapheresis
- Action inhibited by cyclophosphamide.

Preoperative preparation

- Preoperative optimization of cardiovascular and respiratory systems. In particular:
  - Control of hypertension
  - Treatment of angina (e.g. nitrates)
  - Treatment of dysrhythmias
  - Treatment of heart failure
  - Drainage of pericardial/pleural effusions
  - Treatment of intercurrent pneumonia.
- Patients with severe cardiovascular disease may require perioperative invasive haemodynamic monitoring (e.g. central venous and pulmonary artery pressures).
- Perioperative steroid cover will be needed for the patient receiving corticosteriods.
- Take antithrombotic measures perioperatively in patients with anticardiolipin antibody:
  - Antiembolic stockings
  - Avoid dehydration
  - Subcutaneous heparin.
- Patients with the anticardiolipin antibody and a history of thrombotic events require

permanent anticoagulation with either warfarin or aspirin. They should receive heparin as an infusion perioperatively.

PERIOPERATIVE MANAGEMENT

Blood transfusions can exacerbate SLE.

Induction:
- Avoid drugs and techniques likely to cause tachycardia, hypertension, hypotension or reduced myocardial contractility (e.g. ketamine, thiopentone)
- Use a 'cardiac' anaesthetic (e.g. opiate induction ± intravenous lignocaine) to limit the hypertensive response to laryngoscopy
- Preoxygenate prior to induction
- Administer high concentrations of oxygen when there is cardiorespiratory disease.

Airway considerations
There are rare reports of a narrowed airway due to cricoarytenoid arthritis in SLE.

Maintenance:
- Avoid drugs and techniques likely to cause tachycardia, hypertension, hypotension or reduced myocardial contractility
- When plasmapheresis has been recent, the action of ester drugs (e.g. suxamethonium) may be prolonged
- The action of suxamethonium may be prolonged by cyclophosphamide
- Administer high concentrations of oxygen when there is cardiorespiratory disease
- Avoid hypotension and maintain fluid balance, especially in the patient with renal involvement
- Drug metabolism is altered in renal disease; avoid drugs which are metabolized/ excreted by the kidneys
- Hypoalbuminaemia in nephrotic syndrome will affect drug distribution
- Avoid vasoconstrictors in Raynaud's disease.

Regional techniques:
- Be absolutely sure of the patient's coagulation status before embarking upon regional anaesthetic techniques
- Document existing sensorimotor neuropathies prior to use of regional techniques.

Monitoring:
- CM_5 ECG is useful to detect myocardial ischaemia and arrhythmias
- Radial artery cannulation may be inadvisable in the presence of Raynaud's phenomenon
- Transoesophageal echocardiography is helpful intraoperatively in severe cardiac disease
- Neuromuscular junction monitoring is essential if cyclophosphamide or plasmapheresis used.

POSTOPERATIVE MANAGEMENT

Common problems/complications are:

- Deterioration in cardiovascular function
- Deterioration in renal failure
- Risk of arterial or venous thromboses.

Continue systemic steroid supplements.

BIBLIOGRAPHY

Davies S R. Systemic lupus erythematosus and the obstetrical patient – implications for the anaesthetist. Canadian Journal of Anaesthesia 1991; 38: 790–796
Menon G, Allt-Graham J. Anaesthetic implications of the anticardiolipin antibody syndrome. British Journal of Anaesthesia 1993; 70: 587–590
Malinow A M, Rickford W J K, Mokkiski B L K, Saller D N, McGuinn W J. Lupus anticoagulant. Implications for the obstetric anaesthetist. Anaesthesia 1987; 42: 1291–1293

CROSS REFERENCES

Aortic valve disease
Patient Conditions 4: 95
Chronic renal failure
Patient Conditions 6: 158
Inherited coagulopathies
Patient Conditions 7: 178

URTICARIA AND ANGIO-OEDEMA

P. McQuillan

Urticaria is a well demarcated, usually pruritic, skin reaction characterized by erythematous, raised, palpable lesions, often with pale centres, which blanch on pressure. Urticarial lesions result from a transient increase in capillary permeability causing focal oedema of the superficial part of the dermis. *Angio-oedema* describes a condition in which there is circumscribed, nonpitting subepithelial oedema, sometimes with erythema. It may involve the eyelids, lips, tongue, larynx, pharynx, respiratory tract, gastrointestinal tract, renal system and, occasionally, the central nervous system. This may result in airway obstruction, pleural effusions, abdominal pain, vomiting, diarrhoea, hemiplegia and seizures.

Urticaria and angio-oedema often accompany each other; however, in those cases of angio-oedema due to a deficiency of the C_1-esterase deficiency (see below), urticaria does not occur. Individual attacks of urticaria and angio-oedema usually last no longer than 48 h. If episodes of urticaria/angio-oedema occur for more than 2 months, the condition is termed 'chronic'.

PATHOPHYSIOLOGY

Many common forms of urticaria and angio-oedema (Table 1) result from the antigen-induced release of biologically active substances from mast cells which are found in organs rich in connective tissue (e.g. skin, respiratory tract, etc.). Urticaria/angio-oedema may also be caused by drugs which cause direct mast cell degranulation or which activate the arachidonic acid or complement pathways. In all these cases, release or activation of mediators (e.g. histamine, heparin, tryptase, chymase, chemotactic factors, prostaglandins, leucotrienes, platelet activating factor (PAF), adenosine, oxygen radicals) causes altered vascular permeability, smooth muscle contraction and chemotaxis of leucocytes. This results in a spectrum of signs and symptoms ranging from simple urticaria or angio-oedema to fulminant anaphylaxis.

Table 1.
Aetiology of urticaria and angio-oedema

Idiopathic
Foodstuffs and additives
Drugs:
Antibiotics
Muscle relaxants, e.g. D-tubocurare
Opiates, e.g. morphine
Heparin
Protamine
Antihypertensives, e.g. ACE inhibitors
NSAIDs
Psychotropic drugs
Insect bites and stings
Physical:
Dermatographism
Cold/heat
Vibration
Exercise
Delayed pressure urticaria
Infections
Collagen vascular disease
Endocrine disease
Vasculitis
Malignancy
Hereditary and acquired angio-oedema
Miscellaneous

Some forms of angio-oedema result from a functional deficiency of the inhibitor of the first component of the complement cascade (C_1), C_1 esterase inhibitor (C_1EI). Hereditary angio-oedema (HAO) is an autosomal dominant disorder characterized by recurrent spontaneous episodes of oedema of the skin and the mucous membranes of the respiratory tract and gut. Minor trauma, concomitant illness or perioral surgery (e.g. dentistry or tonsillectomy) may precipitate an attack. Attacks may increase during pregnancy (when C_1EI levels are low) or during menstrual bleeding. The major serious complication of an acute attack of HAO is upper airway obstruction, although oedema of bowel wall may be mistaken for an acute abdomen and result in unnecessary, and risky, surgery. Low levels of C_1EI also occur as an acquired disorder (Table 2). Acquired C_1EI deficiency can be distinugished from HAO by the absence of complement abnormalities in other family members, late age of onset and by the reduced level of C_1 seen in the acquired form.

Table 2.
C_1-esterase inhibitor (C_1EI) deficiency

Hereditary C_1EI deficiency
Type 1 (85%)
Impaired synthesis
Mostly autosomal dominant
Type 2 (15%)
Dysfunctional protein
Heterogeneous genetic groups, mostly autosomal dominant
Aquired C_1EI deficiency
Associated with:
B-cell lymphoproliferative disorders
Connective tissue diseases
Monoclonal gammopathies
Antibodies to C_1EI

LONG-TERM TREATMENT OF URTICARIA/ANGIO-OEDEMA

Chronic urticaria/angio-oedema:

- Identify and avoid precipitating factors
- Avoid drugs which may aggravate disease, e.g. salicylates, NSAIDs, opiates
- Treat with H_1-receptor antagonists, e.g. chlorpheniramine
- Add a β-adrenergic agonist, e.g. terbutaline
- Add an H_2-receptor antagonist, e.g. cimetidine
- Consider use of a tricylcic antidepressant, e.g. doxepin (this acts against both H_1- and H_2-receptors)
- Corticosteroids are used only in very severe disease
- Adrenaline is used for severe attacks of anaphylaxis.

C_1EI deficiency (hereditary and acquired)

- Androgens, e.g. stanozolol; stimulate hepatic synthesis of C_1EI
- Antifibrinolytic agents, e.g. tranexamic acid or epsilon aminocaproic acid (EACA); these inhibit plasmin activation (plasmin is a potent catalyst for complement activation)
- Purified C_1EI concentrate (IMMUNO AG).

PREOPERATIVE ASSESSMENT

History and examination

Take a careful history. Specifically ask about:

- Atopy
- Hypersensitivity
- Drug reactions
- Family history
- Previous episodes of urticaria/angio-oedema, including frequency, duration, effect, etc.
- Drug therapy (see above).

Investigations:

- C_1EI function in HAO
- Radioallergosorbent (RAST) tests.

Preoperative preparation:

- Skin testing may be useful, but results are often unreliable and there is a small risk of severe anaphylaxis during test
- Avoid precipitating drugs or factors in chronic urticaria/angio-oedema.

Premedication

- Avoid precipitating drugs or factors in chronic urticaria/angio-oedema
- In all cases of urticaria/angio-oedema, suitable premedication should be used to allay anxiety.

In chronic urticaria/angio-oedema the following premedication may be useful:

- H_1 antihistamines
- H_2 antagonists
- β-Adrenergic agonists
- Corticosteroids.

In HAO attempts should be made to increase C_1EI levels preoperatively using:

- Androgens
- Antifibrinolytics
- Two units of fresh frozen plasma (FFP)
- Purified C_1EI concentrate (IMMUNO AG).

If the patient is not receiving long-term therapy with androgens or antifibrinolytics, these should be administered for several days prior to surgery. Although they start to act within 24 h, they require 1–2 weeks to reach maximum effect. Alternatively, the administration of 2 units of FFP given in the immediate preoperative period will restore the C_1EI to a safe level (40% of normal) for between 1 and 4 days. These measures also seem appropriate for the acquired form of

C_1EI deficiency, although there is little documentation of their use.

PERIOPERATIVE MANAGEMENT

Induction/maintenance:

- Venepuncture has precipitated forearm angio-oedema in a patient with HAO.
- Use the most 'immunologically benign' agents, particularly in atopic patients. Avoid histamine-releasing drugs, where possible.
- Avoid airway manipulation and intubation, where possible.

In *cold urticaria*:

- Use warm fluids
- Use warm laryngoscope
- Use warming blankets
- Use HME.

Monitoring

Monitor core temperature, especially in cold and cholinergic (heat) urticaria.

Positioning

In *pressure urticaria* use extra protection for bony prominences, tourniquets, etc.

Regional techniques

These may allow the avoidance of intubation.

Cardiopulmonary bypass

Cardiopulmonary bypass (CPB) has been undertaken successfully in patients with certain forms of urticaria/angio-oedema.

Management of acute attacks of urticaria and angio-oedema

- Always have facilities available to treat anaphylaxis or airway obstruction, e.g. intubation equipment and tracheostomy facilities.
- Treat acute attacks of chronic urticaria/ angio-oedema with adrenaline, steroids and antihistamines
- Treat attacks of angio-oedema due to C_1EI deficiency with FFP or purified C_1EI concentrate (1000–1500 plasma units)
- *There is no response during an acute attack of HAO to adrenaline, steroids, or antihistamines*
- Monitor coagulation status in HAO

- Remember that C_1EI levels will fall due to haemodilution if patients with C_1EI deficiency undergo CPB.
- CPB in a patient with cold urticaria has led to a rise in arterial histamine levels during rewarming.

BIBLIOGRAPHY

Johnston W E, Moss J, Philbin D M et al. Management of cold urticaria during cardiopulmonary bypass. New England Journal of Medicine 1982; 306: 220–221

Kharasch E D. Angiotensin-converting enzyme inhibitor-induced angioedema associated with endotracheal intubation. Anesthesia and Analgesia 1992; 74: 602–604

Razis P A, Coulson I H, Gould T R et al. Aquired C_1 esterase inhibitor deficiency. Anaesthesia 1986; 41: 838–840

Wall R T, Frank M, Hahn M. A review of 25 patients with hereditary angioedema requiring surgery. Anesthesiology 1989; 71: 309–311

CROSS REFERENCES

Allergic reactions
Anaesthetic Factors 33: 610
Intraoperative bronchospasm
Anaesthetic Factors 33: 632
Intraoperative hypotension
Anaesthetic Factors 33: 638

10

METABOLISM

I. Campbell

GLYCOGEN STORAGE DISEASE

I. Campbell

Glycogen is a polysaccharide made up of glucose units and found in virtually every tissue in the body.

Principal storage sites of glycogen are the liver and muscle:

- Liver glycogen is concerned with maintenance of blood glucose concentrations
- Muscle glycogen comprises the energy store for muscle itself, it does not contribute to blood glucose homeostasis.

Glycogen structure

Chains of 6–12 glucose units are joined at carbon atoms 1 and 4. The chains are joined by 1:6 linkages to form branching structures.

Glycogen metabolism

- Is under the control of a variety of enzymes which synthesize and break glycogen down to its constituent glucose units (liver glycogen) or to pyruvate and lactate in muscle
- Muscle glycogen is principally used in anaerobic metabolism via the relatively inefficient glycolytic pathway
- Metabolism occurs in situations where sudden bursts of activity are required and there is no time for increases in cardiac output and delivery of oxygen
- Lactate diffuses into general circulation; it may then be resynthesized to glucose by the liver
- Muscle and blood lactate also rise in 'shock'; production stimulated by adrenaline.

GLYCOGEN STORAGE DISEASE

Numerous enzymes are required in the synthesis and breakdown of glycogen. In 1952 the deficiency of glucose 6-phosphatase was described in Von Gierke's disease; the enzyme hydrolyses glucose 6-phosphate to glucose and phosphate immediately prior to release of glucose into the general circulation. Since then, 13 types of glycogen storage disease have been described.

Type I glycogenosis: Von Gierke's disease

Diagnosis is by liver or muscle biopsy and enzyme studies.

- Deficiency of glucose 6-phosphatase in the liver, kidney and intestine, with an inability to immobilize liver glycogen to maintain blood glucose
- Autosomal recessive disorder
- Short stature; prominent rounded abdomen due to liver enlargement; kidneys also enlarge; fat deposits in cheeks and buttocks
- Hypoglycaemic, hyperlipidaemic and a tendency to acidosis (keto acidosis and lactic acidosis)
- Prolonged bleeding time due to platelet glucose-6-phosphatase deficiency.

Treatment:

- Frequent or nasogastric feeding to maintain blood glucose
- A porta canal shunt enables absorbed glucose to bypass the liver
- Diazoxide, which inhibits insulin release and raises blood glucose.

Type II glucogenosis: Pompe's disease

- 1:4-α-Glucocidase (acid maltase).
- Lysosomal enzyme; normally breaks 1:4 linkage in glucose chains.
- Glycogen present in excessive quantities in:
  - Liver
  - Heart
  - Muscle
  - Tongue
  - Central nervous system
  - *Especially* anterior horn cells.

Blood sugar, lipid and ketone concentrations and response to glucagon and adrenaline are normal, but the prognosis is poor due to muscle weakness and heart failure.

Type III glycogenosis: Cori's disease

- Deficiency of amylo 1,6-glucosidase (debranching enzyme)
- Features similar to type I but milder; able to mobilize glucose from outer chains of glycogen molecule
- Liver enlarged, growth retardation, hypoglycaemia, elevated blood lipid concentrations and increased hepatic glycogen
- Treatment consists of frequent feeds with a high protein diet (gluconeogenic pathway intact); hypoglycaemia can cause mental retardation.

Type IV glycogenosis: Andersen's disease

- Deficiency of 1,4-glucose-6-glucosyl transferase (brancher) enzyme
- Normal at birth, but fails to thrive
- Enlarged liver and spleen, muscles hypotonic
- Problems are those of liver disease; death in the second year of life.

Type V glycogenosis: McArdle's syndrome

- Lack of muscle phosphorylase which normally removes glucose units from glycogen as glucose 1-phosphate for metabolism to pyruvate and lactate; therefore unable to maintain glucose supply
- Symptoms usually develop in second decade of life
- Muscle of glycogen moderately elevated; severe pain and muscle cramps at start of exercise due to lack of glucose availability, but passes off (second wind) if exercise persists because of increased cardiac output, vasodilatation and availability of circulating glucose and fatty acids; advised to start exercise gradually.

Type VI glycogenosis: Hers' disease

- Reduced hepatic phospharylase
- Clinically mild form of type I; enlarged liver and mild hypoglycaemia.

Type VII to XII glycogenoses

Extremely rare.

ANAESTHESIA IN GLYCOGEN STORAGE DISEASE

Experience is limited. With hepatic glycogenosis (type I and type III) problems are hypoglycaemia and acidosis. Both lactic acidosis in type I and ketoacidosis in type IX have been described along with hyperthermia. It is thus important to provide enteral or parenteral nutrition pre- and post-operatively and to monitor acid–base status.

With type II disease problems are of myocardial involvement with congestive or obstructive cardiomyopathy and skeletal muscle weakness. A large tongue may cause airway problems. Successful surgery has been done with ketamine and vecuronium and obsessional attention to detailed monitoring, particularly oxygenation. Also, an enlarged heart has caused bronchial obstruction.

Anaesthetic experience with type V disease is also very limited. On theoretical grounds suxamethonium should be avoided because of the potential myoglobin release and renal damage. Atracurium and alcuronium have been used uneventfully, as has extradural spinal anaesthesia with bipuvacaine. Any increased metabolic demand on, or diminution in the blood supply to skeletal muscle is a potential problem, e.g. hypotension, hypothermia and shivering. Also, the use of a tourniquet should be avoided.

BIBLIOGRAPHY

Casson H. Anaesthesia for portocaval bypass in patients with metabolic disease. British Journal of Anaesthesia 1975; 47: 969–975

Coleman P. McArdle's disease. Problem of anaesthetic management of Caesarian section. Anaesthesia 1984; 39: 784–787

Cox J M. Anesthesia and glycogen storage disease. Anesthesiology 1968; 29: 1221–1225

Edelstein G, Hershman C A. Hyperthermia and ketoacidosis during anaesthesia in a child with glycogen storage disease. Anesthesiology 1980; 52: 90–92

McFarlane H J, Soni N. Pompe's disease and anaesthesia. 1986; 41: 1219–1224

Samuels T A, Coleman P. McArdle's disease and Caesarian section. Anaesthesia 1988; 43: 161–162

Rajah A, Bell C F. Atracurium and McArdle's disease. Anaesthesia 1986; 41: 93

PORPHYRIA

I. Campbell

10

Porphyria is a group of diseases related to defects in the synthesis of haem which functions in several systems concerned with the transport and utilization of oxygen: haemoglobin, myoglobin and mitochondrial and microsomal enzymes, including hepatic cytochrome P450 (Figure 1).

Haem is essential to life. Its synthesis is regulated by the feedback mechanism of haem itself on the enzyme δ-aminolaevulinic acid (ALA) synthase – the first, and rate-limiting, step in the haem synthetic pathway. ALA activity can be induced directly by:

- Barbiturates
- Steroids
- Alcohol.

In addition, the cytochrome P450 enzyme system in the liver is the main hepatic consumer of haem; induction of the P450 system stimulates ALA synthesis via the resultant fall in haem concentration.

CLINICAL FEATURES

Clinical features are largely neurological. The reasons for this are uncertain. ALA or products of porphyrin may be neurotoxic. ALA also resembles the neurotransmitter α-aminobutyric acid, and so might compete for GABA receptor sites.

Symptoms are nonspecific, comprising scattered lesions in the central and autonomic nervous systems. There are few, or no, physical signs:

- Abdominal pain, possibly colicky
- Vomiting
- Constipation
- Dehydrated/hypovolaemic
- Base disturbances
- Acid–base sensory motor or autonomic abnormalities
- Pain syndromes
- Psychological disturbances
- Impairment of consciousness
- Bulbar palsy
- Convulsions.

Symptoms are provoked by pregnancy, alcohol, dietary restriction and a wide variety of drugs (see below).

Acute intermittent porphyria (Sweden)

All the above-described features are seen, precipitated by lipid-soluble drugs. Diagnosis is by the ALA and porphobilinogen concentrations in urine.

Variegate porphyria (South Africa)

As above, but 80% of cases have photosensitivity/skin fragility, possibly due to photosensitive porphyrins in the skin.

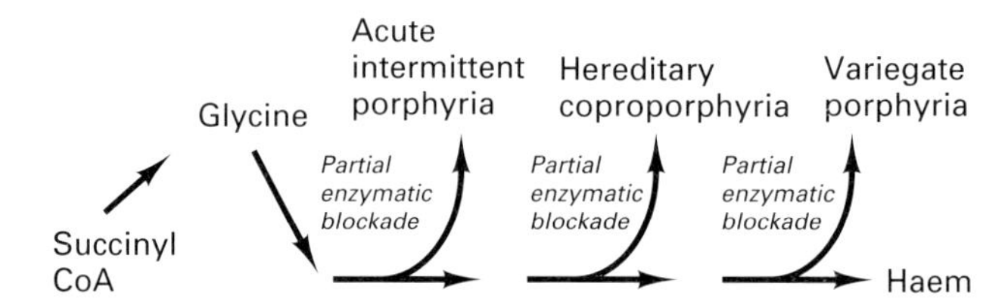

Figure 1
Deficiencies in three enzymes give rise to three types of porphyria; total blocks in one or other of these enzymes would be lethal, but the partial block leads to an accumulation of the various metabolites proximal to the block.

Hereditary coproporphyria

This is very rare. It is similar to the acute intermittent form. It is diagnosed by a pattern of porphyria and porphyrin precursors in urine. Symptoms may also be precipitated by stress, infections, fasting and endogenous hormonal fluctuations.

DIAGNOSIS OF PORPHYRIA

Diagnosis is made on the basis of blood and urinary levels of:

- ALA
- Porphobilinogen
- Total porphyrin.

ANAESTHETIC TECHNIQUE

The porphyrogenicity of drugs is determined by using various types of cell culture and laboratory animals rendered porphyric by infusion of diethoxycarbonylophydrocollidine.

Anaesthetic drugs are high on the list of those that may precipitate an acute attack. No ideal anaesthetic technique has yet been determined; reports about the dangers of different agents are inconsistent and dependent on animal work and clinical experience. Various lists have been produced at various times of drugs that, with uncertain degrees of reliability, have been thought to precipitate or not precipitate attacks. Recently published lists are reproduced in Table 1.

The major problem has been the choice of induction agent. Numerous recent case reports have indicated that propofol may be safe. All the amide local anaesthetics have at various times been implicated, but a recent

Table 1.
Safety of commonly used drugs

Category	Drug group	Drugs
Safe	*Gases and vapours*	Nitrous oxide Cyclopropane Diethyl ether
	Neuromuscular blocking agents	Suxamethonium Curare
	Local anaesthetics	Procaine Procainamide
	Opiates	Pethidine Fentanyl Morphine Buprenorphine
	Oral analgesics	Paracetamol Temazepam
	Major tranquillizers	Droperidol Phenothiazines
	Adrenergic agonists/antagonists	Beta blockers Adrenaline Phentolamine Salbutamol
	Other	Atropine Neostigmine Domperidone
Possibly safe	*Induction agents*	Propofol
	Neuromuscular blocking agents	Vecuronium
	Benzodiazepines	Midazolam Lorazopam
	Other	Metoclopramide Amethocaine Naloxone Corticosteroids
Contentious	*Induction agents*	Ketamine
	Gases and vapours	Halothane
	Neuromuscular blocking agents	Pancuronium
	Local anaesthetics	Lignocaine Prilocaine Bupivacaine
	Benzodiazepines	Diazepam Triazolam Oxazepam
	Other	Disopyramide Ranitidine
No data	*Gases and vapours*	Isoflurane
	Neuromuscular blocking agents	Atracurium
	Opiates	Alfentanyl Sufentanyl
	Parasympathetic agents	Glycopyrronium
	Antidysrhythmia agents	Mexilitine Bretylium
	Vasoactive agents	β Agonists α Agonists
	Vasodilators	Sodium nitroprusside
Unsafe/probably unsafe	*Induction agents*	Barbiturates Etomidate
	Gases and vapours	Enflurane
	Neuromuscular blocking agents	Alcuronium
	Local anaesthetics	Mepivacaine
	Vasoactive agents	Tilidine Verapamil Nifedipine Diltiazem Hydralazine Phenoxybenzamine
	Opiates	Pentazocine
	Other	Aminophylline Cimetidine

report has described the successful and uneventful use of bupivacaine in epidural anaesthesia for Caesarean section.

BIBLIOGRAPHY

Harrison G G, Meissner P N, Hift R J. Anaesthesia for the porphyric patient. Anaesthesia 1993; 48: 417–421

McNeill M J, Bennet A. Use of regional anaesthesia in a patient with acute porphyria. British Journal of Anaesthesia 1990; 64: 371–373

Meissner P N, Harrison G G, Hift R J. Propofol as an IV anaesthetic induction agent in variegate porphyria. British Journal of Anaesthesia 1991; 66: 60–65

WATER AND ELECTROLYTE DISTURBANCES

I. Campbell

The body is roughly 60% water, which is contained almost exclusively in lean tissue. Adipose tissue is virtually anhydrous. The ratio of intracellular/interstitial/intravascular water is 10:3:1, or as a percentage of body weight 40:14:5.

Normal body water turnover is in the region of 2–3 l day^{-1}. On the intake side fluid intake is about 1200 ml; 1000 ml in solid food and about 400 ml day^{-1} is derived from oxidation of foodstuffs. Urine output amounts to 1500 ml, with 600–1000 ml insensible losses via the skin and respiratory tract, and 50 ml via the gut.

The principal extracellular ions are sodium and chloride, with a plasma osmolality of about 300 mOsm. Sodium and chloride ions permeate through the whole of the extracellular fluid.

The intra/extracellular fluid and electrolyte relationships are maintained via the relative permeabilities of sodium and potassium ions and the high protein content of the intracellular fluid with its negative charge. They are also maintained by activity of the Na^+ and K^+ pump.

Movement of fluid between the capillaries and the interstitial fluid is determined by the colloid oncotic and hydrostatic forces across the capillary wall.

REGULATION OF SODIUM AND WATER BALANCE

Total body sodium ion and water are

controlled by a variety of mechanisms involving antidiuretic hormone (ADH) and atrial natriuretic peptide (ANP) – a 'hormone' released by the muscle cells of the heart (plasma levels correlate with right atrial pressures). ANP is thought to affect salt and water secretion via an effect on glomerular filtration and sodium absorption in the proximal tubule.

ADH is secreted in response to changes detected by osmoreceptors in the hypothalamus. An increase in osmolality stimulates ADH secretion and resorption of fluid in the collecting ducts due to an increase in their permeability; less water is excreted and the urine is more concentrated.

The atrial receptors also have an effect on ADH secretion. Stretching, as in hypervolaemia, inhibits ADH secretion; loss of volume, such as following haemorrhage, stimulates it.

Renin–angiotensin system

Sodium and water balance are also controlled by the renin–angiotensin system. The juxtaglomerular cells are sensitive to

- Plasma sodium concentration,
- Blood pressure in afferent arterioles
- Input from sympathetic nerves.

That is, they are sensitive to indicators of plasma sodium concentration and plasma volume.

Renin secretion is stimulated by the three factors listed above. Renin cleaves angiotensin I from angiotensinogen in plasma, which is then converted to angiotensin II by converting enzyme and then to angiotensin III in the adrenal cortex, where it stimulates aldosterone secretion.

Aldosterone controls reabsorption of sodium from the distal tubule but the system responds slowly and is the 'fine tuning' of the sodium and water balance, controlling only the final 3% of the filtered load; its effect may take several days to become evident.

Disorders of the renin–angiotensin system may result in hypertension; failure of the aldosterone system results in sodium loss and hypotension.

ANP acts as a control both on the renin–angiotensin system and by inhibiting the reabsorption of sodium in the distal tubule; it is a vasodilator and thus also affects blood pressure directly.

Water homeostasis

The kidney, via the ADH response, has a huge reserve capacity to clear excess water, so excess intake normally only results in a transient decrease in osmolality. The sensation of thirst and the ADH, ANP and the renal–angiotensin system are all interlinked. Angiotensin II is a powerful thirst-causing substance, and ADH neurones and the thirst centre in the hypothalamus are closely associated.

Extracellular fluid homeostasis

This involves gain or loss of: isotonic sodium chloride (NaCl), pure water, or pure NaCl.

- Cell membranes are effectively impermeable to sodium ions, so addition or loss of isotonic saline results in changes to only the extracellular fluid compartment (75% interstitial, 25% plasma)
- Loss of extracellular water results in an increase in extracellular osmolality which causes water to move from the cells. With a gain in pure water the reverse is true.
- Changes in the extracellular fluid NaCl content alone are compensated for by movement of fluid into or from the intracellular fluid compartment.

Thus a change in pure water or NaCl alone affects both intracellular as well as extracellular fluid, whereas isotonic changes affect only extracellular fluid.

POTASSIUM HOMEOSTASIS

The potential across cell membranes is largely controlled by the differential potassium ion concentrations. Changes in extracellular potassium have a disproportionately marked effect on the size of this potential.

Ninety per cent of potassium is reabsorbed from the kidney in the proximal tubule and the proximal part of the loop of Henle. The remaining 10% arrives in the distal tubule; it is via this 10% that all potassium regulation occurs. Reabsorption of potassium from the distal tubule is via an active pump in the tubular cells; in the presence of hyperkalaemia aldosterone secretion increases in response to the direct effect of potassium on the adrenal cortex (a mechanism not involving the renin–angiotensin pathway). Sodium reabsorbed from this distal tubule is associated with secretion of potassium and hydrogen ions, the two cations being in competition with each other.

10

CALCIUM AND PHOSPHATE HOMEOSTASIS

The normal plasma concentration of calcium ions is 2.5 mM, but the physiologically important part is ionic calcium which constitutes just under 50%: 46% of plasma calcium is protein bound, and 6% is bound to phosphate.

Calcium ions are important in membrane excitability and are sensitive to pH changes, with alkalinity decreasing calcium ion concentration and acidosis increasing it.

Elevated [Ca^{2+}]	Decreased [Ca^{2+}]
Lethargy	Muscle cramps
Fatigue	Convulsions
Sensory loss	Increased neuromuscular excitability

Metabolism and control of calcium ion concentration are inextricably bound up with phosphate metabolism; most calcium ions are contained in bone which acts as a massive reserve in the control of calcium ion concentration. Intestinal uptake of calcium ions is in the range 20–70%, varying in response to changes in plasma concentration. Calcium and phosphate are excreted by the kidney – filtered out then absorbed under hormonal control (Table 1).

DISTURBANCES IN FLUID AND ELECTROLYTES

Probably the commonest abnormality in clinical practice is hypovolaemia, i.e. loss of both fluid and electrolytes, due either to blood loss or fluid loss such as diarrhoea/vomiting, or loss into the gastrointestinal tract in obstruction or burn injury. This is loss of both fluid and electrolytes and is best replaced by balanced salt solution, Ringer's lactate (Hartmann's solution) or 0.9% saline, although the latter provides a large chloride load and tends to produce metabolic acidosis, and lactate is metabolized in the liver to carbon dioxide and water and tends to produce alkalosis. If the hypovolaemia is severe enough to produce problems with cardiac output and peripheral perfusion, intravascular volume is more effectively repleted with colloidal solutions such as albumin, or one of the synthetic colloids, or even blood.

The colloid versus crystalloid debate continues. The objection to the latter is that is takes, on average, three times as much crystalloid to produce a persistent increase in blood volume as it does colloid, because of rapid transfer of the former to the extracellular space. Colloid also eventually leaks into the extravascular space, but more slowly. The objection to colloid is that this type of problem is usually associated with an acute phase response and an increase in capillary permeability, both generally and at the site of injury. Fluid that leaks from the intravascular space is sequestered in this 'third' or 'oedema space', which may include the lung. When the patient recovers this fluid is remobilized and excreted. With colloid this remobilization may be more protracted.

Table 1.
Hormonal control of calcium metabolism

Hormone	Source	Trigger to stimulation	Effect
Calcitonin	Parafollicular cells of thyroid		• Stimulates bone deposition • Decreases plasma Ca^{2+}
Parathormone	Parathyroid glands	Low plasma calcium	• Release of Ca^{2+} from bone • Reabsorption from renal tubule • Decreases renal reabsorption of phosphate
1,25-Dihydroxy-cholecalciferol (1,25-DOHCC)	Derivative of vitamins D_2 and D_3 via metabolic pathways in liver and kidney		• Ca^{2+} and phosphate absorption from the gut

FLUID BALANCE DURING SURGERY AND ANAESTHESIA

Patients arriving for surgery may have been starved for up to 12 h and would be about 1 l in deficit. This deficit is of both fluids and electrolytes, and so can be replaced with balanced salt solution. Fluid requirements during surgery depend on the extent of the surgery. It is conventional practice in the normal individual to transfuse blood when about 20% of the circulating blood volume has been lost. With blood loss, fluid requirements (in addition to blood replacement) are in the range 5–15 ml kg^{-1} h^{-1}, depending on the amount of blood loss and the extent of surgery. Hypotonic (glucose) solutions should not be given for volume replacement, as in the short term they produce significant hyperglycaemia (>20 mol/l^{-1}) and in the longer term persistent hyponatraemia.

Table 2.

Disorder	Causes	Clinical signs	Biochemical signs	Treatment
Water deficiency	Diabetes insipidus Hyperosmolar nonketotic diabetic coma Nephrogenic diabetes insipidus Some types of chronic pyelonephritis	Loss of skin turgor Loss of eyeball tension Dry mucous membrane Low BP Delirium Coma	Plasma Na^+ and Cl^- elevated Plasma hypertonic, Na^+ conserved K^+ and H^+ excreted to produce hypokalaemic acidosis Haematocrit and plasma protein concentration Urine and plasma osmolality increased	Oral rehydration, if possible, or dextrose (5% i.v.)
Water excess	Heart failure Acute renal failure Iatrogenic (administration of 5% dextrose)	Abdominal and skeletal muscular twitching and cramps Stupor Convulsions In severe cases peripheral and pulmonary oedema	Low plasma Na^+ and Cl^- Increased blood and plasma volume Low osmolality Low plasma proteins and haematocrit	
Sodium chloride deficiency	Decreased intake unusual, but may occur in diarrhoea, malabsorption, severe vomiting Increased Na^+ loss in diabetic acidosis Chronic renal disease Excessive sweating Adrenal insufficiency	Symptoms develops as [Na^+] drops below 115 Clouding of consciousness Convulsions Coma	Plasma Na^+ and Cl^- drop after 4 or 5 days Decrease in blood volume K^+ moves out of cells (to maintain tonicity) Na^+ conservation via renin–angiotensin–aldosterone system Metabolic alkalosis Haematocrit and plasma proteins increased (decreased in dilutional hyponatraemia)	
Sodium chloride excess	Iatrogenic (particularly intravenous nutrition) Primary aldosteronism	Oedema Congestive heart failure Fluid retained so osmolality and [Na^+] may be normal		

Table 2 (*contd.*)

Disorder	Causes	Clinical signs	Biochemical signs	Treatment
Potassium deficiency	Gastrointestinal losses Renal disease Diuretics Hormonal (aldosteronism) Cushing's disease Steroids Diabetic acidosis Trauma Burns Intravenous feeding with no added K^+	Drowsy Muscular weakness Paralytic ileus Bradycardia Heart block ST depression Inverted T waves Prolonged QT and PR intervals U waves		
Potassium excess	Renal failure Iatrogenic (administration of K^+) Na^+ conserving diuretics Adrenal insufficiency Acidosis Hypoxia	Anxiety Agitation Stupor Weakness Hyporeflexia Paralysis of extremities Peaked T waves Widened QRS and prolonged PR interval Arrhythmias Cardiac arrest		Acute treatment with Ca^{2+} salts Glucose/insulin Ion exchange resins

11

PATIENT AGE

G. Meakin

THE ELDERLY PATIENT

E. Cheetham

The elderly population is defined as all persons over the age of 65 years. Demographically, this is an increasing proportion of the population.

Preoperative assessment includes:

- Assessment of functional ability
- Assessment of underlying medical illness, with the rational use of special investigations
- Risk assessment for surgery.

Detailed descriptions of the physiological and anatomical alterations of old age, and changes in drug handling are beyond the scope of this section but, where relevant, are mentioned.

ASSESSMENT OF FUNCTIONAL ABILITY

Functional assessment is a vital component of preoperative evaluation, facilitating successful reintegration into society, possibly after major surgery. Comprehensive evaluation is aimed towards baseline assessment, risk-factor screening and planning for rehabilitation. Assessment considers:

- *Physical function.* The ability to perform tasks ranging from activities of daily living (ADL), e.g. basic human functions to more complex tasks of manual performance and housekeeping. Examples are the Barthel ADL scale and the Instrumental ADL scale.
- *Cognitive function.* Impairment in cognitive function is common in elderly patients. Various instruments have been used to assess the degree of impairment, but differentiation of acute confusional states requires further clinical assessment (see below). Examples of such scales include the Short Portable Mental Status Questionnaire, the Wechsler Memory Scale and the Dementia Rating Scale.
- *Emotional status.* This detects the presence of depression, which is common amongst the hospitalized elderly.
- *Social activities and support.*

ASSESSMENT OF UNDERLYING MEDICAL ILLNESS

This should be based upon history, clinical examination and results of investigations (as indicated), with subsequent management guided by the extent and urgency of planned surgery. Clinical examination should include all major organ systems, together with an assessment of nutrition, hydration, vision, hearing and dentition. In the systems enquiry one should look particularly for the following age-related pathology, and drug therapies:

Nervous system:
- Cerebrovascular disease
- Autonomic dysfunction
- Parkinsonism
- Depression
- Impaired vision and hearing
- Dementia or acute confusional states.

Drugs: antiparkinsonian therapy, antipsychotics, anticonvulsants, glaucoma therapy.

Cardiovascular disease:
- Ischaemic heart disease (angina, myocardial infarction, cardiac failure or conduction and rhythm disturbances)
- Hypertension
- Valvular heart disease
- Peripheral vascular disease.

Drugs: antihypertensives, antianginals, diuretics and other antifailure therapy, anticoagulants.

In the case of fall-related trauma in the elderly, the cause of the fall must be ascertained. Although often innocent, such as tripping over, falls can frequently be caused by:

- Cardiac dysrhythmias
- Silent myocardial infarction
- Cerebrovascular disease
- Acute confusional states, possible organic causes of which include drugs, infection,

metabolic (endocrine or electrolyte disturbances), hypoxia and intracranial space-occupying pathology.

Respiratory system:
- Chronic obstructive pulmonary disease
- Acute chest infection.

Drugs: bronchodilators, steroids, antibiotics.

Renal system:
- Urinary tract infection
- Transitional cell malignancy
- Prostatic hypertrophy and malignancy
- Renal failure secondary to cardiovascular, drug, infiltrative or obstructive causes.

Drugs: antibiotics, oestrogens, hormone antagonists.

Endocrine and metabolic systems:
- Diabetes mellitus
- Thyroid disease
- Electrolyte imbalances (drug induced, endocrine or gut tumour secretory).

Drugs: hypoglycaemics, thyroxine or antithyroid therapy, electrolyte supplements.

Connective tissue and bone:
- Osteoporosis, osteomalacia and Paget's disease
- Osteoarthritis and rheumatoid arthritis.

Drugs: anti-inflammatory agents, steroids.

Gastrointestinal system:
- Dysphagia, achalasia and silent aspiration
- Malnutrition
- Inflammatory bowel disease and malignancy.

Haematological system:
- Anaemia – iron deficiency, megaloblastic or anaemia of chronic disease
- Haematological malignancies and paraproteinaemias.

INVESTIGATIONS

These should be guided by the pathology, the extent of planned surgery and the urgency.

Urinalysis
Suspected infection; diabetes.

Plasma electrolytes
Suspected drug-induced, endocrine or gut tumour disruption.

Blood glucose
Diabetes. A formal glucose tolerance test may be useful, if time allows.

Blood gases
Prior to abdominal or thoracic surgery in patients with known respiratory disease.

Predicted P_aO_2 (mmHg) in old age:
Normal: $P_aO_2 = 100 - (\text{Age} \times 0.32)$
Postoperatively: $P_aO_2 = 100 - (\text{Age} \times 0.54)$

Full blood count
Suspicion of anaemia, anticipated blood loss, suspected malignancy or infection.

Chest X-ray
Not a useful predictor of postoperative pulmonary morbidity, but has been shown to be a useful baseline should respiratory or cardiac complications occur.

ECG
Shown to be a useful baseline to aid interpretation of postoperative complications, but again is a poor predictor of cardiac morbidity.

Pulmonary function tests
Indicated prior to pulmonary surgery and, with blood gases, shown to be a predictor of the need for postoperative ventilation for abdominal surgery in patients with severe respiratory impairment.

Values	Implication
$FEV_1 > 1$ l, $P_aO_2 > 7$ kPa, $P_aCO_2 < 6.5$ kPa	Careful monitoring and oxygen therapy
$FEV_1 < 1$ l, $P_aO_2 < 7$ kPa, $P_aCO_2 > 6.5$ kPa	Likely to need postoperative ventilation

Laboratory-based cardiac evaluation
Most useful in revealing occult ischaemic heart disease in patients undergoing peripheral vascular surgery. Indicated in planned cardiac surgery. Tests might include: echocardiography, exercise ECG testing, invasive haemodynamic assessment.

RISK ASSESSMENT

In abdominal and noncardiac thoracic surgery, the commonest postoperative complications are respiratory (14–40%) and cardiac (12–14%) in nature. Most attempts to produce predictors have been directed towards these outcomes.

Also relevant is postoperative stroke which, although rare (0.4–3%), carries a high acute mortality (16–50%).

Useful predictors of cardiac morbidity:
- ASA classification
- Goldman cardiac risk factors (especially a third heart sound and cardiac failure)
- Exercise tolerance – this may be assessed clinically (can the patient leave their own home as a result of their own effort at least two times per week?), or quantified more objectively (using a bicycle ergometer, can the patient pedal for more than 2 min, maintaining a heart rate greater than 99 beats min^{-1}?).

Useful predictors of respiratory morbidity:
- ASA classification III or IV
- Upper abdominal surgery
- High body mass index
- Impaired exercise tolerance (see above).

Predictors of perioperative stroke (noncarotid surgery):
- Transient ischaemic attacks
- Previous cerebral infarction
- Hypertension
- Increasing age
- Atrial fibrillation
- Diabetes.

BIBLIOGRAPHY

Baillière's Clinical Anaesthesiology 1993; 7:
Gerson M C et al. Prediction of cardiac and pulmonary complications related to elective abdominal and noncardiac thoracic surgery in geriatric patients. American Journal of Medicine 1990; 88: 101–107
Kaufman L. Anaesthesia for the elderly. In: Kaufman L (ed) Anaesthesia review 1992, vol 9
Wong D H W. Peri-operative stroke. Part 1: General surgery, carotid artery disease, and carotid endarterectomy. Canadian Journal of Anaesthesia 1991; 38: 347–373

INFANTS AND CHILDREN

G. Meakin

Infants and children differ from adults in size, bodily proportions and maturity. Small size presents practical problems for the anaesthetist, while differences in proportion and the maturation of organ systems have complex effects on the responses to anaesthetic drugs.

SIZE

Size is usually measured by weighing patients. The following formula gives average values for children aged less than 13 years:

$$\text{Weight} = \frac{(\text{Age} + 3) \times 5}{2}\ \text{kg}$$

Many physiological processes are related to *body surface area*. As the surface area/weight ratio of the infant is approximately twice that of the adult (Figure 1), there is a proportionate increase in *metabolic rate, water, electrolyte and ventilation requirements*, and some *drug dosages*. These differences decrease gradually throughout childhood.

RESPIRATORY SYSTEM

Oxygen consumption is 7 ml kg^{-1} min^{-1} in the neonate compared with 3.5 ml kg^{-1} min^{-1} in the adult; similarly, ventilation is increased to 200 ml kg^{-1} min^{-1} compared with 100 ml kg^{-1} min^{-1} in the adult. As tidal volume remains constant at around 7 ml kg^{-1}, the increased ventilation in younger patients is brought about by an increase in respiratory rate; this is

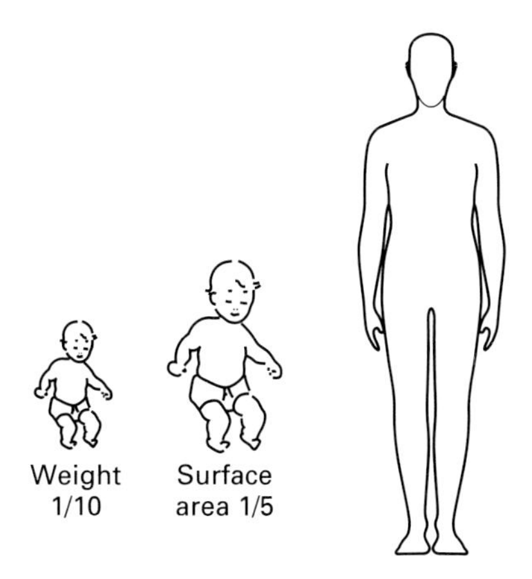

Figure 1
Proportions of an infant aged 6 months relative to an adult, with respect to weight and surface area.

approximately 30 breaths min^{-1} at birth, 24 breaths min^{-1} at 1 year and 12 breaths min^{-1} in the adult.

Lung compliance is reduced in infants, and small airways tend to close at end-expiration. This tendency is increased during anaesthesia, thus increasing the risk of absorption atelectasis and hypoxaemia. In order to prevent these effects, it is customary to control ventilation in infants using large tidal volumes (12 ml kg^{-1}) and applying up to 5 cmH_2O end-expiratory pressure.

Premature infants, especially those with a gestational age of less than 46 weeks and a postnatal age of less than 4 months, are at increased risk of apnoea following anaesthesia. These patients require careful monitoring for 24 h postoperatively and should not be accepted as day-cases.

CARDIOVASCULAR SYSTEM

Changes in the cardiovascular system mirror those in pulmonary ventilation (Figure 2). The increased cardiac output in younger patients is brought about by an increase in heart rate; stroke volume remains constant at 1 ml kg^{-1} throughout life.

Parasympathetic control is well developed at birth, but sympathetic control is incomplete. This may explain the normally reduced blood pressure in infants and their increased susceptibility to reflex bradycardia and hypotension. Bradycardia during anaesthesia can be prevented or treated with intravenous atropine (20 μg kg^{-1}).

WATER AND ELECTROLYTES

Approximately 1 ml of fluid is required per kilocalorie of energy expended. Thus, maintenance fluid rate and metabolic rate may be calculated using the same formula (Table 1).

Maintenance requirements of electrolytes are: 30 mmol sodium, 20 mmol chloride and 20 mmol of potassium per 1000 kcal. These will be supplied by 0.18% saline with 20 mmol potassium chloride per litre.

TEMPERATURE MAINTENANCE

This is a problem in infants because of their

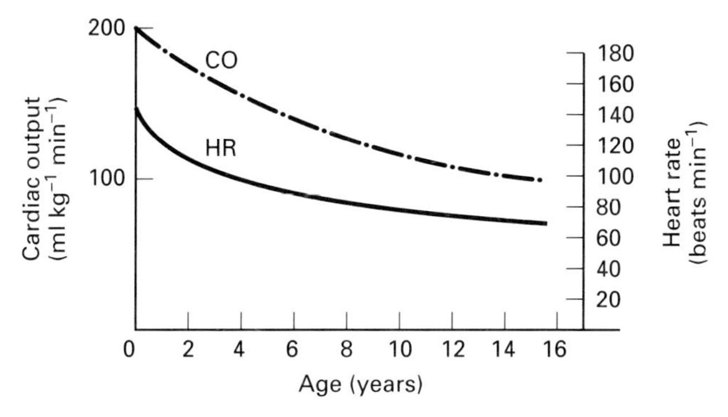

Figure 2
Variation in cardiac output (CO) and heart rate (HR) with age.

Table 1.
Maintenance fluid (and energy) requirements

Body weight (kg)	Amount and rate
0–10	4 ml kg h^{-1}
10–20	40 ml + 2 ml kg^{-1} h^{-1} for each kilogram over 10
>20	60 ml +1 ml kg^{-1} h^{-1} for each kilogram over 20

small size, large surface area/body weight ratio, and lack of subcutaneous fat. During moderate–light anaesthesia, hypothermia increases oxygen demand, which may result in hypoxia, lactic acidosis, bradycardia, hypotension and cardiac arrest. Hypothermia can be prevented by increasing the temperature of the operating room to 24–26°C, and using heating devices such as warming mattresses and warm-air blowers.

PSYCHOLOGICAL FACTORS

Childhood is a period of great emotional lability and impressionability. Stressful experiences in hospital make a more lasting impression on children, and behavioural disturbances frequently occur after they return home. The following may reduce the stress of hospitalization:

- Preadmission visit to the hospital
- Video presentation showing hospital procedures
- Preoperative visit of the anaesthetist
- Parental presence at induction of anaesthesia
- EMLA cream to venepuncture sites 1 h preoperatively
- Oral sedative premedication, e.g.
  - Day-cases: midazolam (0.5 mg kg^{-1}) 45 min preoperatively
  - In-patients: diazepam (0.25 mg kg^{-1}) and droperidol (0.25 mg kg^{-1}) 1 h preoperatively.

DRUG DOSAGE

Paediatric drug dosage is determined by pharmacokinetic and pharmacodynamic variables which are changing independently of one another during development. Consequently, there is no general rule of converting adult doses to paediatric ones. The doses of the following anaesthetic drugs were determined by clinical studies.

Thiopentone

Neonates require 4–5 mg kg^{-1}, infants 7–8 mg kg^{-1} and children 5–6 mg kg^{-1} of thiopentone for induction of anaesthesia. The reduced requirements in neonates can be explained by decreased plasma protein binding. The increased requirements in infants and children compared with adults (usual dose 4 mg kg^{-1}) may be due to their increased cardiac output, as this would be expected to reduce the first-pass concentration of thiopentone arriving at the brain. Doses may be reduced by up to 50% by sedative premedication.

Morphine

Infants aged less than 6 months appear sensitive to the respiratory depressant effects of morphine due to increased permeability of the blood–brain barrier. Balanced anaesthesia in neonates may be supplemented with 25 μg kg^{-1} of morphine followed by maintenance doses of 5–10 μg kg^{-1} h^{-1}. Infants aged more than 6 months and older children may be given a loading dose of 100 μg kg^{-1} with maintenance doses of 25 μg kg^{-1} h^{-1}.

Tubocurarine

The neuromuscular junction of the neonate is three times more sensitive to the effects of tubocurarine than is that of the adult. However, because of the increased volume of extracellular fluid in younger patients, which approximates to the volume of distribution of tubocurarine, dose does not vary significantly with age. This is probably also true of other nondepolarizing muscle relaxants.

In children, as in adults, a dose of 0.5 mg kg^{-1} tubocurarine produces about 45 min of neuromuscular blockade. In infants the duration of action is prolonged due to an increase in half-time of elimination secondary to the increase in volume of distribution.

Atracurium

Atracurium at a dose of 0.5 mg kg^{-1} produces about 30 min of neuromuscular blockade in children and adults. Recovery is slightly faster in neonates and infants, owing to an increase in plasma clearance. This unique and attractive feature probably relates to the fact that 50% of the drug is eliminated by non-organ routes such as Hofmann hydrolysis.

Suxamethonium

Infants require at least 3 mg kg^{-1} and children 2 mg kg^{-1} of suxamethonium to produce reliable conditions for intubation. The duration of action of these doses is about the same as that produced by 1 mg kg^{-1} in adults.

Neostigmine

Neostigmine at a dose of 35 μg kg^{-1} antagonizes nondepolarizing neuromuscular blockade more rapidly in paediatric patients than in adults. Increasing the dose does not increase the rate of reversal, which is unlikely to be satisfactory in the absence of a response to train-of-four stimulation.

Halothane

In neonates, the MAC of halothane is about 0.9%, but it increases rapidly to a maximum of 1.2% at 6 months, after which it declines gradually to about 0.8% in the adult. The reduced requirements of halothane in neonates compared with infants may be due to attenuation of the pain response. The increased requirements in infants and children compared with adults may reflect an increase in brain water. Uptake and elimination is more rapid in children than in adults, because of the larger minute volume of ventilation and lower functional residual capacity in children.

BIBLIOGRAPHY

Harris J S. Special pediatric problems in fluid and electrolyte therapy in surgery. Annals of New York Academy of Science 1957; 66: 966–975

Holliday M A, Segar W E. The maintenance need for water in parenteral fluid therapy. Pediatrics 1957; 19: 823–832

Meakin G. Anaesthesia for infants and children. In: Healy T E J, Cohen P J (eds). A practice of anaesthesia, 6th edn. In press

PART 2

SURGICAL PROCEDURES

12

NEUROSURGERY

M. Smith, N. P. Hirsch

GENERAL PRINCIPLES OF NEUROANAESTHESIA

C. Goldsack

POSITIONING

Supine: reverse Trendelenburg with up to 30 degrees head-up tilt, modest neck flexion and back elevation to help promote venous drainage.

Prone: care with eyes, face, axillae, breasts. Avoid excessive venous pressure.

Sitting: beware hypotension and venous air embolism.

Lateral: ensure head and body are well supported. Avoid pressure on nerves and jugular compression.

CONTROL OF RAISED INTRACRANIAL PRESSURE

- *Cerebral dehydration*
  Osmotic diuretics (mannitol 0.25–1 g/kg)
  Loop diuretics (frusemide 0.5–1 mg/kg): useful if volume overload precludes mannitol or in combination with mannitol if ICP is greatly raised
  Avoid over-hydration.
- *Moderate hyperventilation*
  Approximately 3.8–4.2 kPa. Over-zealous hyperventilation may cause cerebral ischaemia
  Transient effect (up to about 24 hours).
- *Corticosteroids*
  Useful for vasogenic oedema associated with tumours or abscesses; dexamethasone (4 mg q.d.s.) is the drug of choice
  Ineffective in head injury
  Onset of effect takes several hours.
- *Reduction in central venous pressure*
  Slight head-up tilt (up to 30 degrees)
  Avoid compression of neck veins
  Adequate anaesthesia and muscle relaxation
  NB. high levels of PEEP (> 10 cmH_2O) may increase CVP and ICP.
- *Drainage of cerebrospinal fluid*
  In hydrocephalus consider:
  - external ventricular drain
  - ventriculoperitoneal or ventriculoatrial shunt (may lead to ventricular collapse if ongoing brain swelling).

Treatment of acute herniation (coning)

Hyperosmotic agents
Loop diuretics
Hyperventilation.

FLUID MANAGEMENT

Patients are generally run moderately dry to minimize the risks of fluid overload and cerebral oedema. There has been a recent trend away from excessive fluid restriction because it leads to:

- hypovolaemia
- hypotension
- raised haematocrit
- hypernatraemia.

Aim for a haematocrit of 30–35%, which minimizes viscosity but maintains adequate oxygen-carrying capacity.

Circulating volume should be normalized – monitoring CVP and direct arterial BP may help.

Standard fluid replacement is 0.9% saline.

Avoid glucose-containing solutions. Hyperglycaemia is associated with a worse outcome after brain injury as an increase in glucose levels in ischaemic brain results in worsening of lactic acidosis, hyperkalaemia, free-radical formation and intracellular oedema. Hypoglycaemia should be avoided to ensure continued glucose supply to aerobically metabolizing brain. Aim for a blood sugar of 4–9 mmol/l.

Compound sodium lactate should also be avoided – it has a lower osmolality (approx. 250–260 mOsm/l) than calculated (273 mOsm/l) because of the tendency for molecular aggregation of sodium ions.

If blood loss is heavy, large volumes of crystalloid may cause extracellular fluid overload (e.g. pulmonary oedema); colloid solutions, albumin or blood should be considered.

Hypertonic solutions:
'Small volume' resuscitation – hyperosmotic, hypertonic saline–dextran (7.2% saline and 10% dextran 60)
May be more effective than conventional methods at restoring cerebral blood flow and oxygen delivery
Reduce raised intracranial pressure.

ELECTROLYTE DISTURBANCES

Hyponatraemia

See Table 1 for symptoms and causes.

SIADH

Often vague presentation. The hyponatraemia is dilutional due to water retention.
See Table 2 for details.

Cerebral salt wasting

Progressive natriuresis combined with a diuresis, leading to hyponatraemia in association with a reduced extracellular volume. See Table 2.

Hypernatraemia

See Table 1 for a list of causes. The most likely causes in the neurosurgical patient are iatrogenic hypernatraemia and diabetes insipidus.

Iatrogenic causes

Diagnosis
- low urine volume (unless osmotic diuresis)
- high urine specific gravity (>1.020)
- high urine osmolality

Treatment
- administration of isotonic fluids.

Table 1.
Disorders of sodium balance

	Hyponatraemia	Hypernatraemia
Symptoms	Confusion, irritability Nausea, vomiting Progresses to reduced conscious level and coma Seizures, especially if plasma sodium falls below 120 mmol/l	Vague presentation Nausea, vomiting Confusion
Causes	Excessive loss – vomiting – diarrhoea Replacement with sodium-free solutions Syndrome of inappropriate antidiuretic hormone secretion (SIADH) Cerebral salt wasting (CSW)	ADH deficiency (diabetes insipidus, DI) Iatrogenic: (a) hypertonic sodium solutions; (b) excessive fluid restriction Osmotic diuresis TPN Insensitivity to ADH – nephrogenic DI Acute tubular necrosis

Table 2.
Distinguishing SIADH from CSW

	SIADH	Cerebral salt wasting
Diagnosis	Low plasma osmolality Inappropriately high urine osmolality Urinary sodium loss >30 mmol/l Absence of hypotension	Marked hypotension common Derived parameters of sodium and water homeostasis are useful Distinguishing from SIADH is difficult
Treatment	Fluid restriction (500–1000 ml/day) Monitor urine and plasma osmolalities Regular weighing Demethyltetracycline Hypertonic saline (rarely necessary)	Fluid restriction will not help and causes further hypotension Hypertonic saline[a]

[a]Caution is required when using hypertonic saline because rapid correction of hyponatraemia may result in central pontine myelinolysis. Aim to correct plasma sodium by 1 mmol/l/h over 24–48 hours.

Diabetes insipidus (DI)
May occur following surgery to pituitary or hypothalamus, or after head injury.
Diagnosis
- high urine output (>200 ml/h)
- low urine specific gravity (<1.005)
- plasma osmolality >295 mosm/l
- urine osmolality <300 mosm/l

Treatment
- desmopressin acetate (DDAVP)
- dose: 0.04–0.1 μg as required (i.m. or i.v.)
- in conscious patients high fluid loss is best corrected by allowing patient to control fluid intake according to thirst
- in unconscious patients normal maintenance fluid and DDAVP is the best treatment. Water administered via a nasogastric tube is useful.

DI usually resolves within a few days. A minority of patients may need long-term DDAVP, usually administered as a nasal spray.

SEIZURES IN NEUROSURGICAL PATIENTS

Aetiology
- pre-existing epilepsy or documented convulsions
- parietal lobe lesions
- temporal lobe lesions
- middle cerebral artery aneurysm surgery
- post head injury, especially if
  - depressed skull fracture
  - intracerebral haematoma
  - penetrating injury
- following other neurosurgery, especially in the presence of
  - hypoxia
  - electrolyte disturbances
  - infection
  - endocrine disturbance

Treatment
- ensure adequate oxygenation
- terminate the seizure:
  - benzodiazepines are often used (e.g. diazepam in 5 mg increments up to 25 mg) but:
    - may blur neurological examination
    - respiratory depression
    - unpredictable effects
  - thiopentone 25–100 mg is a more suitable agent
    - short acting
- definitive therapy: phenytoin
  - 15–18 mg/kg i.v. loading dose over 60 minutes
  - 300–400 mg daily, thereafter
  - monitor levels

Status epilepticus
Incomplete recovery between fits.
Consider
- termination of seizures as above
- chlormethiazole infusion
- propofol infusion

Monitor EEG
Attenuate excessive muscle activity with neuromuscular blockade (only if EEG monitored)
Add a second-line long-acting agent, e.g. phenobarbitone.

Prophylactic anticonvulsants
Controversial
Some centres use prophylaxis in most 'at risk' cases (see above)
Phenytoin is the agent of choice.

ANALGESIA

Opiates
Codeine phosphate is widely used.
- reportedly less respiratory depressant than other opiates, but this may merely reflect inadequate dosage

Other opiates may be used if patient is monitored on an intensive care unit
Essential to avoid respiratory depression
- elevated P_aCO_2 may cause brain swelling

Short-acting agents (fentanyl, alfentanil) by infusion in those patients requiring ventilation. (*Note*: bolus alfentanil may cause raised intracranial pressure.)

NSAIDs
Useful adjuncts, e.g. diclofenac
Concern about increased bleeding tendency due to antiplatelet action.

THROMBO-EMBOLIC PROPHYLAXIS

There is a high risk of deep venous thrombosis and pulmonary embolism in neurosurgical patients. However, anticoagulation increases the risk of serious haemorrhage.
Hence a compromise is often adopted:
- peri-operative calf compression
- TED stockings in association with peri-operative intermittent calf compression (continue until mobilizing)
- commence subcutaneous heparin on first postoperative day in those at risk.

BIBLIOGRAPHY

Laycock J R D, Walters F J M. Basic anaesthetic technique for intracranial surgery. In: Walters F J M, Ingram G S, Jenkinson J L (eds). Anaesthesia and intensive care for the neurosurgical patient, 2nd edn. Blackwell Scientific Publications, Oxford, 1994

Smith M. Postoperative neurosurgical care. *Current Anaesthesia and Critical Care* 1994; 5: 29–35

Robertson G L, Aycinena P, Zerbe R L. Neurogenic disorders of osmoregulation. *American Journal of Medicine* 1982; 72: 339–353

ANAESTHESIA AND CERVICAL SPINE DISEASE

I. Calder

SURGICAL APPROACHES

An anterior approach to the spine, to left or right of the trachea in the supine position, is the commonest approach, and can be used for most lesions from C3 to C7. Lesions above C3 can be approached through the mouth, or after splitting the chin, mandible and tongue.

The posterior approach is less commonly used although occasionally surgeons still prefer the sitting position.

DISEASES

Cervical spondylosis is the commonest indication for surgery. Osteophytes pressing on nerve roots or the cord are removed microscopically through an anterior cervical approach. The joint is usually fused with iliac crest or artificial bone (Cloward or Smith–Robinson operations).

Cervical disc protrusions are not common, but are approached in the same fashion as spondylosis.

Tumours: primary (of bone or neural tissue – chordoma, glioma, neurofibroma), and secondary.

Fracture/dislocations. It is worth remembering that neurological deterioration can occur at any time, even long after the initial injury.

Rheumatoid arthritis. Cervical involvement is common, but often symptomless, in RA. Important features are:

- Atlanto-axial subluxation (99% on flexion)

rarely causes acute cord damage. Pain in the neck and back of the head is the usual symptom. The extent of subluxation is poorly correlated with neurological signs. Obtaining flexion cervical radiographs before anaesthesia for other surgery is unnecessary, provided the patient is treated as 'at risk' – recovery is perhaps the most dangerous time.
- Cranio-cervical 'settling' – erosion of bone, cartilage and joint space leads to shortening and immobility of the cervical spine. Erosion of C1 and the lateral masses of C2 can cause impaction of the odontoid peg on the high cord/brain stem ('vertical subluxation').
- Staircase spine – multiple joint disease can result in subluxation at several levels.
- Temporo-mandibular joint disease is common and leads to difficulties with airway control (Esmarch–Heiberg manouevre).
- Arytenoid arthritis is present in about one-third of patients. Exacerbations are a well recognized complication of tracheal intubation.

UNSTABLE CERVICAL SPINES

This term can mean anything from a few millimetres difference on radiographs in a symptomless patient, to intermittent quadraparesis.

It is sensible to restrict movements to less than that tolerated by the patient when awake.

There is no convincing evidence to show that direct laryngoscopy is more dangerous than flexible fibre-optic laryngoscopy. However, iatrogenic 'paradoxical' stability (fixation devices) may make direct laryngoscopy difficult.

CONDUCT OF ANAESTHESIA

A drying premed is valuable if flexible fibre-optic laryngoscopy is required.

Indications for awake fibreoptic intubation include: metal fixation device in place, class C mandibular protrusion, and an absent atlanto-axial gap (on lateral flexion C spine radiograph).

Fibreoptic-assisted intubation through the LMA (6.0 mm Mallinkrodt armoured tube) is a valuable technique. Extubation can be performed with the patient deep.

Elective tracheostomy should be considered if intubation will be needed for more than a few days.

Elective percutaneous gastrostomy is useful if swallowing will be impaired and there is a pharyngeal wound, since nasogastric tubes predispose to sinusitis.

Hypotension should be avoided. The cervical cord is less vulnerable than the thoracic cord, which has less generous blood supply (artery of Adamkiewicz).

Neurophysiological monitoring is often applied. Median nerve sensory evoked potentials are tolerant of volatile agents. Tibial nerve SEPs, and motor-evoked potentials are not. The best conditions are produced with infusions of propofol and fentanyl or alfentanyl.

Extubation is often better delayed after prolonged surgery until hypothermia and metabolic acidosis have resolved.

POSTOPERATIVE COMPLICATION – AIRWAY OBSTRUCTION

Haematoma. Any anterior cervical operation may have this complication, usually some hours after surgery. The swelling may be hidden by surgical collars. Presentation is with difficulty in breathing and voice changes, frank stridor is unusual (differential: unilateral recurrent laryngeal nerve palsy, the patient has a weak voice and cough on awakening, no treatment).

Tissue swelling. Swelling sufficient to obstruct the airway is unusual, except after tongue and mandible splitting approaches. Swelling is minimal after trans-oral surgery. Postoperative infection may cause obstruction.

Arytenoid arthritis. Rheumatoid patients commonly have a degree of arytenoid involvement, some have intermittent stridor. Intubation should be atraumatic – fibre-optic-assisted if direct laryngoscopy is difficult, with a small (6.0 mm) tube.

MANAGEMENT

- If any suspicion, nurse in high-dependency area – deterioration can be sudden. Oximetry is not a good guide.
- Intervention should be contemplated earlier if direct laryngoscopy is likely to be difficult.

- Obtain surgical assistance.
- Do not assume that opening the wound will necessarily improve obstruction.
- In complete obstruction, the alternatives are direct laryngoscopy and gum elastic bougie, or tracheostomy. Percutaneous tracheal cannulation is likely to be difficult.
- When obstruction is partial, decisions can be more difficult. Glycopyrrolate should be given to reduce secretions. Awake fibre-optic intubation, with the patient sitting, is ideal. Careful inhalational (halothane) or intravenous (propofol) induction with 'quick look' laryngoscopy or LMA insertion has been successful. The LMA usually allows easy fibre-optic intubation (6.0 mm Mallinkrodt). Lignocaine often causes laryngospasm if sprayed onto the glottis, unless the patient is awake or very deeply anaesthetized. It is probably better to paralyse the patient before attempting to pass the tube.
- Extubation should not be considered for at least 24 hours. Glottic oedema can persist for several days after drainage of a haematoma. There should be an air leak around the tube before extubation.

ANAESTHESIA FOR STEREOTACTIC SURGERY

M. Smith

There is an increasing need in neurosurgery to obtain biopsies from, or make discrete lesions in, central nervous system tissue which is deep in the brain or so intricately associated with eloquent areas that the risks of an open approach are unacceptable. Stereotactic surgery has now found an established place in the diagnosis and treatment of neurological disease.

PRINCIPLES OF STEREOTACTIC SURGERY

Instruments may be accurately directed to a specific area of the brain using the relationship between the three-dimensional space occupied by an intracranial structure or lesion and an extracranial reference system. Imaging of the brain with CT or MRI provides information about the structure or lesion in the horizontal plane and a knowledge of the spatial relationship between slices allows the position in the vertical plane to be described. This is usually achieved by application of a stereotactic headframe which remains outside the image but is included in every slice. Using this three-dimensional information, computer programs generate detailed coordinates for trajectory and depth of specialized instrumentation. Using stereotactic methods the biopsy needle or lesion generator can be placed with an accuracy of about 1 mm.

INDICATIONS FOR STEREOTACTIC SURGERY

- *Biopsy* is the commonest stereotactic procedure in the UK. It allows tissue samples to be obtained from tiny, deep-seated lesions inaccessible by open surgery.

- *Aspiration of haematoma, cyst or abscess* allows decompression and cytological or microbiological diagnosis.

  Stereotactic resection. Deep-seated tumours or those intimately involved with eloquent areas may not be suitable for free-hand resection.
- *Stereotactic implantation of radioactive seeds* to a deep-seated inoperable tumour.
- *Functional surgery*: ablation of nervous pathways to alter the function of specific parts of the nervous system. Lesions generated in the thalamus or basal ganglia may control intractable tremor in Parkinson's disease. Chronic pain conditions may be alleviated by lesions in the midbrain and nuclei of the thalamus or by implantation of stimulation electrodes in the peri-aqueductal grey matter.

12

APPLICATION OF THE HEADFRAME

Application of the stereotactic headframe occurs just prior to the imaging studies and takes 15–20 minutes. Some frames obstruct the mouth and prevent access to the airway, whereas others allow airway access at any stage during the procedure. This has obvious implications for the anaesthetic technique.

When the headframe obstructs the airway, general anaesthesia with an endotracheal tube in place prior to headframe application is the preferred technique in many centres in the UK. Alternatively, the whole procedure may be carried out under local anaesthesia.

Complications of headframe application
- Scalp haematoma
- Venous air embolism
- Subdural/extradural haematoma.

IMAGING STUDIES

These may be carried out under general or local anaesthesia, but patients must be continually monitored and accompanied by an anaesthetist, even if awake. Incremental sedation may be administered to awake patients but over-sedation must be avoided if airway access is impossible. The problems of conducting general anaesthesia during CT or MRI scanning are dealt with elsewhere.

ANAESTHETIC TECHNIQUE

This may involve local or general anaesthesia or a combination of the two. The choice of technique will depend upon the condition and wishes of the patient, the type of stereotactic headframe and, to a lesser extent, the preference of the surgeon.

Premedication

Benzodiazepines may be prescribed if premedication is indicated by heavy sedation must be avoided, especially in those with intracranial hypertension. Drugs which inhibit tremor and rigidity are contraindicated in patients undergoing stereotactic procedures for Parkinson's disease, but small doses of benzodiazepines appear to be safe.

Local anaesthesia

This is the method of choice in many countries, and is gaining popularity in the UK. Some procedures must be carried out under local anaesthesia and include those in whom somatotrophic localization is required (e.g. thalamotomy, pallidotomy).

Monitoring during local anaesthesia
- ECG
- Oxygen saturation
- Non-invasive blood pressure – uncomplicated biopsy
- Invasive blood pressure – complicated procedures, or when degree of hypotension required
- ± End tidal Co_2 (see text).

Technique

An intravenous infusion and arterial line (if applicable) must be inserted using local anaesthetic. An anaesthetist must be present at all times from application of the headframe until the end of the procedure. The frame is applied to the head by means of small pins screwed into the outer table of the skull, and the area of the scalp and periosteum underlying the pin sites must be adequately anaesthetized with local anaesthetic. A mixture of 1% lignocaine and 0.5% bupivacaine with 1:200 000 adrenaline allows rapid onset of action with prolonged duration of action. Scalp anaesthesia between 8 and 12 hours has been reported using this technique. Anaesthesia for the small scalp incision and burr hole required for passage of the stereotactic instrumentation is carried out in a similar manner. The burr hole can be drilled without pain, but the dura must be separately anaesthetized with plain lignocaine (1%) prior to dural incision.

Incremental sedation may be administered as required using small doses of midazolam and fentanyl with 0.5 mg of droperidol (for anti-emesis). Infusion of a subanaesthetic dose of propofol is now a useful alternative. Over-sedation must be avoided because of the difficulty of airway access. In patients with raised intracranial pressure, sedation without airway control must be avoided, and general anaesthesia should be employed if the patient cannot tolerate an awake procedure.

If mild sedation is employed, airway control may be enhanced by the use of a soft nasopharyngeal airway inserted after 'cocainization' of the nasal airway. End tidal Co_2 monitoring is also possible by side-stream sampling from the end of the airway. Supplemental oxygen should be administered to all sedated patients via the contralateral nostril.

If the stereotactic frame obstructs the mouth, it may be impossible to ventilate and intubate the patient in an emergency without removing the whole frame. Equipment for emergency airway control must be to hand and should include a laryngeal mask airway and intubating fibreoptic laryngoscope.

General anaesthesia

Advantages:

- Provision of optimal operating conditions – control of P_aco_2 and blood pressure
- Control of intracranial hypertension
- Comfortable conditions for the patient.

Requirements:

- Rapid wake-up
- Prevention of brain swelling
- Presence of a 'full' brain during biopsy procedures
- Usual precautions for patients with space-occupying lesions.

Patient position:

- Head-up tilt and prevention of neck vein obstruction ensures unimpeded intracranial venous outflow and optimal conditions
- The headframe may prevent ideal positioning but it is essential to avoid excessive compression of neck veins.

Monitoring during general anaesthesia

- ECG
- Oxygen saturation
- Invasive arterial blood pressure
- End tidal CO_2

Technique:

- As for other intracranial surgery
- Modest hypotension may be required – small doses of labetolol are usually sufficient.

POSTOPERATIVE CARE

Although the complication rate after stereotactic surgery is less than that for open procedures, patients should be nursed in a high-dependency unit in the immediate postoperative period. There is a reported mortality rate of less than 0.5%, with the risk of significant neurological morbidity of just over 2%. The risk of haemorrhage is greatest within the first few hours but other complications are rare. Some, such as seizures, may occur because of the underlying pathology.

BIBLIOGRAPHY

Girvin J P. Neurosurgical considerations and general methods for craniotomy under local anaesthesia. International Anesthesiology Clinics 1986; 24: 89–114

Perkins W J, Kelly P J, Faust R J. Stereotactic Surgery. In: Cucchiara R F, Michenfelder J D (eds) Clinical neuroanaesthesia. Churchill Livingstone, New York, 1990, pp 379–419

Thomas D G T, Nouby R M. Experience in 300 cases of CT directed stereotactic surgery for lesion biopsy and aspiration of haematoma. British Journal of Neurosurgery 1989; 3: 321–326

Smith M. Epilepsy and stereotactic surgery. In: Walters F J M, Ingram G S, Jenkinson J L (eds) Anaesthesia and intensive care for the neurosurgical patient. Blackwell Scientific Publications, Oxford, 1994, pp 318–344

12

ANAESTHESIA FOR TRANS-SPHENOIDAL HYPOPHYSECTOMY

J. Dziersk and
N. P. Hirsch

ANATOMY

The pituitary gland lies within the hypophyseal fossa of the body of the sphenoid bone. The optic chiasma lies anteriorly and the cavernous sinus on each side of the fossa. The diaphragma sellae forms the roof. Although traditionally performed via a craniotomy, pituitary surgery is now more commonly carried out using the trans-sphenoidal route.

PATHOLOGY

Pituitary tumours account for 15% of all intracranial tumours and may present with either:

- Hypersecretion of hormones
  Increased secretion of growth hormone resulting in acromegaly
  Increased adrenocorticotrophic hormone resulting in Cushing's disease
  Prolactin-secreting tumours resulting in infertility
- Mass effects
  Headache, visual field defects, hypopituitarism, cranial nerve palsies (III, IV, VI) and obstructive hydrocephalus.

Tumours of non-pituitary origin in this region (e.g. craniopharyngiomas) may disrupt pituitary function.

PRE-OPERATIVE ASPECTS

Acromegalic patients

- Tissue hypertrophy in mouth, tongue and larynx may pose airway problems
- Obstructive sleep apnoea occurs in 40% of patients
- Hypertension occurs in 30% and may require pre-operative treatment
- Left ventricular hypertrophy and coronary artery disease is common
- Impaired glucose tolerance or frank diabetes mellitus occurs in 25% and requires pre-operative treatment.

Cushing's disease

- Truncal obesity in 95%
- Hypertension occurs in 85% and often requires pre-operative treatment
- Impaired glucose tolerance or diabetes mellitus in 60% and requires pre-operative treatment
- Metabolic disturbances (especially hypokalaemia)
- Increased susceptibility to infection
- Increased skin and blood vessel fragility
- Steroid cover will be necessary pre- and postoperatively.

Prolactin-secreting tumours

- These tumours are usually small and do not normally result in anaesthetically important endocrine problems.

Premedication is usually avoided although an oral benzodiazepine is acceptable. Antihypertensive treatment should be continued up to the time of surgery.

PERI-OPERATIVE MANAGEMENT

- Having established full monitoring (including direct arterial blood pressure measurement), anaesthesia is induced with thiopentone and fentanyl (1–2 μg/kg).
- Following administration of a non-depolarizing neuromuscular blocking agent, the trachea should be intubated using a flexometallic (non-kinkable) tracheal tube. If intubation problems are anticipated, fibre-optic intubation may be indicated.
- Following intubation, the patient should be moderately hyperventilated (P_aCO_2 3.5–4.0 kPa) with nitrous oxide, oxygen and isoflurane.
- After placing a throat pack, Moffett's solution (or xylometazoline) should be instilled into each nostril to shrink the nasal mucosa and improve surgical conditions.
- If there is suprasellar extension of the pituitary tumour, a lumbar drain should be inserted into the subarachnoid space.

- Patient is placed supine on the operating table with a slight head-up tilt.
- Under X-ray control, the surgeon enters the sphenoid air sinuses and reaches the pituitary fossa by removing the floor of the fossa. The pituitary tumour is then removed, the nasal mucosa sutured and nasal packs inserted.
- If there is suprasellar extension to the tumour, the anaesthetist may be asked to inject a 10–30 ml volume of saline into the lumbar drain. The increased pressure produced 'delivers' the tumour extension into the operative field.
- At the end of the procedure neuromuscular block is reversed, the throat pack removed and the trachea extubated following thorough suction of pharynx and return of airway reflexes.
- The major potential peri-operative complications are haemorrhage from the cavernous sinus or carotid arteries and leakage of cerebrospinal fluid.

POSTOPERATIVE MANAGEMENT

- Patients should be nursed in a high-dependency area. Routine neurological observation must be performed.
- Codeine phosphate (0.6–0.9 mg/kg i.m.) is the analgesic drug of choice.
- Obstructive sleep apnoea may occur in acromegalic patients.
- Diabetes insipidus occurs in up to 50% of patients undergoing pituitary surgery. Characterized by polyuria (>250 ml/h for >4 hours) with a urine specific gravity <1005. Management requires meticulous fluid balance. If persistent, desmopressin (0.4 μg i.v. repeated as necessary) should be given.
- If a CSF leak has been produced during surgery, drainage via the lumbar drain may be required for 24–48 hours.

BIBLIOGRAPHY

Jewkes D. Anaesthesia for pituitary surgery. Current Anaesthesia and Critical Care 1993; 4: 8–12

Levy A, Lightman S L. Diagnosis and management of pituitary tumours. British Medical Journal 1994; 308: 1087–1091

ANAESTHESIA FOR VASCULAR SURGERY

C. Goldsack

ANAESTHESIA FOR INTRACRANIAL VASCULAR SURGERY

Intracranial vascular lesions can be categorized into aneurysms or vascular malformations.

Aneurysms

Saccular (Berry) aneurysms usually occur at branching points in the circle of Willis and proximal cerebral arteries. The commonest site is on the anterior communicating artery complex (40%). Multiple aneurysms occur in 25% of cases.

Micro-aneurysms occur secondarily to hypertension and resulting disruption of the vessel wall.

Clinical features

Relate to compression effects, seizures, haemorrhage and their sequelae. Details are shown in Table 1.

Intracranial vascular malformations

Arteriovenous malformations (AVMs). A fistulous connection between a hypertrophied feeding artery (often several) and a dilated draining vein(s). May enlarge to several centimetres.

Venous malformations. Collection of venous channels and (usually) a large draining vein.

Cavernous malformations (angiomas). Collection of abnormal dilated sinusoidal vessels.

Telangiectasias. A collection of dilated capillaries.

12

Table 1.
Clinical features of intracranial vascular lesions

Aneurysms	Vascular malformations
1. Haemorrhage subarachnoid intracerebral	1. Asymptomatic
2. Mass effects optic nerve and chiasm 3rd, 4th and 5th cranial nerves brainstem	2. Intracerebral haemorrhage ± ventricular extension
3. Ischaemia TIA stroke	3. Ischaemia secondary to steal TIA stroke
4. Seizures	4. Seizures
5. Hydrocephalus secondary to haemorrhage	

Clinical features
Often asymptomatic, but may cause seizures or haemorrhage. Details are shown in Table 1.

Associated pathology

Saccular aneurysms are associated with several other disorders:

Familial
Polycystic kidney disease
Marfan's syndrome
Ehlers–Danlos syndrome
Pseudoxanthoma elasticum
Hereditary haemorrhagic telangiectasia (also associated with cerebral telangiectasias)

Non-familial
Fibromuscular dysplasia
Coarctation of the aorta
Klinefelter's syndrome
Progeria

GRADING OF SUBARACHNOID HAEMORRHAGE (SAH)

(World Federation of Neurosurgeons)
This has prognostic implications.

Grade	GCS	Motor deficit
I	15	–
II	13–14	–
III	13–14	+
IV	7–12	±
V	3–6	±

COMPLICATIONS OF SAH

Vasospasm

This is angiographically demonstrable in 70% of aneurysmal SAH and is a significant cause of morbidity and mortality. Vasospasm begins about 3 days after SAH, peaking at 10 days, and has generally subsided by day 21. It is due to blood products released into the CSF, especially oxyhaemoglobin. Treatment should be aggressive and early:

Calcium channel blockers (nimodipine)
enteral: 60 mg NG or orally, 4-hourly
i.v. 1 mg/h increasing to 2 mg/h if no adverse effects (e.g. hypotension)
The i.v. route offers no advantage and is much more expensive.
Hypervolaemic hypertensive haemodilution therapy, HHH or 'triple-H therapy'. Volume loading and inotropes. Aim for:
MAP >110 mmHg
PAWP 18–20 mmHg
haematocrit 30–35%
cardiac index >3.0
Angioplasty.

Hydrocephalus

Subarachnoid blood may obstruct CSF drainage, causing hydrocephalus and raised intracranial pressure. It may be necessary to insert an external ventricular drain (EVD) but a rapid reduction in pressure may increase the risk of re-bleeding.

ECG changes

These are common after SAH but do not reflect myocardial disease. They may be due to raised circulating catecholamines. Changes include:

ventricular and supraventricular arrhythmias

Table 2.
Early versus late surgery following SAH

	Early surgery	**Late surgery**
Advantages	Reduces risk of re-bleeding HHH therapy for vasospasm is safer	Technically easier Reduced operative mortality Self-selects better prognostic group
Disadvantages	Technically more difficult May worsen cerebral oedema and ischaemia	Vasospasm difficult to treat Risk of re-bleeding

ST depression
T inversion and Q waves.

Check cardiac enzymes if there is real concern about myocardial infarction.

ANAESTHETIC TECHNIQUES

There is controversy over whether surgery after subarachnoid haemorrhage should be performed early (within 24–48 hours) or late (after 10 days). See Table 2.

The anaesthetic techniques for aneurysm surgery depend upon whether the operation is urgent (acute SAH) or elective.

Premedication

Should not be given routinely as sedative effects may be hazardous, leading to respiratory depression with ensuing arterial hypertension, increased P_aCO_2, increased cerebral blood volume and raised intracranial pressure. The effects of premedication may also persist into the postoperative period, leading to drowsiness at a time when the assessment of conscious levels is important.

Monitoring

Standard monitoring for all patients
ECG, pulse oximetry, end-tidal CO_2, FiO_2, etc.
Arterial line for IBP and blood gases
Nasopharyngeal and peripheral temperature probes
Consider CVP line or long-line via antecubital fossa.

Additional monitoring for patients with vasospasm or after acute SAH
CVP monitoring obligatory
Pulmonary artery catheters helpful, especially if HHH therapy used
Jugular bulb catheters for SjO_2 and jugular bulb lactate
Urinary catheter.

Anaesthesia for aneurysm clipping following SAH

Induction
Stability is more important than the actual agents used
Avoid large swings in arterial blood pressure (prevent haemorrhage; avoid ischaemia)
Thiopentone 4–7 mg/kg, or propofol 2–3 mg/kg are suitable
Cardiostable muscle relaxants (e.g. atracurium or vecuronium) should be used
Fentanyl 3–5 μg/kg may be given to reduce the pressor response to intubation.

Maintenance
Nitrous oxide and a volatile agent are most commonly used for maintenance. However, some authorities avoid nitrous oxide because it may increase intracranial pressure. Isoflurane is the preferred volatile agent because it does not increase cerebral blood flow at concentrations below 1.1 MAC. Supplementary doses of fentanyl 0.5–1 μg/kg may be administered.
Increasingly, propofol and alfentanil infusions are used.
Neuromuscular blockade is maintained with atracurium or vecuronium.
Ventilation should be controlled to a P_aCO_2 of 3.8–4.2 kPa.
Glucose-containing intravenous fluid should be avoided because of the risks of worsening cerebral oedema and ischaemia.

Position
Anterior circulation aneurysms: supine, head slightly turned
Basilar aneurysms: lateral (park bench) or supine, head turned further (do not to obstruct neck veins)
Posterior fossa aneurysms: prone.

Reduction in brain bulk
Position: 30 degrees head-up tilt
Moderate hyperventilation to a P_aCO_2 of 3.8–4.2 kPa. An excessive reduction in P_aCO_2

causes an increased risk of ischaemia in the presence of vasospasm
Mannitol 0.5 g/kg followed by frusemide 0.5 mg/kg (requires a urinary catheter)
Removal of CSF at surgery.

Deliberate hypotension
Only if surgery is impossible without hypotension or if the aneurysm ruptures during surgery
Temporary clipping is safer and is preferred if rupture occurs
Aim for a systolic pressure of 60–80 mmHg using:
increased isoflurane concentrations
thiopentone 3–5 mg/kg
labetolol in increments of 5–10 mg
a mixture of trimetaphan 0.1% (1 mg/ml) and sodium nitroprusside 0.01% (0.1 mg/ml) in 500 ml of saline titrated against response.
(The last is rarely advised today.)
NB. Do not induce hypotension in the presence of vasospasm.

Anaesthesia for elective aneurysm clipping
Similar techniques are used.
Less risk of vasospasm and raised intracranial pressure.

Anaesthesia for AVMs
Many are now treated by interventional neuroradiology (see below).
Surgery may be urgent if an expanding haematoma is causing pressure effects.
Substantial blood loss may occur during open surgery.

Anaesthetic technique
Standard techniques as above particular attention to maintaining perfusion and reducing brain bulk.

Postoperative hyperperfusion
Shunting of blood through an AVM may cause chronic ischaemia in the surrounding brain tissue, with arteriolar dilatation and loss of autoregulation. Following excision of the AVM, there is a sudden increase in perfusion through the surrounding area because blood flow through the AVM has been cut off. This may cause cerebral oedema, haemorrhage and raised intracranial pressure. Postoperative hyperperfusion occurs especially with large AVMs. It can be prevented by maintaining hyperventilation and moderate hypotension into the postoperative period radiological techniques to embolize large AVMs prior to surgery. This reduces the vascularity of the lesion and increases the flow in surrounding arteries, thus enabling the restoration of autoregulation pre-operatively.

Postoperative care
- High-dependency unit for elective aneurysms and AVMs.
- Intensive care unit for post-SAH patients and those requiring treatment for vasospasm.

INTERVENTIONAL NEURORADIOLOGY

Increasingly employed for the treatment of cerebrovascular pathology, including lesions that are difficult to treat by open surgery.

Uses include:
Flow reduction prior to surgery:
reduction in the vascularity of AVMs
to control proximal flow to cerebral aneurysms, especially giant aneurysms
Test occlusion:
temporary occlusion of a vessel to determine the effects of proposed surgical ligation
Definitive treatment:
balloon or coil occlusion of aneurysms
embolization of AVMs
Angioplasty:
to dilate carotid or vertebral artery constrictions
to treat vasospasm following subarachnoid haemorrhage.

BIBLIOGRAPHY

Mahla M E. Neurologic surgery. In: Gravenstein N, Kirby R R (eds). Clinical anesthesia practice. W B Saunders, Philadelphia, 1994
Moss E. Anaesthesia for cerebrovascular surgery. Current Anaesthesia and Critical Care 1994; 5: 2–8
Moss E. Anesthesia for vascular surgery. In: Walters F J M, Ingram G S, Jenkinson J L (eds). Anaesthesia and intensive care for the neurosurgical patient, 2nd edn. Blackwell Scientific Publications, Oxford, 1994
Pickard J D, Murray G D, Illingworth R, Shaw M D W et al. The effect of oral nimodipine after cerebral infarction and outcome after subarachnoid haemorrhage: British aneurysm nimodipine trial. British Medical Journal 1989; 298: 636–642
Warlow C. Disorders of cerebral circulation. In: Walton J (ed.). Brain's diseases of the nervous system, 10th edn. Oxford University Press, Oxford, 1993

ANAESTHESIA FOR SUPRATENTORIAL SURGERY

S. Wilson

SUPRATENTORIAL SURGERY

Procedure

Surgery involves:

- Burr-hole biopsy for histological diagnosis
- Craniotomy for tumour excision or debulking
- Aspiration of cerebral abscess for debulking and antibiotic sensitivities.

Patient characteristics

Patients are usually otherwise fit

- All ages
- ASA 1
- Possible primary tumour in lung, breast, thyroid and bowel
- Primary sites for abscesses may be middle ear, paranasal sinuses or lung.

Pre-operative assessment and investigations

- Raised intracranial pressure (ICP) is from peritumour oedema treated with dexamethasone (4 mg q.d.s.) given with an H_2 antagonist
- Prophylactic or therapeutic anticonvulsants may be required for temporoparietal or subfrontal lesions
  Phenytoin (100 mg t.d.s.) following loading dose (15 mg/kg^{-1}).
- Intravenous fluids restricted to 30 ml kg^{-1} per day if cerebral oedema present
- Patients on regular mannitol may have hypernatraemia
- Blood transfusion availability
- Check CT or MRI scan for tumour size, site and signs of raised intracranial pressure.

Premedication

Patients often extremely anxious, careful explanation essential. Anxiolysis with benzodiazepines, unless intracranial pressure is raised.

Theatre preparation

- Personnel to help with positioning, patient supports and padding for pressure areas
- Maintain normothermia (warming mattress, space blanket, blood warmer and humidification)
- Prevention of deep vein thrombosis (TED stockings, intermittent calf compression).

Peri-operative management

Monitoring

For all cases:

- ECG
- Invasive BP
- Sa_{O_2}
- ET_{CO_2}
- Core temperature.

May also require:

- CVP
- Urine output (long procedures, possibility of giving mannitol).

Anaesthetic technique

Induction

- Smooth induction with no coughing, straining or rapid changes in BP
- Fentanyl (1–3 μg kg^{-1})
- Thiopentone or propofol
- Non-depolarizing muscle relaxant (atracurium/vecuronium)
- Intubate with armoured cuffed endotracheal tube fixed securely
- Cover and protect eyes (eye pads, not eye shields which may themselves cause damage)
- Large-bore intravenous cannula and arterial line (consider patient position)
- Central venous catheter if risk of large blood loss (meningioma or metastatic tumour).

Positioning the patient

Patient position is dictated by the surgical approach:

- Supine for most procedures
- Lateral (park bench) for some temporoparietal approaches.

For all patients ensure:

- Head-up tilt (15–25°)
- Good venous drainage by avoiding extreme flexion and rotation of the neck.

- Head secured with a horseshoe headrest or three-point pin fixator (may need bolus dose of fentanyl to prevent hypertension on securing pins).
- Before patient draped check for kinks in the endotracheal tube, ensure monitors and vascular cannulae unimpeded.

Maintenance of anaesthesia
- Maintain $ETco_2$ at 3.8–4.2 kPa
- Humidification of dry gases
- FIo_2 of 0.3–0.5 with nitrous oxide or air. Nitrous oxide should be avoided in the presence of severe cerebral oedema
- Isoflurane and/or propofol infusion supplemented with fentanyl.

Control of blood pressure
Normotension or modest hypotension maintained for most procedures. With large vascular tumours moderate hypotension may improve the surgical field. Usually achieved by deepening anaesthesia, but may require:

- labetalol/β-blockers
- sodium nitroprusside.

Fluid balance
- Use normal saline for maintenance fluids
- Replace blood loss with colloid and blood
- Avoid 5% dextrose.

Intra-operative management of a tight brain
Bulging dura on removal of the craniotomy flap indicates a 'tight' brain. Intracranial hypertension is often secondary to peri-tubular oedema. Various manoeuvres may improve operating conditions (see Table 1).

Table 1.
Anaesthetic measures to reduce intra-operative oedema

- Check patient position (tilt, head rotation)
- Ensure moderate hypocarbia (3.8–4.2 kPa)
- Control BP
- Discontinue N_2O
- Mannitol (0.25–0.5 g kg^{-1})
- Frusemide (0.5–1.0 mg kg^{-1})
- Dexamethasone (12–16 mg) for tumours

Swelling may also be due to bleeding into the tumour, causing resistant hypertension and a tachycardia followed by bradycardia. To preserve cerebral perfusion pressure, normotension is maintained prior to opening the dura, despite the risk of bleeding.

POSTOPERATIVE MANAGEMENT

Once haemostasis is achieved:

- Return blood pressure to normal
- Restore normocapnia and spontaneous breathing
- Give analgesia (codeine phosphate or fentanyl)
- Treat hypertension on emergence with labetalol, hydralazine or small bolus propofol
- Extubate 'deep'
- Return to high-dependency area or intensive care unit for postoperative monitoring.

Consider postoperative sedation and ventilation if:

- Patient severely obtunded pre-operatively
- Massive haemorrhage
- Acute brain swelling.

Postoperative intracranial pressure monitoring will be necessary if the patient is to be sedated and ventilated.

Postoperative analgesia is achieved with an adequate dose of codeine phosphate given 3 hourly. Intravenous fluids are restricted to 30 ml kg^{-1} of normal saline in 24 hours until drinking. Mechanical methods for preventing DVT should be continued postoperatively as the use of low-dose heparin may increase the risk of postoperative haematoma.

BIBLIOGRAPHY

Michenfelder J D. Anaesthesia and the Brain, 1st edn. Churchill Livingstone, London, 1988, pp 52–29
Miller J D, Leech P. Effects of mannitol and steroid therapy on intracranial volume – pressure relationships in patients. Journal of Neurosurgery 1975; 42: 274–81
Pickard J D, Czosnyka M, Management of raised intracranial pressure. Journal of Neurology, Neurosurgery and Psychiatry 1993; 56: 845–858
Thromboembolic Risk Factors Consensus Group. Risk of and prophylaxis for venous thromboembolism in hospital patients. British Medical Journal 1992; 305: 567–74

ANAESTHESIA FOR POSTERIOR FOSSA SURGERY

G. S. Ingram

ANATOMY AND PHYSIOLOGY

The posterior fossa is bounded by the tentorium above, the foramen magnum below, the occiput behind and the clivus in front. Even a small amount of swelling and oedema can create major neurological change because:

- the pons and medulla contain the major sensory and motor pathways, the vital vascular and respiratory centres, and the lower cranial nerve nuclei. Pressure on these structures may result in decreased levels of consciousness, rising BP and falling pulse, respiratory depression and impairment of the reflexes that protect the airway.
- CSF flows from the 3rd through the 4th ventricle and out onto the surface of the brain. Obstruction of this pathway will result in hydrocephalus.

Gross swelling will cause coning, either upwards through the tentorium, or more commonly downwards through the foramen magnum. Because the respiratory centre lies in the lower medulla, the latter will result in slow irregular respiration progressing to apnoea which may be sudden.

PATHOLOGY

Malignant tumours
  Primary – particularly astrocytomas in children
  Secondary – often metastasize to cerebellum
Benign tumours
  Acoustic neuromas in cerbellopontine angle
  Meningiomas less common than supratentorial

Vascular
  Uncommon but angiomas, arteriovenous malformations and aneurysms can occur. Also, nerve decompression for hemifacial spasm and trigeminal pain. Haematomas and trauma.

PRE-OPERATIVE ASPECTS

Particular attention to

- Assessment of ICP, clinically from conscious state, headache and vomiting, together with response to steroids. Examination of CT/MRI to assess lesion size and oedema.
- Fluid status – may be depleted due to vomiting and/or poor intake.
- Electrolytes and glucose, particularly if on steroids.
- General physical status – CVS with reference to ability to tolerate prone or sitting positions and respiratory status including gag reflex.

In severe cases pre-op ICP monitoring and if hydrocephalus is present, ventricular drainage, will be needed.

CHOICE OF POSITION

Prone

Good surgical access to midline structures, but excessive bleeding may obscure surgical field. Careful positioning with avoidance of increased venous pressure essential.

Lateral (Park bench)

Used for laterally placed lesions, especially those in cerebellopontine angle. Good compromise, particularly in older patients. Body well supported, head on horseshoe headrest or clamped. *Avoid* pressure damage to peripheral nerves; jugular compression due to excessive flexion/rotation of the neck; pressure on lower eye with horseshoe.

Sitting – see below

SITTING POSITION

Carries additional risks and should only be used when specifically indicated and in experienced hands.

Generally, the sitting position is achieved by using the standard operating table – removing

Table 1.
Advantages and disadvantages of the sitting position

Advantages	Disadvantages
• Spatial orientation • Easy access • Good venous and CSF drainage (all surgical)	• Postural hypotension • Air embolism (all anaesthetic)

12

the head portion, placing the back part vertically and arranging for the legs to be slightly flexed to ensure the buttocks remain firm against the vertical portion. The head is then held against a horseshoe headrest mounted on a frame across the table. *Avoid* too much head flexion which can cause jugular compression, swelling of the tongue and face and cervical cord ischaemia. A minimum gap of two fingers should be maintained between the chin and suprasternal notch. The ulnar, sciatic and lateral peroneal nerves are particularly at risk.

AIR EMBOLISM

Causes

Venous air embolism (VAE) is a potential risk whenever the operation site and open veins are above the level of the heart. The greater the distance, the greater the negative hydrostatic pressure and the rate at which air will tend to enter. In posterior fossa surgery the danger is increased as cut veins in the bone may be held open by surrounding structures; there are large veins in the neck muscles and large venous sinuses within the skull.

Incidence

Variously quoted as between 25 and 40%, dependent on sensitivity of monitoring, precautions taken and surgical skill.

Pathophysiology

Small amounts may have little clinical significance. Air will be drawn down through the right atrium and ventricle into the pulmonary arterioles. The pulmonary vascular resistance increases, the PA pressure rises, cardiac output falls and ECG abnormalities are seen. Gas exchange is impaired as physiological deadspace increases causing V/Q mismatch and a fall in CO_2 excretion.

Detection

Precordial *Doppler* is the most sensitive method of monitoring for VAE, but problems include positioning the probe, diathermy interference and need for continuous monitoring by a trained person of the sounds emitted. *Capnography* is generally regarded as the most useful monitor, a fall in $ETCO_2$ being an indication for immediate action. *Oximetry*, although later in detecting the presence of air, is very valuable in the management of an established case. *PA pressure* measurement, *transoesophageal echocardiography* and *end-tidal nitrogen* have all been advocated.

Prevention

- Volume loading is helpful in reducing the risk of a fall in BP when the patient is sat up. It assists in raising venous pressure and reducing the risk of VAE.
- PEEP has been widely used, levels up to 10 cmH_2O being employed.
- Compression of the abdomen and/or lower limbs raises venous pressure, this may be by the use of bandages, a G-suit or medical antishock trousers (MAST).
- CVP catheters, as well as allowing measurement of the effectiveness of attempts to raise venous pressure and reduce the hydrostatic gradient, can be used to aspirate air that has entered the circulation. For optimum recovery it has been shown that the tip of the catheter should be close to where the SVC enters the right atrium and that catheters with multiple orifices are more effective.
- As N_2O may cause problems if air enters, its use has been questioned.

VAE – management

In order, as indicated:

- Notify the surgeons
- Occlude the wound with a wet swab
- Turn to 100% oxygen – stop N_2O
- Raise the venous pressure – level table/neck compression
- Aspirate CVP line.

If there is cardiovascular collapse:

- Turn patient on to left side with head down
- Commence CPR.

Prompt diagnosis and action will limit the need for the last two steps, which are barely practical and are unlikely to result in a successful outcome when the posterior fossa is exposed.

PARADOXICAL AIR EMBOLISM

From post-mortem studies it is known that approximately 25% of the general population have a probe patent foramen ovale. A potential route therefore exists for air to pass from the right to the left atrium. Whereas the presence of small amounts of air in the venous circulation and pulmonary vascular bed may not be dangerous to the patient, the presence of minimal volumes of air in the systemic circulation can be lethal. Even a small air embolism in the circulation of the brain or heart will result in irreversible damage. A gradient of 4 mmHg is all that is required to reverse flow across a shunt. When air enters the pulmonary circulation the obstruction to flow that results causes pressure to rise on the right side of the heart and fall on the left, thus increasing the potential gradient. Apart from the foramen ovale, other anatomical routes exist such as arteriovenous shunts and the pulmonary circulation whereby air can pass from the right to left side of the circulation.

OTHER PEROPERATIVE CONCERNS

Interference with the midbrain, vital centres and cranial nerves through direct intervention, retraction or occlusion of the blood supply may result in sudden alteration of monitored readings. As the patient is paralysed and ventilated, respiratory changes will not be seen but cardiovascular changes may be abrupt and dramatic. *The anaesthetist's first responsibility is to warn the surgeon*; drugs such as atropine and β-blockers will mask midbrain responses and should be used only when it is essential. The occurrence of changes is generally an indication of the limits of surgery. More sensitive monitoring techniques, such as evoked potentials, are increasingly used and may assist in defining what is surgically feasible.

The facial nerve (VII) is stretched across the capsule of acoustic neuromas. The need for neuromuscular monitoring to identify and preserve the nerve may limit the degree of muscle relaxation available to the anaesthetist.

Blood pressure should be brought close to normal, prior to closure, in order to assess the adequacy of haemostasis.

If N_2O is continued once the skull is closed, there is a potential risk that air trapped in the skull will lead to an increasing gas volume through diffusion of N_2O and the development of pneumocephalus.

The choice of anaesthetic drugs is not critical, and most well managed techniques will suffice. However, the importance of relating the effect of anaesthetic drugs and other manoeuvres to BP and ICP so as to ensure that cerebral perfusion pressure (CPP) is maintained at all times, is essential.

If the head is to be held in a headclamp with pins into the skull rather than in a padded horseshoe headrest, analgesia and anaesthesia must be sufficiently deep to avoid too marked cardiovascular response.

POSTOPERATIVE MANAGEMENT

- Postoperative swelling in the posterior fossa is a potential danger. The small anatomical space, the tendency of the cerebellum to swell following prolonged retraction, and bleeding, all add to the threat. In addition reduced respiration may result from, and in its turn increase, such swelling. Sedative and respiratory depressant drugs must be used with great caution, if at all. There is much to be gained from elective ventilation following prolonged posterior fossa surgery.
- Swelling can be delayed, sometimes developing some hours after an initially good recovery.
- If the patient does deteriorate, an immediate scan (CT/MRI) is usually indicated.
- Hydrocephalus, following on occlusion of the CSF pathway, may also raise ICP and lead to deterioration of conscious level.
- Damage to the lower cranial nerves may impair the gag reflex. If not recognized aspiration into the lungs may take place. An NG tube and nil by mouth are indicated.
- Following major postoperative surgery, patients should go to an appropriately equipped ITU to be looked after by nursing staff experienced in the care of neurosurgical patients.

BIBLIOGRAPHY

Albin M S, Baninski M, Maroon J C, Jannetta P J. Anesthetic management of posterior fossa surgery in the sitting position. Acta Anaestheseologica Scandinavica 1976; 20: 117–128

Artru A A, Cucchiara R F, Messick J M. Cardiorespiratory and cranial nerve sequelae of surgical procedures involving the posterior fossa. Anesthesiology 1980; 52: 83–86

Bedford R F. Posterior fossa procedures. In: Newfield P, Cottrell J E. (eds). Neuroanesthesia: handbook of clinical and physiologic essentials, 2nd edn, 1991, Little, Brown & Co, Boston, pp 249–263

Ingram G S, Walters F J M. Anaesthesia for posterior fossa surgery. In: Walters F J M, Ingram G S, Jenkinson J L (eds), Anaesthesia and intensive care for the neurosurgical patient, 2nd edn, 1994, Blackwells, Oxford, pp 212–238

Losasso T J, Muzzi D A, Dietz N M, Cucchiara R F. Fifty percent nitrous oxide does not increase the risk of venous air embolism in neurosurgical patients operated on in the sitting position. Anesthesiology 1992; 77: 21–30

Perkins-Pearson N A K, Marshal W K, Bedford R F. Atrial pressure in the seated position: implications for paradoxical air embolism. Anesthesiology 1982; 57: 493–497

ANAESTHESIA FOR NEURORADIOLOGY

S. A. Bew

The development and widespread availability of CT and MRI scanners has led to a big increase in the number of neuroradiological investigations and procedures performed. Most investigations are elective, and performed on awake patients, but general anaesthesia is sometimes desirable or essential for:

- Cerebral or spinal cord angiography
- CT scan
- MRI scan
- Interventional Neuroradiology.

GENERAL CONSIDERATIONS

- X-ray departments are usually isolated from main theatres
- Not designed for provision of anaesthesia (cramped, no piped medical gas and vacuum)
- Dark during many procedures
- Radiation hazard to staff and patient
- X-ray tables cannot be tipped head down, but may move horizontally during scans
- Access to the patient may be limited, so all i.v. lines, tubes etc. must be secure.
- Communication with radiologists and radiographers is essential
- Anaesthesia should not be provided without adequate equipment, monitoring, trained assistance and recovery facilities.

PATIENT ASSESSMENT

As for any neurosurgical case, noting neurological defect, level of consciousness and presence of raised intracranial pressure (ICP).

ANAESTHETIC MANAGEMENT

Basic principles of neuro-anaesthesia with control of ICP. Specific requirements are detailed below.

ANGIOGRAPHY

Few general anaesthetics are given for elective angiography as the use of non-ionic contrast media greatly reduced the discomfort of the procedures. Anaesthesia is required for urgent/emergency investigations post intracerebral bleed in patients with reduced level of consciousness, raised ICP and frequently cardiovascular instability. Anaesthetic management should include control of intracranial pressure, and invasive monitoring and control of arterial pressure as for aneurysm surgery.

Specific points

- Risk of further bleed during procedure
- Reactions to iodine-based contrast. Less frequent (×10) with newer non-ionic media, 0.004% incidence of life-threatening reaction
- Osmotic diuresis. Non-ionic media have osmolality of 411–796 mOsm/kg H_2O, thus urinary catheter and attention to fluid balance required
- Radiation hazard.

CT SCAN

The collection of tomographic images requires the patient to lie still whilst a rotating gantry containing the X-ray source takes a series of axial 'cuts', each of which takes only a few seconds with the new generation of scanners.

Indications for general anaesthesia

- Claustrophobia
- Movement disorder
- Confusional state
- Already intubated/ventilated for control of airway and ICP.

Many patients for elective scans who do not have ICP/airway protection problems can be safely managed using a laryngeal mask airway and a spontaneously breathing technique. For ventilated patients basic principles of neuro-anaesthesia apply.

Specific points

- Patients are relatively inaccessible during the scan and the airway must be secure
- Iodine-based contrast may be used (see above)
- Radiation hazard.

MRI

In magnetic resonance scanning, pulsed radiofrequency energy is delivered to tissues in a powerful magnetic field, requiring the patient to lie still within the narrow core of the magnet. Indications for general anaesthesia are as for CT scan, but the patient is in a much narrower inaccessible tunnel during the scan, and some find this and the loud noise of the scanner disturbing, even with ear plugs.

The powerful magnetic field (0.5–1.5 Tesla) is turned off only as a planned event, and it is time-consuming and expensive to re-establish the field. Thus, the magnet is on at all times and in the event of an emergency the patient must be removed not just from the magnet but also from the scanning room, before further management.

Specific points

- The magnetic field contraindicates scanning in certain patients and most units have a checklist which must be completed before a patient enters the magnet. Cardiac pacemakers and other electrically operated implants may be inactivated, and are an absolute contraindication to a scan. Any ferromagnetic implants (aneurysm clips, flexometallic endotracheal tubes, cochlear implants, prosthetic heart valves, metallic intra-ocular foreign bodies) may be dislodged and cause heating or induction of electrical current. Degradation of the image quality by ferromagnetic objects may cause misinterpretation of scans or render them diagnostically useless.
- 'Missile effect' of any ferromagnetic object e.g. oxygen cylinder, pair of scissors; if brought within the magnetic field can accelerate towards the core of the magnet
- Monitoring equipment using electric cables (ECG pulse oximetry) will not function due to interference
- Metallic monitoring cables, armoured tracheal tubes etc. will degrade image quality and cause induction currents and heating.
- Patient is inaccessible and the head is not

visible during scanning. The airway must be secure
- Contrast, if used, is gadolinium-based and is generally safe and well tolerated, though there are reports of anaphylactoid reactions.

Anaesthetic management
Induction of anaesthesia outside the scanning room on a non-ferromagnetic trolley avoids many problems. There are several approaches to management during the scan, and many of the monitoring difficulties have been overcome by the development of MRI compatible equipment.

The anaesthetist may stay in the scan room using a completely non-ferromagnetic ventilator, or a normal ventilator in fixed position as far from the magnet as possible, and shielded ECG leads and fibre-optic saturation monitor.

More usually, anaesthetist and equipment stay outside the scan room using long ventilator tubing and monitoring cables which pass through specially shielded holes in the scan room wall.

Monitoring
ECG – shielded cables do not interfere with imaging

Pulse oximetry – fibre-optic cables do not cause or suffer from interference

Blood pressure – cuffs with plastic connectors and up to 10 m of tubing give clinically adequate readings

Capnography – sampling tubing up to 10 m long causes minimal waveform distortion but a delay of about 5 s

Invasive pressure – tubing of 5–6 m causes some damping of the waveform but without substantial error in systolic and diastolic pressures.

INTERVENTIONAL NEURORADIOLOGY

In these procedures, fluoroscopically guided catheters inserted through a 7.5Fr sheath, usually in the femoral artery, access the cerebral or spinal circulation. Microcatheters of variable stiffness and with steerable guidewires allow superselective catheterization of distal vessels in the arterial circulation for procedures including:

- occlusion of aneurysms with balloons or Guglielmi electrolytically detachable coils
- embolization of AVM using glue or sclerosants, either as sole therapy or as an adjunct to surgery
- angioplasty for vasospasm post SAH
- thrombolysis.

These procedures may be performed awake, but often take several hours and require the patient to be absolutely still, especially during subtraction or roadmapping imaging sequences, and anaesthesia is usually required. A neurolept technique allows for frequent assessment of neurological status, but a standard neurosurgical anaesthetic allows control of ICP and arterial pressure if needed.

Specific points
- Patients are heparinized prior to catheter insertion. A baseline ACT is taken post induction and when required heparin 5000 U/70 kg given to achieve an ACT 2× normal. The ACT should be checked hourly and additional heparin given as needed to maintain anticoagulation. Reverse with protamine at the end of the procedure and confirm that the ACT has returned to baseline before removal of the femoral catheter sheath
- Hypotension may be required during embolization to slow blood flow through an AVM
- Haemorrhage due to aneurysm or vessel rupture requires immediate reversal of heparinization
- Arterial spasm, embolization or haemorrhage may require rapid manipulation of the blood pressure
- Cerebral oedema may be caused or exacerbated particularly by the preferential embolization of venous rather than arterial vessels in an AVM
- Large volumes of contrast are used, and a urinary catheter is essential to manage fluid balance
- The swinging C-arm fluoroscope may pull on leads, lines and tubes if not well secured out of reach
- Postoperatively, careful attention must be paid to control of blood pressure as after aneurysm surgery and patients may require nursing in a neurosurgical ICU.

BIBLIOGRAPHY

Menon D K, Peden C J, Hall A S, Sargentoni J, Whitwam J G. Magnetic resonance for the anaesthetist, Parts I and II. Anaesthesia 1992; 47: 240–255

Young W L, Pile-Spellman J. Anaesthetic considerations for interventional neuroradiology. Anaesthesiology 1994; 80: 427–456

ANAESTHESIA FOR MINOR NEUROSURGICAL PROCEDURES

S. Wilson

MINOR PROCEDURES

Evacuation of intracranial haematoma

Extradural haematoma:

- Usually results from middle meningeal artery tear
- May be associated with skull fracture
- Patient may have a lucid period
- Primary brain injury often minimal
- Early evacuation essential.

Intracerebral haematoma:

- Secondary to head injury or bleed from intracranial aneurysm or arteriovenous malformation
- Spontaneous, secondary to anticoagulation therapy
- Haematoma evacuated only if further deterioration in neurology occurs.

Acute subdural haematoma:

- Occurs from veins between cerebral cortex and dura
- Primary brain damage may be severe
- Early evacuation improves outcome.

Chronic subdural haematoma:

- Seen in the elderly after apparent trivial injury
- Signs slow in onset, involving clumsiness and confusion
- Haematoma evacuated via burrholes
- May be performed under local anaesthetic.

Patient characteristics

All ages.

May have associated injuries if secondary to trauma (chest, pelvis, abdomen)
ASA 2–4 E
Elderly may be on warfarin.

Preoperative assessment and investigations

- Assess airway and intubate if GCS <8 (protect cervical spine, assume full stomach)
- Resuscitate and treat associated major injuries
- Assess level of consciousness with Glasgow Coma Scale, pupil size and reaction
- Check blood clotting profile
- Blood products available
- Give mannitol (0.25–0.5 g kg^{-1}) if needed.

Premedication

Contraindicated in patients with intracerebral haematoma. Explain procedure to patient if possible.

Perioperative monitoring

Monitoring

- ECG
- BP (invasive for all but chronic subdural)
- Sao_2
- $ETco_2$
- Core temperature
- CVP (trauma patients, large blood loss)
- Urine output.

Anaesthetic technique

- Smooth induction and intubation
- May need rapid sequence induction if full stomach
- Cover and pad eyes
- Hyperventilate to P_aco_2 3.8–4.2 kPa
- Keep normotensive or above to maintain cerebral perfusion pressure (CPP)
- Maintain muscle paralysis
- Keep volatile agents to minimum
- Tilt table 15–30°, head up
- Avoid nitrous oxide if cerebral oedema severe or intracranial air present
- Avoid surges in blood pressure with bolus of fentanyl
- Give mannitol or frusemide (0.5 mg kg^{-1}) as required
- Maintain circulating blood volume with colloid or blood
- Maintain patient's body temperature (humidification, warming mattress, space blanket, warm intravenous fluids)
- Prophylaxis for deep vein thrombosis (TED stockings, compression boots).

Intraoperative hypotension

Once surgical decompression occurs there may be rapid decrease in BP as drive to hypertension is removed. Treat with volume replacement.

Intracranial pressure monitor

May be inserted pre-operatively on ITU or postoperatively if there is:

- Pre-operative coma
- Tight brain at craniotomy after haematoma evacuated
- Ventilation required postoperatively for other injuries.

Intracranial pressure is now routinely monitored with fibre-optic intraparenchymal catheters (Camino).

POSTOPERATIVE MANAGEMENT

- All patients in coma pre-operatively or with tight brain at craniotomy are ventilated on ITU for 12–24 hours postoperatively
- Others extubated with care to avoid coughing or hypertension
- Analgesia is maintained with codeine phosphate or fentanyl infusions if ventilated
- Maintain CPP by controlling ICP and maintaining BP (inotropes may be needed).

Postoperative management of raised intracranial pressure:

- Nurse head up (15–30°)
- Moderate hyperventilation (P_aco_2 3.8–4.2 kPa)
- Sedation with propofol or midazolam (may need analgesia for associated injuries)
- Control hypertension
- Treat raised ICP with mannitol as required
- Aim to keep CPP above 70 mmHg

SHUNT PROCEDURES

Procedure

Shunts are inserted for hydrocephalus:

- Ventriculoperitoneal (VP)
- Ventriculo-atrial (VA)
- Lumboperitoneal (LP).

Indications

In childhood:

- Primary hydrocephalus

- Secondary to spina bifida (Arnold–Chiari malformation) intraventricular haemorrhage or meningitis.

In adults:

- Inoperable brain tumours
- Subarachnoid haemorrhage.

Shunts often block or become infected, needing revision.

Patient characteristics
- May have signs of raised intracranial pressure
- All ages
- Neurological signs associated with the cause of hydrocephalus.

Pre-operative assessment and investigations
- Emergency cases may have full stomach
- May be dehydrated
- Assess for ease of positioning on table (contractures)
- Antibiotic treatment or prophylaxis (opinions vary).

Premedication
Many patients will have had previous surgery and be anxious. Benzodiazepines can be used, but are contraindicated with raised intracranial pressure.

Peri-operative management

Monitoring
- ECG
- Non-invasive BP
- Sa_{O_2}
- ET_{CO_2}

Anaesthetic technique
- As for evacuation of intracranial haematomas, but uncover area of abdomen on ipsilateral side as shunt.

Complications
- Watch for signs of pneumothorax or haemothorax as trocar placed subcutaneously.

POSTOPERATIVE MANAGEMENT

- Wake patient with minimal coughing and straining
- Analgesia provided by intramuscular codeine phosphate.

12

BIBLIOGRAPHY

Dearden M. Intracranial pressure monitoring. Care of the Critically Ill 1985; 1: 8–13
Finch M D, Morgan G A R. Traumatic pneumocephalus following head injury. Anaesthesia 1991; 46: 385–387
Rose J, Valtonen S, Jennett B. Avoidable factors contributing to death after head injury. British Medical Journal 1977; 2: 615–618
Seelig J M, Becker D P, Miller J D, Greenberg R P, Ward J D, Choi S C. Traumatic acute subdural haematoma. Major mortality reduction in comatose patients treated within four hours. New England Journal of Medicine 1981; 304: 1511–1518
Teasdale G M, Murray G, Anderson E, Mendelow A D, MacMillan R, Jennett B, Brookes M. Risks of acute traumatic intracranial haematoma in children and adults: implications for managing head injuries. British Medical Journal 1990; 300: 363–367

13

OPHTHALMIC SURGERY

R. K. Mirakhur

13

CATARACT SURGERY

J. H. Gaston

PATHOLOGY

- Opacification of the lens by a proteinaceous precipitate.

PATIENT CHARACTERISTICS

- Generally elderly, 60–90+ years old (ASA I–IV) or newborn to 10 years old (ASA I–III).

POSSIBLE ASSOCIATED PROBLEMS IN CHILDREN

- Prematurity
- Poor temperature control
- Upper respiratory tract infection
- Up to 50% may be associated with specific conditions of pregnancy and/or associated congenital conditions.

POSSIBLE ASSOCIATED PROBLEMS IN ADULTS

- Predominantly senile
- Strong possibility of coexistent disease, in particular:
  - hypertension
  - ischaemic heart disease
  - chronic obstructive airways disease
  - diabetes mellitus
  - renal disease
  - hypothyroidism.

PROCEDURE

Congenital:
- Best results with early surgery
- Lensectomy by an aspiration–irrigation technique using a suction-cutter instrument.

Adult:
- Extracapsular lens extraction via a limbal incision
- Phacomemulsification – a rapidly developing technique requiring a much smaller incision
- Intraocular lens implant is now routine
- Intracapsular lens extraction quite uncommon now.

PREOPERATIVE ASSESSMENT AND INVESTIGATIONS

- Assessment and optimization of any medical conditions if required
- Haematological and biochemical investigations; ECG and chest X-ray, if necessary.

PREMEDICATION

- Heavy sedation to be avoided, particularly in those having a local anaesthetic
- Anxiolysis with benzodiazepines, e.g. temazepam.

MONITORING AND PREPARATION FOR ANAESTHESIA

- See Table 1.

Table 1.
Monitoring and preparation

General anaesthesia
ECG
Arterial pressure
Spo_2
$ETco_2$
Peripheral nerve stimulator
Temperature (particularly in children)
Intravenous cannulation
Local anaesthesia
ECG
Spo_2
Intravenous cannulation

ANAESTHETIC TECHNIQUES

- Must ensure a low IOP
- Lack of movement and vascular congestion
- Anaesthesia and akinesia of globe, eyelids and the orbicularis muscle.

LOCAL ANAESTHESIA

Advantages of local anaesthesia:
- Avoidance of general anaesthetic side-effects (particularly nausea and vomiting)
- Some postoperative analgesia
- Attenuation of stress response.

Techniques of local anaesthesia:
- Particularly good for day-case surgery.
- Topical anaesthesia with 1% amethocaine or 0.4% benoxyprocaine.
- *Retrobulbar block* – 4–5 ml of local anaesthetic (either 2% lignocaine with adrenaline, or 2% lignocaine with adrenaline in combination with 0.5% bupivacaine), with hyaluronidase 5–10 units per millilitre of solution. Inject 3–4 ml inferolaterally into the muscle cone. Must be accompanied by a facial nerve block; 3–5 ml of same local anaesthetic solution by the van Lint, O'Brien or Nadbath techniques.
- *Peribulbar block* – local anaesthetic solution (5–10 ml) with hyaluronidase, as for retrobulbar block, injected medially through the midpoint of caruncle using a 25-gauge 2.5-cm needle, followed by a second injection (5–7 ml) of the same solution injected inferolaterally. The solution is deposited more anteriorly than in a retrobulbar block. Safer than a retrobulbar block; does not need a facial nerve block and is less painful to institute.
- Pressure over the eye for 10–15 min with Honan's balloon or mercury bag following block.

Complications of local analgesia:
- *Chemosis* – normally clears with pressure and is less with the use of hyaluronidase
- *Retrobulbar haemorrhage* – very low incidence, more frequent with retrobulbar block; treated with a pressure bandage, generally requires postponement of surgery but may occasionally require exploration
- *Perforation of the globe* – associated with both blocks, more common with axial lengths of greater than 2.6 cm and following previous retinal surgery
- *Ptosis* – normally corrects postoperatively
- *Extraocular muscle paresis* – avoid direct injection into extraocular muscles; usually recovers in the postoperative period
- *Neurological* – convulsions, trauma to optic nerve, subarachnoid injection or brain-stem anaesthesia leading to cardiorespiratory arrest.

GENERAL ANAESTHESIA

- Intravenous induction – propofol is particularly suitable (lowers IOP more than thiopentone), or inhalational induction in children
- Intubation and ventilation – atracurium or vecuronium are ideal agents. Modify the pressure response to intubation by deepening anaesthesia, additional dose of the induction agent, injecting lignocaine (1.5 mg kg^{-1} i.v.) or fentanyl (1 μg kg^{-1} i.v.) prior to intubation or using laryngeal mask airway
- Maintenance – oxygen or nitrous oxide/oxygen combination with a volatile agent and/or analgesic, e.g. fentanyl; or a propofol infusion
- Moderate hyperventilation
- Smooth anaesthesia avoiding straining, coughing or patient movement
- Reversal of neuromuscular block.

Complications of general anaesthesia:
- Coughing and straining, but these cause little problem with modern surgical techniques and are attenuated by lignocaine (1–1.5 mg kg^{-1} i.v.) before extubation
- Postoperative acetazolamide for control of IOP; this may cause emetic symptoms
- Nausea and vomiting – use prophylaxis such as droperidol 1.0 mg or ondansetron 4 mg.

POSTOPERATIVE PAIN

- Usually alleviated by mild oral analgesics such as paracetamol.

BIBLIOGRAPHY

Akhtar T M, McMurray P, Kerr W J, Kenny G N C. A comparison of laryngeal mask airway with tracheal tube for intraocular ophthalmic surgery. Anaesthesia 1992; 47: 668–671

Barker J P, Vafidis G C, Robinson P N, Burrin J M, Hall G M. The metabolic and hormonal response to cataract surgery. Anaesthesia 1993; 48: 488–491

Hamilton R C, Gimbel H V, Strunin L. Regional anaesthesia for 12,000 cataract extraction and intraocular lens implantation procedures. Canadian Journal of Anaesthesia 1988; 135: 615–623

Katsev D A, Drews R C, Rose B T. An anatomic study of retrobulbar needle path length. Ophthalmology 1989; 96: 1221–1224

Mirakhur R K, Elliott P. Anaesthesia for ophthalmic surgery. Current Anaesthesia and Critical Care 1992; 3: 212–217

Roberts F L, Dixon J, Lewis G T R, Tackley R M, Prys-Roberts C. Induction and maintenance of propofol anaesthesia. A manual infusion scheme. Anaesthesia 1988; 43 (suppl): 14–17

CROSS REFERENCES

The elderly patient
Patient Conditions 11: 252

Day-case surgery
Anaesthetic Factors 29: 542

Total intravenous anaesthesia
Anaesthetic Factors 32: 606

Local anaesthetic toxicity
Anaesthetic Factors 33: 642

CORNEAL TRANSPLANT

J. C. Stanley

PROCEDURE

- Patient positioned supine
- Either full thickness (penetrating keratoplasty) or occasionally partial thickness (lamellar keratoplasty) grafts may be used
- May be performed as a repeat procedure
- Often combined with cataract extraction and intraocular lens implantation.

PATIENT CHARACTERISTICS

Patients for corneal transplant are generally:

- Of any age, depending on the underlying condition
- Are likely to have one of the conditions listed in Table 1.

INDICATIONS

- Central opacification of the cornea
- Abnormality of the cornea which seriously limits vision and is unsuitable for other management
- In general, most of these conditions do not have any associated anaesthetic problems, but the patients may have other coexisting diseases.

PREOPERATIVE ASSESSMENT AND INVESTIGATIONS

- Identification and treatment of associated medical conditions.

Table 1.
Conditions expected to benefit from keratoplasty

Hereditary and acquired dystrophies
- Keratoconus (may have associated atopy)
- Stromal, e.g. mucopolysaccharidosis, amyloid deposits
- Endothelial, e.g. Fuchs dystrophy, secondary post-traumatic and postsurgical, bullous keratopathy

Keratitis
- Interstitial
- Herpetic
- Rosaceal
- Trachomatous

Trauma
- Thermal
- Chemical

Neoplasia

PREMEDICATION

- Anxiolysis (if required) with benzodiazepines in adult patients and benzodiazepines or trimeprazine in children
- Avoidance of postoperative nausea and vomiting is very important; consideration should be given to an antiemetic prophylaxis
- Therapeutic premedication if indicated, e.g. salbutamol nebulizer in asthmatic patients, or nitrates to patients with angina
- If parents accompany children to theatre, full explanation is necessary.

PERIOPERATIVE MANAGEMENT

Monitoring:
- ECG
- Blood pressure
- SpO_2
- $ETCO_2$
- Peripheral nerve stimulator
- Core temperature.

Anaesthetic technique:
- Either local or general anaesthesia
- Avoid any patient movement, coughing, or straining which results in a rise in intraocular pressure (IOP) because, as the eye is totally open for a period, this could have catastrophic results
- Because the operation is often combined with cataract extraction and lens implantation (triple procedure) the duration of the procedure may be excessive to maintain the patient's cooperation for a local block. In the absence of any serious systemic disease, many prefer general anaesthesia.

Local anaesthesia:
- Peribulbar anaesthesia using a lignocaine/ bupivacaine (2%/0.5%) mixture with added hyaluronidase (50–150 units). Total volume of injection is 5–15 ml. An ocular compression device should be applied and inflated to a pressure of 40 mmHg for a minimum of 15–20 min.
- Retrobulbar anaesthesia using the same mixture. Total volume of injection is 3–6 ml. Facial nerve block is usually necessary to prevent blepharospasm.

General anaesthesia:
- As with cataract extraction or any other intraocular procedure, a careful technique is necessary to avoid any rise in IOP
- Intravenous induction with thiopentone or propofol; inhalational induction in children
- Tracheal intubation using a non-depolarizing relaxant (e.g. vecuronium or atracurium) with relatively deep neuromuscular block to ensure no sudden movement
- Maintenance of anaesthesia with nitrous oxide in oxygen, and a volatile agent or using a total intravenous technique
- Additional analgesia with fentanyl, as required
- Moderate hyperventilation to ensure a low IOP
- Routine use of an antiemetic is recommended
- Antagonism of neuromuscular block with neostigmine and glycopyrrolate
- Atropine or glycopyrrolate may be required to counter the oculocardiac reflex.

Emergence and recovery:
- Extubate while deeply anaesthetized if possible, although not absolutely essential
- Lignocaine (1.0–1.5 mg kg^{-1} i.v.) before extubation reduces coughing.

POSTOPERATIVE MANAGEMENT

- More painful than other intraocular procedures requiring narcotic analgesia in the immediate postoperative period
- Antiemetics, as required
- Acetazolamide (Diamox) may be required postoperatively to control IOP

- Patient can usually be discharged from hospital the following day.

BIBLIOGRAPHY

Casey T A, Mayer D J. Corneal grafting: principles and practice. Saunders, London, 1981
Morrison J D, Mirakhur R K, Craig H J. Anaesthesia for eye, ear, nose, and throat surgery, 2nd edn. Churchill Livingstone, London, 1985
Roper-Hall M J. Stallard's eye surgery, 7th edn. Butterworth, London, 1989
Van den Berg A A, Lambourne A, Clyburn P A. The oculoemetic reflex. Anaesthesia 1989; 44: 110–117

CROSS REFERENCES

Infants and children
Patient Conditions 11: 252
Intraocular pressure
Surgical Procedures 13: 294
Local anaesthetic toxicity
Anaesthetic Factors 33: 642

DETACHMENT AND VITREOUS SURGERY

R. K. Mirakhur

PATHOLOGY

- Collection of fluid between the layers of retina leading to the inner photosensitive layer becoming detached; retina may develop big holes and tears
- Vitreous may become fibrosed and develop traction bands which pull off the retina from its outer layers
- There may be proliferation of blood vessels and haemorrhages into the vitreous
- Retina and vitreous may have become damaged as a result of trauma.

PROCEDURE

Detachment surgery is essentially extraocular, but vitrectomy is an intraocular procedure. Detachment repair and vitrectomy:

- Are performed with the patient supine and head in the midposition
- Are performed in a theatre with a lot of equipment and in darkness for part of the time
- Take much longer than the more common ophthalmic surgical procedures
- May require treatment with a laser
- May need to be repeated at short intervals
- May involve insufflation of air, sulphur hexafluoride or silicone oil into the eye.

PATIENT CHARACTERISTICS

- Likely to be elderly
- Many are insulin-dependent diabetics of long duration

- Some patients, particularly those having suffered trauma, may be having repeat anaesthetics.

PREOPERATIVE ASSESSMENT AND PREPARATION

- Assessment and treatment of associated medical conditions
- Stabilization of the diabetic status and control of hyperglycaemia and any ketosis (surgery for diabetic retinopathy can usually wait)
- Assess any propensity to hypoglycaemia
- Assess autonomic dysfunction in diabetics
- Haemoglobin estimation unnecessary unless clinically indicated
- Measure urea and electrolytes in the elderly
- Measure blood sugar in diabetics
- ECG (where indicated, or in patients above 50 years of age)
- Routine chest X-ray considered unnecessary unless indicated.

PREMEDICATION

- Anxiolysis, if required, with oral temazepam
- Anticholinergic premedication not required, although intravenous atropine may be required later during surgery for prevention and treatment of oculocardiac reflex
- Measurement of blood glucose early in the morning in the diabetic patients and commence intravenous dextrose infusion with appropriate amounts of actrapid insulin on a sliding scale. (Addition of potassium is rarely required as these patients are able to resume oral intake and their usual insulin regime within a few hours after the end of surgery.)

ANAESTHETIC MANAGEMENT

- Vitreous surgery is carried out on a table with a special head-piece and arm rests for the surgeon
- Care of the pressure areas, as usual
- Carefully secure the airway because access to the airway is virtually impossible once surgery has started, without causing damage to the eye.

Monitoring:

- ECG
- Noninvasive BP
- Sp_{O_2}
- ET_{CO_2}
- Peripheral nerve stimulator when administering a general anaesthetic
- Special attention to ventilation disconnection alarms (dark theatre)
- Intravenous fluids at 2–3 ml kg^{-1} h^{-1} until resumption of oral intake.

Anaesthesia:

General anaesthesia is the technique of choice because of the long duration of surgery.

- Intravenous induction with thiopentone or propofol
- Analgesia with fentanyl (2–3 μg kg^{-1})
- Muscle relaxation with vecuronium or atracurium followed by increments. Relatively deep block required until near the end of surgery. Monitor the block to prevent any sudden movement of the patient
- Maintenance with oxygen in air and isoflurane, or with continuous intravenous infusion of propofol
- Avoid nitrous oxide if sulphur hexafluoride or air are being insufflated into the eye; if nitrous oxide has been used in the beginning, it should be discontinued 20 min before insufflation of these agents (maintain communication with the surgeon)
- Reverse neuromuscular block appropriately
- Antiemetic prophylaxis.

General anaesthesia is advantageous because it provides absolute immobility during a long operation and avoids any increase in intraocular pressure and vascular congestion.

Local anaesthesia may be used and administered in the same way as for a cataract operation.

POSTOPERATIVE CARE

- Analgesia with opioids (together with an antiemetic), if required, in the early postoperative period, followed by oral analgesics subsequently
- Early recovery from anaesthesia desirable as the patient may need to be positioned differently for optimal placement of the gas bubble and successful surgery
- Antiemetics may be required for 24 h.

BIBLIOGRAPHY

Mirakhur R K. Anaesthetic management of vitrectomy. Annals of the Royal College of Surgeons of England 1985; 67: 34–46

Mirakhur R K, Stanley J C. Propofol infusions for maintenance of anaesthesia for vitreous surgery: comparison with isoflurane. Anesthesia and Analgesia 1989; 68: S197

Morrison J D, Mirakhur R K, Craig H J L. Anaesthesia for eye, ear, nose and throat surgery, 2nd edn. Churchill Livingstone, London, 1985

Stinson T W, Donlon J V. Interaction of intraocular air and sulfur hexafluoride with nitrous oxide: a computer simulation. Anesthesiology 1982; 56: 385–388

Wolf G L, Capuano C, Hartung J. Nitrous oxide increases intraocular pressure after intravitreal sulfur hexafluoride injection. Anesthesiology 1983; 59: 547–548

CROSS REFERENCES

Diabetes mellitus
Patient Conditions 2: 42, 2: 44
The elderly patient
Patient Conditions 11: 252
Cataract surgery
Surgical Procedures 13: 288
Intraocular pressure
Surgical Procedures 13: 294
Total intravenous anaesthesia
Anaesthetic Factors 32: 606

INTRAOCULAR PRESSURE

R. K. Mirakhur

Control of intraocular pressure (IOP) is important both in health and in an open eye.

NORMAL VALUES

- 10–22 mmHg with a lower value in infants and young children
- Diurnal variation with the pressure being 5–7 mmHg higher on waking up.

PHYSIOLOGY

- Maintained by balance between production and drainage of the aqueous
- Produced from the epithelium of the ciliary processes
- Drained into the episcleral veins through the trabecular meshwork and the canal of Schlemm
- Factors contributing to the maintenance of IOP are the volumes of the vitreous, aqueous and the choroidal blood and elasticity of the sclera.

FACTORS AFFECTING IOP

Arterial pressure:
- Minimal effect within physiological variations because of autoregulation
- Sudden increases in arterial pressure may cause a transient increase in IOP
- Decrease in IOP more pronounced below 80–90 mmHg systolic pressure.

Venous pressure:
- IOP and venous pressure have a close parallel relationship (Figure 1)

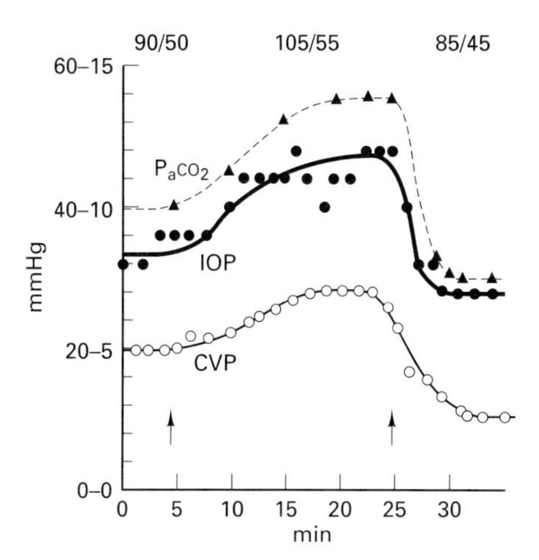

Figure 1
Influence of $P_a co_2$ and venous pressure on IOP; the left-hand arrow indicates the beginning of hypoventilation and the right hand arrow the beginning of hyperventilation. (Reproduced with permission from Hvidberg et al 1981.)

- Increase in venous pressure, such as by coughing, straining, breath holding or obstructed respiration, leads to a sustained increase in IOP
- The effect is mediated by changes in the choroidal blood volume.

Posture:
- A 15° head-up tilt reduces IOP to the same extent as hyperventilation to a $P_a co_2$ of 3.5–4.0 kPa
- A head-up position enhances venous drainage and reduces the venous pressure.

Respiration and $P_a co_2$:
- Changes in $P_a co_2$ affect the IOP very markedly (Figure 1)
- Hyperventilation with a consequent reduction in $P_a co_2$ results in a marked decrease in IOP
- Hypoventilation increases IOP
- The changes are mediated by changes in the choroidal blood volume
- Changes in arterial oxygen tension, as happen during anaesthesia, have minimal effect.

Anaesthetic agents:
- Intravenous opioids and benzodiazepines produce some reduction in IOP
- Anticholinergic agents have little effect
- The intravenous anaesthetics thiopentone, methohexitone, etomidate and propofol reduce IOP, the last producing a more pronounced decrease
- Ketamine may increase IOP
- Total intravenous anaesthesia using propofol is associated with a low IOP
- The inhalational agents halothane, enflurane and isoflurane reduce IOP significantly, but without a dose-related effect
- Nitrous oxide has little effect.

Muscle relaxants:
- Suxamethonium increases IOP markedly. The effect is maximal in 1–2 min and lasts 5–6 min. Suxamethonium can therefore be used during induction of anaesthesia
- The effect of suxamethonium is due to a sustained contracture of the fibres of the extraocular muscles and an increase in choroidal blood flow
- The use of suxamethonium is therefore contraindicated when the eye is open
- Pretreatment with intravenous acetazolamide, nondepolarizing relaxants, benzodiazepines, opioids, nitrates and supplementary doses of induction agents all attenuate the increase in IOP, but never completely or reliably prevent it from rising
- Among the nondepolarizing relaxants, tubocurarine and vecuronium reduce IOP, while others have no effect.

Other agents:
- Mannitol, sucrose and glycerol reduce IOP by withdrawing fluid from the vitreous body
- The carbonic anhydrase inhibitor acetazolamide reduces IOP by inhibiting the secretion of aqueous
- Timolol, adrenaline, nitrates, α_2 agonists and calcium entry blockers reduce IOP and are used in preoperative treatment of raised IOP; these may interact with the agents used in anaesthesia
- Although induction of anaesthesia is associated with a reduction in IOP, laryngoscopy and tracheal intubation often cause an increase in IOP
- Judicious combination of many of the agents and techniques often attenuates this increase (Table 1).

Table 1.
Methods of maintaining low IOP

Methods
Smooth induction and maintenance of anaesthesia (avoiding coughing and straining)
Moderate hyperventilation
Unobstructed respiration
Deep anaesthesia
Slight head-up tilt
Maintaining a low venous pressure
Reducing arterial pressure (may be limited by patient's condition)
Use of specific drugs

BIBLIOGRAPHY

Cunningham A J, Barry P. Intraocular pressure – physiology and implications for anaesthetic management. Canadian Anaesthetists' Society Journal 1986; 33: 195–208

Hvidberg A, Kessing S V, Fernandes A. Effect of changes in $P\text{co}_2$ and body positions on intraocular pressure during general anaesthesia. Acta Ophthalmologica 1981; 59: 465–475

Mirakhur R K. Use of relaxants in eye surgery. In: Rupp S M (ed) Problems in anesthesia: neuromuscular relaxants. J B Lippincott, Philadelphia, 1989, vol 3, p 510–521

Mirakhur R K, Gaston J H Anaesthesia for ophthalmic surgery. In: Healy T E J, Cohen P (eds) A practice of anaesthesia. Edward Arnold, London, 1994, 1995, pp 1265–1281

Murphy D F. Anesthesia and intraocular pressure. Anesthesia and Analgesia 1985; 64: 520–530

CROSS REFERENCES

Hypertension
Patient Conditions 4: 111

PENETRATING EYE INJURY

J. H. Gaston

PROCEDURE

- Repair of laceration varying from minor corneal injury to complete disruption of the globe
- Degree of damage to the eye frequently diagnosed following induction of anaesthesia
- Removal of foreign body, generally through a second separate incision.

PATIENT CHARACTERISTICS

- All age groups
- May have coincidental disease.

PROBLEMS

- Sometimes there is only isolated eye injury
- There may be multiple injuries, particularly to head and neck
- Full stomach (with possible alcohol intake)
- When eye is open the pressure of the contents equals atmospheric pressure and any external pressure or increase in IOP may lead to extrusion of eye contents.

AIMS

- Prevention of aspiration of gastric contents
- Limiting the increase in IOP and preventing further damage to the eye.

PREOPERATIVE ASSESSMENT AND CONSIDERATIONS

- Systemic assessment and management of any associated injuries

- Assessment of airway for any potential difficulties
- Resuscitation as required
- Optimization of coincidental conditions (time-limited)
- Discussion with the surgeon
- Delay surgery if necessary (often possible for isolated eye injury); this does not always guarantee an empty stomach.

PREMEDICATION

- May not be required or appropriate
- Anxiolytic (temazepam) where appropriate.

MONITORING

- ECG
- Arterial pressure
- Spo_2
- $ETco_2$
- Peripheral nerve stimulator
- Fluid balance, as appropriate.

ANAESTHETIC TECHNIQUE

- Regional anaesthesia is unsuitable; it may aggravate the injury and both peribulbar and retrobulbar blocks may initially increase intraocular pressure
- Rapid sequence induction required in most cases
- Consider whether to use suxamethonium or a nondepolarizing relaxant for intubation
- Suxamethonium provides the best intubating conditions most rapidly, but raises IOP
- Nondepolarizing relaxants do not raise IOP but are slower in onset
- Since laryngoscopy and tracheal intubation also raise IOP, the use of suxamethonium may be justified
- Although not always reliable, the rise in IOP due to suxamethonium may be attenuated by prior administration of i.v. lignocaine (1–1.5 mg kg^{-1}), or a nondepolarizing relaxant (10–15 mg gallamine, or 3–5 mg tubocurarine)
- Routine rapid sequence induction
- An alternative modified rapid sequence induction is favoured by some clinicians where vecuronium (0.15 mg kg^{-1}) (the newer agent rocuronium, when available, may be more appropriate) is substituted for suxamethonium
- Use suxamethonium if inexperienced, or if there is any doubt about the success of intubation
- Intravenous induction and muscle relaxant preferable even in children, because it is not easy to judge the depth of anaesthesia suitable for intubation when using an inhalational technique of induction, and children may also have sustained more damage than is initially obvious.

COMPLICATIONS

- Further injury to eye
- Oculocardiac reflex; prevent or treat with atropine (10–15 μg kg^{-1}).

POSTOPERATIVE MANAGEMENT

- Analgesics for pain: non-steroidal analgesics, or opioids
- Antiemetics for nausea and vomiting
- Appropriate treatment of other injuries.

OUTCOME

- Related to initial injury and successful prevention of secondary injury.

BIBLIOGRAPHY

Lavery G G, McGalliard J N, Mirakhur R K, Shepherd W F I. The effects of atracurium on intraocular pressure during steady state anaesthesia and rapid sequence induction. A comparison with succinylcholine. Canadian Anaesthetists' Society Journal 1986; 33: 437–442

Lerman J, Kiskis A A. Lidocaine attenuates the intraocular pressure response to rapid intubation in children. Canadian Anaesthetists' Society Journal 1985; 32: 339–345

Libonati M M, Leahy J J, Ellison N. The use of succinylcholine in open eye surgery. Anesthesiology 1985; 62: 637–640

Mirakhur R K, Elliott P, Shepherd W F I, Archer D B. Intraocular pressure changes during induction of anaesthesia and tracheal intubation; a comparison of thiopentone and propofol following vecuronium. Anaesthesia 1988; 43: 54–57

Mirakhur R K, Shepherd W F I, Darrah W C. Propofol and thiopentone: effects on intraocular pressure associated with induction of anaesthesia and tracheal intubation (facilitated with suxamethonium). British Journal of Anaesthesia 1987; 59: 437–439

CROSS REFERENCES

Infants and children
Surgical Procedures 11: 255
Emergency surgery
Anaesthetic Factors 29: 547
Trauma
Anaesthetic Factors 33: 672

STRABISMUS CORRECTION

J. C. Stanley

PROCEDURE

- Recession and/or resection of one or more extraocular muscles
- Performed with the patient supine
- May be performed as a day-case procedure
- Relatively short duration (20–60 min)
- May be performed as a repeat procedure.

PATIENT CHARACTERISTICS

Patients for strabismus correction are generally:

- Between 6 months and 8 years old; older children and adults may also present
- Usually ASA status 1–2
- May occasionally be part of a congenital syndrome with other system disorders
- Very rarely may have an association with other muscle disorders and malignant hyperthermia.

PROBLEMS

- Intraoperative bradycardia (oculocardiac reflex)
- High incidence of postoperative nausea and vomiting
- Need for postoperative analgesia.

PREOPERATIVE ASSESSMENT AND INVESTIGATIONS

- Most patients are fit and healthy
- Exclude upper respiratory tract infections in children.

PREMEDICATION

- Anxiolysis (if required) with benzodiazepines or trimeprazine syrup
- Anticholinergic premedication may be indicated for prevention of the oculocardiac and oculoemetic reflexes; this can be given orally, but is more reliable when given intravenously
- EMLA cream to the proposed venepuncture site
- Explanation to parents, if appropriate.

PERIOPERATIVE MANAGEMENT

Monitoring:
- ECG
- Arterial pressure
- Spo_2
- $ETco_2$
- Core temperature
- Peripheral nerve stimulator (if appropriate).

Anaesthetic technique:
- General anaesthesia is usually the method of choice as most patients are children, although regional anaesthesia with peribulbar or retrobulbar block can be used, if required, in adults
- Intravenous induction with thiopentone or propofol, or inhalational induction with nitrous oxide in oxygen and halothane, enflurane or isoflurane
- Intravenous anticholinergic agent such as atropine (15 μg kg^{-1}) or glycopyrrolate (7.5 μg kg^{-1}) to prevent intraoperative bradycardia
- Facilitation of intubation with suxamethonium or vecuronium (pretreat for suxamethonium pains)
- A laryngeal mask may be used without a relaxant (experience limited with this)
- Maintenance of anaesthesia with nitrous oxide in oxygen, and a volatile agent
- Ventilation and reversal of block if a nondepolarizing relaxant has been used
- Analgesia with fentanyl may be given
- Useful to administer an antiemetic routinely.

EMERGENCE AND RECOVERY

- Can be extubated deep or laryngeal mask left in situ until awake.

POSTOPERATIVE MANAGEMENT

- Topical amethocaine at the end of surgery
- Opioids rarely needed
- Oral paracetamol usually satisfactory
- NSAIDs may be used
- Antiemetic drugs may be required.

BIBLIOGRAPHY

Broadman L M, Ceruzzi W, Patane P S et al. Metoclopramide reduces the incidence of vomiting following strabismus surgery in children. Anesthesiology 1990; 72: 245–248

Fenelly M E, Hall G M. Anaesthesia and upper respiratory tract infection – a non-existent hazard? British Journal of Anaesthesia 1990; 64: 535–536

Levy L, Pandit U A, Randel G I, Lewis I H, Tait A R. Upper respiratory tract infections and general anaesthesia in children. Anaesthesia 1992; 47: 678–682

Mirakhur R K, Jones C J, Dundee J W, Archer D B. I.m. or i.v. atropine or glycopyrrolate for the prevention of the oculocardiac reflex in children undergoing squint surgery. British Journal of Anaesthesia 1982; 54: 1059–1063

Watson D M. Topical amethocaine in strabismus surgery. Anaesthesia 1991; 46: 368–370

CROSS REFERENCES

Malignant hyperthermia
Patient Conditions 2: 57
Infants and children
Patients Conditions 11: 255
Premedication
Anaesthetic Factors 29: 549
Malignant hyperthermia
Anaesthetic Factors 33: 644

14

ENT SURGERY

B. J. Pollard

14

LARYNGOSCOPY AND MICROSURGERY OF THE LARYNX

I. S. Chadwick

The development of techniques of laryngoscopy and laser surgery have led to the development of techniques of anaesthesia for these procedures. The procedures involve direct visualization of the vocal cords under general anaesthesia, often with biopsy or surgery to lesions, sometimes using a laser. Either the Kleinasser laryngoscope and suspension system or the ventilating laryngoscope, are used.

Close cooperation between surgeon and anaesthetist is essential. This is not a field for the novice.

PATIENT CHARACTERISTICS

- Often older age groups.
- Commonly smokers because vocal cord lesions are associated with tobacco smoking. Associated medical problems are likely, related to age and smoking history, e.g. cardiac and respiratory disease.

PREOPERATIVE ASSESSMENT

- Routine assessment of pre-existing medical conditions
- Appropriate investigations depending upon the history and examination
- Assessment of the airway is important – there may be a degree of airway restriction from any lesion in upper airway or larynx; stridor may be present
- Preliminary assessment of the airway, using indirect laryngoscopy with topical local anaesthesia by the ENT surgeon may be required.

PREMEDICATION

- Light anxiolysis without excessive respiratory depression
- Antisialogogue may be beneficial in some circumstances.

THEATRE PREPARATION AND MONITORING

- Full access to difficult intubation and emergency tracheostomy facilities is essential
- Monitoring should include the routine standards of ECG, noninvasive BP, Sa_{O_2}, ET_{CO_2}, airway pressure, disconnect alarm and neuromuscular blockade
- Position is as for most head and neck work, resulting in restricted access for the anaesthetist.

GENERAL PRINCIPLES OF ANAESTHETIC TECHNIQUE

The main problem concerns the sharing of the airway with the surgeon, in order to provide surgical access. To overcome this, several techniques have been developed.

Lesions in the larynx may cause significant stridor and a gaseous induction or even tracheostomy under local anaesthesia before induction may be required.

Meticulous attention to anaesthetic detail is essential. Full relaxation of the patient and immobile vocal cords are required. There should be a rapid return of consciousness and protective reflexes after what can vary between a very short to a quite prolonged period of anaesthesia.

Occasionally the surgeon may need to observe the movements of the vocal cords, at the end of the procedure.

Manipulation of the larynx can cause a hypertensive response and cardiac arrhythmias.

Aspiration of blood and surgical debris into the trachea can occur.

Avoidance of hypoxia and awareness can be difficult.

ANAESTHETIC TECHNIQUE

The choice of anaesthetic technique depends

on the predisposing condition of the patient and individual preference of the anaesthetist.

Essentials are cardiovascular stability, avoidance of awareness and a smooth and rapid recovery.

An intravenous induction is suitable for most patients followed by maintenance using a balanced type of anaesthesia with oxygen, nitrous oxide and a volatile agent with or without an opioid. A total intravenous technique is a useful alternative, particularly if administration of a volatile agent is not possible. Muscle relaxation using one of the shorter acting relaxants, e.g. atracurium, vecuronium or mivacurium, is required. Propofol should be used carefully in the elderly. Occasionally a spontaneous breathing technique may be required.

The anaesthetic technique depends to a great extent on the method of airway maintenance.

AIRWAY MAINTENANCE

This can be managed in four ways:

- Tracheal intubation
- Tracheal catheter
- Venturi jet ventilation
- High-frequency ventilation.

Tracheal intubation

This facilitates general anaesthesia, but interferes with surgical access. A small diameter (5.0–6.0 mm) cuffed flexible microlaryngeal (Pollard) type tube can be used. This can be placed either orally or nasally. The narrow diameter offers increased resistance to flow, and controlled ventilation is required. In difficult cases some anaesthetists have used large diameter urinary Foley-type catheters with the 30-ml balloon acting as a cuff.

Tracheal catheter

These are usually used with a spontaneous breathing technique. A 14 French gauge or similar catheter is threaded down to the carina and a mixture of oxygen and a volatile anaesthetic insufflated. Disadvantages include movement of the cords and no protection of the lower airway from aspiration. Surgical access is good.

Jet ventilation

The principal of the Sanders Venturi injector is employed with either oxygen or oxygen/nitrous oxide from a blender as the driving gas. There is variable air entrainment, depending on the position of the tip of the injector and the duration of gas flow. A ventilating laryngoscope is commonly used. The axis of the jet must be in line with the trachea and it is imperative that there is no mechanical obstruction to the outflow of air. Alternatives are to place the tip of the injector below the cords, by passing the catheter through the mouth. This has the advantage of reducing the risk of blowing debris down the trachea. The catheter could also be inserted directly into the trachea through a crico-thyroid puncture. Awareness is a potential risk because full muscle paralysis is required for this technique and a total intravenous anaesthetic technique is required.

Jet ventilation techniques may not ensure adequate ventilation in patients with poor lung compliance or obesity. There is a danger of barotrauma and surgical emphysema with jet ventilators. Only experienced operators should use this technique.

High-frequency ventilation techniques

These techniques may be used, through a catheter passed well below the vocal cords with a driving pressure of 40–140 kPa, and a rate of 60–100 breath min^{-1}. Advantages of this technique are lower airway pressure, less risk of barotrauma and good cardiovascular stability. Operating conditions for the surgeon are good.

High-frequency ventilation is not widely available and conventional jet ventilation is the more frequently used technique.

AIRWAY MAINTENANCE FOR ANAESTHESIA FOR LASER SURGERY

Lasers are used for excision of various laryngeal lesions. Lasers are accurate in focal tissue removal, provide a bloodless field with minimal tissue reaction and little post-operative oedema or pain. Carbon dioxide or Nd-YAG type lasers are usually used.

Various safety considerations are essential in order to protect staff and patient from burns, especially to the eyes and skin.

With ENT laser work, the biggest danger is a fire in the airway. The endotracheal tube can ignite and both oxygen and nitrous oxide will support combustion.

14

Special endotracheal tubes have been developed:

- An ordinary tube may be used wrapped in wet muslin or the tube may be wrapped in metal-foil tape; however, these are bulky and the foil may come off and traumatize the airway
- Flexible metallic tubes have been used
- Flexible silicone lined 'laser-proof' tubes have been developed. These can still ignite with prolonged laser exposure, particularly in the region of the cuff.

To overcome the problem of cuff deflation by the laser, various designs of double cuff, saline- or foam-filled cuffs have been developed.

JET VENTILATION AND LASER

Jet ventilation avoids the use of tracheal tubes and provides good surgical access and view. Coordination is required between surgeon and anaesthetist to ensure that the cords are motionless during the firing of the laser.

FIRE PRECAUTIONS AND TREATING A FIRE

Mixtures of 30% oxygen in nitrogen or helium have been used to reduce the fire risk. However, in practice standard anaesthetic gases and extreme caution by the surgeon limiting the laser to short bursts are used.

If a fire occurs the circuit must be immediately disconnected to prevent blowing ignited gases down the trachea. Extinguish the fire with saline, which should always be ready on the scrub trolley in a 50 ml bladder syringe.

Remove the damaged tracheal tube and restore airway control. Assess the degree of tissue damage with bronchoscopy and treat in the ITU as an inhalation burn. The complications are serious and often fatal.

POSTANAESTHETIC AND POSTSURGICAL COMPLICATIONS

Following laryngoscopy and surgery, the common complications are:

- Short term:
  - Aspiration of blood and debris
  - Laryngospasm
  - Oedema
  - Stridor.
- Medium term (24–48 h):
  - Bleeding
  - Oedema
  - Stridor.
- Long term:
  - Tissue scarring
  - Hoarseness
  - Vocal cord paralysis.

BIBLIOGRAPHY

Mayne A, Joucken K, Collard E, Randour P. Intravenous infusion of propofol for induction and maintenance of anaesthesia during endoscopic carbon dioxide laser ENT procedures with high frequency jet ventilation. Anaesthesia 1988; 43 (suppl): 97–100

Mirakhur R K. Advances in ENT anaesthesia. In: Kaufman L (ed) Anaesthesia review. Churchill Livingstone, London, 1988, vol 5, p 196–215

Padfield A, Stamp J M. Anaesthesia for laser surgery. European Journal of Anaesthesiology 1992; 9: 353–366

Shikowitz M J, Abramson A L, Liberatore L. Endolaryngeal jet ventilation: 10-year review. Laryngoscope 1991; 101: 455–461

CROSS REFERENCES

Difficult airway – difficult tracheal intubation
Anaesthetic Factors 30: 564
Awareness
Anaesthetic Factors 33: 614

MIDDLE EAR SURGERY

G. Robson

Middle ear operations started with the invention of the otoscope in 1860. Fenestration was first practised in 1938, and since then middle ear surgery has advanced considerably. Examples of middle ear operations include tympanoplasty and mastoid cavity operations.

For middle ear surgery a smooth anaesthetic is absolutely essential. It is imperative to avoid coughing, straining and bucking because all of these increase venous pressure and cause oozing which may persist for some time and potentially jeopardize the success of the surgery.

PREOPERATIVE ASSESSMENT

- Surgery to the middle ear may be performed on any age group
- Routine assessment should be undertaken according to the patient's general medical condition
- Investigations according to the patient's medical condition
- No specific factors apply to these surgical techniques.

PREMEDICATION

A sedative premedication is valuable to ensure a calm, relaxed patient.

PERIOPERATIVE MANAGEMENT

- A smooth induction of anaesthesia is important
- Thiopentone is recommended because the induction period can be taken more slowly (these patients are not managed as day cases)
- A long-acting relaxant is suitable and time should be allowed for full relaxation to develop before intubation is attempted
- Atropine should be avoided if possible
- A beta blocker adjuvant at induction together with topical lignocaine spray to the larynx and trachea after full relaxation can help avoid the reflex response to intubation
- A nonkinking (armoured) orotracheal tube should be used.

Some anaesthetists favour allowing the patient to breathe spontaneously through a laryngeal mask or tracheal tube so that assessment of potential facial nerve damage can be made by the surgeon. This technique, however, often leads to progressive hypercapnia with increased venous oozing, and so is not recommended.

When using IPPV, moderate hypocapnia should be the aim. Care must be taken in elderly and hypertensive patients whose cerebrovascular autoregulatory mechanism may be impaired.

The middle ear is a closed cavity and nitrous oxide diffuses in rapidly causing an increase in pressure. This reaches a maximum about 40 min after commencement of the nitrous oxide. This increase in pressure may cause grafts to become dislodged and, because of this, many anaesthetists now use an oxygen/nitrogen or oxygen/air mixture to avoid the potential problems of nitrous oxide. This could present a potential awareness problem.

Promotion of a bloodless operating field is desirable. A 10–15° head-up tilt dramatically improves venous drainage and reduces venous ooze, and is considered essential by the author. Induced hypotension also aids the surgeon. This technique should only be attempted by the experienced anaesthetist after careful assessment of the patient. It may be achieved in a variety of ways. Nitroprusside and nitroglycerin are unsuitable due to the length of most middle ear surgery operations (tachyphylaxis and toxic levels would soon be reached). A combination of halothane and tubocurarine has been used to good effect. The author, however, favours the use of isoflurane and a beta blocker, which gives a very easily controlled hypotension.

Bandaging of the ear at the end of the procedure involves movement of the head. This should be supervised by the anaesthetist to prevent undue movement on the tracheal tube which may lead to gagging. Ideally, the patient should be maintained in a fully paralysed state whilst the bandaging is taking place. Unfortunately this results in prolongation of the anaesthetic for 10–15 min after the end of surgery before the muscle relaxant can be safely reversed.

MONITORING

- ECG
- Sao_2
- Noninvasive BP (invasive BP monitoring is preferable if induced hypotension is planned)
- $ETco_2$
- Neuromuscular transmission.

POSTOPERATIVE PROBLEMS

Nausea and vomiting can be a particular problem following these procedures and a suitable antiemetic should be given. A 5-HT_3 antagonist, e.g. ondansetron given intravenously at induction is particularly effective.

CROSS REFERENCES

Induced hypotension during anaesthesia
Anaesthetic Factors 32: 597

OESOPHAGOSCOPY

A. McCluskey

PROCEDURE

Rigid oesophagoscopy may be performed for:

- Removal of a foreign body
- Diagnosis of dysphagia
- Biopsy of neoplastic lesions
- Dilatation of a stricture
- Palliative intubation
- Injection of varices.

PATIENT CHARACTERISTICS

There are two main groups:

- Children – usually fit, for removal of foreign body
- Elderly – ASA II–IV associated diseases (see below).

FACTORS INFLUENCING THE MANAGEMENT OF PATIENTS PRESENTING FOR OESOPHAGOSCOPY

- Often elderly
- Malnutrition
- Dehydration
- Hiatus hernia, achalasia, stricture
- Malignant disease
- Hypoalbuminaemia
- Anaemia
- Retention of food residues above lesion, delayed gastric emptying, increased risk of regurgitation and aspiration
- Co-existent low-grade chest infection or lung abscess secondary to regurgitation
- Smoking habit

- Conditions associated with old age (hypertension, ischaemic heart disease, diabetes, etc.).

PREOPERATIVE ASSESSMENT AND INVESTIGATION

Patients may present in a debilitated state. Aim to optimize condition as far as possible over 24–48 h.

Diagnosis and treatment of co-existent medical conditions, particularly hypovolaemia and chest infection.

Investigations

- Full blood count
- Urea and electrolytes
- Group and save
- Cross-match for varices
- ECG
- Chest X-ray.

PREMEDICATION

Sedation is best avoided as protective reflexes must return promptly after the procedure. An anticholinergic agent is often all that is required.

An H_2 antagonist or omeprazole may be prescribed with the intention of raising intragastric pH, but must be given several hours before the procedure to be effective. Particulate antacids may obscure the surgeon's view.

Metoclopramide and prochlorperazine increase lower oesophageal sphincter pressure and may promote gastric emptying.

INDUCTION OF ANAESTHESIA

Insertion of a large-bore (16 French gauge or greater) intravenous cannula is essential as acute severe haemorrhage may occur. Efficient suction apparatus must be immediately available.

All patients are at increased risk of aspiration and must therefore be intubated following preoxygenation, rapid sequence induction of anaesthesia and application of cricoid pressure. Consider inducing anaesthesia with a steep head-up tilt to reduce the incidence of regurgitation or, alternatively, with the patient in the lateral position and a downward tilt.

An endotracheal tube one size smaller than usual helps to avoid impeding the passage of the oesophagoscope. The tube should preferably be reinforced as the oesophagoscope may otherwise compress it. The patient's eyes should be well protected and the tube fixed to the left side of the mouth to permit the surgeon access.

ANAESTHESIA

Monitoring:

- Continuous ECG
- Noninvasive BP
- Oxygen saturation
- End-tidal CO_2
- Nerve stimulator.

Anaesthetic technique

The aim is to produce deep anaesthesia, as the procedure is highly stimulating, with prompt recovery and return of protective reflexes. Full muscle relaxation helps to permit easy passage of the oesophagoscope through the cricopharyngeal sphincter, and prevents coughing which may cause oesophageal perforation. A balanced technique is best suited to these aims.

Choice of particular drugs is dependent on the condition of the patient and personal preference. Either a volatile agent or total intravenous anaesthesia may be used successfully. Propofol with or without alfentanil by continuous infusion or intermittent bolus is associated with rapid recovery.

Suxamethonium and mivacurium are suitable neuromuscular blocking agents, depending on the length of the procedure.

PROBLEMS AND HAZARDS

- Introduction of the oesophagoscope may damage teeth, lips and mouth
- The cuff of the tracheal tube may need to be deflated to allow passage of the oesophagoscope
- Compression of the tracheal tube by the oesophagoscope is avoided by the use of a reinforced tube
- Arrhythmias are common, but are usually transitory and of no concern
- Haemorrhage following biopsy or injection of varices may be life-threatening
- Pulmonary aspiration
- Cardiovascular collapse due to undiagnosed or untreated hypovolaemia and/or poor general condition of the patient

- Hypertension and tachycardia due to insufficient depth of anaesthesia relative to the stimulation of the procedure may result in myocardial ischaemia in susceptible patients
- Oesophageal perforation has a very high mortality and may occur during an apparently uneventful procedure.

RECOVERY

- The patient should be supervised by an experienced nurse or the anaesthetist
- Patients should be nursed in the lateral position on a tilting trolley; oxygen is administered by mask and suction facilities must be immediately available
- Complaints of painful swallowing must be treated with a high index of suspicion for perforation of the oesophagus
- Intravenous fluids should be prescribed postoperatively as patients remain nil by mouth for some time
- A chest X-ray is mandatory before allowing anything by mouth, to exclude pneumothorax, pneumomediastinum and surgical emphysema.

BIBLIOGRAPHY

Gothard J W W, Branthwaite M A. Anaesthesia for thoracic surgery, 2nd edn. Blackwell Scientific, Oxford, 1993, ch 3

Kestin I G, Chapman J M, Coates M B. Alfentanil used to supplement propofol infusions for oesophagoscopy and bronchoscopy. Anaesthesia 1989; 44: 994–996

Marshall B E, Longnecker D E, Fairley H B. Anesthesia for thoracic procedures. Blackwell Scientific, Oxford, 1988, ch 13

CROSS REFERENCES

Disorders of the oesophagus and swallowing
Patient Conditions 5: 138
Hiatus Hernia
Patient Conditions 5: 141

OPERATIONS ON THE NOSE

B. J. Pollard

With operations on the nose, as with other ENT operations, cooperation between the anaesthetist and surgeon is essential. The surgeon must recognize that the anaesthetist requires access to the airway and the anaesthetist must supply an unhindered operating field and avoid any coughing and straining by the patient.

Procedures on the nose are usually fairly short and straightforward, e.g. removal of polyps, submucous diathermy to the septum, or submucous resection of nasal cartilage. Reduction of a fractured nose is also not a long procedure, unless it is an old fracture which requires the nose to be broken and reset. Septorhinoplasty may, however, be more prolonged.

PATIENT CHARACTERISTICS

- Patients with polyps are often of an atopic disposition
- Patients with fractured noses may have suffered a recent head injury
- If there has been recent significant blood loss, the patient may have swallowed much of it.

PREOPERATIVE ASSESSMENT AND INVESTIGATIONS

- Routine history and examination
- State of hydration if the patient has been bleeding significantly; rehydrate intravenously if necessary

- Chest X-ray; ECG in the older age groups
- Other investigations as indicated by the history and examination.

PREMEDICATION

- None necessary in many patients
- If in pain, a suitable dose of an opioid will suffice.

NASAL VASOCONSTRICTORS

The nose is a very vascular organ and the application of a topical vasoconstrictor is considered essential by many surgeons. The following are used in various centres:

- Topical cocaine solution – this has fallen in popularity because of the additional adverse effects of cocaine
- Topical cocaine paste – this is rarely used now
- Commercially available topical vasoconstrictor drops or sprays, e.g. ephedrine, oxymetazoline, etc.
- Direct injection of local analgesic with 1:100 000 or 1:200 000 adrenaline at the start of the procedure
- Felypressin solution.

PERIOPERATIVE MANAGEMENT

Monitoring:

- ECG
- Noninvasive BP
- Spo_2
- $ETco_2$
- Disconnection alarm.

Anaesthetic technique

- Preoxygenation is recommended, if only because nasal patency may be compromised.
- If there has been bleeding from the nose, the risk of regurgitation of swallowed blood is high and so a rapid sequence induction technique is recommended.
- The choice of induction agent depends upon the patient's general medical condition.
- Intubation of the trachea is mandatory using a cuffed tube in an adult to protect the airway because bleeding into the back of the pharynx is not uncommon.
- It will be difficult to gain access to the tracheal tube once surgery is in progress. All connections must be absolutely secure. The use of preformed tubes is helpful.
- Two techniques are commonly used:
  - Intubate using suxamethonium and then allow the patient to breathe spontaneously
  - Intubate using either suxamethonium followed by a nondepolarizing agent or intubate using a nondepolarizing relaxant and then control ventilation.
- Choice of technique for maintenance is not usually important. Controlled ventilation with a muscle relaxant, volatile agent and narcotic is suitable. Halothane is best avoided because of the potential arrythmias associated with the use of vasoconstrictors in the nose.
- The eyes should be taped closed and protective pads used to cover them.

Safe use of a pharyngeal pack

A pharyngeal pack should be inserted after intubation and before surgery is commenced. Wet gauze strip is the commonest type of pack, but various preformed sponge or gauze packs are favoured by some anaesthetists. The pack should be placed under direct vision using a laryngoscope and Magill's forceps. It is imperative to either leave a 'tail' of the pack protruding from the mouth, or to place an adhesive label on the patient as a reminder so that the pack cannot be accidentally left in the pharynx at the end of the operation.

At the end of the operation the pharynx should be aspirated under direct vision to ensure that the pack has been removed intact and that no foreign bodies or blood clots remain in the back of the pharynx.

POSTOPERATIVE MANAGEMENT

- A pack is commonly placed in the nose at the termination of surgery; no airway is therefore possible through the nose in the majority of cases
- It is important not to press on the nose with a face-mask because this may distort the shape
- The patient should be extubated in the lateral position
- Administer oxygen in recovery in a routine fashion
- Bleeding may occur from the nose, necessitating repacking
- Analgesia will be required; a NSAID is often sufficient but opioids are needed following more extensive surgery.

TONSILLECTOMY AND ADENOIDECTOMY

D. Greenhalgh

PROCEDURE

Adenotonsillectomy is performed through the mouth using a gag. Specific problems are:

- Shared airway with the surgeon
- Difficult intubation, especially when marked lymphoid hypertrophy or infection is present
- The gag (Boyle–Davis) may obstruct the endotracheal tube
- Postoperative bleeding:
  - Airway embarrassment
  - Hypotension.

PATIENT CHARACTERISTICS

Patients for adenotonsillectomy are usually:

- ASA I or II
- Children or young adults
- Have chronic infection
- May have sleep apnoea
- Adults may have associated medical conditions including chronic hypoxia and cor pulmonale.

Many centres are treating selected patients as day-cases.

PREOPERATIVE ASSESSMENT AND INVESTIGATIONS

History:

- Particularly of snoring and airway problems
- Bleeding tendencies (routine coagulation studies are not indicated unless the history suggests a problem)
- Patients are often snuffly; check if they are worse than normal
- Look for any associated medical conditions, e.g. Down's syndrome, deafness.

Investigations:

- Full blood count
- Relevant tests as indicated by the preoperative assessment.

PREMEDICATION

- In younger children, trimeprazine syrup (2–4 mg kg^{-1}) or diazepam syrup (0.3 mg kg^{-1}) given 2 h preoperatively
- At present, midazolam is not available in an oral preparation in the UK, but would be a suitable alternative if available
- EMLA cream to venepuncture sites at least 1 h preoperatively
- For older children and adults an anxiolytic of choice, e.g. temazepam, may be prescribed
- **Do not give sedation if there is any airway obstruction.**

PERIOPERATIVE MANAGEMENT

The anaesthetic room and theatre should be warm to minimize heat loss. The length of surgery varies, but is usually between 20 and 45 min.

Monitoring:

- ECG
- Sao_2
- Noninvasive BP
- $ETco_2$
- Core temperature – rectal
- Blood loss.

Anaesthetic technique

- Induction can be by either the inhalational or intravenous route, whichever is preferred or appropriate for the patient and anaesthetist
- Endotracheal intubation is performed, facilitated by either suxamethonium (1–2 mg kg^{-1}) or a nondepolarizing muscle relaxant, e.g. atracurium or vecuronium
- A smaller tube than expected may be necessary and a selection should be available
- An oral RAE tube is most suitable, as it is easily positioned centrally in between the jaws of the gag – check that it is not too long before starting

- The patient may breathe spontaneously through a T-piece or coaxial circuit, or have ventilation assisted, depending on the patient's, surgeon's and anaesthetist's preferences or circumstances
- Maintenance of anaesthesia with oxygen, nitrous oxide and a volatile agent is a suitable technique
- The patient is positioned supine with the head extended on a ring; a roll or pad is placed under the shoulders if extension is insufficient; the eyes need to be protected by tape or, preferably, pads
- Bradycardia may occur when the surgeon palpates the postnasal space during adenoidectomy; this usually resolves on cessation or if atropine is administered
- Analgesia should be given intraoperatively so that the patient is pain free on emergence, e.g. intramuscular (pethidine 1 mg kg^{-1}) or morphine (0.1 mg kg^{-1})
- Blood loss can be deceptive, especially in smaller infants, though it is not routinely measured
- Extubation should be performed with the patient head down and in the lateral position.

POSTOPERATIVE MANAGEMENT

Analgesia:

- Intramuscular opioids can be given via a cannula placed intraoperatively into a muscle, thereby providing analgesia without the trauma of an injection
- NSAIDs e.g. diclofenac suppositories, have been found to be opioid sparing, especially when given prior to surgery, and do not increase bleeding complications
- Paracetamol elixir.

Intravenous fluids are rarely required routinely because oral intake usually commences when the patient returns to the ward and has recovered adequately.

DISCHARGE

Many recent studies have shown that this procedure can be performed as a day-case.

Careful evaluation of the patients reduces the readmission rate for complications. Most episodes of haemorrhage occur prior to discharge or later than 24 h after operation. With careful selection the reoperation rate can be as low as 0.33%. The overall complication rate was 7.9% in one study (in-patients 11.8%; out-patients 4.1%), reflecting the selection of the patients. This was thought to be acceptable for day-cases.

MANAGEMENT OF THE BLEEDING TONSIL

Problems:

- Potentially the stomach may be full of blood, with risk of aspiration
- Hypovolaemia
- Potentially difficult airway, oedematous and obscured by blood
- Recent anaesthesia from which the patient may not yet have made a full recovery.

Preoperative management:

- Intravenous resuscitation with fluids and blood is mandatory
- Experienced anaesthetist must be present.

Anaesthetic management:

- Full resuscitation prior to induction
- Full monitoring instituted and effective suction available
- Head-down position
- Rapid sequence induction with thiopentone and suxamethonium (only use thiopentone if resuscitation is complete)
- Intubation may require a smaller endotracheal tube than previously used
- Maintenance as before
- Prior to extubation, wash the stomach out via a nasogastric tube
- Extubate head-down and on the side
- Inhalational induction may be preferred and performed with cricoid pressure, followed by intubation under deep volatile anaesthesia.

Use the technique with which you are familiar and with which you can secure the airway as rapidly as possible.

Postoperative management:

- Check haemoglobin
- If the throat has been packed, beware:
  - Heavy sedation may result in airway obstruction
  - Hypoxia may present as restlessness
- Remember that further bleeds may occur.

Resuscitation prior to anaesthesia is essential.

BIBLIOGRAPHY

Bolger W E, Parsons D S, Potempa L. Preoperative assessment of the adenotonsillectomy patient. Otolaryngology, Head and Neck Surgery 1990; 103: 396–405

Nordbladh I, Ohlander B, Bjorkman R. Analgesia in tonsillectomy: a double-blind study on pre- and post-operative treatment with diclofenac. Clinics in Otolaryngology 1991; 16: 554–558

Reiner S A, Sawyer W L, Clark K F, Wood M W. The safety of outpatient tonsillectomy and adenoidectomy. Otolaryngology, Head and Neck Surgery, 1990; 102: 161–168

Steward D J. The manual of pediatric anaesthesia. The Hospital for Sick Children, Toronto, Canada, p 100–102

Tewary A K. Day-case tonsillectomy: a review of the literature. The Journal of Laryngology and Otology 1993; 107: 703–705

CROSS REFERENCES

Infants and children
Patient Conditions 11: 255
Difficult airway
Anaesthetic Factors 30: 558
Difficult airway – aspiration risk
Anaesthetic Factors 30: 558

TRACHEOSTOMY

H. StJ. Gray

PROCEDURE

Tracheostomy is usually performed:

- Under general anaesthesia
- With the neck extended (sandbag under the shoulders and a headring)
- By cutting an elliptical disk.
- At the third tracheal ring
- Using a vertical slit in a child
- Inserting a tracheostomy tube after careful retraction of the endotracheal tube.

Percutaneous techniques are developing in the ITU. The tracheostomy tube is initially plastic with a high volume, low pressure cuff.

INDICATIONS

- Relief of respiratory obstruction
- Protection of the tracheobronchial tree
- Treatment of respiratory failure exceeding 2 weeks.

PATIENT CHARACTERISTICS

- General debility is common
- Associated respiratory, cardiovascular, neurological and/or metabolic disease
- ASA III–V
- Oro- or naso-tracheal intubation often difficult.

PREOPERATIVE ASSESSMENT

History:
- Full assessment as for the critically ill patient

- Look for the effects of persistent aspiration
- Assess the severity of airway obstruction
- Obtain information from any recent general anaesthesia (tube size/problems).

Examination:
- Cyanosis
- Stridor
- The use of accessory muscles of respiration
- Patient position.

Investigations:
- Chest X-ray
- Neck X-rays (aneroposterior and lateral)
- Arterial blood gases
- Pulmonary function tests.

THEATRE PREPARATION

- Assemble equipment for difficult intubation
- Prepare pressure transducers for monitoring
- Obtain a ventilator with PEEP facility
- Assemble a range of tracheostomy tubes and a sterile catheter mount and tubing
- A second anaesthetist may be useful.

PERIOPERATIVE MANAGEMENT

Premedication
Sedatives are not usually required; they may actually be dangerous. Anticholinergics may be helpful.

Induction:
- This is ideally performed in theatre; a gas induction is the preferred mode in the presence of obstruction
- A surgeon should be scrubbed and instruments prepared for urgent tracheostomy
- Intravenous induction is suitable when other indications for tracheostomy are present
- The tube should be fixed so that retraction is easy
- Careful oral toilet is essential.

Maintenance
Balanced anaesthesia with IPPV is preferable to spontaneous breathing. Note the inflation pressure. Use 100% oxygen.

TUBE INSERTION

- A tracheotomy is performed above the cuff
- Ventilation is stopped
- The tube is withdrawn to just above the tracheotomy
- The tracheostomy tube is placed
- Ventilation is re-started
- Note the CO_2 trace and inflation pressure.

POSTOPERATIVE MANAGEMENT

Nursing care
Nurse in the sitting position and ensure that the tube fixation is secure. Continue humidified oxygen and perform regular suction.

Tracheostomy tubes should not be removed for at least 5 days initially, when a track will have formed. Changes can be made over a catheter if desired.

Tracheal dilators, smaller tracheostomy tubes and reintubation equipment should always be available.

COMPLICATIONS

Early:
- Haemorrhage
- Tube displacement
- Surgical emphysema
- Pneumothorax
- Luminal occlusion (blood, sputum, tracheal wall).

Late:
- Tube occlusion
- Mucosal ulceration or deep erosion
- Perichondritis
- Tracheal stenosis.

EMERGENCY TRACHEOSTOMY

- Needle tracheotomy
- Cricothyroidotomy (mini-tracheostomy)
- Formal tracheostomy under local analgesia.

BIBLIOGRAPHY

Gray R F, Hawthorne M. Synopsis of otolaryngology, 5th edn. Butterworth-Heinemann, Oxford, 1992

Oh T E. Intensive care manual, 2nd edn. Butterworth, London, 1985

CROSS REFERENCES

Artificial airway
Anaesthetic Factors 30: 554
Difficult airway
Anaesthetic Factors 30: 558

15

HEAD AND NECK SURGERY

B. J. Pollard

DENTAL ABSCESS

C. Littler

Dental abscess is usually caused by dental or periodontal disease or by dental cysts. The abscess usually points into the buccal cavity or externally onto the skin, but may point intraorally. Most abscesses are localized, causing pain and local swelling, but spread can occur via lymphatics and tissue planes, leading to cellulitis, oedema and trismus.

Occasionally, but fortunately rarely nowadays, the infection can spread to the pharynx and neck, leading to gross swelling and oedema and possible airway problems (Ludwig's angina). This may present as an acute anaesthetic emergency.

Although pyrexia and malaise occur, progression to septicaemia is rare. Dental abscess was once a common occurrence, but due to better dental hygiene and better dental services, the incidence is now much lower. Most abscesses can be managed in dental surgeries with the use of antibiotics and local anaesthesia.

The indications for general anaesthesia are:
- Severe trismus and/or airway compromise
- Children
- Mental handicap or uncooperative patients
- Failed local anaesthesia.

PROCEDURE

Incision and drainage of the abscess either intraorally or extraorally, depending where the abscess is pointing.

PATIENT CHARACTERISTICS

Patients of all age groups present, but most are young adults. Special groups are:

- Children
- Mentally handicapped.

PREOPERATIVE ASSESSMENT

Full routine assessment and management of any concurrent medical conditions. Assessment of the airway is the main priority, looking for:

- Swelling
- Trismus, which may limit mouth opening
- Pus in the airway
- Excess salivation and difficulty swallowing in severe cases.

PREMEDICATION

- Usually none
- Antisialagogue if excess secretions
- Mild sedation in children and mentally handicapped if there are no airway problems
- Starvation (rarely an 'emergency' procedure)
- H_2 antagonists and metoclopramide may be used to reduce acidity and promote gastric emptying.

THEATRE PREPARATION

- Routine monitoring equipment, including a capnograph
- Trained assistance
- Essential equipment for an anticipated difficult intubation, including a fibre-optic flexible laryngoscope.

PERIOPERATIVE MANAGEMENT

Establish good intravenous access.

Induction

Depends on airway:

- *No airway problem anticipated* – intravenous induction with a muscle relaxant, as required.
- *Possible airway problems* – inhalational induction, maintaining spontaneous respiration with assessment of the airway and the ability to ventilate. A muscle relaxant may be given if it is then safe to do so. Otherwise, consider blind nasal or fibre-optic intubation with the patient breathing spontaneously.

- *Severe cases* – consider awake fibre-optic intubation.

Airway
A laryngeal mask may be used for external incision, provided that there is no trismus, the patient is starved and there is no chance of the abscess rupturing into the mouth. Oral intubation should otherwise be performed, unless this might impede surgical access, when nasal intubation may be required.

Maintenance
Inhalation agent or TIVA with or without a muscle relaxant are all suitable techniques.

A throat pack should be inserted if surgery will be performed in the mouth, to absorb any pus or blood.

Problems
Once the airway is secured the problems are few. Arrhythmias may occur with any dental surgery, therefore care should be taken with halothane and local infiltration with solutions containing adrenaline. Enflurane or isoflurane may be better choices.

POSTOPERATIVE MANAGEMENT

Extubate when awake in the lateral head-down position. Problems are those of foreign material, such as blood or pus gaining access to the airway, and possibly laryngospasm. Analgesia may be provided by opioids. Consider NSAIDs, unless contraindicated.

OUTCOME

Full recovery is to be expected. The patient may need to return to theatre for definitive treatment at a later date.

BIBLIOGRAPHY

Atkinson R S, Rushman G B, Lee J A. Dental anaesthesia. In: A Synopsis of anaesthesia, 10th edn, ch 25, 1987; Wright, Bristol, p 493–504

Moore J R, Gillbe G V. Principles of oral surgery, 4th edn. Manchester University Press, Manchester, 1991, ch xii, p 144–159

CROSS REFERENCES

Difficult airway
Anaesthetic Factors 30: 558

DENTAL SURGERY

M. S. Chetty

PROCEDURE

Dental surgery includes relatively simple procedures:

- Simple extractions – for caries or orthodontic treatment
- Surgical removal of wisdom teeth
- Dental clearance
- Surgical excision of apical roots
- Drainage of intraoral abscesses
- Lifting of fractured zygoma.

and more complex procedures:

- Maxillary osteotomy
- Mandibular reconstruction with or without bone grafting
- Plating of mandibular fractures.

Operative location can vary, and depends on the procedure planned, patient, and anaesthetic technique required (Table 1). Over the past 25 years, there has been a progressive decline in the number of patients undergoing general anaesthesia, reflecting better dental hygiene and acceptance of other techniques available. New recommendations on training and equipment have reduced the number of general dental surgeons practising general anaesthesia. Such cases should be restricted to sites specially designed, equipped and staffed for general anaesthetic procedures. A second skilled assistant and monitoring are required if anything other than straightforward local anaesthesia is administered.

PATIENT CHARACTERISTICS

- Often children
- A number of young adults
- Possibly mentally handicapped, with poor dental hygiene
- May have a phobia of dental treatment.

SPECIFIC PROBLEMS

- Airway shared with surgeon
- Intubation usually required, despite brief procedure
- Bleeding is common
  - Surgical
  - Nasal, following intubation
- Intraoral dental debris
- Often day-cases – select patients and anaesthetic agents accordingly
- Increased risk of laryngospasm postextubation
- Increased risk of ventricular arrhythmias, especially with halothane.

PREOPERATIVE ASSESSMENT

- Cardiac lesions require antibiotic prophylaxis
- Identify bleeding diatheses, or anticoagulant medication
- Fulfil criteria for day-case procedure and ensure that the patient is fully aware of the problems
- Assess the airway
  - Loose dentition
  - Trismus
  - Spasticity from cerebral palsy

Table 1.

Patient	Technique	Location
Cooperative adult	Local anaesthetic alone	Dental surgery
Uncooperative adult	Local anaesthetic with sedation	General anaesthesia department in dental hospital
Child	General anaesthetic	Operating theatre in hospital

- Request appropriate laboratory results, depending upon the findings in the history and examination; there are no specific requirements for these procedures.

INDICATIONS FOR GENERAL ANAESTHESIA

- Failed local technique or sedation
- Multiple extractions in three or four quadrants
- Prolonged procedure, heavy retraction and bone work
- Trismus or pain restricting access
- Sepsis at local-anaesthetic injection site
- Child, or patient with emotional or physical handicap where there is poor compliance.

PREMEDICATION

- Generally inappropriate for day-cases
- Benzodiazepine, if patient is specially anxious
- EMLA cream 1 h preoperatively for children
- Antisialogogue if anticipate inhalational induction
- Nasal vasoconstrictor in anaesthetic room for nasal intubation.

INTRAOPERATIVE MANAGEMENT

Monitoring:
- ECG
- Noninvasive BP
- Spo_2
- $ETco_2$
- Disconnect alarm.

Children

Induction:
- Intravenous induction preferred (thiopentone or methohexitone); inhalational (N_2O/O_2/halothane), if above difficult.

Maintenance:
- Simple procedures:
  - Nasal mask (Goldman)
  - Spontaneous breathing – N_2O/O_2/volatile agent
  - Support jaw
  - Oropharyngeal pack to collect debris and act as a gas seal.
- Multiple/complex extractions:
  - Intubate with preformed endotracheal tube (e.g. RAE)
  - Throat pack
  - IPPV (N_2O/O_2/volatile agent/opioid if required).

Adults

Induction:
- Airway compromised (e.g. by trismus):
  - Pre-oxygenate
  - Inhalational induction (N_2O/O_2/ halothane)
  - Avoid muscle relaxant until cords visualized
- Airway not compromised:
  - i.v. induction and relaxant.

Intubation:
- Nasal if surgical access limited
- Oral if access satisfactory.

Maintenance:
- N_2O/O_2/volatile agent/opioid/NSAID
- Controlled ventilation.

Note: The use of the laryngeal mask remains controversial.

EMERGENCE AND RECOVERY

- Ensure adequate surgical haemostasis
- Full neuromuscular reversal
- Remove throat pack!
- Full nasopharyngeal toilet including postnasal space
- Extubate awake, with reflexes intact, in lateral position.

POSTOPERATIVE MANAGEMENT

Oral analgesics usually sufficient. NSAIDs are analgesic and reduce swelling. Assess fitness for discharge with a responsible adult.

BIBLIOGRAPHY

Commission on the provision of surgical services. Guidelines for day case surgery. Royal College of Surgeons of England, 1985

Report of an expert working party on GA, sedation and resuscitation in dentistry. Department of Health, Dental Division, 1991

CROSS REFERENCES

Infants and children
Patient Conditions 11: 255
Dental chair
Surgical Procedures 28: 534
Day-case surgery
Anaesthetic Factors 29: 542
Difficult intubation (Difficult airway)
Anaesthetic Factors 30: 558

15

FACE AND JAW FRACTURES

M. J. Beech

PROCEDURE

Fractures may involve the zygoma, maxilla and mandible. Fractures of the maxilla may be classified according to the LeFort system. The procedure will consist of open or closed reduction of the fracture and, if necessary, transdental intermaxillary fixation (IMF) or internal fixation with metalwork.

PATIENT CHARACTERISTICS

The patients are often male with fractures due to trauma, e.g. car accidents, sports injuries, assault. Conditions may be present which predispose the patient to accidents, e.g. dysrhythmias, epilepsy, a cerebrovascular event, intoxication with alcohol or drugs. Pathological fractures due to diseased bone can occur.

Patients may present acutely for emergency treatment if fractures are life-threatening due to a compromised airway or haemorrhage. The patient may have a full stomach from food, drink and swallowed blood. Aspiration of blood, gastric contents, teeth and debris may have occurred, especially if the patient is unconscious. Other injuries may also be present, e.g. head injury, damage to the cervical spine, major bone fractures, chest and abdominal injuries.

In some patients definitive surgery may be delayed because of:

- Necessity to treat other injuries or conditions first
- Presentation with a full stomach if surgery can be postponed
- Late presentation to hospital.

PREOPERATIVE ASSESSMENT AND INVESTIGATIONS

These should be directed towards assessment of:

- The extent of compromise to the airway
- Haemorrhagic shock
- Respiratory insufficiency from aspiration
- Other injuries (cervical spine injuries of relevance to airway management)
- Coexisting medical conditions.

PREMEDICATION

An antisialogogue may be given if an awake intubation is planned. A benzodiazepine can be given for anxiolysis, and an analgesic if there is pain. Respiratory depressants should be used with great caution in the presence of a compromised airway. An H_2 antagonist is indicated if IMF is to be used.

PERIOPERATIVE MANAGEMENT

Airway management (nasal intubation, oral intubation, or tracheostomy) should be planned taking into account:

- Any compromise to the airway and the possible effect of anaesthesia
- The presence of a full stomach
- The required surgical access.

If the airway is compromised the options are:

- Awake intubation
- Tracheostomy under local anaesthesia
- Inhalational induction.

Trismus due to pain from a fractured mandible is usually alleviated by general anaesthesia. Preoxygenation may be difficult due to inability to obtain a gas-tight seal with the face-mask. A similar difficulty may occur during an inhalational induction.

Nasal intubation or the insertion of a nasogastric tube can be dangerous if there is a basal skull fracture or CSF rhinorrhoea.

Maintenance of anaesthesia:

- Definitive muscular relaxation is not usually a surgical requirement
- Prophylactic antiemetics are indicated if IMF is applied
- Regional blockade is useful for postoperative analgesia. Either wound infiltration or nerve blocks using bupivacaine are suitable techniques.

Urinary catheterization is indicated in shocked patients, or if the procedure is expected to last many hours.

IMMEDIATE POSTOPERATIVE PERIOD

If there is significant swelling of tissues and resultant compromise of the airway, extubation may be delayed until the swelling has subsided. Under these circumstances, the patient will need to be transferred to an ITU or high-dependency environment.

If IMF has been applied, extubation should be delayed until laryngeal reflexes have returned. A nasopharyngeal airway may be inserted. A one-to-one staff/patient ratio must be maintained while there is a risk of aspiration. Attending staff must know the location of the fixation, and wire-cutters must be available for immediate use. If the patient is in danger, the wires should be cut without hesitation. Antiemetics and H_2 antagonists may be given.

Narcotics are indicated for analgesia. Intravenous fluids will be needed until feeding has been re-established by the oral route (either enteral tube feeding or a normal diet self-administered).

COMPLICATIONS

The NCEPOD 1991/92 report found that over half of the complications leading to death after maxillofacial surgery were associated with respiratory or cardiovascular problems.

BIBLIOGRAPHY

Bogdanoff D L, Stone D J. Emergency management of the airway outside the operating room. Canadian Journal of Anaesthesia 1992; 39: 1069–1089

Ochs M W, Tucker M. Current concepts in management of facial trauma. Journal of Oral and Maxillofacial Surgery 1993; 51(suppl 1): 42–55

Campling E A, Devlin H B, Moile R W, Lunn J N. The Report of The National Confidential Enquiry into Perioperative Deaths 1991/1992; The National Confidential Enquiry into Perioperative Deaths, London, 1993

CROSS REFERENCES

Difficult airway
Anaesthetic Factors 30: 558
Trauma
Anaesthetic Factors 33: 672

MAJOR RECONSTRUCTIVE SURGERY

S. Deegan

PROCEDURES

Major reconstructive surgery of the head and neck is performed:

- After ablative cancer surgery
- To correct congenital craniofacial and maxillofacial deformity
- To correct acquired facial deformity, e.g. following facial trauma.

These procedures may involve several surgical specialities working separately or as part of a multidisciplinary team. This type of surgery has been revolutionized in the past two decades with the bicoronal approach to the anterior cranial fossa, the orbits and nasoethmoid complex, the use of pedicled myocutaneous flaps and, more recently, the microvascular free transfer of tissue, including bone. These techniques have allowed single-stage reconstruction to be carried out. Additional technical developments which include titanium reconstruction plates have improved mandibular reconstruction, and mini-bone-plating systems which allow internal fixation have reduced the need for complex external fixation frames and intermaxillary fixation.

These operations have many common features:

- They are complex procedures of long duration
- Blood loss may be considerable
- There is sharing of and limited access to the airway

- Potential airway difficulties may exist
- There is the potential for difficult intubation
- There may be a request for induced hypotension, particularly during tumour resection.

PATIENT CHARACTERISTICS

- Variable age range
- Infants and children with congenital craniofacial deformity, who may have upper airway obstruction, raised intracranial pressure and other spine anomalies
- Young healthy adults having orthognathic surgery, primarily for cosmetic reasons
- Older patients with cancer who may be malnourished chronic smokers with a high incidence of related cardiovascular and respiratory disease; these patients may also have had preoperative chemotherapy and radiotherapy.

PREOPERATIVE ASSESSMENT

This is influenced by the underlying pathology, the surgery to be performed and the presence of associated medical conditions. Of particular importance is the assessment of potential airway and intubation difficulties. The following should be evaluated:

- Facial asymmetry/deformity
- Restriction of mouth opening
- Limitation of neck movement
- Evidence of upper airway obstruction due to altered anatomy or the presence of tumour
- Previous surgery or radiotherapy which may cause difficulties with the airway and intubation
- Tests predicting difficult intubation, e.g. assessment of visible oropharyngeal structures (Mallampati)
- Radiographs of the cervical spine and CT scan of the head and neck, which are often part of the surgical assessment, may also be of use.

A full assessment is essential because it allows a planned approach to the management of the airway and a strategy for difficult intubation if necessary. Consideration should also be given to the availability of blood and the need for deep vein thrombosis prophylaxis.

Routine investigations should include:

- Full blood count
- Urea and electrolytes
- Blood group and cross-match
- Chest X-ray
- ECG.

PREMEDICATION

- Anxiolysis or sedation is useful
- Oral premedication with a short-acting benzodiazepine, e.g. temazepam, is suitable
- Intramuscular opioids may also be used
- Antisialogogues are not routinely required but are useful for operations within the mouth or when awake intubation is planned
- Antiemetics should be considered to prevent postoperative vomiting with the added risk of aspiration if the jaws are wired
- Heavy sedation and intramuscular opioids should be avoided in patients with raised intracranial pressure or with upper airway obstruction.

THEATRE PREPARATION

- Skilled assistance and equipment for the management of the difficult airway, including a fibre-optic laryngoscope
- Suitable padding for pressure areas when positioning the patient
- Prevention of heat loss by raising theatre temperature, warming mattress, intravenous fluid warmer, humidification of inspired gases.

PERIOPERATIVE MANAGEMENT

Difficult airway or intubation

Management involves anticipation of problems and includes:

- Gaseous induction
- Awake intubation with or without the fibre-optic laryngoscope
- Bypassing upper airway obstruction using transtracheal cannulation and jet ventilation, or tracheostomy performed under local anaesthetic.

Tracheostomy will be required for resection of the tongue, pharynx and larynx, or if there is a need for prolonged postoperative ventilation.

Airway control

Endotracheal intubation is mandatory, via the oral or nasal route depending on the requirements of the surgery and the need for intermaxillary fixation (IMF). A securely fixed reinforced tube is advisable because of the proximity of the surgery.

Correct placement is important to avoid endobronchial displacement with movement of the head or dislodgement, e.g. with maxillary advancement. A throat pack will help to stabilize the tube and prevent pharyngeal soiling. Lightweight coaxial circuits with taping of connections helps reduce the risk of disconnection.

Monitoring

- ECG.
- Intra-arterial BP
- Sa_{O_2}
- ET_{CO_2}
- Core and peripheral temperature
- Fluid balance
- Blood loss
- Urine output
- Central venous pressure (CVP)
- Nerve stimulator
- Disconnection alarm.

The site of the arterial line has to be considered in relation to the surgery, e.g. the use of a radial free flap. The dorsalis pedis artery is a useful alternative.

Monitoring of CVP is not always required. The use of neck veins may be restricted by the surgery and also carries the risk of pneumothorax when access to the patient is limited.

ANAESTHETIC TECHNIQUE

General anaesthesia

- Balanced technique using opioids, neuromuscular blockers and a volatile agent is common
- Consider the avoidance of nitrous oxide during prolonged procedures
- Monitoring of the end-tidal concentration of volatile agent can be helpful when conventional assessment of depth of anaesthesia is difficult due to limited access to the patient
- Total intravenous anaesthesia may be used.

Local anaesthesia

- Has a limited role in reconstructive surgery of the head and neck
- Nerve blocks and infiltration of the donor graft site can help in postoperative pain relief.

Control of bleeding

- Smooth induction with avoidance of coughing
- Head-up tilt
- Careful surgical technique
- Use of local vasoconstrictors by the surgeon
- Induced hypotension.

Procedures with intracranial involvement may require controlled hyperventilation, osmotic diuretics and drainage of CSF to shrink the brain tissue and facilitate the surgery.

Free-flap surgery

Graft survival may be optimized with maintenance of blood flow to the flap. Good anaesthetic management includes the maintenance of:

- Normal cardiac output and blood pressure
- Satisfactory tissue oxygenation
- Fluid balance, thus avoiding hypovolaemia
- Normal body temperature
- Normocapnia
- Adequate analgesia.

POSTOPERATIVE MANAGEMENT

Following major head and neck surgery admission to a high-dependency unit or ITU is required. Continued monitoring allows the provision of adequate analgesia using an opioid infusion or PCA. NSAIDs are also of use after maxillofacial surgery.

Extubation is delayed until the patient is awake, protective reflexes have returned and postoperative bleeding or oozing has settled. Prolonged periods of ventilation are rare unless there is coexisting respiratory disease. Dexamethasone has been used successfully to reduce postoperative swelling.

If IMF is used, wire cutters should be readily available. Where there has been major surgery to the mouth or upper airway, anticipation of severe postoperative swelling or bleeding dictates the need for tracheostomy.

Early postoperative complications include airway difficulties, bleeding, compromised blood supply to flaps, and haematoma formation under the flap. All of these may result in an early return to theatre.

In the long term, many of these patients, particularly those with severe facial deformity and those with malignancy, often require repeat procedures.

BIBLIOGRAPHY

Barham C J. Anaesthesia for maxillofacial surgery. In: Patel H (ed) Anaesthesia for burns, maxillofacial and plastic surgery. Edward Arnold, London, 1993, p 53–77

Goat V A. Anaesthesia for craniofacial surgery. In: Atkinson R S, Adams A P (eds) Recent advances in anaesthesia and analgesia. Churchill Livingstone, Edinburgh, 1989, p 139–153

Inglis M, Robbie D S, Edwards J M, Breach N M. The anaesthetic management of patients undergoing free flap reconstructive surgery following resection of head and neck neoplasms – a review of 64 patients. Annals of the Royal College of Surgeons of England 1988; 70: 235–238

Sweeney D B, Sainsbury D A. Anaesthesia for cranio-maxillary-facial surgery. Current anaesthesia and critical care 1992; 3: 11–16

CROSS REFERENCES

Induced hypotension
Anaesthetic Factors 32: 597
Prolonged anaesthesia
Anaesthetic Factors 32: 604
Trauma
Anaesthetic Factors 33: 672

OPERATIONS ON THE SALIVARY GLANDS

B. J. Pollard

Operations on the salivary glands may be simple procedures, e.g. for a stone blocking a duct, or more complex and radical procedures, e.g. glandular excision for malignancy. The salivary glands include the parotid, sub-mandibular and submaxillary glands.

The operative approach may be either through a skin incision or through the mouth.

The patients may be of any age, but are more usually from about 40 years onwards.

PREOPERATIVE ASSESSMENT

- Routine history and examination
- Investigations as indicated from the history and examination
- If massive swelling or limited mouth opening is present, there may be difficulties with the airway; assessment of the airway is therefore important in all patients
- Any coexisting medical conditions should be fully evaluated.

PREMEDICATION

- An antisialogogue is useful if an awake intubation is planned or if the surgeon is operating within the mouth
- A benzodiazepine can be given for anxiolysis, and an analgesic if there is pain.

PERIOPERATIVE MANAGEMENT

Induction of anaesthesia

Induction is usually undertaken using an

intravenous agent, as dictated by the patient's medical history and the anaesthetist's choice.

Tracheal intubation will need to be performed in most patients, facilitated by either suxamethonium or a nondepolarizing muscle relaxant, e.g. atracurium or vecuronium. A laryngeal mask may be suitable for shorter procedures in which the surgeon does not require access to the inside of the mouth. It will be difficult to gain access to the tracheal tube or laryngeal mask once surgery is in progress. The tube must therefore be carefully fixed and all connections must be absolutely secure.

A preformed oral or nasal tube (e.g. RAE type) is most suitable as it is easily positioned out of the surgeon's way. Check that it has not entered either main bronchus before surgery begins. If any surgery is to be performed inside the mouth, a pharyngeal pack should be inserted after intubation and before surgery is commenced. Wet gauze strip is the commonest type of pack, but various preformed sponge or gauze packs are favoured by some anaesthetists. The pack should be placed under direct vision using a laryngoscope and Magill's forceps. It is imperative to either leave a 'tail' of the pack protruding from the mouth, or to place an adhesive label on the patient as a reminder, so that the pack cannot be accidentally left in the pharynx at the end of the operation.

At the end of the operation the pharynx should be aspirated under direct vision to ensure that the pack has been removed intact and that no foreign bodies or blood clots remain in the back of the pharynx.

Maintenance of anaesthesia

The patient may be allowed either to breathe spontaneously through a coaxial circuit, or to have ventilation assisted, depending on the preferences or circumstances of the patient, the surgeon and the anaesthetist.

Maintenance of anaesthesia with oxygen, nitrous oxide and a volatile agent is a suitable technique, with additional opioid analgesics as required. The eyes will need to be protected by using tape to hold the lids shut if necessary, and the eyes then covered with pads.

Monitoring

- ECG
- SaO_2
- Noninvasive BP
- $ETCO_2$
- NMT if a relaxant is in use.

POSTOPERATIVE MANAGEMENT

- Analgesia will be required using standard techniques, e.g. intramuscular opioids or patient-controlled analgesia
- A NSAID, e.g. ketorolac or diclofenac, may be adequate alone; they also have an opioid sparing action, especially when given prior to surgery
- Intravenous fluids are not often required routinely.

THYROIDECTOMY

S. P. Roberts

PROCEDURE

Thyroidectomy is performed for a number of indications (Table 1). Most thyroid pathology presents as solitary nodules or goitre, with 10% of solitary nodules being malignant.

Table 1.
Surgical indications for thyroidectomy

Thyrotoxicosis • Graves' disease • Multinodular goitre • Toxic solitary nodule
Malignancy • Papillary carcinoma • Follicular carcinoma • Medullary carcinoma • Anaplastic carcinoma
Bilateral nontoxic goitre
Autoimmune thyroiditis

Incision is made via a transverse cut 3–4 cm above the sternum and extended laterally. The recurrent laryngeal nerves are located and preserved, as are the four parathyroid glands. Following resection, haemostasis is achieved and a suction drain left in the neck. Retrosternal goitres can usually (82%) be excised via a standard incision, though a sternal split may be required occasionally.

PATIENT CHARACTERISTICS

The patient types depend on the pathology. Graves' disease is common in females aged 20–40 years. Toxic nodular goitre occurs in an older age group. Thyroid malignancies vary in their distribution, papillary carcinoma occurring in the 30–40 year age group, and follicular and medullary carcinoma occurring in an older group.

Hyperthyroidism is associated with:
- Graves' disease (diffuse toxic goitre)
- Thyroiditis
- Thyroid toxic nodule
- Multinodular toxic goitre.

PREOPERATIVE PATIENT ASSESSMENT

Apart from the general examination and investigations appropriate to the age of the patient, there are important considerations relating to the specific pathology of the patient.

Clinical assessment:
- Cardiovascular features of hyperthyroidism, heart failure, tachyarrythmias, atrial fibrillation, mitral valve prolapse and papillary muscle dysfunction
- Eye features of hyperthyroidism, especially lid retraction and conjunctivitis
- State of hydration
- Assess the airway clinically for tracheal deviation and signs of stridor
- Check cord movement with indirect laryngoscopy (there is a 1% incidence of preoperative recurrent laryngeal nerve palsy)
- Look for clinical evidence of anaemia and thrombocytopenia
- Look for clinical signs of hypercalcaemia
- Look for evidence of other conditions associated with thyroid disease, especially diabetes mellitus and myasthenia gravis.

PREOPERATIVE INVESTIGATIONS

Evaluation of thyroid function

Thyroid function is usually evaluated by the measurement of the free levels of thyroxine (T4) or the measurement of total T4 and the free T4 index (which corrects for variation in the number of serum protein binding sites available).

A thyroid releasing factor (TRF) stimulation test can be performed. TRF is administered and the levels of thyroid stimulating hormone (TSH) are measured. The absence of a rise in TSH indicates hyperthyroidism.

Normal values	
Total T4	64–160 nmol l^{-1}
Free T4 index	17–47
Free T4	10–40 pmol l^{-1}

Other investigations:
- Haemoglobin, platelet count
- Urea and electrolytes, baseline calcium and phosphate levels
- ECG
- Radiographs of chest and thoracic inlet (to assess airway)
- A CT scan of the neck can be useful to look for retrosternal goitre
- Blood group and cross-match.

PREOPERATIVE PREPARATION

Hyperthyroid patients are at risk of 'thyroid storm' and must be rendered euthyroid. Beta blockade should be continued even on the day of operation.

- Carbimazole for 3–6 weeks
- Potassium iodide for 10 days (this suppresses thyroid-gland function)
- Propranolol 160 mg day^{-1} to control the cardiovascular effects
- Anxiolytic premedication.

ANAESTHETIC TECHNIQUE

- Patient fully monitored on induction
- Preoxygenation
- Intravenous infusion sited
- Consider gas induction/awake intubation if airway difficult (rarely necessary)
- Intravenous induction and controlled ventilation with isoflurane or enflurane (halothane is not recommended because of the risk of arrhythmias)
- Intubation with an armoured endotracheal tube
- Hypertension and tachycardia should be avoided
- Position the patient supine with the neck extended and a head-up tilt to reduce blood loss
- Eye protection is very important in patients with lid retraction
- Perform direct laryngoscopy prior to extubation to assess cord movement.

POSTOPERATIVE CARE

- Continue beta blockers
- Check serum calcium and thyroxine levels
- Monitor airway for evidence of obstruction.

UPPER AIRWAY COMPLICATIONS

- *Haematoma formation* – causes tracheal compression. Manage by removal of skin clips (sutures are not often used because clips can be removed faster) and evacuation of haematoma.
- *Recurrent laryngeal nerve palsy* – causes the vocal cords to rest in adduction and hence obstruct the airway. Management may necessitate reintubation or tracheostomy.
- *Laryngeal oedema* – can cause respiratory obstruction. Even if bilateral cord palsy is present, complete airway obstruction will only occur if there is a degree of laryngeal oedema present.
- *Tracheal collapse* – can follow resection for massive carcinomas or goitres. This can happen intra- or post-operatively.
- *Tracheal kinking* – can occur following excision of a massive goitre.

Reintubation of patients with respiratory obstruction following thyroid surgery is occasionally hazardous due to laryngeal oedema and tracheal compression or deviation. Ideally, a surgeon capable of performing emergency tracheotomy should be present. Anaesthetic technique is contentious. Though gas induction has advantages, some anaesthetists recommend the use of muscle relaxants to prevent spasm of the vocal cords.

OTHER COMPLICATIONS

- *Pneumothorax* occurs with extensive surgery and should be managed with a chest drain.
- *Thyroid storm* is very rare. It involves massive release of thyroid hormones, hyperpyrexia, cardiac arrhythmias and cyanosis (see Table 2 for management). It may initially be difficult to distinguish from malignant hyperthermia.
- *Hypocalcaemia* presents with the features of tetany. Management is with intravenous calcium therapy.

Table 2.
Management of thyroid storm

- Beta blockers to control heart rate and blood pressure. Digoxin and verapamil may be needed in some cases
- Cool patient with cooling blankets, cold intravenous fluids, gastric and colonic lavage.
- Inhibit further thyroid hormone release with iodine, propylthiouracil and adrenocortical steroids

BIBLIOGRAPHY

Gravenstein N. Manual of complications during anesthesia. J B Lippincott, London, 1993, p 596–601

Hilary Wade J S. Respiratory obstruction in thyroid surgery. Annals of the Royal College of Surgeons of England 1980; 62: 15–24

Mercer D M, Eltringham R J. Anaesthesia for thyroid surgery. Ear, Nose and Throat Journal 1985; 64: 342–375

Wheeler M H. Malignant goitre/thyroidectomy. Surgery 1984; 9: 200–209

CROSS REFERENCES

Hyperthyroidism
Patient Conditions 2: 48
Hypothyroidism
Patient Conditions 2: 52
Endocrine surgery – general considerations
Surgical Procedures 25: 487

16

PLASTIC SURGERY

R. Greenbaum

16

OVERVIEW

R. Greenbaum

Plastic surgery began as a specialty with the aim of improving reconstructive surgery of the skin and soft tissues. Plastic surgeons have since developed many techniques which have widespread applications in all fields of surgery. Although plastic surgery is mainly concerned with the head and neck, overlapping with ENT and maxillofacial surgery, it has pioneered methods of repairing tendons and nerves and restoring hand function after injury or congenital abnormality. Plastic surgeons were also initiators of 'free-flap' microvascular surgical techniques and are involved in the latest major reconstructive craniofacial operations.

The scope of plastic surgery and the consequent problems for the anaesthetist are described in this chapter in which some of the more common or more hazardous conditions are covered.

It can be seen that there is a full spectrum of patient age and health, and type, severity and duration of surgery. Moreover, plastic surgeons often decide on the exact surgery required on the day of operation. The posture(s) and operative requirements are therefore unknown preoperatively.

THE AIRWAY

Many conditions are associated with difficult airway and intubation problems. A careful operative assessment must include:

- History of sleep apnoea, snoring or partial airway obstruction
- Mouth opening, dentition, inspection of the fauces, cervical spine movement and atlanto-occipital movement
- Previous anaesthetic problems
- Chest infections
- Other defects.

Many patients will have predictable airway problems and certain rules should be followed:

- Antisialogogue premedication and 2 h fasting from clear fluids
- Mild sedation
- Avoid a point of 'no return' during induction of anaesthesia
- Have available several intubation aids:
  - Various laryngoscopes
  - Wands, bougies
  - Retrograde method
  - Transtracheal jet
  - Transcricothyrotomy cannulation
  - Fibre optic available to 4–5 mm tracheal tubes
  - Blind nasal.

During surgery problems may arise with a previously satisfactory tracheal tube, so beware of:

- Accidental extubation
- Endobronchial intubation (with neck flexion or mandibular shortening)
- Surgical transfixion of the tracheal tube
- Surgical transection of the tracheal tube
- Obstruction of the tracheal tube.

THE SURGICAL FIELD

In both major surgery for tumour resection or congenital abnormalities and minor cosmetic operations on the face, plastic surgeons appreciate a relatively bloodless field.

Induced hypotension is generally used. It can be slow onset and moderate (systolic pressure maintained above the normal diastolic pressure). The retum of blood pressure to normal levels can be gradual, as this probably reduces the risk of reactionary haemorrhage and haematoma formation. If the resection is followed by free-flap reconstruction, the circulation must be restored to prioritize the survival of the flap.

When prolonged or profound hypotension is required or rapidly acting vasodilators such as sodium nitroprusside are used, direct continuous arterial blood pressure monitoring is mandatory.

In all cases the use of posture, local vasoconstrictors, adequate analgesia and avoidance of tachycardia are essential. The $P_{a}CO_2$ should be kept in the normal range because the combination of hypocapnoea and hypotension can produce severe cerebral ischaemia. Hypercapnoea produces skin vasodilation, which is clearly undesirable.

Where surgery is prolonged, certain other considerations should be taken into account:

- Nitrous oxide administration for more than 6 h is undesirable
- Pressure areas should be protected by at least 4 in. of foam, and pressure points carefully padded
- The patient should lie on a heated mattress; insulation blankets (or polythene sheets) should also be used
- Transfusion and other fluids should be warmed
- Inspired gas must be humidified
- The theatre temperature should be 22–24°C
- There must be adequate teams of anaesthetists and anaesthetic nurses.

THE POSTOPERATIVE PHASE

The results of plastic surgery may be influenced by the quality of the patient's recovery from anaesthesia and by the early postoperative care. Coughing and straining increase the risk of haemorrhage and haematoma. Cold, shivering, hypoxic patients hazard the viability of free flaps and skin pedicle grafts. In general:

- Extubate awake or leave intubated and ventilated in an ITU until warm and stable
- Use antiemetics to prevent vomiting
- Dexamethasone and, possibly, diclofenac reduce postoperative swelling.

BURNS

P. Broderick

PROCEDURE

Burns surgery is usually required for deep dermal and third-degree burns. The aim is to harvest skin, excise the burn and cover the burn site with fresh skin. As a quick assessment of burn size, the patients palm area represents 1% total body surface area (TBSA) (Table 1).

Table 1. Assessment of burns

1st degree	Superficial, blisters, painful, heals in 3–4 days
2nd degree	Partial thickness, heals 2–3 weeks, deep dermal burns may scar
3rd degree	Full thickness, anaesthetic, dermis destroyed, dry, leathery, white or brown in colour

Burns surgery

- Is usually performed in the supine position, occasionally prone
- May involve repeated procedures
- May require tourniquet(s) to reduce blood loss
- Major burn is defined as:
  - adult >20% TBSA, second or third degree
  - child >10%.

PATIENT CHARACTERISTICS

Patients for burns surgery:

- Can be any age, but extremes of ages are common

- May have associated injuries
- May have associated medical conditions such as epilepsy
- May have an alcohol induced injury.

See Table 2.

Table 2.
Associated injuries

Associated injuries
Smoke inhalational injury • Cyanide and carbon monoxide poisoning • Airway involvement, swelling
Electrical burn • Myocardial damage
Chemical burn
Renal/hepatic damage • Difficult access to veins, due to burn injury

PREOPERATIVE ASSESSMENT AND INVESTIGATIONS

- Has there been any history of exposure to smoke, or inhalational injury?
- Has resuscitation been completed?
- Check availability of blood for transfusion.
- Full blood count, urea and electrolytes, chest X-ray, arterial blood gases, clotting screen, urine output.

Theatre preparation:

- Ideally, two surgical teams, as well as two anaesthetists
- Prewarm operating theatre
- Warming mattress; intravenous-fluid warmer
- Humidifier for breathing system.

See Table 3.

Table 3.
Resuscitation of burns patients

Mount Vernon regime	0.5 × weight (kg) × %TBSA (ml) of 4.5% human albumin in each of six periods over 36 h
Lactated ringers (USA)	4 ml kg^{-1} per %TBSA in 24 h
Hypertonic saline	0.3 ml kg per %TBSA in first hour, then adjust to urine output

PREMEDICATION

- Anxiolysis may be required, especially in children (e.g. trimeprazine); in adults an opioid analgesic may be desirable
- Anticholinergic premedication can be useful, particularly in children, but also in anticipated cases of difficult intubation.

PERIOPERATIVE MANAGEMENT

Monitoring:

- ECG
- Spo_2
- $ETco_2$
- Noninvasive BP
- Central venous pressure
- Fluid balance and blood loss
- Urine output
- Core temperature.

Access to limbs during surgery may be restricted, and an intra-arterial pressure line may be necessary. Central venous pressure measurement may also be useful for in the management of fluid therapy.

ANAESTHETIC TECHNIQUE

General anaesthesia is almost always the chosen technique. For change of burns dressing it is quite common practice to use ketamine (i.v. or i.m.), especially for children. Pretreatment with a benzodiazepine or equivalent is helpful.

Intravenous induction of anaesthesia (propofol or thiopentone are suitable), with a muscle relaxant (atracurium or vecuronium are suitable) and an opioid with or without an inhalational agent. Harvesting split skin grafts is intensely painful and care must be taken to use a sufficient dosage of opioid. There may be a large blood loss and large volumes of fluid administered during the procedure.

- Avoid suxamethonium, except within the first 24 h postburn
- Anticipate blood loss. Intraoperative Hb measurement may be useful (e.g. Hemocue). Beware of dilutional effect on clotting factors.

POSTOPERATIVE MANAGEMENT

- Common complications: bleeding, infection
- Return to burns unit: nurse supine on low air loss bed

- Large TBSA burn patients or inhalationally injured patients are best ventilated postoperatively
- Postoperative pain relief may be provided by intravenous infusions of opioids or by means of a patient-controlled analgesia (PCA) device, which can be modified for use by means other than fingers if necessary
- Feeding: basal metabolic rate is increased by up to 100%. Early nutritional supplement is essential; 3000–5000 calories day^{-1} in an adult.

OUTCOME

- Age related – decreasing survival with increasing age over 30 years
- Is worse in the presence of respiratory injury
- Major reconstructive surgery may be required in the future
- Prognosis for burns over 70% TBSA is very poor, with the cut-off level for survival being about 40%. Women have a worse prognostic index compared to men (6.3% mortality compared with 5.1%).

The trend in numbers of burns is declining, but increasing in severity and decreasing mortality. This may be due to earlier nutritional replacement, topical silver sulphadiazine cream and earlier surgery.

BIBLIOGRAPHY

Barisone D, Peci S, Governa M, Sanna A, Furlan S. Mortality rate and prognostic indices in 2615 burned patients. Burns 1990; 16: 373–376

Muir I F K, Barclay T L. Burns and their treatment, 2nd edn. Lloyd Luke, London, 1974

Rylah L T A (ed). Critical care of the burned patient. Cambridge University Press, Cambridge, 1992

CROSS REFERENCES

Prolonged anaesthesia
Anaesthetic Factors 32: 604
Blood transfusion
Anaesthetic Factors 33: 616
Fluid and electrolyte balance
Anaesthetic Factros 33: 626
Postoperative pain management
Anaesthetic Factors 33: 655

COSMETIC SURGERY

E. M. Grundy

PROCEDURE

Primarily surface surgery is involved, but this is not synonymous with minor surgery. Procedures can take several hours. Multiple procedures are increasingly undertaken. Some procedures are undertaken as day-cases; rarely is more than one night in hospital required.

PATIENT CHARACTERISTICS

- Patients are sensitive about an aspect of their appearance
- Mostly young or middle-aged women
- Becoming increasingly popular as the public at large become aware as to what is available.

PREOPERATIVE ASSESSMENT AND CONSIDERATIONS

- Standards of preoperative assessment should not differ because this population of patients are young and fit
- History, examination and investigations as indicated
- DVT prophylaxis should be considered for prolonged cases.

PREMEDICATION

Premedication is usually not required.

THEATRE PREPARATION

- A warming blanket is useful

- For surgery around the head and neck, the surgeon will expect full access, and thus the anaesthetist will be at the patient's feet.

PERIOPERATIVE MANAGEMENT

Increasingly, procedures are being performed under local anaesthesia with sedation. Standards of monitoring should be maintained. Transition from heavy sedation to light general anaesthesia occurs only too easily and should be anticipated.

Intraoperatively the surgeon can be expected to inject local anaesthetic solution into the surgical field. This reduces the amount of surgical stimulation and allows a lighter level of anesthesia to be employed. It will also provide good quality postoperative analgesia.

Intraoperative bleeding can be reduced by:

- Addition of a vasoconstrictor to the local anaesthetic (usually 5 μg ml^{-1} of adrenaline)
- Head-up tilt in the case of upper body surgery
- Induced hypotension – most anaesthetists are prepared to bring the BP down to the low end of the physiological range (around 80 mmHg systolic), but in some centres much more profound hypotension is employed on a regular basis.

Head and neck surgery

Head and neck surgery – procedures:
- Blepharoplasty
- Browlift
- Facelift
- Necklift
- Rhinoplasty
- Surgery for baldness

A secure airway is mandatory and induced hypotension will be expected as part of the control of intraoperative bleeding. At the end of surgery the head and neck will often be moved around significantly during the application of the dressings: the patient should neither buck nor become hypertensive during this period. Shortly afterwards, the anaesthetist will have to extubate the patient and must ensure that the patient is left with a safe airway. Pharyngeal suction is necessary after rhinoplasty or where an intraoral incision has been made. This sequence requires expertise.

Abdominoplasty

This can be a treacherous operation in the grossly obese who undergo a major reduction. Postoperative retention of secretions and postoperative respiratory failure can occur. Preoperative assessment of respiratory function is important and should not be overlooked.

Body contouring surgery

Invariably to the trunk, buttocks or lower limbs and utilizing liposuction (haemo-liposuction would be a more appropriate, if more provocative, description). This may be done 'dry' (without injection) or 'wet' (with injection). Care must be exercised to ensure that 'the injection' is made up according to an acceptable formula and that the patient is not injected with a toxic dose of drugs. The volume aspirated will contain fat (the desired effect) some of the injectate (thus reducing the dose available for systemic absorption) and blood. The volume of blood can be considerable and perioperative fluid infusion and a check on Hb the next morning are both recommended. It is considered unwise to suck out more than 2 l, but if this is exceeded blood transfusion may well be required.

POSTOPERATIVE MANAGEMENT

Postoperative haematomas are usually obvious because of the superficial site of the surgery and may well require draining (Table 1).

Table 1.
Causes of postoperative haematomas

Stormy emergence from anaesthesia
Rebound hypertension after intraoperative hypotension
Bucking on tracheal tube
Obstructed airway
Shivering from hypothermia or other cause
Straining from postoperative vomiting

Postoperative pain is usually not great as the surgery is superficial and the surgeon will have injected local anaesthetic. Elevation of the surgical site will also help to reduce swelling, and hence pain.

OUTCOME

Almost all patients will be mobile and out of hospital within 24 h of surgery. Postoperative pain and swelling settles within a few days; however, bruising can take 7–14 days to settle.

CROSS REFERENCES

Obesity
Patient Conditions 5: 148
Operations on the nose
Surgical Procedures 14: 308
Free-flap surgery
Surgical Procedures 16: 335
Day-case surgery
Anaesthetic Factors 29: 542
Induced hypotension during anaesthesia
Anaesthetic Factors 32: 597
Local anaesthetic toxicity
Anaesthetic Factors 33: 642
Thrombotic embolism
Anaesthetic Factors 33: 664

FREE-FLAP SURGERY

D. K. Patel

PROCEDURE

Free-flap surgery involves:

- Repair of a large skin or compound (skin, muscle and bone) defect, termed the 'recipient site'
- The use of a distant tissue flap complete with it own arterial and venous (and sometimes nerve) supply, termed the 'donor site'
- The use of an operating microscope
- prolonged anaesthesia (6–12 h, or even longer)
- Provision of an adequate perfusion pressure and a hyperdynamic circulation
- Reimplantation of limbs or digits.

PATIENT CHARACTERISTICS

Free-flap surgery involves patients who are:

- Young children
- Adults and the elderly
- ASA status grade I–IV
- Treated for cancer ablation, trauma or cosmetic defects; the majority of these patients present for cancer resection in the head and the neck (including the oral) region.

PREOPERATIVE ASSESSMENT AND CONSIDERATIONS

- Systemic review of likely diseases of old age
- Assessment of cardiac and respiratory reserves and the ability to safely respond to provide a hyperdynamic circulation

- Assessment of the airway and the likelihood of difficult intubation
- Need for elective tracheostomy
- DVT prophylaxis
- Blood transfusion availability
- Antibiotic prophylaxis and drug allergy
- Discussion with the surgeon regarding nonaccessibility of arm or leg for donor site.

PREMEDICATION

Patients who are anticipated to be difficult to intubate should be given a full and repeated explanation of the local anaesthetic technique for intubation. Anxiolysis with a benzodiazepine is useful.

THEATRE PREPARATION

- Skilled manpower, patient supports and padding to pressure areas
- Anaesthetic room and theatre temperature at 22–24°C and relative humidity of 50%
- Maintenance of body temperature (warming blanket, fluid warming, humidifier and Gamgee or polythene sheets)
- Equipment for difficult intubation, including a tracheostomy set.

PERIOPERATIVE MANAGEMENT

Monitoring:
- ECG
- BP, invasive or noninvasive as appropriate
- Central venous pressure (CVP)
- SpO_2
- $ETCO_2$
- Core and peripheral temperature
- Urine output and blood loss.

ANAESTHETIC TECHNIQUE

General anaesthesia is preferred because of prolonged surgery and the need to keep the patients absolutely still for microsurgery. Adjuvant local anaesthetic techniques are used to promote blood flow through the flap.

Hypotensive anaesthesia is often employed during the preparation of the recipient and donor site, for ease of surgery and minimization of blood loss.

Following arterial and venous anastomosis, blood flow through the flap is promoted by maintenance of:

- Arterial pressure at near-normal values by:
  - Maintenance of anaesthesia with isoflurane with its beneficial vasodilatory effects
  - Adequate hydration with crystalloid infusion at 7 ml kg^{-1} h^{-1}
  - Replacement of blood loss.
- A high cardiac output and alteration in rheology by:
  - Maintaining the CVP at about 2–3 mmHg above the baseline and a haematocrit of 30–35% by an infusion of colloid solutions. Dextran 40 in 0.9% sodium chloride is commonly used, though the hydroxyethyl starch (HES) solutions have a longer plasma half-life. The efficacy of various colloid solutions in causing changes in blood viscosity and the organization of erythro-aggregates is, in decreasing order, Dextran 40 > Hes = albumin > Dextran 110 > gelatins. Dextrans and HES also have antithrombotic effects and lead to improvements in patency of flaps.
- Peripheral vasodilatation by:
  - Meticulous attention to maintaining body temperature (Note: the greatest drop in body temperature occurs in the first hour of anaesthesia)
  - Provision of adequate analgesia
  - Maintenance of normocapnia and oxygenation
  - Vasodilating drugs: isoflurane for maintenance or anaesthesia is a direct vasodilator with minimal effect on cardiac output. A variety of drugs including sodium nitroprusside, glyceryl trinitrate, phenoxybenzamine, phentolamine and calcium channel blockers have been used with success. Whichever drug is used, it is desirable for its vasodilatory effect to last into the postoperative period.

POSTOPERATIVE MANAGEMENT

Transfer to the high-dependency unit is advisable for continued monitoring of circulatory control and adequate analgesia. Colloid solution is infused at 7 ml kg^{-1} day^{-1} for 3 days. The flap is monitored with impedance or photoplethysmography or laser Doppler flowmetry. Common complications are flap arterial thrombus and haematoma requiring re-exploration.

BIBLIOGRAPHY

Green D. Anaesthesia for microvascular surgery. In: Patel H (ed) Anaesthesia for burns. Maxillofacial and plastic surgery. Edward Arnold, London, 1993, p 93–108

Macdonald D J F. Anaesthesia for microvascular surgery: a physiological approach. British Journal of Anaesthesia 1985; 57: 904–912

CROSS REFERENCES

Difficult intubation (Difficult airway)
Anaesthetic Factors 30: 558

Induced hypotension during anaesthesia
Anaesthetic Factors 32: 597

Blood transfusion
Anaesthetic Factors 33: 616

Complications of position
Anaesthetic Factors 33: 618

PERIPHERAL LIMB SURGERY

J. Anderson

PROCEDURES

- Involve the repair of bones, tendons, nerves and vessels; may be elective or urgent (trauma)
- Elective surgery includes surgery for correction of acquired abnormalities, e.g. Dupuytren's contracture, carpal tunnel syndrome, reconstructive surgery for rheumatoid disease, and excision of tumours or skin lesions
- A tourniquet is usually used to secure a bloodless field
- Prolonged surgery may be involved, e.g. reimplantation surgery.

PATIENT CHARACTERISTICS

- Can be any age
- May have other trauma associated, e.g. head injury or chest trauma
- May have alcohol-related injury
- Congenital anomalies may be multiple.

PREOPERATIVE ASSESSMENT AND INVESTIGATIONS

- Exclude concomitant abnormalities or injuries
- Look for other associated medical conditions, e.g. rheumatoid arthritis
- Haematological and biochemical investigation, as indicated
- ECG, chest X-ray and other investigations, as indicated
- Remember the sickle cell screen, especially if a tourniquet is to be applied.

PREMEDICATION

- Give a full explanation of the procedure and warn the patient about temporary postoperative limb numbness and weakness
- An anxiolytic drug, e.g. a benzodiazepine, is useful.

PERIOPERATIVE MANAGEMENT

Monitoring:
- ECG
- Spo_2
- Noninvasive BP
- $ETco_2$ (not necessary for regional blocks).

Technique

Regional or local block, with or without sedation is the technique of choice:

- Venous access should be established prior to block
- Suitable for a wide range of procedures
- Associated sympathetic block provides optimum perfusion for reimplantation surgery
- Check suitability for block before starting (Table 1)
- For details on technique the reader is referred to a suitable major text. Regular practice with regional blocks greatly increases the success rate.

Table 1.
Contraindications to regional block

Sepsis
Anticoagulation therapy
Coagulopathy
Physical or mental inability to cope

General anaesthesia, with or without a local or regional block is also suitable:

- Useful for children
- Useful for prolonged procedures
- Useful for uncooperative patients
- If a regional block is used in addition, the associated sympathetic block provides optimum perfusion for reimplantation surgery.

UPPER LIMB SURGERY

Brachial plexus block:
- The most common block for upper limb surgery
- Performed by the subclavian, perivascular or axillary approaches (Table 2).

Practical points when performing a brachial plexus block
- Use a blunt needle to decrease risk of nerve damage and increase success rate
- Use of a nerve stimulator will increase success rate
- Use of adrenaline with the local analgesic agent will increase the intensity and duration of block
- A catheter can be inserted for prolonged surgery and postoperative pain relief
- Speed for onset is increased by carbonation and warming the solution
- Avoid peripheral nerve blocks in unconscious patients

Peripheral nerve blocks:
- Ulnar, median and radial nerve blocks at the elbow and wrist may be used to supplement a brachial plexus block

Table 2.
Common approaches to brachial plexus block

Area blocked	Advantages	Disadvantages
Axillary		
Hand and foream	Minimal complications Ideal for out-patients	Radial and musculocutaneous nerves may be missed
Subclavian perivascular		
Whole arm	Rapid reliable block	Risk of pneumothorax
Interscalene block		
Shoulder and arm	Easy access	Risk of inadvertent dural puncture or vertebral artery puncture. C8–T1 area may be missed

- There is a small risk of nerve damage at the elbow
- Digital nerve blocks may be needed – avoid adrenaline-containing solutions.

Intravenous regional anaesthesia (IVRA)
- Easy to perform for small or closed procedures
- The principal disadvantage is the rapid loss of analgesia on cuff deflation, which prevents further surgery to secure haemostasis should this be necessary
- Tourniquet pain may be a problem.

LOWER LIMB SURGERY

Lumbar and caudal epidural blocks and also spinal blocks are ideal for unilateral or bilateral lower limb surgery.

Peripheral nerve blocks
Mainly used for pain relief in knee surgery and fractures of the lower leg:

- Femoral nerve block
- Three-in-one block (femoral, obturator, and lateral cutaneous nerve of the thigh)
- Sciatic nerve block.

Ankle blocks:
- Useful for surgery to the foot not requiring a tourniquet
- Nerves blocked are the sural, saphenous, posterior tibial, superficial peroneal and deep peroneal nerves.

THE USE OF A TOURNIQUET

- Maximum pressure in the leg 300 mmHg
- Maximum pressure in the arm 200 mmHg
- Maximum tourniquet time 1–2 h
- Avoid in sickle cell disease; if use is necessary, discuss with a haematologist.

BIBLIOGRAPHY

Winnie A P. Perivascular techniques of brachial plexus block. In: Winnie A P (ed) Plexus anaesthesia. Schultz I, 1983, Copenhagen

Wildsmith J A, Armitage E N. Principles and practice of regional anaesthesia, 1993, Churchill Livingstone

Thompson A M, Newman R J, Semple J C. Brachial plexus anaesthesia for upper limb surgery: a review of eight years experience. Journal of Hand Surgery 1988; 13:

CROSS REFERENCES

Sickle cell syndrome
Patient Conditions 7: 188
Day-case surgery
Anaesthetic Factors 29: 542
Prolonged anaesthesia
Anaesthetic Factors 32: 604
Local anaesthetic toxicity
Anaesthetic Factors 33: 642

PAEDIATRIC PLASTIC SURGERY

S. Berg

Children of all ages present for corrective surgery, from the neonate to the adolescent. Procedures range from minor day-case operations to major restorative surgery.

GENERAL FEATURES

- Most operations are elective. Children with features of a recent or current chest infection should be delayed.
- Many children require multiple surgical procedures. It is important to establish a rapport with the child and the parents. Anxiolytics are rarely required and, increasingly, many procedures are being conducted on a day-stay basis.
- Halothane hepatitis appears much more rarely in children than in adults. Several authors feel that repeat administration of halothane is justified, although any previous history of postoperative hepatitis associated with a pyrexia should preclude its use.
- Operations on the skin and superficial tissues are painful. Appropriate analgesia including local infiltration, nerve blocks and epidurals will facilitate a lighter plane of anaesthesia and prevent a straining, restless child in the postoperative phase, which could increase bleeding and jeopardize the surgery.
- Local infiltration by adrenaline is used routinely by many plastic surgeons; up to 10 μg kg^{-1} can be used safely. Volatile agents may potentiate dysrhythmias.
- Some children may present for surgery for conditions associated with syndromes which include features of anaesthetic significance (e.g. difficult intubation).

CLEFT LIP AND CLEFT PALATE

Patient characteristics:

- Common conditions (1 in 600 births). Polygenic inheritance. Some association with maternal corticosteroid therapy.
- 30% of clefts are limited to lip; 25% to palate; 45% involve both.
- Range of deformity.
- Average age of correction:
  - Cleft lip, neonate to 3 months;
  - Cleft palate, 6 months to 1 year.
- Cleft palate is often associated with other congenital anomalies which may be of anaesthetic significance (Table 1).

Table 1.
Syndromes of anaesthetic significance associated with cleft palate

Syndrome	Significant features
Klippel–Feil	15% associated with cleft palate. Short, webbed neck. Fused cervical vertebrae. Congenital cardiac disease
Pierre Robin	80% associated with cleft palate. Severe micrognathia. Congenital cardiac disease. Intubation easier with age
Treacher Collins	28% associated with cleft palate. Micrognathia. Maxillary hypoplasia. Ear malformations. Intubation more difficult with age

Preoperative assessment and investigations:

- Assess the airway
- Exclude associated cardiac disease
- Blood should be available for transfusion.

Premedication

- Atropine 20 μg kg^{-1} i.m.
- Avoid opioid or sedative premedication in patients under 6 months, or if airway is compromised.

Theatre preparation

Maintain body temperature by warming

theatre to 22–24°C, using a warming mattress and aluminium foil, warming fluids and humidifying gases.

Perioperative management

Monitoring:

- ECG
- $ETco_2$
- Noninvasive BP
- Sao_2
- Nerve stimulator
- Precordial stethoscope
- Core temperature
- Fluid balance and blood loss.

Induction of anaesthesia

Use inhalational induction if difficulty with the airway is anticipated. Halothane is quicker than enflurane or isoflurane, with fewer complications. Sevoflurane may prove to be a suitable alternative. Judicious use of CPAP may assist maintenance of the airway.

Intubation following administration of suxamethonium (1–2 mg kg^{-1}). Care should be taken that the laryngoscope blade does not get caught in the cleft. The tube should be centrally positioned and checked to prevent kinking or endobronchial intubation before inserting a pharyngeal pack.

Maintenance of anaesthesia

Spontaneous ventilation or, more commonly, IPPV. Local infiltration of up to 2–5 mg kg^{-1} of lignocaine with adrenaline (1:200 000) produces good analgesia, an improved operating field and reduced blood loss. Intravenous fentanyl (1–2 μg kg^{-1}) can be used to supplement anaesthesia, but should be given cautiously in neonates or in the presence of upper airway problems.

Postoperative management

The patient should be extubated only when fully awake, breathing adequately and in the tonsillar position. The insertion of a tongue stitch to allow the tongue to be pulled forward is a useful, although uncommonly used, technique.

Codeine phosphate (1 mg kg^{-1} i.m.) is usually sufficient analgesia. Reuniting mother and baby is a more important step, and feeding can commence 2 h postoperatively.

CRANIOFACIAL SURGERY

- This constitutes major reconstructive surgery
- Problems include major blood loss, hypothermia and difficult intubation
- Arterial and central venous pressure (via the femoral vein) are usually measured.

HAEMANGIOMA

- May be complicated by major blood loss and air embolism
- A cutaneous haemangioma around the face and neck may be associated with a subglottic haemangioma.

CYSTIC HYGROMA

- Multiloculated cystic swelling in the neck that may invade the oropharynx and tongue; can present as an upper airways obstruction in the neonate
- Intubation can be hazardous; spontaneous ventilation must be maintained until intubation has been achieved
- Postoperative problems include bleeding and respiratory obstruction.

BURNS

See page 331. Similar principles apply as in adult practice. Analgesia is often inadequate; epidurals and ketamine can be useful.

BIBLIOGRAPHY

Battersby C F, Bingham R, Facer E et al. Halothane hepatitis in children. British Medical Journal 1987; 295: 117

Johnston R R, Eger II E I, Wilson C. A comparative interaction of epinephrine with enflurane, isoflurane and halothane in man. Anaesthesia and Analgesia 1976; 55: 709–712

Michael S, Barker J, Henderson P, Griffiths R W, Reilly C S. Pharmacokinetics of lignocaine in children after infiltration for cleft palate surgery. British Journal of Anaesthesia 1992; 69: 577–579

Tobias J D. Indications of applications of epidural anaesthesia in a paediatric population outside the perioperative period. Clinical Pediatrics 1993; 82: 8–15

Whitburn R H, Sumner E. Halothane hepatitis in an 11-month-old child. Anaesthesia 1986; 41: 611–613

CROSS REFERENCES

Infants and children
Patient Conditions 11: 255
Difficult airway
Anaesthetic Factors 30: 558
Local anaesthetic toxicity
Anaesthetic Factors 33: 642

17

THORACIC SURGERY

J. Gothard

17

OVERVIEW

J. W. W. Gothard and L. Murdoch

Only 20% of patients with lung cancer have resectable tumours at presentation. The vast majority of lung resections in the UK are carried out for the treatment of lung cancer (Table 1). The operative mortality following pneumonectomy and lobectomy remains high at 6.5% and 2.5%, respectively. This is a result of the extensive nature of the surgery involved and intercurrent disease of the patients.

Bronchoscopy, mediastinoscopy and pleurectomy (Table 1) are carried out in relatively large numbers with low mortality. Bronchoscopy and mediastinoscopy often precede a more major procedure which will present a greater operative risk. Pleurectomy is, in the main, carried out in relatively fit young patients with spontaneous pneumothoraces, so the mortality in this type of operation is very low.

ANAESTHESIA FOR THORACIC SURGERY

Endobronchial intubation

Anaesthesia for thoracic surgery has evolved steadily since the early 1930s when Gale and Waters (USA) and subsequently Magill (UK) introduced single-lumen endobronchial tubes for selective endobronchial intubation. The double-lumen endobronchial tube of Carlens, which was originally introduced for differential spirometry in 1949, was redesigned by Robertshaw in 1962 and produced in right and left forms. More recently, plastic disposable double-lumen endobronchial tubes have been introduced by several manufacturers.

The 'blind' placement of endobronchial tubes has always been difficult. The introduction of relatively cheap and robust (yet slim) fibreoptic bronchoscopes now enables the thoracic anaesthetist to place endobronchial tubes under direct vision, or at least to check their position following blind placement.

One-lung anaesthesia

The majority of major thoracic surgery is carried out with the patient in the lateral position. When ventilation to the upper lung is discontinued to aid surgery, pulmonary blood flow continues to that lung. A 'true' shunt is therefore created and hypoxia may occur.

A variety of steps can be taken to improve oxygenation during one-lung anaesthesia. Assuming that the endobronchial tube is in the correct place and that secretions have been removed, it may be neccessary to take some of the following measures:

- Keep the same MV for one-lung as two-lung ventilation (CO_2 removal is rarely a problem)

Table 1.
UK thoracic surgery 1991: operative figures with 30-day hospital mortality (from UK Thoracic Surgical Register)

Procedure	No. of patients	Mortality (%)
Pneumonectomy*	1041	6.5
Lobectomy*	1846	2.5
Thoracotomy + pleurectomy	813	0.61
Bronchoscopy	7858	0.23
Mediastinoscopy	1231	0.24

*These figures relate to primary lung tumours.

- Ventilate the lower lung adequately with the lowest possible intra-alveolar pressures (high pressure will divert pulmonary blood flow to the upper lung)
- Reduce TV slightly if inflation pressure is more than 30–35 cmH_2O
- Increase F_IO_2 up to 100% (some authors advocate this from the outset)
- Insufflate oxygen to the upper lung under pressure (CPAP 5–10 cmH_2O) – rarely necessary
- Combine CPAP to upper lung with PEEP to lower lung – rarely necessary. (Note: PEEP to lower lung alone usually diverts pulmonary blood flow and does not improve oxygenation.)

Hypoxic pulmonary vasoconstriction (HPV) on current evidence, seems to play little part in reducing hypoxaemia during the time it takes to complete a pneumonectomy or lobectomy. Thus, although many inhalational agents inhibit HPV, they do not appear to significantly impair arterial oxygenation during one-lung anaesthesia.

High frequency jet ventilation (HFJV) has been advocated for use during thoracic surgery, but is not in widespread use. HFJV may be of benefit in patients with lung cysts and bronchopleural fistulae, but even in these conditions its use remains controversial.

Postoperative pain relief
Operations carried out through a lateral thoracotomy incision can be extremely painful in the postoperative period. There have been a number of advances in the provision of pain relief following thoracic surgery in recent years. These include the application of extrapleural and intrapleural analgesic techniques and the use of epidural opioid drugs.

BIBLIOGRAPHY

Gothard J W W. Anaesthesia for Thoracic Surgery. 1993, Blackwells, Oxford

CROSS REFERENCES

Preoperative assessment of cardiovascular risk in noncardiac surgery
Anaesthetic Factors 34: 692
Preoperative assessment of pulmonary risk
Anaesthetic Factors 34: 697

BRONCHOPLEURAL FISTULA

J. W. W. Gothard and L. Murdoch

A bronchopleural fistula (BPF) is a direct communication between the tracheobronchial tree and the pleural cavity. Causes of BPF include:

- Trauma
- Neoplasm
- Inflammatory lesion
- Dehiscence of bronchial stump.

In developed countries, dehiscence of the bronchial stump following pneumonectomy is the commonest reason for patients to present for surgical repair of BPF. The incidence of BPF following pneumonectomy is, however, extremely low in specialized surgical centres.

PROCEDURE

Minor forms of postpneumonectomy BPF can be cauterized at bronchoscopy with sodium hydroxide or, alternatively, may be sealed with a fibrin glue.

Large fistulas require surgical repair (resuture of the bronchial stump) via a lateral thoracotomy through the previous incision.

PATIENT CHARACTERISTICS

- Often postpneumonectomy (3–15 days)
- ASA status IV or V.

PREOPERATIVE ASSESSMENT AND INVESTIGATIONS

Symptoms
Symptoms relate to fluid from the infected space flowing over to the remaining lung:

- Malaise
- Low-grade fever
- Cough
- Haemoptysis
- Wheeze/dyspnoea

or, in acute onset with a large BPF:

- Severe dyspnoea
- Coughing up copious amounts of thinnish brown fluid.

Investigations

Chest X-ray shows:

- Loss of pneumonectomy space fluid
- Consolidation/collapse of remaining lung.

Arterial blood gas analysis demonstrates:

- Hypoxia
- Hypercarbia
- Metabolic acidosis.

PREMEDICATION

None required if acute onset, otherwise the anaesthetist's routine premedication is suitable.

THEATRE PREPARATION

- General resuscitation including oxygen by face-mask
- Sit patient up to prevent further 'spillover'
- Insert chest drain on pneumonectomized side
- Transport patient to theatre in sitting position with drain open.

PERIOPERATIVE MANAGEMENT

Monitoring:

- ECG
- BP – preferably invasive
- Sao_2
- $ETco_2$
- Central venous pressure or PCWP
- Core temperature
- Urine output.

Anaesthetic technique

Classically it has been advocated that a postpneumonectomy fistula should be isolated with an endobronchial tube before IPPV is employed. A double-lumen endobronchial tube (DLT) is inserted in the remaining bronchus. To secure airway prior to the administration of a muscle relaxant, two methods were previously advocated:

- Awake endobronchial intubation using local analgesia of the upper respiratory tract
- Inhalational induction and intubation under deep inhalational anaesthesia.

The above techniques should be discussed at examinations, but in practice both are fraught with difficulty. Most experienced anaesthetists now use the following technique:

- Patient sitting upright, with drain open
- Preoxygenation
- Slow intravenous induction
- Intravenous suxamethonium
- Insertion of DLT – use of fibre-optic bronchoscope useful
- Administer further muscle relaxant
- IPPV via endobronchial portion of tube
- Patient placed in lateral position for thoracotomy.

POSTOPERATIVE MANAGEMENT

Re-establish spontaneous respiration, in the sitting position where possible, and transfer the patient to an ITU for further management. Respiratory failure is common after this type of procedure and this should be treated conventionally where indicated, with IPPV via an endotracheal tube. High-frequency jet ventilation has been advocated for the pre- and post-operative management of bronchopleural fistulae because of the low peak airway pressures employed. The evidence that this mode of ventilation is significantly better than conventional techniques remains conflicting.

OUTCOME

Morbidity is high following this type of surgery. Mortality is probably in the region of 10–20%, but national figures are not available.

BIBLIOGRAPHY

Feeley T W, Keating D, Nishimura T. Independent lung ventilation using high-frequency ventilation in the management of a bronchopleural fistula. Anesthesiology 1988; 69: 420–422

Lauckner M E, Beggs I, Armstrong R F. The radiological characteristics of bronchopleural fistula following pneumonectomy. Anaesthesia 1983; 38: 452–456

Ryder G H, Short D H, Zeitlin G L. The anaesthetic management of a bronchopleural fistula with the Robertshaw double-lumen tube. British Journal of Anaesthesia 1965; 37: 861–865

CROSS REFERENCES

Bronchiectasis
Patient Conditions 3: 71
Bronchial carcinoma
Patient Conditions 3: 73
Pneumonectomy
Surgical Procedures 17: 355
Postoperative analgesia for thoracic surgery patients
Surgical Procedures 17: 358
One-lung anaesthesia
Anaesthetic Factors 32: 602
Preoperative assessment of pulmonary risk
Anaesthetic Factors 34: 697

INHALED FOREIGN BODY

J. W. W. Gothard and L. Murdoch

Foreign bodies can be inhaled at any age but are more common in children under 3 years of age. Foreign bodies within the tracheobronchial tree require removal at bronchoscopy. The rigid bronchoscope is by far the best instrument for this procedure, as it allows grasping forceps of an adequate size to be used.

Peanuts are of a size easily inhaled by children and they are liable to fragment in the airway, releasing an irritant oil that causes severe inflammation. Inorganic objects can also be inhaled, however, and will also require removal at bronchoscopy.

PATIENT CHARACTERISTICS

Inhalation of foreign bodies is more common in the following groups:

- Children
- The elderly
- Debilitated subjects
- Drunks.

PREOPERATIVE ASSESSMENT AND INVESTIGATIONS

Symptoms

There may be a specific history of inhalation such as a bout of coughing whilst eating peanuts. Alternatively, a chronic cough with wheeze, stridor and fever may be the presenting symptoms some time after the original inhalation. A persistent chest infection in an otherwise healthy child may warrant investigation for an inhaled foreign body.

Investigations

A variety of chest X-ray changes may be present:

- Obstructive emphysema (seen best on expiratory film)
- Radio-opaque object (e.g. pin) in tracheobronchial tree
- Nonspecific changes (atelectasis/ consolidation)
- Normal X-ray.

Other investigations:

- Full blood count in children
- Standard investigations relating to age and medical condition of adult, e.g. ECG, urea and electrolytes, LFT.

PREMEDICATION

- Anaesthetist's preferred standard regime in adults and children
- Anticholinergics not essential
- Omit premedication if any question of *upper airway obstruction.*

PERIOPERATIVE MANAGEMENT

Monitoring:

- ECG
- Noninvasive BP
- Sao_2

Anaesthetic technique

General anaesthesia is preferred for rigid bronchoscopy in both adults and children.

- Preoxygenation
- Intravenous induction in adults and bigger children (use EMLA cream)
- Inhalational induction in smaller children
- Consider inhalational induction in all patients with upper airway obstruction.

If upper airway obstruction is present because of a foreign body lodged in the upper trachea or larynx, it may be safer to perform initial bronchoscopy under deep inhalational anaesthesia. In the majority of circumstances it will be safe to introduce the bronchoscope after the administration of suxamethonium. If the procedure is likely to be prolonged, intermittent suxamethonium can be used (N.B. use an anticholinergic to prevent bradycardia), but it is preferable to use a longer acting drug such as atracurium.

Anaesthesia can be maintained by a propofol infusion in adults, whilst a volatile agent is ideal for use with a ventilating bronchoscope in children. Ventilation in adults can be carried out satisfactorily with a venturi system, but care must be taken not to blow fragments of foreign body further down the tracheobronchial tree.

POSTOPERATIVE MANAGEMENT

After a relatively short atraumatic procedure, the patient can be allowed to wake up in the usual manner, once the bronchoscope has been removed and muscular relaxation reversed. Oxygen is then administered by face-mask. If the procedure has been long and difficult the instrumentation may cause upper airway oedema, especially in small children. It is prudent, therefore, to take the following precautions:

- Remove bronchoscope and reintubate with a small oral endotracheal tube
- Allow patient to awake on side, breathing a high $F_{I}O_2$
- Suction, as required
- Extubate when fully awake
- Be prepared for emergency reintubation.

Postextubation, children should be nursed in humidified, oxygen enriched air and monitored in a high-dependency area. In the presence of severe laryngeal oedema a period of postoperative ventilation may be required until a gas leak appears around the endotracheal tube. The use of steroids and nebulized adrenaline at this stage is controversial.

BIBLIOGRAPHY

Baraka A. Bronchoscopic removal of foreign bodies in children. British Journal of Anaesthesia 1974; 46: 124–126

CROSS REFERENCES

Rigid bronchoscopy
Surgical Procedures 17: 360
Preoperative assessment of pulmonary risk
Anaesthetic Factors 34: 697

LOBECTOMY

J. W. W. Gothard and
L. Murdoch

PROCEDURE

Lobectomy is the surgical excision of one lobe of a lung. Usual indications are:

- Malignant and benign tumours
- Bronchiectasis
- TB and fungal infections.

PATIENT CHARACTERISTICS

Lobectomy for malignant tumours:
- Elderly
- Smokers
- ASA grade II–IV.

Lobectomy for benign tumours:
- Younger age group.

Lobectomy for bronchiectasis:
- Children and adults
- Resection indicated if disease confined to one or two lobes
- If lung disease is generalized:
  - Indicates high risk
  - Patients often debilitated.

PREOPERATIVE ASSESSMENT

As for Pneumonectomy (p. 355). CT scan and bronchogram used to evaluate extent of any bronchiectasis.

Patients unable to tolerate pneumonectomy may withstand lobectomy.

PREMEDICATION

- Continue cardiac and respiratory medications until surgery
- Conventional opioid or benzodiazepine premedication is satisfactory
- Anticholinergic drugs not essential
- Low-molecular-weight heparin for DVT prophylaxis.

Patients with bronchiectasis are admitted several days preoperatively for postural drainage, physiotherapy and antibiotic medication. This is intended to reduce the volume and purulence of secretions.

PERIOPERATIVE MANAGEMENT

Monitoring:
- ECG
- BP, preferably invasive
- Sao_2
- $ETco_2$
- Core temperature
- Central venous pressure
- TV and AWP
- Arterial blood gases
- Urine output (if epidural analgesia employed).

ANAESTHETIC TECHNIQUE

General anaesthesia with muscle relaxation and mechanical ventilation is the technique of choice. Intravenous opioids can be used to supplement analgesia; alternatively, epidural techniques can be employed (see section on Postoperative analgesia for thoracic surgery patients (p. 358).

A double-lumen endobronchial tube is placed in the nonoperative lung to provide one-lung ventilation and control of secretions. An unacceptable degree of hypoxaemia may occur during one-lung ventilation in patients with generalized pulmonary disease who are judged capable of withstanding lobectomy, although this is uncommon. It may be necessary to use an inspired gas concentration of 100% oxygen, possibly in combination (rarely) with oxygen insufflated at a positive pressure to the operative lung.

In bronchiectasis the remaining lobe or lobes on the nonoperative side are unprotected from the spread of secretions if a double-lumen tube is used, and infected material can seep past the endobronchial cuff into the opposite lung. Repeated suction to both lungs limits this contamination. Spread of secretions from lobe to lobe can be reduced by using bronchial blockade (e.g. a Fogarty embolectomy catheter used as blocker or the 'Univent Tube', a blocker combined with an endotracheal tube) to block specific bronchi whilst continuing to ventilate the remaining lobes. The main drawback of blocking techniques is that if they fail (e.g. by dislodgement), all protection from the spread of secretions is lost.

PERIOPERATIVE MANAGEMENT

One-lung anaesthesia is used when requested. The integrity of bronchial suture lines is tested prior to chest closure. The bronchial stump is covered with sterile water (malignant disease) or saline (benign disease) and a pressure of 30–40 cmH_2O is exerted by manual compression of a rebreathing bag. Any leak is then detected. Leaks from raw lung surfaces are detected in a similar manner, but at a pressure of approximately 20–25 cmH_2O. Any significant leaks require suturing, or may be sealed with tissue glue sprayed onto the surface.

Chest drainage
- Apical and basal drains
- Suction at 5 kPa via under water seal
- Anterior and posterior drains are occasionally used.

POSTOPERATIVE PERIOD

- Extubate patient in the sitting position, breathing spontaneously
- Administer humidified oxygen by face-mask
- Management of other complications as for pneumonectomy (p. 355)
- Persistent air leak can be a problem.

OUTCOME

The 30-day operative mortality for lobectomy in primary malignant tumours of the lung is currently 2.5% in the UK.

BIBLIOGRAPHY

Eisenkraft J B, Neustein S M. Anesthethic management of therapeutic procedures of the lungs and airway. In: Kaplan A J (ed) Thoracic anesthesia, 2nd edn, 1991, Churchill Livingstone, New York, pp 419–440

CROSS REFERENCES

Bronchiectasis
Patient Conditions 3: 71
Pneumonectomy
Surgical Procedures 17: 355
One-lung anaesthesia
Anaesthetic Factors 32: 602
Preoperative assessment of respiratory risk
Anaesthetic Factors 34: 697

MEDIASTINAL OPERATIONS

J. W. W. Gothard and L. Murdoch

PROCEDURES

Mediastinal surgery can be split into two categories:

- Diagnostic – mediastinoscopy, mediastinotomy
- Therapeutic – excision of tumours and cysts.

Mediastinoscopy and mediastinotomy are commonly carried out to assess mediastinal lymph node involvement in the staging of lung cancer. These patients are in the categories outlined for pneumonectomy and lobectomy and are in a relatively low-risk category for the staging procedure. Patients with mediastinal tumours are in a very different category. Some are low risk, e.g. those with mediastinal cysts, small intrathoracic thyroids or thymomas. Many, particularly those with large anterior mediastinal tumours, are high risk. These high-risk patients may present for a histological diagnosis to be determined. If this is the case, the problems outlined for major mediastinal surgery must also be taken into account for the lesser procedures.

MEDIASTINOSCOPY/MEDIASTINOTOMY

In mediastinoscopy, a mediastinoscope is passed into the pretracheal area via a small incision above the suprasternal notch. Biopsies can then be taken and nodes palpated digitally. A mediastinotomy allows direct surgical access to the anterior mediastinum via an incision through the bed of the second costal cartilage.

- Rigid bronchoscopy is usually performed first
- Position the patient supine with a sandbag under the shoulders, the head on a ring, and the neck extended.

Patient characteristics

As for pneumonectomy (see p. 355) and lobectomy (see p. 349).

Preoperative assessment and considerations

As for pneumonectomy (see p. 355) and lobectomy (see p. 349).

Premedication

As for pneumonectomy (see p. 355) and lobectomy (see p. 349).

Perioperative management

Monitoring:

- ECG
- Noninvasive BP
- Sao_2
- $ETco_2$
- Intravenous infusion is essential – vascular structures may be biopsied in error.

Anaesthetic technique

- Intravenous induction
- Muscular relaxation (atracurium, vecuronium, mivacurium)
- Maintenance – volatile agent
- Low to moderate dose opioid.

Perioperative management

Mediastinotomy is often on the left side. Pleura may be breached surgically. This is drained via a wide-bore nasogastric tube which is removed as the anaesthetist applies continuous positive pressure to the lungs and the surgeon completes the suture line to prevent reoccurrence of the pneumothorax.

Postoperative management

- Extubate
- Sit up
- Check chest X-ray for pneumothoraces.

MEDIASTINAL TUMOURS

Mediastinal tumours are rare. The tumours that more commonly present for surgical excision are:

- Retrosternal thyroid

- Thymectomy for myasthenia gravis
- Neurogenic tumours
- Reduplication cysts
- Thymoma without myasthenia.

Procedure
Most resectable mediastinal tumours are removed surgically via a median sternotomy, with the patient in a supine position. Anterior mediastinal tumours are particularly likely to cause problems during anaesthesia. The major problems encountered are:

- Airway obstruction
- Compression of intrathoracic vascular structures
- Effects of radiotherapy and chemotherapy (N.B. bleomycin lung)
- Intraoperative bleeding
- Section of phrenic and recurrent laryngeal nerves at operation.

Patient characteristics
Mediastinal tumours appear more commonly in young adults.

Preoperative assessment and considerations
As for other major thoracic surgery, such as pneumonectomy (see p. 355). Further investigations will depend on symptoms.

- Respiratory symptoms (cough, dyspnoea, orthopnoea):
  - CT or MRI scan of airway
  - Lung function with flow volume loop.
- SVC obstruction:
  - CT or MRI scan of airway.
- Cyanosis with reasonable lung function (? pulmonary artery occlusion):
  - Consider echo investigation in addition to CT or MRI scans.

Premedication
Omit in airway obstruction.

Perioperative management
Monitoring:
- Standard monitoring as for pneumonectomy (p. 355) and lobectomy (p. 349)
- Additional venous access required in lower limb in the case of major surgical disruption of superior vena cava.

Anaesthetic technique
General anaesthesia with muscle relaxation and mechanical ventilation. Major problems relate to external compression of airway at induction of anaesthesia. To circumvent this:

- Splint airway with bronchoscope following intravenous induction and intravenous suxamethonium
- Pass long endotracheal or endobronchial tube through the compression
- Consider the use of cardiopulmonary bypass, especially in the presence of pulmonary artery compression (very rare)
- Note: inhalational induction is very difficult if there is gross external compression of the airway.

Perioperative management
- IPPV
- Replace blood loss, which can be substantial (N.B. lower limb intravenous access)
- Use lowest $F_{I}O_2$ compatible with adequate arterial oxygen saturation if patient has had recent bleomycin therapy.

Postoperative management
Consider mechanical ventilation following:
- A long operation
- If major nerves (e.g. phrenic) sectioned
- Airway patency still a problem.

Outcome
Good results if tumours resectable. Very low operative mortality in the UK, despite potential difficulties. Reoccurrence a problem with some tumours, but these may respond to chemotherapy or radiotherapy. Some tumours (e.g. secondary teratomata) may require reoperation.

BIBLIOGRAPHY

Gothard J W W. Anaesthesia for thoracic malignancy. In: Filshie J, Robbie D S (eds) Anaesthesia and malignant disease. Edward Arnold, London, 1989

Mackie A M. Anaesthesia and mediastinal masses. Anaesthesia 1984; 43: 864–866

CROSS REFERENCES

Bronchial carcinoma
Patient Conditions 3: 73
Sarcoidosis
Patient Conditions 3: 82
Lobectomy
Surgical Procedures 17: 349
Pneumonectomy
Surgical Procedures 17: 355

PLEURECTOMY

J. W. W. Gothard and L. Murdoch

PROCEDURE

- Parietal pleura is stripped over all but the diaphragmatic and mediastinal surfaces of the lung
- Carried out as an open procedure via a lateral thoracotomy, or as an endoscopic procedure via a thoracoscope, also in the lateral position. Additional small wounds may be necessary for instrumentation during the endoscopic procedure
- Treatment of choice for fit patients with recurrent pneumothoraces
- Lesser procedures (e.g. pleurodesis) indicated in debilitated patients and those with malignant disease.

PATIENT CHARACTERISTICS

Spontaneous pneumothorax commonly occurs in:

- Young fit adults
- Tall and thin subjects
- More frequently in males and smokers.

Secondary pneumothorax occurs in:

- Chronic bronchitis and emphysema
- Tuberculosis
- Cystic fibrosis
- Lung cancer.

PREOPERATIVE ASSESSMENT AND INVESTIGATIONS

- General medical condition – particularly with secondary pneumothorax

- Size of existing pneumothorax, presence of functioning drain, etc.
- Rarely possible to obtain meaningful lung function studies.

PREMEDICATION

- Conventional opioid or benzodiazepine premedication satisfactory
- Anticholinergic drugs not essential
- Low-molecular-weight heparin for DVT prophylaxis.

PERIOPERATIVE MANAGEMENT

Monitoring:
- ECG
- BP (preferably invasive)
- Sao_2
- $ETco_2$
- TV and AWP.

Problems of pneumothorax during anaesthesia:
- Size of pneumothorax will increase with uptake of nitrous oxide
- Positive pressure ventilation may create tension pneumothorax
- Both of the above are unlikely with a functioning chest drain
- Safer to drain a large pneumothorax preoperatively (a minor air space is usually tolerated).

ANAESTHETIC TECHNIQUE

Endoscopic and open pleurectomy
General anaesthesia with muscle paralysis and mechanical ventilation is the preferred technique. Postoperative pain relief is a much greater problem after open surgery. In general:

- Safer to avoid nitrous oxide
- Minimize inflation pressures
- Potential for pneumothorax on nonoperative side (bilateral disease)
- Endotracheal intubation satisfactory if:
  - Either no pneumothorax present
  - Or functional drain present
- Double-lumen endobronchial tube (in left lung) mandatory for endoscopic technique and in presence of a large air leak for open operation
- Facility to collapse operative lung may be requested for open technique by some surgeons
- Blood loss can be significant, particularly if pleura is diseased
- Surgeon may ligate bullae or seal leaks with tissue glue
- Test for air leaks as described for lobectomy (p. 349).

Bilateral pleurectomy
Usually performed through a median sternotomy. A double-lumen endobronchial tube is indicated for intraoperative management. Continuous arterial blood pressure monitoring is essential as the heart and great vessels can be distorted at surgery. This operation causes less postoperative pain than does bilateral thoracotomy, but there is substantial interference with lung function, and adequate analgesia is essential. A short period of postoperative ventilation via an endotracheal tube may be beneficial to reinflate the lungs and allow controlled weaning.

POSTOPERATIVE MANAGEMENT

- Generally possible and desirable to establish spontaneous respiration
- Patients after bilateral pleurectomy and those with generalized lung disease may need a period of mechanical ventilation
- Sit patient up as soon as possible
- Administer humidified oxygen by face-mask
- Pleural cavity usually drained postoperatively, as for lobectomy (p. 349)
- Adequate pain relief essential.

OUTCOME

Incidence of recurrence of pneumothorax after open pleurectomy is very low. The long-term results of endoscopic pleurectomy have yet to be determined.

BIBLIOGRAPHY

Millar F A, Hutchinson G L, Wood R A B. Anaesthesia for thoracoscopic pleurectomy and ligation of bullae. Anaesthesia 1992; 47: 1057–1060

CROSS REFERENCES

Bronchial carcinoma
Patient Conditions 3: 73
Chronic obstructive airways disease
Patient Conditions 3: 75
Cystic fibrosis
Patient Conditions 3: 78
Postoperative analgesia for thoracic surgery patients
Surgical Procedures 17: 358
One lung anaesthesia
Anaesthetic Factors 32: 602

PNEUMONECTOMY

J. W. W. Gothard and L. Murdoch

PROCEDURE

- Usual indication is carcinoma of the lung
- Performed via a lateral thoracotomy.

PATIENT CHARACTERISTICS

Patients for pneumonectomy are generally:

- Elderly
- Smokers (past or present)
- ASA status II–IV.

PREOPERATIVE ASSESSMENT AND INVESTIGATIONS

Assessment of cardiac and respiratory function:

- Clinical examination
- ECG
- Chest X-ray
- CT scan
- Full blood count
- Urea and electrolytes
- Arterial blood gases (breathing air)
- Lung function tests
- Cross-match (4 units of blood or packed cells).

Evaluate the risk of pneumonectomy:

- Cardiac dysfunction common
- Cardiac risk index (e.g. Goldman) may be valuable
- No clear-cut criteria exist for selection of patients who will tolerate pneumonectomy
- FEV_1 and FVC are essential baseline measurements

- Good preoperative exercise tolerance indicates patient probably in low-risk group
- Can identify high-risk group with full lung function testing (Table 1).

Table 1.
Criteria indicating high risk for pneumonectomy

Age over 70 years
Abnormal ECG
FVC less than 50% of predicted value
FEV_1 less than 50% of FVC or less than 2 l
Maximum breathing capacity less than 50% predicted
T_Lco less than 50% predicted
P_aco_2 more than 6 kPa

PREMEDICATION

- Continue cardiac and respiratory medications
- Conventional opioid or benzodiazepine premedication is satisfactory
- Anticholinergic drugs not essential
- Low-molecular-weight heparin for DVT prophylaxis.

PERIOPERATIVE MANAGEMENT

Monitoring:
- ECG
- BP (preferably invasive)
- Sao_2
- $ETco_2$
- Core temperature
- Central venous pressure
- TV and AWP
- Arterial blood gases
- Urine output (if epidural analgesia employed).

ANAESTHETIC TECHNIQUE

General anaesthesia with muscle paralysis and mechanical ventilation is the technique of choice. Intravenous opioid drugs can be used to provide intra- and post-operative analgesia; alternatively, epidural analgesia can be employed. A double-lumen endobronchial tube is used to separate both lungs and provide one-lung ventilation when required.

PERIOPERATIVE MANAGEMENT

- Blood loss may be substantial
- During one lung ventilation
  - Monitor Sao_2 and arterial blood gases
  - Adjust TV, RR, F_Io_2, as necessary
- Test integrity of bronchial suture line when requested by surgeon; release clamp on double-lumen tube to the operated side and slowly apply inflation pressure up to 40 cmH_2O with the bronchial stump immersed in water.

CHEST DRAINAGE FOLLOWING PNEUMONECTOMY

If air leak does not occur, chest drainage is not mandatory.

No chest drain sited

Air is aspirated from the pneumonectomy space at the end of operation, via a cannula placed through the chest wall, with the patient in a supine position. Air is aspirated until there is a negative pressure within the space. The mediastinum will then be approximately central or slightly towards the side of surgery. This is confirmed on chest X-ray.

Chest drain sited

Usually a single basal chest drain is left clamped but connected to an underwater seal drain. The drain is unclamped for 1–2 min every hour to reveal excess blood loss and centralize the mediastinum by releasing trapped air. Never apply suction to a pneumonectomy drain. This will pull the mediastinum across and severely impair venous return to the heart.

POSTOPERATIVE MANAGEMENT

Most patients are allowed to breathe spontaneously immediately following surgery.

- Sit the patient up as soon as possible to encourage expansion of remaining lung
- Administer humidified oxygen by face-mask
- Chest drain is usually removed 12–24 h after surgery, if there is no significant bleeding
- Careful attention to fluid balance is essential.

COMPLICATIONS OF PNEUMONECTOMY

Haemorrhage

Perioperative bleeding can be substantial. Excess accumulation of fluid in the pneumonectomy space can cause hypovolaemia and respiratory distress. The latter is relieved by chest drainage, or by release of the drain clamps.

Sputum retention, infection and respiratory failure

More likely to occur in patients with poor lung function. Treat as follows:

- Physiotherapy and antibiotics
- Consider minitracheotomy if cough is poor
- Consider mechanical ventilation if there is severe deterioration in respiratory function (high mortality)
- Infection in pneumonectomy space:
  - Requires draining
  - Associated with a bronchopleural fistula in some cases.

Dysrhythmias:

- More common postoperatively
- Usually atrial in origin
- Treated by digitalization (or other suitable drug therapy) rather than cardioversion
- Some surgeons favour prophylactic digitalization.

OUTCOME

- Mortality up to 6% (UK figures)
- Cardiorespiratory dysfunction is the major cause of death.

BIBLIOGRAPHY

Entwistle M D, Roe P G, Sapsford D J, Berisford R G, Jones J G. Patterns of oxygenation after thoracotomy. British Journal of Anaesthesia 1991; 67: 704–711

Goldman L. Assessment of the patient with known or suspected ischaemic heart disease for non-cardiac surgery. British Journal of Anaesthesia 1988; 61: 38–43

Goldstraw P. Post-operative management of the thoracic surgical patient. In: Gothard J W W (ed) Thoracic anaesthesia. Clinical Anaesthesiology, Baillière Tindal, London, 1987, vol 1, p 207–231

CROSS REFERENCES

Bronchial carcinoma
Patient Conditions 3: 73
Smoking and anaesthesia
Patient Conditions 3: 85
Lobectomy
Surgical Procedures 17: 349
One-lung anaesthesia
Anaesthetic Factors 32: 602
Preoperative assessment of cardiovascular risk in noncardic surgery
Anaesthetic Factors 34: 692
Preoperative assessment of pulmonary risk
Anaesthetic Factors 34: 697

17

POSTOPERATIVE ANALGESIA FOR THORACIC SURGERY PATIENTS

B. A. Sutton

Aim of analgesia
- Reduce distress to patient
- Improve lung function
- Allow early mobilization
- Reduce incidence of postoperative complications, and hospital stay

Sources of pain
- Chest wall and most of pleura via intercostal nerves
- Diaphragmatic pleura via phrenic nerves
- Mediastinal pleura via the vagus nerve
- Shoulder joint via spinal nerves C5–C7

ANALGESIC TECHNIQUES

Regional:
- Intercostal nerve block
- Extrapleural block
- Intrapleural block
- Paravertebral block
- Epidural block.

Opioid:
- Parenteral
- Epidural
- Intrathecal
- Patient-controlled analgesia (PCA).

Other:
- Cryoanalgesia
- Nonsteroidal anti-inflammatory drugs (NSAIDs).

REGIONAL ANAESTHESIA

Intercostal nerve block
Simple to perform. Main disadvantages are short duration of action (unless indwelling intercostal catheters used), and failure to ameliorate pain from diaphragmatic pleura, mediastinal structures and areas supplied by the posterior primary rami.

Extrapleural block
Indwelling catheter is placed in a pocket of retracted pleura so that the tip lies against a costovertebral joint. Local anaesthetic spreads to paravertebral space providing anaesthesia of both anterior and posterior primary rami. Increasingly popular due to promising analgesic results.

Intrapleural block
Local analgesic agent deposited between visceral and parietal pleura via indwelling catheter. Analgesic action due to widespread intercostal nerve block. Does not spread to paravertebral space. Analgesia unpredictable due to variable loss of drug into chest drains, binding with blood in thorax, and rapid systemic absorption.

Paravertebral block
Percutaneously inserted catheter at one level allows considerable spread of drug between adjacent paravertebral spaces. Provides good analgesia of both anterior and posterior primary rami, with less side-effects than epidural. Main disadvantages are problems of accurate siting and easy displacement.

Epidural
Height of required block necessitates thoracic approach if local analgesic drug alone is used. Can provide excellent analgesia, but side-effects of extensive sympathetic block, motor weakness and urinary retention limit its usefulness.

OPIOID ANALGESIA

Parenteral
Intermittent intramuscular opioids provide inadequate pain relief. Analgesia is improved by continuous infusion, but at the expense of excessive sedation, respiratory depression, nausea and vomiting.

Epidural
Improved pain relief compared to intravenous route, with decreased total opioid requirement and less sedation, nausea and vomiting. Main disadvantage is respiratory depression (may be delayed), urinary retention and pruritus. Combined local analgesic and opioid epidural provides superior analgesia with decreased side-effects and is probably achievable by the lumbar route.

Intrathecal
Produces profound but short-term analgesia, unless indwelling catheter used. Risk of respiratory depression greater than with epidural opioids.

Patient-controlled analgesia
Either intravenous or epidural. Analgesia generally superior to continuous infusions with reduced sedation and respiratory depression. Requires patient and staff education to achieve optimum effect.

OTHER

Cryoanalgesia
Application of extreme cold (–20 to –60°C) to intercostal nerves, under direct vision. Produces disruption of impulse transmission lasting several months. Decline in popularity due to poor analgesic results and possible association with chronic post-thoracotomy pain syndrome.

NSAIDs
Inadequate when used alone but have synergistic action when combined with opioids and regional techniques. Adverse side-effects of platelet dysfunction, gastrointestinal bleeding and renal dysfunction precludes their use in all patients.

BIBLIOGRAPHY

Stevens D S, Edwards W T. Management of pain after thoracic surgery. In: Kaplan J A (ed) Thoracic anesthesia, 2nd edn, 1991; Churchill Livingstone, New York, pp 563–592

CROSS REFERENCES

Bronchopleural fistula
Surgical Procedures 17: 345
Lobectomy
Surgical Procedures 17: 349
Pleurectomy
Surgical Procedures 17: 353
Pneumonectomy
Surgical Procedures 17: 355
Local anaesthetic toxicity
Anaesthetic Factors 33: 642

RIGID BRONCHOSCOPY

J. W. W. Gothard and L. Murdoch

PROCEDURE

Isolated rigid bronchoscopy has largely been superseded by flexible fibre-optic bronchoscopy for the initial diagnosis of airway and lung disease. Rigid bronchoscopy remains the procedure of choice for surgical assessment of the airway before staging procedures such as mediastinoscopy or prior to thoracotomy. The rigid bronchoscope is also the preferred instrument for therapeutic manoeuvres such as removal of a foreign body, stent insertion and diathermy resection of airway tumour.

PREOPERATIVE ASSESSMENT AND INVESTIGATIONS

Investigations similar to those described for pneumonectomy (p. 355) (especially if bronchoscopy is carried out immediately prior to thoracotomy). Cardiac and respiratory dysfunction are both common in this group of patients.

- ECG
- Chest X-ray
- Full blood count, urea and electrolytes
- Arterial blood gases (breathing air)
- Lung function tests.

It is particularly important to assess the degree of upper airway obstruction (if any) when rigid bronchoscopy is carried out as an isolated procedure. Further investigations of upper airway obstruction following clinical examination may include:

- Flow-volume loop
- Lateral X-ray of the trachea
- CT or MRI scan showing main airways.

Rigid bronchoscopy may entail a degree of neck extension

- Check lateral neck X-ray in rheumatoid arthritis.

PREMEDICATION

- Continue all cardiac and respiratory medication
- Anticholinergic medication not essential, but may be administered if preferred
- Anxiolysis with short-acting oral benzodiazepine, if required
- Omit sedatives if there is evidence of significant airway obstruction.

PERIOPERATIVE MANAGEMENT

Monitoring:
- ECG
- Noninvasive BP
- Sa_{O_2}.

Ventilation
The airway is 'shared' with the surgeon during rigid bronchoscopy. Main methods of providing adequate gas exchange are:

- *Venturi injector.* A high-pressure source of oxygen is intermittently injected through a needle at the proximal end of the bronchoscope. Air is entrained and positive pressure ventilation produced via the distal end of the bronchoscope. *Using this technique it is essential that there is always an adequate opening at the proximal end of the bronchoscope to allow entrainment of air during inspiration and egress of gas during expiration.* It is also essential to match the injector needle size to the type of bronchoscope and oxygen pressure used (Table 1). This method of ventilation is usually used in adults.
- *Ventilating bronchoscope.* A glass slide device at the proximal end of the bronchoscope allows manual positive pressure ventilation with a suitable anaesthetic gas mixture via a side port built into the bronchoscope. This technique is ideal for infants and children. A T-piece circuit can be attached to the side port and anaesthesia is maintained with noncumulative gaseous agents. This

Table 1.
Maximum inflation pressure achieved with various Venturi bronchoscope injector systems (oxygen driving pressure 410 kPa)

Negus bronchoscope	Injector needle (SWG)	Approx maximum pressure (cmH_2O)
Adult	14	50
Adult	16	25–30
Child	19	14–18*
Suckling	19	15*

*Manual ventilation technique with Storz-type bronchoscope preferred in this age group.

method avoids the use of injector techniques, which are more likely to cause barotrauma in children.
- *High-frequency jet ventilation.* Not used widely in the UK, but popular in some other countries.

ANAESTHETIC TECHNIQUE

- Intravenous induction
- Short-acting muscle relaxant (suxamethonium, mivacurium)
- Inhalational induction
  - Children
  - Upper airway obstruction

Maintenance of anaesthesia is usually with intermittent bolus doses of an intravenous agent. Awareness during bronchoscopy is a real problem and it is preferable to use a constant infusion for all but the shortest procedures. Propofol is a particularly suitable agent in this respect. If the bronchoscopy is prolonged or to be followed by a surgical procedure a longer acting muscle relaxant such as vecuronium or atracurium can be used.

POSTOPERATIVE MANAGEMENT

- Reverse the muscle relaxant
- Administer oxygen by mask
- Allow patient to awaken
- Lie patient with suppurative side down if secretions are present
- Be prepared to reintubate in the presence of airway obstruction.

BIBLIOGRAPHY

Hill A J, Feneck R O, Underwood S M, Davis M E, Marsh A, Bromley L. The haemodynamic effects of bronchoscopy. Comparison of propofol and thiopentone with and without alfentanil pretreatment. Anaesthesia 1991; 46: 266–270

CROSS REFERENCES

Bronchial carcinoma
Patient Conditions 3: 73
Inhaled foreign body
Surgical Procedures 17: 347
Mediastinal operations
Surgical Procedures 17: 351
Preoperative assessment of pulmonary risk
Anaesthetic Factors 34: 697

18

ABDOMINAL SURGERY

B. J. Pollard

OVERVIEW

B. J. Pollard

General anaesthesia is usually the technique of choice for surgery within the abdominal cavity. Operations on the lower quadrants may, however, be readily undertaken using a regional block; a spinal or an epidural block is suitable. The slightly more superficial operations, e.g. hernia repair, may also be performed using nerve blocks and field blocks, although not every surgeon is willing to attempt this. Surgery in the upper quadrants of the abdominal cavity has been performed under a high spinal or epidural block, although this is technically more difficult and the height of the block results in marked cardiovascular effects. An epidural placed in the upper lumbar or lower thoracic region is commonly used for postoperative analgesia.

Surgery within the abdominal cavity carries with it a number of considerations, in particular alterations of:

- Respiratory function
- Cardiovascular function
- Thermoregulation
- Fluid and electrolyte balance.

THE RESPIRATORY SYSTEM

There is some impairment of pulmonary gas exchange following the induction of general anaesthesia in the majority of patients. This may be seen with both spontaneous ventilation and controlled ventilation. In cases of surgery in the abdominal cavity, upward pressure on the diaphragm caused by packs and retractors will exacerbate this problem. The V/Q mismatch which occurs peri-operatively can be considerable. If the patient had pre-existing ascites, surgical drainage will result in a temporary improvement in ventilation.

Respiratory problems are not confined to the operative period. There is good evidence to demonstrate impairment of pulmonary function for up to 1 week after abdominal surgery, with the maximum impairment occurring on the second or third postoperative day. This impairment is more marked the higher in the abdomen the surgery is, i.e. procedures close up under the diaphragm result in the highest incidence of problems.

Postoperative respiratory insufficiency is improved by adequate analgesia, but exacerbated by oversedation or larger doses of parenteral opioid analgesics. Regional techniques, e.g. epidural or intercostal nerve blocks, do not suffer from this disadvantage, and have therefore much to recommend them.

THE CARDIOVASCULAR SYSTEM

Approximately 20% of the blood volume is in the splanchnic circulation at rest, and the splanchnic circulation (including the liver) accounts for about 25% of the cardiac output, although this increases markedly following a meal. This whole is under a complex system of autoregulation. Handling the intestines together with the stress of surgery can produce significant sympathetic stimulation, which causes splanchnic vasoconstriction. This will displace a significant volume of blood into the systemic circulation. The liver receives about 70% of its supply from the portal venous system and, therefore, any reduction in portal flow has the potential to deprive the liver of a significant proportion of its oxygen supply.

THERMOREGULATION

A consideration in all anaesthetized patients, thermoregulation is a particular problem in intra-abdominal surgery. When the intra-abdominal viscera are exposed, heat loss, which is mainly by evaporation and radiation, can be considerable. This is in addition to other losses encountered during anaesthesia, which result from peripheral vasodilatation and airway evaporation.

Prevention of heat loss during intra-abdominal surgery can be difficult. Placing displaced intestines into a sterile plastic bag, or wrapping them in saline-soaked packs will minimize, but not completely prevent, the problem. Consideration should be given to increasing the ambient temperature of the operating theatre and all irrigation solutions should be prewarmed. The patient should also be placed on a warming mattress on the operating table, intravenous fluids should be warmed, and a humidifier used in the airway.

FLUID AND ELECTROLYTE CHANGES

Intra-abdominal surgery may be associated with conditions where there has been diarrhoea, vomiting, or a reduction in preoperative fluid intake. Preoperative bowel preparation with laxatives or enemas can cause large fluid losses. The patient's fluid status can therefore be markedly deranged and this should be assessed carefully before anaesthetizing the patient. Hypovolaemia in particular should be ruled out if a spinal or epidural block is being considered.

When intestines are handled at surgery, mild trauma can produce localized tissue oedema. This increase in extracellular fluid, the so-called 'third space' fluid, is lost to the circulation. If there is severe inflammation, e.g. bacterial or chemical peritonitis, or temporary ischaemia of the bowel, then several litres of fluid can be sequestered into this third space.

If there was pre-existing ascites, then this will be drained at operation. If the ascitic collection was large, with significant intra-abdominal pressure, venous return from the lower part of the body may have been impaired. There will be a temporary haemodynamic advantage to drainage of the ascites under these circumstances. It must be remembered that this ascites may recollect in the early postoperative period, resulting in the removal of fluid, electrolytes and protein from the circulating volume.

Preoperative diarrhoea or vomiting, or losses through fistulae or a nasogastric tube, will produce electrolyte and acid–base abnormalities, as well as fluid balance problems. The exact biochemical picture will depend upon the nature of the fluid lost. For example, loss of gastric contents will result in loss of hydrogen and chloride ions, tending to produce a hypochloraemic alkalosis. Generally speaking, patients who have suffered any gastrointestinal losses tend to have a reduced total body potassium concentration.

SPECIFIC POINTS

Opioids and anastomoses

There has been much debate over the years with respect to the benefit or harm of using opioids in gastrointestinal surgery. All of the commonly used opioids decrease intestinal transit time and increase gut contraction and sphincter activity. Morphine causes spasm of the sphincter of Oddi and is thus avoided in biliary colic. Recent evidence has implicated morphine in an increase in leaks of anastomoses. Pethidine would therefore appear to be the parenteral opioid of choice for these patients at present.

Anticholinesterases

Drugs of this family increase gut motility and also increase intraluminal pressure. The effect is not reliably prevented by treatment with either atropine or glycopyrrolate in normal clinical doses. The suggestion has been made that the use of an anticholinesterase to reverse a nondepolarizing neuromuscular block may increase the chance of anastomotic breakdown. The evidence is, however, inconclusive. The known serious risk to the patient of partial paralysis in recovery is regarded by most anaesthetists as far outweighing the possible unproven risk to the anastomosis.

Antibiotics

These are frequently requested by the surgeon during the perioperative period. A cephalosporin with metronidazole is a popular combination. If an aminoglycoside is used, the potentiating action of such drugs on a nondepolarizing neuromuscular block must be remembered. Irrigation of the abdominal cavity with a dilute solution of an aminoglycoside may result in sufficient absorption to markedly potentiate a neuromuscular block. This combination may not reverse well with an anticholinesterase; calcium chloride may help, but should not be relied upon.

Venous thromboembolism

Surgery in the abdomen and pelvis is a risk factor for the development of a deep vein thrombosis. Patients with malignant disease are at a particularly high risk. Appropriate prophylaxis should be considered.

CROSS REFERENCES

Postoperative pain management
Anaesthetic Factors 33: 655
Thrombotic embolism
Anaesthetic Factors 33: 664
Preoperative assessment of cardiovascular risk in noncardiac surgery
Anaesthetic Factors 34: 692
Preoperative assessment of pulmonary risk
Anaesthetic Factors 34: 697

HAEMORRHOIDECTOMY

D. Stott

PROCEDURE

Surgical excision of haemorrhoids is indicated where:

- Conservative treatment has failed
- Internal haemorrhoids are large and prolapsing.

The standard operation in the UK is excision and ligation by the Milligan Morgan technique. This necessitates:

- The lithotomy position with Trendelenburg's tilt
- Blunt dissection from the anal mucosa and internal anal sphincter
- Maximal relaxation of the anal sphincter.

Some surgeons prefer a degree of tone to be retained in the anal sphincter and may therefore be averse to intraoperative regional analgesia.

PATIENT CHARACTERISTICS

Any adult can be affected, but patients are generally:

- 40–70+ years old
- May have a variety of disorders associated with ageing
- May be pregnant
- ASA grades I–IV.

During pregnancy, palliative treatment is usually indicated. The situation usually improves once the pregnancy is over, and surgery may be avoided altogether.

PREOPERATIVE ASSESSMENT

- Symptomatic patients with chronic disease need preoperative investigations, as indicated by the history and examination
- Younger, asymptomatic patients need only a full blood count to eliminate the possibility of anaemia due to bleeding.

PREMEDICATION

An anxiolytic, such as a benzodiazepine, is normally adequate for this procedure.

PERIOPERATIVE MANAGEMENT

Surgery in the region of the anus causes severe pain and can precipitate adverse responses such as:

- Reflex laryngeal spasm (Brewer–Luckhardt reflex)
- Tachyarrhythmias and/or potentially serious ventricular arrythmias from sympathetic stimulation
- Reflex movement of the patient.

The choice of anaesthetic technique lies between regional anaesthesia or deep general anaesthesia. A combination approach is employed by some anaesthetists.

ANAESTHETIC TECHNIQUE

Regional anaesthesia

Regional anaesthesia is frequently the method of choice because:

- It avoids general anaesthesia
- It provides good postoperative analgesia
- It attenuates the stress response.

A low spinal anaesthetic aiming to block the S2–S5 nerve roots produces adequate analgesia and is best performed in the sitting position using 0.6–1.4 ml of 0.5% bupivacaine (heavy). Spinal techniques can be difficult in the elderly, and positioning may be impeded by pain.

Alternatively, a caudal extradural block using 15–20 ml of 0.5% bupivacaine also provides satisfactory perioperative analgesia.

General anaesthesia

Deep general anaesthesia obtained via any of:

- Face-mask
- Laryngeal mask
- Endotracheal tube.

Reference to the following should be considered:

- An endotracheal tube protects the airway from regurgitation and/or laryngeal spasm in the at-risk patient; the patient is also positioned with the head tilted downwards
- A potent analgesic (e.g. alfentanil 5–10 μg kg^{-1}) prior to surgical assault on the anal canal reduces the adverse effects of stimulation
- Close monitoring of the ECG is essential because of the possibility of arrhythmias.

Should arrhythmias occur, asking the surgeon to stop temporarily is normally sufficient to cure the problem and allows time for the patient to become more deeply anaesthetized.

POSTOPERATIVE MANAGEMENT

Pain can be excruciating in the early postoperative period, and a caudal injection provides excellent analgesia for several hours. This can be repeated if necessary or, alternatively, generous doses of opioids can be used for the first 48 h. Other complications include:

- Retention of urine
- Primary haemorrhage (early) or secondary haemorrhage (late)
- The formation of a fistula
- The development of a perianal abscess (rare).

The last three complications will require further surgical treatment under anaesthetic.

CROSS REFERENCES

The elderly patient
Patient Conditions 11: 252

Epidural and spinal anaesthesia
Anaesthetic Factors 32: 594

Complications of position
Anaesthetic Factors 33: 618

HERNIA REPAIR

N. El. Mikatti

PROCEDURE

- Surgical treatment with repair of the defect and excision of the sac, if present
- Inguinal hernia – direct or indirect (75–80% of abdominal wall hernias)
- Incisional hernia through any previous abdominal or thoracic incision
- Less common hernias, e.g. umbilical, periumbilical, femoral
- Diaphragmatic hernia in a neonate (see p. 499)
- A synthetic mesh may be used in recurrent or large hernias
- Laparascopic techniques are gaining in popularity
- Treatment of complications, e.g. resection and anastomosis, may be required.

PATIENT CHARACTERISTICS

- Any age from neonates and infants (e.g. inguinal and diaphragmatic hernias) up to old age
- Patient may present as an elective case, as an in-patient or as a day-case
- Patient may present as a complicated emergency case, e.g. with strangulation.

Possible associations with complicated hernias:

- Intestinal obstruction with distension, vomiting, dehydration and hypovolaemia
- Electrolyte and fluid imbalance and acid–base disorders.

PREOPERATIVE ASSESSMENT AND INVESTIGATIONS

Elective cases:

- Routine history and examination
- Investigations according to findings and local policy; baseline value for full blood count and urinalysis are common with further investigations (e.g. ECG, chest X-ray) as indicated.

Complicated cases:

- The degree of distension and dehydration, vomiting and urine output should be assessed
- Additional investigations will be required (full blood count, urea and electrolytes, ECG, chest X-ray, arterial blood gases)
- Correction of fluid and electrolyte imbalance with appropriate fluid and insertion of nasogastric tube
- Many anaesthetists remove the nasogastric tube before induction of anaesthesia.

PREMEDICATION

- A benzodiazepine or a narcotic analgesic if required.
- Antacids or H_2-receptor antagonists may be used for emergency cases (ranitidine 150 mg orally or 50 mg i.v., 2 h before operation).

PERIOPERATIVE MANAGEMENT

- Establish intravenous infusion
- Routine monitoring:
  - ECG
  - Noninvasive BP
  - $Sa{O_2}$
  - $ETCO_2$
  - Core temperature.

General anaesthesia

If there is no risk of vomiting or regurgitation, either spontaneous (e.g. using LMA) or controlled ventilation (following muscle relaxation and tracheal intubation) is appropriate, depending on the requirements of surgery.

General anaesthesia is indicated in reluctant, anxious and obese patients, children, and certain surgical approaches.

- Ensure prevention of pulmonary aspiration in at-risk patients by using rapid sequence induction

- Maintain adequate muscle relaxation with smooth recovery, without bucking or coughing during extubation
- Rapid return of consciousness and upper respiratory tract reflexes is recommended
- Preserving the anastomosis line, during reversal of muscle relaxants, is achieved by maintaining the base-line pulse rate by giving intravenous atropine as required
- Use of nitrous oxide is not recommended, except in short procedures, because it causes bowel distension.

Regional anaesthesia

- Spinal or epidural block or local infiltration are all suitable
- Sedation, e.g. propofol infusion (1–2 mg kg^{-1} h^{-1}), may be required
- Oxygen administration via nasal cannula or face-mask should be provided
- Regional anaesthesia is suitable because it avoids the complications of general anaesthesia, reduces the stress response, and provides good postoperative analgesia
- Spinal anaesthesia is not recommended in the acute abdomen; severe hypotension may result and there may be bowel-wall contraction, with increased risk of rupture.

POSTOPERATIVE MANAGEMENT

- Chest complications frequently follow these operations, especially in fit, young, male smokers, irrespective of the anaesthetic technique used. The patient should stop smoking one month before operation, and be taught to breathe deeply and cough effectively
- Respiratory embarrassment may result from repair of a large ventral hernia, requiring mechanical ventilation in the ITU
- Pain relief may be provided by opioids either by the intramuscular route, intravenously using patient-controlled anaesthesia, or via a spinal or epidural cannula using intermittent doses. Continuous epidural infusion of bupivacaine (0.125%) and diamorphine (0.5 mg in 15 ml of 0.9% saline) mixture at a rate of 15 ml h^{-1} provides better analgesia than either alone
- Maintenance of electrolyte and fluid balance is important.

Comment

With the present advances in out-patient surgery, day-case hernia repair is no longer restricted to young, healthy patients. Higher risk (ASA III and IV) patients may be considered acceptable if their systemic disease is well controlled preoperatively.

BIBLIOGRAPHY

Apfelbaum J L. Outpatient anesthesia for adult patients. Annual refresher course lectures of the American Society of Anesthesiologists, 1992, p 412

Atkinson R S, Rushman G B, Lee J A. Surgical operations and choice of anaesthetic. A synopsis of anaesthesia, 10th edn. Wright, Bristol, 1987, p 444–493

Kaufman L. Anaesthesia for abdominal surgery. In: Gray T C, Utting J E, Nunn J E (eds) General anaesthesia, 4th edn. Butterworths, London, 1979, vol 2, p 1431–1452

Lee A, Simpson D, Whitfield A, Scott D B. Postoperative analgesia by continuous extradural infusion of bupivacaine and diamorphine. British Journal of Anaesthesia 1988; 60: 845–850

McClure J H, Wildsmith J A W. Aspects of spinal anaesthesia. In: Kaufman L (ed) Anaesthesia review. Churchill Livingstone, Edinburgh, 1988, vol 5, p 269–285

CROSS REFERENCES

Smoking and anaesthesia
Patient Conditions 3: 85
Day-case surgery
Anaesthetic Factors 29: 542
Emergency surgery
Anaesthetic Factors 29: 547

LAPAROSCOPIC CHOLECYSTECTOMY

J. Shaw

PROCEDURE

Laparoscopic cholecystectomy is performed as follows:

- With the patient in a head-down position (to avoid trauma to the viscera), an insufflator is introduced into the peritoneal cavity to produce a pneumoperitoneum (usually using CO_2)
- The patient is then positioned head-up, possibly with a slight left-lateral tilt, and a laparoscopic camera is inserted close to the umbilicus through a 10-mm incision
- Other subcostal puncture sites (3 mm in size), usually totalling three, are used for the introduction of instrumentation
- The operative dissection may be performed using either diathermy or a Nd-YAG laser via a gas-cooled contact tip
- May be performed as a day-case.

PATIENT CHARACTERISTICS

- Ratio of female/male patients is approximately 1.5:1
- Average age is early 50s, but risk of cholelithiasis increases with increasing age
- ASA status I–IV (day-cases should only include ASA I and II)
- Patients have an increased incidence of hiatus hernia and reflux disease
- Obesity is more common.

It is important to note that, unlike open cholecystectomy, laparoscopic surgery is feasible, from a surgical standpoint, in morbidly obese patients.

PREOPERATIVE ASSESSMENT AND INVESTIGATIONS

- Exclusion of associated medical conditions
- Laparoscopic technique may be contraindicated in patients with severe respiratory or cardiovascular problems
- Peritonitis is an absolute contraindication to this technique
- Deep vein thrombosis (DVT) prophylaxis, as indicated
- There is a significant move away from routine antibiotic prophylaxis compared with open surgery; check for allergy if antibiotics are used.

PREMEDICATION

- Anxiolysis with a benzodiazepine, if required
- Consider drugs to reduce gastric acidity.

PERIOPERATIVE MANAGEMENT

Monitoring:

- ECG
- Noninvasive BP
- Spo_2
- $ETco_2$ – this is mandatory
- Core temperature
- Blood loss may be difficult to assess

Anaesthetic technique

General anaesthesia is almost invariably the technique of choice.

- A relatively large pneumoperitoneum is required to facilitate this type of surgery
- A raised pco_2 due to absorption from the peritoneum may occur
- Raised intra-abdominal pressure will embarrass respiration and increase the risk of gastric aspiration
- A regional technique would require a very high block to avoid pain and/or discomfort
- The procedure is, on average, 50% longer than the open operation, and may take several hours.

General anaesthesia

All patients should have an intravenous infusion established prior to induction, and any preoperative fluid deficit should be corrected. This will help to reduce any potential complications from circulatory embarrassment.

Anaesthesia may be induced using any suitable intravenous induction agent. A rapid sequence induction may be indicated. The airway should be secured using endotracheal intubation and IPPV facilitated with a non-depolarizing muscle relaxant. Perioperative analgesia is normally provided using an opioid analgesic. Isoflurane may reduce the incidence of arrhythmias secondary to hypercarbia.

Special precautions

- A nasogastric tube may be required if the stomach is distended
- If a Nd-YAG laser is to be used, the usual safety precautions should be stringently applied.

Table 1.
Complications of laparoscopic cholecystectomy

Cardiovascular collapse
May be due to raised intra-abdominal pressure (IAP) – keep IAP below 15 mmHg. Venous return and cardiac output reduced. Systematic vascular resistance increased

Gas embolism
Consider in differential diagnosis of above. Diagnose by changes in $ETco_2$

Visceral damage
May go unrecognized and lead to subsequent peritonitis

Haemorrhage
Difficult to assess blood loss because of magnification. Gas may disperse blood through abdominal cavity. Retroperitoneal bleeding may not be visible

Hypercarbia
Monitor $ETco_2$. Change ventilatory pattern if necessary

Hypothermia
Large volumes of dry gas may be instilled into the peritoneum and cause cooling. Maintain body temperature (warming blanket, fluid warming and humidification)

POSTOPERATIVE MANAGEMENT

- Postoperative pain is usually less than with the open operation; many patients do not require potent opioid analgesics
- Some patients complain of shoulder-tip pain caused by gas trapped under the diaphragm
- Oxygen therapy may be required, especially in obese patients and patients with significant pulmonary atelectasis.

OUTCOME

The quoted reopening rate ranges from 1 to 6% in different series. The mortality rate is less than 0.4%, as opposed to 2% with open cholecystectomy.

An increasing number of selected patients are now being managed as day-cases, and laparoscopic cholecystectomy is now on the day-case agenda.

18

BIBLIOGRAPHY

Cunningham A J, Brull S J. Laparoscopic cholecystectomy: anesthetic implications. Anesthesia and Analgesia 1993; 76: 1120–1133

Lew J K L, Gin T, Oh T E. Anaesthetic problems during laparoscopic cholecystectomy. Anaesthesia and Intensive Care 1992; 20: 91–92

Marco A P, Yeo C J, Rock P. Anaesthesia for a patient undergoing laparoscopic cholecystectomy. Anesthesiology 1990; 73: 1268–1270

CROSS REFERENCES

Obesity
Patient Conditions 5: 148
Day-case surgery
Anaesthetic Factors 29: 542
Blood transfusion
Anaesthetic Factors 33: 616
Complications of position
Anaesthetic Factors 33: 618
Thrombotic embolism
Anaesthetic Factors 33: 664

OBSTRUCTION OR PERFORATION

B. J. Pollard

18

Perforation of the bowel results in the spillage of bowel contents into the peritoneal cavity. This might include proteolytic enzymes, bile, acid gastric contents, partially digested food, etc. The result is a rapidly developing chemical peritonitis.

Obstruction may present in a more insidious way, with intermittent abdominal pain, vomiting and either diarrhoea or constipation. Obstruction due to strangulation of the bowel is a more urgent situation.

Laparotomy for any of these conditions is an urgent or emergency situation. The aim is to explore the peritoneal cavity, discover the source of the problem, and repair any leaks or relieve any obstruction. Obstructed or strangulated sections of bowel may have to be resected. The peritoneal cavity is then usually washed out with warm saline before closure.

PATIENT CHARACTERISTICS

- More often older age groups, but can affect anyone
- Unless the patient has presented early, may be shocked and in urgent need of fluid resuscitation
- Will be in pain
- The actual diagnosis may not be certain
- There may be underlying malignancy, Crohn's disease or ulcerative colitis.

PREOPERATIVE ASSESSMENT AND INVESTIGATIONS

- Routine history and examination
- State of hydration – rehydrate intravenously as necessary
- Hb, white cell count, haematocrit
- Urea and electrolytes
- Chest X-ray; ECG in the older age groups
- Blood group and save serum or cross-match as indicated
- Arterial blood gases in the more severely ill patients
- Other investigations as indicated by the history and examination.

PREMEDICATION

None necessary in many patients. If in pain, a suitable dose of an opioid will suffice.

PERIOPERATIVE MANAGEMENT

Monitoring:

- ECG
- BP – noninvasive BP is adequate in most patients, but direct arterial pressure monitoring is advisable in the poor-risk patient, particularly if going to an ITU or high-dependency unit for postoperative care
- Sp_{O_2}
- ET_{CO_2}
- Fluid balance – a central venous pressure line is recommended to assist fluid replacement; a pulmonary artery flotation catheter should be considered in the more severely ill or poor-risk patient; a urinary catheter should be inserted.

Anaesthetic technique

A general anaesthetic technique is recommended. Regional anaesthesia should only be considered if general anaesthesia is contraindicated or otherwise highly undesirable. A spinal or epidural block should not be considered without full rehydration.

- Use a rapid sequence induction technique with tracheal intubation.
- If the patient has a nasogastric tube in situ, it is not usually necessary to remove it, but it should be aspirated before induction.
- Choice of technique for maintenance is not usually important; controlled ventilation with a muscle relaxant, volatile agent and narcotic is suitable.
- The use of nitrous oxide may be detrimental as it diffuses into gas-filled spaces in the body. Obstructed bowel may contain considerable volumes of trapped

gas, the volume of which will be increased if nitrous oxide is used. This introduces the risk of rupture of anastomoses or additional perforations. Many anaesthetists avoid nitrous oxide in these patients.
- Antibiotics are commonly requested by the surgeon. The use of an aminoglycoside may lead to difficulty with reversal of a neuromuscular block.
- It should be remembered that the stomach may not be empty at the completion of surgery and the patient should be extubated in the lateral position once airway reflexes have returned.

POSTOPERATIVE MANAGEMENT

- Good analgesia should be prescribed
- Oxygen by face-mask for at least 24 h
- A 24-h stay on the high-dependency unit is sensible for all but the most straightforward procedures in a previously fit patient.
- The more severely ill patient may need overnight ventilation on an ITU
- The occasional patient may develop septicaemia with the risk of adult respiratory distress syndrome and multiple organ failure.

OUTCOME

- Most patients can expect a satisfactory recovery from the acute episode, unless complications are present
- Mortality and morbidity is considerable in those patients who develop septicaemia unless this is treated aggressively
- The principal determinants of outcome are the underlying pathology which precipitated the acute incident and the severity of soiling of the peritoneal cavity.

CROSS REFERENCES

Emergency surgery
Anaesthetic Factors 29: 547
Postoperative pain management
Anaesthetic Factors 33: 655

OESOPHAGO-GASTRECTOMY

A. A. Khan

18

PROCEDURE

These cases should only be undertaken by senior and experienced anaesthetists and surgeons.

The operation is undertaken for the removal of neoplasms involving the oesophagus and stomach.

Carcinoma of the oesophagus
- Incidence in males (UK) 5.9–6.8 per 100 000 (Waterhouse 1976)
- 60% of neoplasms are in the lower third of the oesophagus
- Operative mortality >20% (Matthew 1986)

SURGERY

Resection and organ replacement by specialist surgeon.

Procedures:
- *Lower third* – left thoracoabdominal approach.
- *Middle third* – supine abdominal, then right thoracotomy (Lewis 1946).
- *Upper third* – 'triple approach': supine with paramedian incision, followed by a right thoracotomy, followed by a right anterior cervical incision.

PATIENT CHARACTERISTICS

- ASA II–IV

- Age 60–80 years
- Male/female ratio 3:1
- Alcohol- and tobacco-related in UK
- Cachexia and anaemia.

PREOPERATIVE ASSESSMENT

- Associated chronic obstructive airways disease, ischaemic cardiac disease and hypertension are common (NCEPOD 1991/92)
- Tracheal involvement possible; may require further investigation with CT or MRI scan
- Lung function assessment for one-lung anaesthesia
- Full blood count, urea and electrolytes, ECG and chest X-ray as a minimum
- Group and cross-match blood (at least 2 units).

PREPARATION

- Optimize treatment of intercurrent disease
- Correct anaemia and electrolyte imbalance
- Deep vein thrombosis (DVT) prophylaxis
- Night sedation may be needed on the night preceding surgery
- Premedication with a benzodiazepine and/or an opioid
- Discuss and arrange postoperative-care plan.

ANAESTHETIC PROCEDURES

- Warn ODA of positional requirements
- Warming blanket and intravenous fluid warmer
- Suitable range of double-lumen endobronchial tubes
- Humidifier for inspired gases
- Monitoring resource appropriate to a thoracic case:
  - ECG
  - Sao_2
  - $ETco_2$
  - BP (invasive – arterial line)
  - Airway pressures
  - Central venous pressure – internal jugular or antecubital fossa
  - Temperature – core (rectal) and peripheral (skin)
  - PCV Hb measurement facilities, e.g. microcentrifuge
  - Urinary catheter
  - Nerve stimulator for neuromuscular block assessment
- A general anaesthetic technique with, for example, thiopentone, atracurium, isoflurane, opioid is suitable
- In view of intraoperative positioning of the patient, particular care should be taken with the placement and securing of double-lumen tube and all invasive lines
- Intercostal block with 0.5% bupivacaine and/or a thoracic epidural catheter inserted before surgery
- A nasogastric tube may be requested by the surgeon; this will be repositioned gently after anastomosis is complete
- Antibiotic prophylaxis, depending on local policy (commonly metronidazole and a cephalosporin)
- Pneumatic anti-DVT boots
- Average duration of surgery is 3–4 h.

PERIOPERATIVE HAZARDS

- Haemorrhage – average blood loss is 300–1000 ml
- Ventilation – one-lung anaesthesia may be compromised in the respiratory cripple
- Cardiac arrhythmia or impaired filling due to surgical activity
- Cooling in the cachectic, elderly exposed patient.

POSTOPERATIVE MANAGEMENT

- ITU or a high-dependency unit
- Oxygen therapy, or elective ventilation in high-risk patients
- Suitable analgesic regimen:
  - Intercostal block, and/or
  - Thoracic epidural analgesia, or
  - Patient-controlled analgesia
- Continual monitoring
- Early physiotherapy
- Continued assessment of blood loss and thoracic underwater seal drain (average postoperative blood loss 200–1000 ml)
- Close observation for anastomotic leaks
- Antibiotic prophylaxis – septicaemia is a significant factor in morbidity.

It is common surgical practice to assess anastomotic competence by radio-opaque swallow and X-rays 48 h postoperatively. Substantial leakage may necessitate repeat thoracotomy.

OUTCOME

The overall mortality is high. The morbidity is compounded by the associated disease, in particular ischaemic heart disease and chronic obstructive airways disease in the older age group.

AUDIT

Medical audit has consistently shown perioperative mortality to be due to the following causes, in descending order of importance:

Respiratory infection	>30%
Septicaemia and adult respiratory distress syndrome	>28%
Myocardial infarction and heart failure	>20%
Anastomotic leak	>20%
Haemorrhage	>15%
Renal failure	>15%

CONCLUSION

Before embarking on this procedure a careful assessment should be made of whether the benefits of surgery outweigh the disadvantages.

This operation should only be carried out at centres equipped with an ITU, and scheduled for weekday surgery when full back-up facilities for this major operation are available.

BIBLIOGRAPHY

Waterhouse. IARC Scientific Publication No. 15, 1976

Lewis I. The surgical treatment of carcinoma of the oesophagus. British Journal of Surgery, 1946; 34: 18–31

Mathews H R, Powell D J, McConkey C C. Effect of surgical experience on the results of resection for oesophageal carcinoma. British Journal of Surgery, 1986; 73: 621–623

Campling E A, Devlin H B, Moile R W, Lunn J N. The Report of the National Confidential Enquiry into Perioperative Deaths 1991/1992. Published by the National Confidential Enquiry into Perioperative Deaths, London (1993)

CROSS REFERENCES

Postoperative anaesthesia for thoracic surgery patients
Surgical Procedures 17: 358

One-lung anaesthesia
Anaesthetic Factors 32: 602

Complications of position
Anaesthetic Factors 33: 618

Thrombotic embolism
Anaesthetic Factors 33: 664

Preoperative assessment of pulmonary risk
Anaesthetic Factors 34: 697

OPEN CHOLECYSTECTOMY

P. Bunting and R.G. Rowlands

This is an open abdominal procedure. The usual access is via an oblique subcostal (Kocher's), right paramedian or midline incision. The frequency of this procedure is declining due to laparoscopic techniques. It is still important for:

- The emergency situation
- Where laparoscopy proves difficult or complications occur.

PATIENT CHARACTERISTICS

- Any age in either sex, but more frequent in 'fat, fertile, females of forty'
- Associated with hypercholesterolaemia and haemolytic disease
- Patients may present on elective general surgical lists or as acute abdominal emergencies
- The patient may be jaundiced.

PREOPERATIVE ASSESSMENT

Depends upon the mode of presentation of the patient.

Elective surgical patient:

- Full history and examination
- Full blood count, urea and electrolytes
- Group-and-save serum
- Additional investigations according to any abnormal findings
- Where indicated (diabetics, obese, smokers, ischaemic heart disease, patients over 60 years) an ECG and chest X-ray should be performed.

Emergency surgical patient
- The likely presentation is with vomiting, dehydration and toxaemia
- Full history and examination; investigations as above
- Pain control with opioids
- Vomiting may require antiemetics and nasogastric tube
- Cardiovascular resuscitation may be required with intravenous fluid replacement therapy, as appropriate. If the patient has hypovolaemic shock then colloid should be used. If less than 5% dehydration, crystalloid can be given. Electrolyte abnormalities should be corrected, as appropriate
- Antibiotic therapy should be instituted as early as possible, according to local protocols.

JAUNDICED PATIENT

Jaundice is usually caused by obstruction to flow of bile in the common bile duct. There is impairment of liver function results. Plasma proteins and clotting factors are low; bilirubin levels are high. Coagulation studies are required. Vitamin K (1 mg) may be administered. Hepatorenal syndrome may occur.

ANAESTHETIC TECHNIQUE

Preinduction of anaesthesia:
- Routine minimal monitoring (ECG, noninvasive BP, $Sa{O_2}$, $ET{CO_2}$)
- The toxic patient may require central venous pressure monitoring.
- Patients undergoing emergency surgery are at risk of aspiration pneumonitis, and rapid sequence induction is mandatory.
- The icteric patient and the toxic hypovolaemic patient is at risk of developing renal failure. A diuresis should be induced with mannitol (1 g. kg^{-1} body weight). Dopamine (2–4 $\mu g\ kg^{-1}\ min^{-1}$) may also be used to maintain urine flow.

Induction and maintenance:
- Induction: a standard dose of any intravenous induction agent.
- Maintenance: nitrous oxide in oxygen with a volatile agent, tracheal intubation and IPPV with a nondepolarizing muscle relaxant
- Analgesia: an opioid analgesic, e.g. fentanyl (1–10 $\mu g\ kg^{-1}$)
- A regional anaesthetic technique, e.g. an epidural, may be considered (remember the possibility of a coagulopathy)
- Reversal of residual neuromuscular block on completion of surgery using standard agents.

Recovery – early:
- Oxygen by face-mask.
- Intravenous fluid therapy should be continued.
- Analgesia is necessary. This may be achieved by:
  - Opioids by the intramuscular route or, better, by a patient-controlled analgesia method
  - A regional technique. Epidural or intrapleural analgesia can be maintained by infusion pumps for both early and later postoperative recovery. Analgesia by paravertebral and intercostal block as a single shot can be used for the early postoperative phase.

Recovery – late
Complications specific to this upper abdominal procedure are basal atelectasis with concomitant hypoxia and hypostatic pneumonia subsequent to poor chest expansion secondary to pain. Patients may be obese, and therefore have a higher risk of deep vein thrombosis (DVT) and pulmonary embolism. The further management of these patients includes good analgesia, physiotherapy and early mobilization. Prophylaxis against DVT should be used as indicated.

BIBLIOGRAPHY

Engberg G. Respiratory performance after upper abdominal surgery. A comparison of pain relief with intercostal blocks and centrally acting analgesics. Acta Anaesthesiologica Scandinavica 1985; 29: 427–433
Moore D C. Intercostal nerve block for postoperative somatic pain following surgery of the thorax and upper abdomen. Bristish Journal of Anaesthesia 1975; 47: 284–286
Murphy D F. Interpleural analgesia. British Journal of Anaesthesia 1993; 71: 426–434

CROSS REFERENCES

The jaundiced patient
Patient Conditions 5: 142
Emergency surgery
Anaesthetic Factors 29: 547
Local anaesthetic techniques
Anaesthetic Factors 32: 600
Thrombotic embolism
Anaesthetic Factors 33: 664

SURGERY OF THE RECTUM AND ANUS

P. F. S. Lee and A. Sanchez-Capuchino

Patients for anaesthesia for this type of surgery have a wide age distribution and can be seriously debilitated. Rectal surgery will be largely due to malignancy and occur in a middle-aged to elderly age group who can also be suffering from concomitant disease. Bleeding, either occult or otherwise, can also be present, with the problem of blood transfusion.

Surgery to the colon, besides malignancy, also includes ulcerative colitis and Crohn's disease, which can occur in a much younger age group and who can present *in extremis*. Some of the ulcerative colitis patients may be severely toxic with a very low albumin. They can also be receiving steroid therapy which brings with it further possibilities for complications.

PREOPERATIVE ASSESSMENT

- General health, with particular attention to:
  - Ischaemic heart disease
  - Chronic bronchitis
  - Diabetes mellitus.
- Specific to pathology of the colon and rectum:
  - Weight loss
  - Anaemia
  - Intestinal obstruction
  - Present medication, e.g. steroids
  - Evidence of metastases.
- Investigations:
  - Routine biochemistry
  - Routine haematology
  - ECG, if indicated
  - Chest X-ray, if indicated
  - Other investigations, as indicated.

Many older patients will be on regular medication for a variety of conditions, e.g. antihypertensive treatment. A suitable regime for the continuation of these treatments should be determined.

PREMEDICATION

An oral dose of a benzodiazepine has proven very successful. Some patients can be somewhat disturbed by the bowel preparation, and allowance should be made for this. Opioids have also been widely employed, but may increase intraluminal pressure. A nasogastric tube should be inserted if there are any signs of obstruction.

ANAESTHETIC TECHNIQUE

Both general anaesthesia and regional techniques (spinal or epidural) have been widely employed. General anaesthesia using muscle relaxants and controlled ventilation has proven very successful. Because the patients are often required to be placed in a steep head-down position, controlled ventilation has significant advantages. Acute or obstructed patients should be intubated using a rapid sequence induction technique. Choice of induction agent lies between thiopentone or propofol for the majority of patients. Great care must be exercised when inducing anaesthesia in a shocked or toxic patient; etomidate may be more appropriate for these patients.

In addition to the routine intravenous access, a central line is extremely valuable. An arterial line can also offer increased safety, especially for the poor-risk patient.

The choice of muscle relaxants is wide. One of the intermediate acting agents is suitable, e.g. atracurium or vecuronium. Careful attention to dose may permit recovery without the routine use of neostigmine. This may be advantageous because it has been suggested that the incidence of colonic dehiscence may be increased by the use of neostigmine. Conclusive evidence to support or refute this is, however, lacking. The use of atropine or glycopyrrolate does not prevent the increase in peristalsis from neostigmine, and so the availability of a technique which does not employ neostigmine might be valuable.

Debate has recently centred around the choice of opioid. The use of morphine during and after colonic anastomosis has been linked by some authors to increases in intraluminal pressure. It is generally recommended that morphine should be avoided and pethidine used instead.

These patients can require large volumes of fluid during the operation and also in the postoperative period. Their fluid balance should be monitored carefully.

Routine use of prophylactic antibiotics has become standard practice; a combination of a cephalosporin with metronidazole is popular at present because it covers anaerobic gastrointestinal bacteria.

The employment of spinal and/or epidural anaesthesia has increased in popularity during recent years. There are considerable advantages to using these techniques in this type of surgery:

- Excellent analgesia during and after surgery
- Very good operative conditions; reduced bleeding and contracted intestine
- Reduction in blood loss
- Reduced incidence of thromboembolic complications.

The block is usually combined with a light general anaesthetic, and ventilation is controlled. Any fall in blood pressure can be controlled with the use of vasopressors (e.g. phenylephrine or methoxamine) and intravenous fluids.

An elegant technique is the spinal/epidural combination. The epidural space is first located, following which a fine spinal needle (a little longer) is introduced through the epidural needle and felt to pass through the dura. With the demonstration of free-flowing CSF, 3–4 ml of 0.5% hyperbaric bupivacaine is injected, after which the spinal needle is withdrawn and an epidural catheter inserted. Top-ups can be given if required during the operation. A suitable regime for postoperative analgesia might be 50 ml of 0.125% marcain with 5 mg of diamorphine at a rate of 4–6 ml h^{-1}. If an epidural is not employed postoperatively, then adequate analgesia must be provided by another technique, e.g. using a patient-controlled analgesia pump.

BLOOD TRANSFUSION

This subject has been debated intensely recently. Evidence suggests that there might be an increased incidence of carcinoma associated with blood transfusion. This is probably related to an immunosuppressive effect of the blood transfusion. To withhold a transfusion which is necessary would be clearly incorrect. On the other hand, it would appear that there is enough evidence to support a policy of not giving blood to these patients unnecessarily.

BIBLIOGRAPHY

Sene A, Walsh S, Jeocock J, Kingston R D, Robinson C. Blood transfusion does not have an adverse effect on survival after operation for colorectal cancer. Annals of the Royal College of Surgeons of England 1993; 75: 261–267

McKenzie P J. Deep venous thrombosis and anaesthesia. British Journal of Anaesthesia 1991; 66: 4–7

CROSS REFERENCES

Epidural and spinal anaesthesia
Anaesthetic Factors 32: 594
Blood transfusion
Anaesthetic Factors 33: 616
Local anaesthetic toxicity
Anaesthetic Factors 33: 642
Postoperative pain management
Anaesthetic Factors 33: 655

19

GYNAECOLOGY

D. Bogod

CANCER SURGERY/ PELVIC EXENTERATION

M. Heining

PROCEDURES AND INDICATIONS

- Vulvectomy, including radical vulvectomy for cancer of the vulva. Radical vulvectomy includes excision of the femoral and inguinal lymph nodes and may involve removal of parts of the urethra, vagina and bowel.
- Wertheim's and other forms of radical hysterectomy for advanced cancer of the uterine cervix. Wertheim's hysterectomy includes removal of the upper half of the vagina, broad ligaments and often the iliac and pelvic wall lymph nodes.
- Ovarian cystectomy and oophorectomy for cancer of the ovary; omentectomy may be done at the same time.
- Pelvic exenteration (excision of all pelvic viscera, fascia and lymphatics) as a rare 'last resort' for very advanced or recurrent cancer of the uterine cervix; or, more rarely, for severe radiation damage; very rarely for cancer of the vagina. In anterior exenteration the rectum is preserved, while in posterior exenteration the bladder and ureters are preserved.
- Vaginectomy, which may include excision of the bladder or rectum, for cancer of the vagina.
- Palliative surgery, such as colostomy or urinary diversion for obstruction.

PATIENT CHARACTERISTICS

- Often elderly, frail and cachectic (but patients with cancer of the cervix may be young)
- Cancer of the endometrium is significantly associated with diabetes and obesity (but rarely requires radical surgery)
- Specific associations with cancer of the ovary:
  - Complications of the malignant process (ascites and pleural effusions)
  - Complications of the large intra-abdominal mass (aortocaval compression and reduced lung compliance)
  - Systemic effects (anaemia, hypovolaemia).

PREOPERATIVE ASSESSMENT AND INVESTIGATIONS

- Exclude associated conditions including anaemia, pleural effusions
- Ensure blood available for transfusion
- Optimize chronic medical conditions
- Consider deep vein thrombosis (DVT) prophylaxis: the incidence of DVT is 40% in operations for gynaecological malignancy
- Assess nutritional state where appropriate, e.g. plasma proteins, albumin.

PREMEDICATION

These patients are commonly anxious, so a sedative premedication such as a benzodiazepine is usually indicated.

THEATRE PREPARATION

- Especially with more major surgery, maintenance of body temperature is important (fluid warmer, warming mattress, warm theatre, humidification of inspired gases)
- May require elective ITU admission
- Preparations for elective hypotension if required
- Invasive monitoring if indicated.

PERIOPERATIVE MANAGEMENT

General anaesthesia is almost invariably used for these major procedures.

- For less radical operations, a straightforward relaxant/opioid/volatile agent technique is appropriate
- When induced hypotension is required, e.g. for Wertheim's hysterectomy, an epidural (single shot or continuous) may be added

- With massive ascites or a huge ovarian cyst, induction of anaesthesia may precipitate profound hypotension or difficulty with ventilation; it is advisable to ensure that the surgeon is scrubbed and ready to perform immediate laparotomy to relieve the pressure
- Rapid sequence induction is indicated when there is raised intra-abdominal pressure, or where cancer of the ovary has caused intestinal adhesions leading to obstruction.

MONITORING

In addition to standard monitoring the following are necessary:

- Core temperature
- Blood loss
- Urine output
- Invasive haemodynamic monitoring (intra-arterial pressure monitoring and central venous pressure (CVP)) is desirable for major procedures such as pelvic exenteration or excision of a massive ovarian cyst or in the high-risk patient.

PATIENT POSITIONING

Prolonged operations in the lithotomy or Lloyd–Davies positions require particular attention to pressure points. The anaesthetist must be alert to the possibility of massive and/or very rapid blood loss. A considerable proportion of this may be 'occult', in the sense that it remains hidden in the abdominal cavity. If necessary, appropriate arrangements must be made with the blood bank and haematology department for assessment of clotting status and provision of fresh frozen plasma, platelets, etc.

POSTOPERATIVE MANAGEMENT

- Analgesia may be a major problem. Patient-controlled analgesia, continuous intravenous infusions and continuation of an epidural block with opioids and/or local anaesthetics all have a place.
- Fluid balance is important following these extensive intra-abdominal operations; CVP monitoring may need to be continued.
- ITU admission, with or without elective ventilation, may be indicated.
- Postoperative vomiting may be a major problem as in any gynaecological surgery.

OUTCOME

Prognosis is poor following most of these operations (Table 1). It must be remembered, however, that many of these operations are carried out for relief of symptoms (e.g. pressure symptoms of an ovarian mass) or in young women who often have young families (especially cancer of the cervix).

Table 1.
Five-year survival following surgery for gynaecological cancer

Operation	5-year survival (%)
Radical vulvectomy	60–65
Cancer of the vagina (any treatment)	30–35
Wertheim's hysterectomy	55–60
Cancer of the ovary (any treatment)	30–35
Pelvic exenteration	25–35

CROSS REFERENCES
Epidural and spinal anaesthesia
Anaesthetic Factors 32: 594
Induced hypotension during anaesthesia
Anaesthetic Factors 32: 597
Complications of position
Anaesthetic Factors 33: 618
Postoperative pain management
Anaesthetic Factors 33: 655
Thrombotic embolism
Anaesthetic Factors 33: 664

D&C/TOP

D. Knights

PROCEDURE

Dilatation and curettage (D&C) and suction termination of pregnancy (TOP) are common, minor surgical procedures. Diagnostic D&C is the most commonly performed surgical procedure in England and Scotland (26.2 per 10 000 population). D&C may include hysteroscopy which may lengthen the procedure.

Characteristics of these procedures are as follows:

- Short, often suited to the day-case situation
- Performed in lithotomy or, less commonly, Lloyd–Davies position
- Involves short periods of intense surgical stimulation at cervical dilation requiring deep anaesthesia
- D&C may be diagnostic (e.g. for postmenopausal bleeding) or therapeutic (e.g. for evacuation of retained products of conception (ERPC)).

PATIENT CHARACTERISTICS

- *D&C*: patients may be of any age from puberty onwards. Few diseases are directly linked to the need for surgery.
- *TOP*: patients are generally young and fit. Although rare, surgery may be required because of pre-existing disorders, e.g. cardiac abnormalities.

Patients for TOP or ERPC who are beyond the first trimester of pregnancy or who have symptomatic gastro-oesophageal reflux require precautions against aspiration of gastric contents.

PREOPERATIVE ASSESSMENT AND INVESTIGATIONS

- Assess and adjust adequacy of resuscitation if patient for ERPC has vaginal bleeding, as this may be considerable and continuing
- If urgent ERPC, then ascertain time since last oral intake and what analgesia has been given, as this may indicate the possibility of a full stomach
- Ascertain length of gestation and any symptoms of reflux, if appropriate
- Investigations as clinically indicated, especially Hb if bleeding
- Exclude coexisting disease and any limitation of knee and hip movement (need for lithotomy position)
- Explanation and reassurance
- Assess suitability for day-case care.

PREMEDICATION

- Anxiolysis rarely required with adequate reassurance, but a short-acting benzodiazepine may be given even to the day-case patient if necessary.
- H_2 antagonists and sodium citrate, if at risk of regurgitation.
- Ascertain if prostaglandin pessary is to be given as this may increase requirements for postoperative analgesia. Prostaglandins are used to soften the cervix, especially in primiparous patients, to allow a less traumatic dilatation of the cervix.

THEATRE PREPARATION

- Routine equipment and machine check
- Adequate personnel to ensure simultaneous lifting or lowering of legs to avoid injuries to hips and knees
- Position to avoid nerve injury, particularly that due to pressure on the medial or lateral lower leg from lithotomy poles.

PERIOPERATIVE MANAGEMENT

Monitoring:

- F_IO_2
- SpO_2
- ECG
- Noninvasive BP.
- $ETCO_2$.

Anaesthetic technique

Although the short nature of each of these procedures is well suited to general anaesthesia, there are no surgical contraindications to regional techniques.

- For TOP or ERPC, avoid uterine relaxation due to high alveolar volatile agent concentrations by using a TIVA technique or low concentration of volatile agent
- Intravenous induction and spontaneous ventilation with nitrous oxide/oxygen/ volatile and a short-acting opioid, e.g. alfentanil or fentanyl, to obtund response to cervical dilation is otherwise suitable.
- Rapid sequence induction and endotracheal intubation if at risk of regurgitation
- Oxytocics may be requested by the surgeon. Synthetic oxytocin (e.g. Syntocinon) is preferable to ergometrine containing products (e.g. Syntometrine) as these may cause hypertension, bronchospasm, nausea and vomiting, especially if given intravenously. Oxytocin may cause a transient fall in arterial pressure.
- NSAIDs may be useful for postoperative analgesia, especially if prostaglandin pessaries have been used as these cause significantly more pain due to uterine contractions.
- Antiemetics may be appropriate in view of the high incidence of postoperative nausea and vomiting in patients undergoing gynaecological surgery.

There is little evidence that concentrations of volatile agents of 0.5 MAC or less lead to clinically significant increase in blood loss during TOP or ERPC and any uterine relaxation will be rapidly reversed by discontinuing the agent. It should also be borne in mind that it will take a considerable time for a given concentration of a volatile agent in the inspired gas to rise to the same concentration in the uterus.

POSTOPERATIVE MANAGEMENT

- Recover in lateral position with supplemental oxygen until awake. If trachea was intubated, then extubate awake in the lateral position.
- Male recovery staff should have chaperones in view of the possibility of inappropriate patient behaviour during recovery, especially from propofol/alfentanil anaesthesia.
- Simple analgesics are usually adequate. Postoperative pain is usually minimal, but may be greater in those patients who normally experience painful menstruation or who received a prostaglandin pessary.
- If patient condition allows and domestic circumstances are suitable, most patients may be allowed home on the day of surgery, with appropriate advice with regard to residual effects of anaesthesia.

BIBLIOGRAPHY

Department of Health. Office of Population, Censuses and Surveys. Hospital Inpatient Enquiry 1985 (Ser MB4). HMSO, London, 1987

Information and Statistics Division, Common Services Agency for the Scottish Health Service. Scottish Health Statistics. Common Services Agency, Edinburgh, 1990

Nelson V M, Young P N, Smyth D G et al. Hallucinations after propofol. Anaesthesia 1987; 43: 170–171 (letter)

CROSS REFERENCES

Day-case surgery
Anaesthetic Factors 29: 542

Complications of position
Anaesthetic Factors 33: 618

FERTILITY SURGERY

I. F. Russell

19

PROCEDURE

The procedures range from diagnostic hysteroscopy and laparoscopy through various forms of laparoscopic surgery to laparotomies for tubal reconstruction or for pelvic adhesiolysis in the hope of creating access for future laparoscopic treatments. Procedures may form part of an in vitro fertilization programme; these include egg collection (transvaginally or laparascopically) and gamete intrafallopian transfer (GIFT). An operating microscope may be used during the tubal surgery. Many purchasers no longer feel able to fund fully this type of service, so it is likely that the patient has made a major contribution to the costs of the procedure. Patients are generally highly motivated and knowledgeable about their treatment, and as such often request further information and an explanation of the anaesthetic procedure.

Except for the laparotomies, the procedure is most likely to be performed:

- As an elective day-case
- Laparoscopically
- Within a 'therapeutic time window' – due to ovarian or endometrial stimulation by carefully controlled hormonal preparation
- One of a series of diagnostic/therapeutic interventions
- Note that, depending on the findings, and/or time available, a 15 min diagnostic procedure may suddenly become (intraoperatively) a therapeutic procedure (60–90 min).

PATIENT CHARACTERISTICS

- The patients are generally young, physically fit women (ASA I or II)
- Infertility may be associated with specific psychological problems ranging from anxiety/stress disorders to compulsive/obsessive neurosis, and the women need a sympathetic and understanding approach
- Occasionally there may be associated endocrine problems
- Be aware of the sedative/analgesic cocktail used if the patient is an 'emergency' case following a failed 'office' procedure.

PREOPERATIVE ASSESSMENT

- There may be a history of a recent large (1 l) oral fluid intake preoperatively to fill the bladder for purposes of pelvic ultrasound scan
- Previous multiple anaesthetic history
- Increased risk of postoperative nausea and vomiting; level of risk may be indicated by response to previous anaesthesia and surgery
- Teeth (crowns/caps).

PREMEDICATION

Should take account of:

- Day-case surgery
- Patient's psychological state
- High level of motivation
- Rarely need sedative premedication
- Need to pre-empt postoperative pain with oral/rectal NSAID
- A nurse from the ward, with whom the patient is familiar, can provide valuable psychological support for the patient while awaiting induction of anaesthesia.

THEATRE PREPARATION

The anaesthetist should understand the equipment needs for the procedure and should ensure the presence of:

- Appropriate padded leg supports/stirrups; laparoscopy and video equipment with appropriate connectors and adaptors
- The insufflation equipment and be aware of its particular characteristics, e.g. gas used, flow rates, flow restriction and pressure limits (if any)
- Laser equipment and appropriate eye protection.

For diagnostic laparoscopic procedures nitrous oxide may be used as the insufflating gas. For operative work where diathermy or laser use may be a possibility, then carbon dioxide must be used.

ANAESTHETIC TECHNIQUE

There is no evidence that any anaesthetic technique is associated with higher conception rates, but gynaecologists are reducing the demand on theatre and anaesthetic time by increasing their use of analgesic/sedative methods in 'office' procedures. Unlike ophthalmology and dentistry, there are no guidelines on the use of such sedative/analgesic drugs.

If anaesthesia is required, then it should be appropriate for day-case surgery in young women:

- Avoid suxamethonium
- Be aware of the cumulative nature of some common anaesthetic agents, especially if the procedure is prolonged (>30 min); use short-acting agents
- TIVA should be considered since nitrous oxide is reputed to increase nausea and vomiting by over 30%
- Spinal (≤26 French gauge or pencil point needle) or epidural may be used; motivated patients with an active interest in the proceedings may like to see what is going on
- Ensure removal of peritoneal gas at end of procedure to reduce incidence and severity of postoperative shoulder-tip pain.

PERIOPERATIVE MANAGEMENT

During surgery, a previously correctly placed endotracheal tube may become displaced (endobronchial) due to the head-down position and elevation of the diaphragm secondary to intraperitoneal gas.

Routine monitoring with special attention to:

- Heart rate (audible indication of heart rate is valuable)
- Inspiratory pressure
- Intra-abdominal pressure
- $ETCO_2$
- Surgeon's video screen (to assess operating conditions), but do not be distracted from anaesthetic monitoring.

UNEXPECTED COLLAPSE

May be due to:

- Sudden extreme bradycardia/cardiac standstill secondary to peritoneal distension or traction on pelvic structures
- Blood loss from unrecognized laceration to a major pelvic blood vessel; blood loss may be retroperitoneal and thus unseen
- Venous gas embolism
- Tension pneumothorax.

19

POSTOPERATIVE MANAGEMENT

Pain relief

Ideally oral, with different mechanism of action from that given as premedication. Narcotics may be required; these are best given earlier rather than later.

Antiemetic/nausea prophylaxis

Appropriate use of antiemetic drugs, either prophylactically or in the treatment of nausea and vomiting.

BIBLIOGRAPHY

Robinson J S, Thompson J M, Wood A W. Fire and explosing hazards in operating theatres: a reply and new evidence. British Journal of Anaesthesia 1979; 51: 908

CROSS REFERENCES

Day-case surgery
Anaesthetic Factors 29: 542
Complications of position
Anaesthetic Factors 33: 618

19

HYSTERECTOMY AND LASER SURGERY

D. Phillips

PROCEDURE

Optical examination of the uterine cavity with or without surgical intervention.

UTERINE DISTENSION

Uterine distension is for:
- Visualization
- Removal of blood and detritus
- Dissipation of heat.

It is achieved with:
- Fluid (saline, glycine, dextran)
- CO_2.

Complications

Fluid:
- Absorption and circulatory overload
- Dilution – hyponatraemia, hypoproteinaemia, TUR syndrome
- DIC
- Anaphylaxis.

Carbon dioxide:
- Abdominal distension during long procedures (leak via the Fallopian tubes)
- CO_2 absorption – acidosis, arrhythmias
- CO_2 embolism.

THE LASER

The commonest lasers in gynaecological use are the Nd-YAG and CO_2 lasers. All staff concerned should be familiar with both the Department of Health guidelines on the safe operation of medical lasers and local policies.

Although the laser should only be operated in the surgical field, precautions must be taken to protect against injury from inadvertent operation:

- Patient eye protection
- Staff eye protection
- Designated theatre with locked doors and covered windows (if any)
- Removal/covering of reflective surfaces
- No casual access
- Extra eye protection outside in case of need.

Intrauterine laser surgery is carried out under fluid uterine distension.

Hysteroscopic laser procedures include:
- Endometrial destruction
- Elimination of menses
- Removal of benign intrauterine pathology
- Sterilization.

Complications are:
- Uterine perforation
- Haemorrhage (usually controlled with the laser, but may necessitate laparotomy if uterus is perforated)
- Heat transmission (not clinically important at typical power settings for intrauterine surgery).

PATIENT CHARACTERISTICS

May be any age from mid-teens onwards. No particular medical disorder is associated with the need for hysteroscopic laser surgery, except for anaemia. The procedure may be performed as a day-case, therefore check suitability (medical status, home circumstances, etc.).

PREOPERATIVE ASSESSMENT

- Check for anaemia
- Other investigations, as indicated by patients' medical status.

PREMEDICATION

- Anxiolysis (if required) with a benzodiazepine
- Consider an antiemetic
- Antibiotic prophylaxis, e.g. coamoxyclav or a cephalosporin with metronidazole may be given with the premedication or on induction of anaesthesia.

THEATRE PREPARATION

- Familiarity with policies on the use of the laser
- Availability of patient eye protection (pads, foil)
- Availability of staff eye protection (goggles).

PERIOPERATIVE MANAGEMENT

Monitoring:
- ECG
- Noninvasive BP
- Pulse oximetry
- Fluid balance (including uterine distension fluid)
- Capnography
- Airway pressure
- Core temperature.

Position patient in the lithotomy position.

Anaesthetic technique
Resuscitation equipment should be available.

- General:
  - Spontaneous or controlled respiration
  - Free choice of maintenance technique.
- Regional
  - Epidural or spinal
  - Light sedation may be needed (e.g. midazolam)
  - Oxygen via face-mask.
- Local:
  - Paracervical, intracervical and intrauterine local block may be given by the surgeon; not favoured by all gynaecologists
  - Light sedation may be needed (e.g. midazolam)
  - Analgesia, e.g. ketorolac or alfentanil.

FLUID BALANCE

Measurement of fluid instilled and retrieved can be difficult, but should be attempted because of the possible effects of fluid absorption.

Sample protocol:

1000 ml absorbed	– continue surgery
1500 ml absorbed	– end surgery as soon as possible
2000 ml absorbed	– stop surgery

Excessive blood loss is rarely a problem, therefore keep intravenous fluids to a minimum.

Watch for signs of TUR syndrome, especially with extensive surgery and high intrauterine pressures.

POSTOPERATIVE PERIOD

Any postoperative discomfort may be eased by NSAIDs, e.g. ketorolac.

Gynaecological procedures are associated with an increased incidence of nausea and vomiting, and an antiemetic should be prescribed.

BIBLIOGRAPHY

DHSS. Guidelines On The Safe Use of Lasers In Medical Practice. DHSS, London, 1984

Morrison L M M, Davis J, Sumner D. Absorption of irrigating fluid during laser photocoagulation of the endometrium in the treatment of menorrhagia. British Journal of Obstetrics and Gynaecology 1989; 96: 346–352

Osborne G A, Rudkin G E, Moran P. Fluid uptake in laser endometrial ablation. Anaesthesia and Intensive Care 1991; 19: 217–219

Studd J (ed). Progress in obstetrics and gynaecology. Churchill Livingstone, Edinburgh, 1991, vol 9

Van Boven M J, Singelyn F, Donnez J, Gribomont B F. Dilutional hyponatraemia associated with intrauterine endoscopic laser surgery. Anesthesiology 1989; 71: 449–450

CROSS REFERENCES

Day-case surgery
Anaesthetic Factors 29: 542
Complications of position
Anaesthetic Factors 33: 618
TUR syndrome
Anaesthetic Factors 33: 675

LAPAROSCOPY

S. Piggott

PROCEDURE

Gynaecological laparoscopy may be diagnostic (e.g. dye studies) or therapeutic (e.g. tubal ligation).

Carbon dioxide is insufflated at pressures of 20–40 mmHg to create a pneumoperitoneum. This allows the pelvic organs to be visualized via a telescope passed through a small subumbilical incision.

Lithotomy position with a Trendelenberg tilt is required.

Instrumentation of the vagina is needed to manipulate uterus or inject dye.

PATIENT CHARACTERISTICS

Most patients presenting for gynaecological laparoscopy are relatively healthy. A high proportion are day-cases.

PREOPERATIVE ASSESSMENT AND INVESTIGATION

All patients should have a full blood count; other investigations need only be performed if indicated.

PREMEDICATION

Oral benzodiazepines, if required.

PERIOPERATIVE MANAGEMENT

Problems associated with laparoscopy:

- Hypercapnia – carbon dioxide is absorbed from the peritoneum. This is compounded by a reduction in FRC and compliance secondary to the pneumoperitoneum and Trendelenberg position. $P(\text{a-E}')CO_2$ rises during laparoscopy, but there is good correlation between $PaCO_2$ and $PE'CO_2$. $ETCO_2$ reflects changes in arterial CO_2 tension.
- Regurgitation is a risk because of raised intragastric pressure and head-down tilt.
- Altered haemodynamics – intraabdominal pressures in excess of 40 cmH_2O compresses the inferior vena cava and restricts venous return, with a consequent fall in cardiac output of up to 40%. Blood pressure and heart rate may be unaffected because total peripheral resistance increases.
- Arrythmias – manipulation of the pelvic organs often causes significant bradycardia.
- Perforation of abdominal viscera or major blood vessels by trocar.
- Pneumothorax.
- Carbon dioxide embolism is a rare but potentially fatal complication of laparoscopy, although successful resuscitation has been reported (Table 1).

Table 1.
Carbon dioxide embolism

Diagnosis
Sudden decrease in $ETCO_2$
ECG changes
Hypotension
Decrease in saturation
Management
Stop CO_2 insufflation
100% oxygen
Left lateral decubitus position
Place central line and attempt aspiration of gas from right atrium
CPR as required

Monitoring:

- ECG
- Noninvasive BP
- $ETCO_2$
- Pulse oximeter
- Airway pressure
- Intra-abdominal pressure.

General anaesthesia

General anaesthesia with muscle relaxation, endotracheal intubation and IPPV is the preferred technique because it guarantees airway protection and adequate ventilation. A recent report, however, suggests that in selected patients spontaneous ventilation via a laryngeal mask may be satisfactory.

If the Bain circuit is used for IPPV, higher than normal gas flows are needed to prevent rebreathing; a fresh gas flow of 110 ml kg^{-1} min^{-1} and minute ventilation of 175 ml kg^{-1} min^{-1} should be used. Analgesia is best achieved with an opioid combined with a NSAID. The latter reduces the requirements for opioids which exacerbate PONV and sedation. The choice of opioid is influenced by the duration of surgery and whether the patient is an in-patient or a day-case. An antiemetic should be given before reversal.

The brevity of some procedures could make reversal of nondepolarizing neuromuscular block difficult. Mivacurium, or a small dose of atracurium or vecuronium, are suitable.

Regional techniques

An epidural block over T5–S5 can provide satisfactory anaesthesia for laparoscopy.

It is also possible to perform laparoscopy under local anaesthesia, with or without sedation.

POSTOPERATIVE MANAGEMENT

Pain arises because of:

- Visceral trauma, particularly to the fallopian tubes after sterilization. This is usually short-lived.
- Residual carbon dioxide which causes diaphragmatic irritation and referred shoulder-tip pain. The surgeon should ensure that as much gas as possible leaves the peritoneal cavity at the end of the procedure.
- Peritoneal inflammation has been demonstrated two to three days after laparoscopy and is probably responsible for any persistent discomfort.
- A combination of an opioid and a NSAID provides effective analgesia. Take-home medication should be prescribed for day-patients.
- PONV is frequently associated with laparoscopy. Varying incidences are quoted, and other factors, including the administration of opioids and phase of menstrual cycle, are involved but at least 50% of patients can be expected to have symptoms after gynaecological surgery.

BIBLIOGRAPHY

Gillberg L E, Harsten A S, Stahl L B. Preoperative diclofenac sodium reduces post-laparoscopy pain. Canadian Journal of Anaesthesia 1993; 40: 406–408

Goodvin A P, Rowe W L, Ogg T W. Day case laparoscopy. A comparison of two anaesthetic techniques using the laryngeal mask during spontaneous breathing. Anaesthesia 1992; 47: 892–895

CROSS REFERENCES

Day-case surgery
Anaesthetic Factors 29: 542
Complications of position
Anaesthetic Factors 33: 618

20

OBSTETRICS

D. Brighouse

OVERVIEW

D. Brighouse

This section deals with the major problems encountered by the anaesthetist with responsibility for the obstetric patient. Most women embarking upon pregnancy are young and healthy, and encounter no problems during childbirth other than the need for analgesia. A minority either have significant pathology present before becoming pregnant, or develop such pathology during pregnancy or delivery. The anaesthetist must be equipped to deal with these women.

Hypertensive disease of pregnancy and pulmonary embolism are the leading causes of maternal death. Although anaesthetic-related deaths have reduced in number during the last decade, they still occur, and are usually avoidable.

The role of the obstetric anaesthetist:
- Understanding of the physiological and pathophysiological changes occurring in pregnancy
- Awareness of the effects of analgesic and anaesthetic interventions on the fetus
- Involvement in antenatal assessment of risk
- Provision of antenatal education about analgesia and anaesthesia for childbirth
- Provision of analgesia and anaesthesia for labour, delivery, and the puerperium
- Provision of cardiovascular monitoring and fluid balance management during the peripartum period, where indicated
- Identification and further management of complications arising from anaesthetic intervention
- Organization of teaching and clinical audit (and research when appropriate).

Factors associated with anaesthetic-related maternal mortality:
- Failure to intubate the trachea
- Aspiration of gastric contents
- Haemorrhage
- Severe pre-eclampsia
- Failure of postoperative care
- Complications of regional anaesthesia
- Adult respiratory distress syndrome
- Inadequate preanaesthetic assessment.

Many of the contributors to this section reiterate very basic principles of obstetric anaesthesia, but it is failure to follow these principles that leads to maternal morbidity and mortality.

Basic principles of obstetric anaesthesia:
- Understanding of physiological changes of pregnancy
- Early identification of potential problems
- Early provision of epidural analgesia for high-risk women
- Avoidance of aortocaval compression
- Use of appropriate antacid prophylaxis
- Use of regional rather than general anaesthesia when possible
- Use of rapid sequence induction of general anaesthesia
- Skilled assistance for the anaesthetist.

Principles of resuscitation of the pregnant woman:
- Adopt the modified lateral position – resuscitation is impossible in the supine position if the woman is undelivered
- Safeguard the airway
- Support the circulation
- Deliver the woman as rapidly as possible.

Regional analgesia and anaesthesia

The use of epidural infusions of local anaesthetics, with or without additional opioids has increased the consumer acceptability and reduced the unwanted side-effects of epidural analgesia for labour.

Combined intrathecal and epidural fentanyl/bupivacaine mixtures may allow ambulation to continue for a short time in labour, and may reduce the likelihood of instrumental delivery.

Regional anaesthesia is the technique of choice for Caesarean section. Many obstetric units in the UK now perform at least 70% of all Caesarean sections under regional blockade. Spinal anaesthesia, with or without the back-up of an epidural catheter, is now more popular in the UK for elective section than is epidural anaesthesia alone. Epidural analgesia is frequently extended for urgent Caesarean section.

The use of intrathecal catheters is unlikely to become widespread in obstetric anaesthesia.

CURRENT CONTROVERSIES

Aspirin

The multicentre CLASP trial has failed to demonstrate that low-dose aspirin is universally effective in the prophylactic treatment of pre-eclampsia, although selected high-risk mothers may benefit from treatment. The study did not show an increased incidence of bleeding complicatons associated with the use of regional analgesia and low-dose aspirin. Nevertheless, opinion about the safety of regional techniques in patients taking aspirin remains divided. Use of the bleeding time as a reliable predictor of risk is disputed.

Coagulopathy

Known coagulopathy or full therapeutic anticoagulation are clear contraindications to regional anaesthetic techniques. Many anaesthetists would not consider treatment with prophylactic heparin a contraindication to epidural or spinal blockade, although care should be taken with the timing of anaesthetic procedures in relation to heparin treatment.

The lower limit of platelet count for administration of regional anaesthesia is empirical. A cut-off of 80 000 is generally agreed prudent by the majority of obstetric anaesthetists, although isolated case reports have been published of uneventful regional blockade in women with platelet counts in single figures.

Pre-eclampsia

A policy of fluid restriction for severe pre-eclamptics continues to find popularity with many obstetricians and anaesthetists. However, there is an increasing trend towards use of volume replacement accompanied by vasodilating drugs; the so-called 'volume expansion' regime. The increasing use of a multidisciplinary approach to the management of this group of women, with written protocols and appropriate use of invasive monitoring, may clarify the optimum method of management.

The role of prophylactic anticonvulsants for women who have not fitted is unclear. There are no reliable prognostic indicators of eclampsia. Magnesium sulphate significantly reduces the incidence of fit recurrence after a woman has fitted. Its use as a prophylactic anticonvulsant is not yet proven. Phenytoin does not reliably prevent fit recurrence. Diazepam may be useful in terminating fits, but does not prevent fit recurrence. The use of chlormethiazole involves administration of large volumes of fluid, and the accompanying sedation may compromise the patient's airway. It should not be used in the obstetric unit.

Epidurals and backache

Prospective studies are in progress. Retrospective work appears to suggest an association between epidural analgesia and backache after delivery. The issue is unresolved.

The need for careful follow-up of all women receiving regional analgesia and anaesthesia is clear. The true incidence of early and late complications of regional techniques is not known.

Postdural puncture headache

Management of postdural puncture headache (PDPH) remains controversial; large multicentre studies are required to demonstrate the optimal time for epidural blood patching, and to collect follow-up data on this group of women.

Gastric emptying

It is clear that gastric emptying is delayed by the administration of opioids, regardless of the route of administration. Gastric emptying appears to have returned to normal by 48 h after delivery, but speed of emptying during and immediately after delivery is still unknown. The routine administration of clear antacids and H_2 antagonists to all women during labour is practised by some, but not all, obstetric anaesthetists.

Amniotic fluid embolism

This is still a cause of sudden unavoidable

maternal death. The aetiology is unclear, and positive diagnosis can only be made at postmortem examination. An increased index of suspicion in women presenting with dyspnoea and cardiovascular collapse, and early use of invasive monitoring may improve supportive treatment and elucidate future management strategies.

Many issues in obstetric anaesthesia remain unproven. The contributors in this section present current opinions about their topics, with suggestions for safe management. This does not preclude other management strategies.

BIBLIOGRAPHY

Barker P, Callender C C. Coagulation screening before epidural analgesia in preeclampsia. Anaesthesia 1991; 46: 67–69
Carrie L E S. Post dural puncture headache and extradural blood patch. British Journal of Anaesthesia 1993; 71: 179
Collis R E, Baxandall M L, Srikantharajah I D, Edge G, Kadim M Y, Morgan B M. Combined spinal epidural analgesia with ability to walk throughout labour. Lancet 1993; 341: 767–768
Davison J M, Lindheimer M D. Volume homeostasis and osmoregulation in human pregnancy. Baillières Clinical Endocrinology and Metabolism 1989; 3(2)
de Swiet M. Aspirin and its relevance to pre-eclampsia. International Journal of Obstetric Anesthesia 1992; 1: 178
Gibbs C P, Modell J H. Management of aspiration pneumonitis. In: Miller R D (ed) Anesthesia, 3rd edn. Churchill Livingstone, New York
MacArthur C, Lewis M, Knox E G, Crawford J S. Epidural anaesthesia and long term backache after childbirth. British Medical Journal 1990; 301: 9–12
Ostheimer G W (ed). Manual of obstetric anesthesia, 2nd edn. Churchill Livingstone, New York, 1992
Report on Confidential Enquiries into Maternal Deaths in the UK 1985–87. HMSO, London 1991
Reynolds F. Placental transfer of drugs. Current Anaesthesia and Critical Care 1991; 2: 108–116
Stacey R G W, Watt S, Kadim M Y, Morgan B M. Single space combined spinal–extradural technique for analgesia in labour. British Journal of Anaesthesia 1993; 71: 499–503
Russell R, Groves P, Taub N, O'Dowd J, Reynolds F. Assessing longterm backache after childbirth. British Medical Journal 1993; 306: 1299–1303
Whitehead G M, Smith M, Dean Y, O'Sullivan G. An evaluation of gastric emptying times in pregnancy and the puerperium. Anaesthesia 1991; 48: 53–57

CROSS REFERENCES

Pre-eclampsia
Surgical Procedures 20: 424
Amniotic fluid embolism
Anaesthetic Factors 33: 612
Cardiopulmonary resuscitation
Anaesthetic Factors 34: 687

ANAESTHESIA FOR FIRST AND SECOND TRIMESTERS

J. Goddard

PROCEDURE

The incidence of nonobstetric surgery is approximately 1–1.5% of pregnancies (much lower than in the general population – incidence 5%).

Surgery may be elective or emergency. It may be related to the pregnancy (e.g. cervical cerclage, torsion of ovary), or incidental to the pregnancy. Most common emergency surgery is for trauma and appendicectomy.

Spontaneous abortion occurs most frequently following gynaecological surgery, or where the uterus is manipulated. Postpone elective surgery until at least 6 weeks postpartum. Urgent operations should be delayed until the second trimester.

THE PATIENTS – MOTHER AND FETUS

Fetal considerations:

- Organogenesis most susceptible during days 14 to 56. CNS development continues into the neonatal period.
- Maintenance of placental blood flow.
- Gestational viability:
  - Increased risk of spontaneous abortion
  - IUGR and prematurity.

Maternal considerations:

- Remember the physiological changes of pregnancy:
  - Hormonal from 6 weeks
  - Mechanical from second trimester.
- Increased sensitivity to general and local anaesthetics:
  - MAC decreased by 25–50%
  - Dose of local anaesthetics decreased by one-third.

ANAESTHETIC MANAGEMENT

- Provide safe anaesthesia for the mother
- Maintain the pregnant state
- Ensure the best fetal outcome.

Placental blood flow is reduced by maternal hypotension, hyperventilation, pain or apprehension. Intraoperative hypoxia, shock, infection and postoperative complications increase the incidence of prematurity and fetal loss.

PREOPERATIVE ASSESSMENT

First trimester

Premedication:

- Acid aspiration prophylaxis advisable – incidence of heartburn is approximately 30% in the first trimester
- Ranitidine (150 mg orally; 50 mg i.m. in emergency; no reported teratogenicity)
- Benzodiazepines associated with a four-fold increase in cleft lip with or without cleft palate
- Opiates may be used.

Second trimester

- More marked physiological changes
- Uterus intra-abdominal.

Premedication:

- Acid aspiration prophylaxis mandatory. Ranitidine as above, with 30 ml 0.3 M sodium citrate orally, immediately preoperatively.

Liaise with obstetric staff for fetal monitoring peri- and post-operatively; external heart monitoring feasible after 18–20 weeks.

From second trimester, aortocaval compression is a possibility. Patients should be transported in the left-lateral position. Graduated compression stockings are advisable, as hypercoagulability and venous stasis predispose to thromboembolism.

PERIOPERATIVE MANAGEMENT – GENERAL ANAESTHESIA

First trimester

Some elective minor procedures may be

possible using inhalational anaesthesia (beware the obese patient or multiple pregnancy).

Second trimester and all emergencies in the first trimester
Rapid sequence with good preoxygenation and cricoid pressure. IPPV using opioid and a relaxant plus a volatile agent. None of the anaesthetic drugs have been conclusively proven to be either teratogenic or safe. No particular regimen is therefore safer than any other.

Intraoperative monitoring:
- Routine standards
- Pulse oximetry essential
- $ETco_2$ helpful (maintain at around 4.0 kPa)
- Invasive monitoring may be required for major procedures, or where maternal condition dictates
- Fetal monitoring after 20 weeks, where practical.

Positioning of patient
Uterine displacement is essential after 20 weeks (15° lateral tilt or wedge).

Emergence and recovery
- Awake extubation in the left-lateral position
- Ensure good oxygenation
- Continue fetal monitoring.

Analgesia
- Opioids (intravenous or intramuscular)
- The use of NSAIDs is controversial; they are best avoided due to theoretical risk of premature ductus closure in utero.

PERIOPERATIVE MANAGEMENT – REGIONAL TECHNIQUES

This is the preferred technique where the surgery is suitable and the patient consents:

- Avoids risks of general anaesthesia to mother
- Lower spontaneous abortion rate
- Improved postoperative analgesia.

POSTOPERATIVE MANAGEMENT

- Maintain good oxygenation
- Maintain adequate analgesia
- Fetal monitoring
- Tocolytics controversial (maternal deaths)
- Early mobilization.

NOTES ON PARTICULAR DRUGS

Anticholinergics
Atropine causes maternal and fetal tachycardia. No effect with glycopyrrolate.

Induction agents
Thiopentone may decrease uterine blood flow (UBF) by up to 35% secondary to maternal hypotension.

Ketamine causes an increase in uterine tone and a decrease in UBF in the first and second trimesters.

Opioids
Morphine and pethidine are associated with animal teratogenicity only.

Fentanyl appears to be safe.

Muscle relaxants
Do not readily cross the placenta.

Suxamethonium may show prolonged action in later pregnancy.

Nitrous oxide
Remains controversial, but no substantive evidence of adverse effects in human studies

Note that the manufacturer lists the first 16 weeks of pregnancy as an *absolute* contraindication, so avoid if possible.

Volatile agents
All tend to decrease uterine tone, dilate uterine arteries, and increase UBF at less than 1.5 MAC.

UBF will be decreased secondary to hypotension in higher concentrations.

Vasopressors
α Adrenergic agents decrease UBF, and can increase uterine activity.

Ephedrine improves UBF.

Adrenaline and dopamine can reduce UBF.

BIBLIOGRAPHY

James F M. Anaesthesia for nonobstetric surgery during pregnancy. Clinics in Obstetrics and Gynaecology 1987; 30: 621–628

Ostheimer G W (ed). Manual of obstetric anesthesia. Churchill Livingstone, Edinburgh, 1992

Folb P I, Graham Dukes M N (eds). Drug safety in pregnancy. Elsevier, Amsterdam, 1990

CROSS REFERENCES

Antacid prophylaxis
Surgical Procedures 20: 400

Complications of position
Anaesthetic Factors 33: 618

ANALGESIA FOR LABOUR

M. Bellman

Women in labour are amongst the healthiest patients that anaesthetists will meet. Physiological changes in pregnancy are described in detail elsewhere (Crawford 1984), but important in this context are supine hypotension, the venous drainage of the epidural space, reduced, FRC and twin delivery. Common conditions of concern to the anaesthetist include haemorrhagic conditions which contraindicate epidurals, PET, diabetes, drug addiction and obesity.

PRELIMINARY COUNSELLING

It is much easier to discuss obstetric analgesia at a planned meeting in the antenatal clinic. This commonly defuses emotional tensions that may run high when labour pains reach their peak. Anaesthetists should be prepared to discuss issues, including alternatives to epidurals, and be prepared to answer questions. There are several excellent video recordings to demonstrate epidurals. Advice on the risks of epidurals varies, but most people would warn about accidents: dural puncture (1%), hypotension (2%), incomplete block (3%),* and the need to keep still. A discussion on backache and the alleged increase in incidence of forceps delivery is also appropriate. The high success rate of epidurals (85% completely satisfied and 11%

* These figures are based on the Maternity Unit at Withington Hospital over a year's reports. They have not been published, but have been the subject of hospital audit discussions.

partly satisfied*) compared to entonox and opioids should be discussed.

NARCOTIC ANALGESICS

Narcotic analgesics have a long tradition in obstetric analgesia, but poor efficacy. Pethidine is the most commonly used, but diamorphine might be better. The adverse effects of nausea, vomiting, respiratory depression, drowsiness and variable analgesia are visible. More insidious is the delayed gastric emptying, resulting in a full stomach.

ENTONOX

Entonox is now piped to most units. It is useful for short periods, but exhausting for long periods. The alleged improvement in oxygen delivery to the fetus, caused by an increased inspired oxygen concentration (50%) does not occur. Maternal hyperventilation shifts the oxygen dissociation curve to the left reducing P_ao_2.

TRANSCUTANEOUS ELECTRICAL NERVE STIMULATION (TENS)

TENS has not lived up to early hopes. There is no scientific evidence that it closes the pain gate and it probably acts as a distraction only. Trials in obstetric patients have not been successful.

EPIDURALS

Before performing any epidural, the anaesthetist should take a brief history. This should include a general medical history, any clotting problems, back problems, neurological disease or back sepsis. The anaesthetist should also determine the reason for the request. For details of how to perform an epidural, see p. 594. The commonest serious complications that a trainee may have to deal with are:

- Dural puncture (Stride & Cooper 1993) (Table 1)
- Incorrect placement of solution (Table 2)
- Hypotension.

HYPOTENSION

Hypotension commonly occurs because the sympathetic nerves leave the spine between TI and L2. Pain fibres to the body of the

Table 1.
Dural punctures

Cause
- Tuohy needle puncture
- Epidural catheter puncture
- Epidural catheter migration.

Predisposing factors
- Very fat patients (average depth of space is 5 cm)
- Very thin patients (average depth of space is 5 cm)
- Inexperienced anaesthetist
- Use of new technique or equipment
- Patient movement

Management
- Repeat at different space
- Careful test dose
- Epidural infusion of saline for 24 h
- Offer blood patch 24 h postpuncture

Table 2.
Incorrect placement of solution

Location	Reaction	Manifestation	Treatment
Intravascular (test doses may not detect this)	Toxicity	Convulsions	Oxygen anticonvulsants; intubate if necessary
Intrathecally (test doses will usually detect)	Total spinal	CVS collapse; respiratory collapse	Inotropes; intubate and ventilate
Into ligaments	No effect	No analgesia; no BP change; no motor loss; no sensory change	Repeat epidural

uterus are at T10–L1 and these must be blocked to relieve pain in the first stage of labour. The vaginal canal is innervated by S2–S4 which must be blocked for the second stage of labour. The combination of reduced venous return caused by the supine hypotensive syndrome and hypotension induced by epidural block is potentially dangerous to the fetus. There is a greatly reduced cardiac output and a redistribution of blood flow resulting in fetal hypoxia. All pregnant mothers should be nursed in either the sitting or lateral position and the blood pressure checked regularly. Position has very little effect on the spread of epidural blocks. Hypotension should be treated by placing the mother head-down with a quick intravenous infusion of crystalloid. If hypotension persists, 5–10 mg ephedrine should be given intravenously and the height of the block reassessed.

SELECTION OF PATIENTS FOR EPIDURAL

Suitable mothers include those expecting a long labour, forceps delivery or twins. It is particularly valuable for mothers with PET (improves placental blood flow) and diabetes (improves stability).

Unsuitable subjects include those with back sepsis, existing hypotension, clotting disorders and reluctant patients. Caution should be exercised in patients with pre-existing back problems, neurological disease and those who are psychologically disturbed or unable to remain still.

There are many individual local anaesthetic regimes. Many units institute epidural blockade using either low concentration bupivacaine (0.125–0.25%) alone, or a combination of bupivacaine and fentanyl (0.1–0.125% bupivacaine with fentanyl 2–2.5 μg/ml), in volumes of 10–15 ml. The epidural may then be maintained with intermittent boluses of the local anaesthetic and opioid solution, or with an infusion (0.0625–0.1% bupivacaine with fentanyl 2–2.5 μg/ml). These regimens provide analgesia without significant motor block. The mother may therefore be able to ambulate or sit out of bed if she wishes.

POSTDELIVERY PERIOD

Every maternity unit should operate a follow-up scheme to assess success and complication rates and institute appropriate therapy. Common residual effects are headache (2%), backache (4%), micturition difficulties (1%) and numbness (0.7%), but these will not all be due to an epidural, particularly if the patient had an instrumental delivery in the lithotomy position.

Persistent headache may be due to dural puncture. Classic symptoms include a bilateral headache exacerbated by sitting up. Photophobia is common and the patient feels generally miserable. A blood patch has over 90% success rate and should be offered. If headache returns, repatching until the cure is permanent is suggested (Brownridge 1983).

Epidurals have many benefits. They do work, resulting in healthier, less exhausted mothers and babies with good Apgar scores. They also enable obstetric intervention, if necessary.

BIBLIOGRAPHY

Brownridge P. The management of headache following accidental dural puncture in obstetric patients. Anaesthesia and Intensive Care 1983; 11: 4–15

Crawford J S. Principles and practice of obstetric anaesthesia, 5th edn. Blackwell Scientific, Oxford, 1984

Stride P C, Cooper G M. Dural taps revisited: a 20 year survey from Birmingham Maternity Hospital. Anaesthesia 1993; 48: 247–255

CROSS REFERENCES

Epidural and spinal anaesthesia
Anaesthetic Factors 32: 594
Local anaesthetic toxicity
Anaesthetic Factors 33: 642
Total spinal anaesthesia
Anaesthetic Factors 33: 667

ANTACID PROPHYLAXIS

G. O'Sullivan

20

The classic description of the acid pulmonary aspiration syndrome by Mendelson in 1946, focused the anaesthetist's attention on the gastrointestinal tract. Prophylaxis became mandatory when successive maternal mortality reports implicated Mendelson's syndrome as one of the commonest anaesthetic-related causes of maternal death (Report 1964–1966, 1967–1969). Antacid administration, every 2 h during labour, with a further bolus before surgery was for many years the cornerstone of prophylaxis. Within 10 years of the wide acceptance of antacid prophylaxis it was obvious that the regimes used had made little or no difference to the maternal mortality from aspiration, and particulate antacids themselves were acknowledged to be toxic if inhaled (Gibbs et al 1979). The increasing use of regional anaesthesia for Caesarean section and the introduction of H_2 antagonists are factors to which the current decrease in incidence of aspiration during pregnancy can be attributed (Report 1985–1987). Thus the obstetric anaesthetist must strive to use regional block as often as possible for both elective and emergency surgery.

GASTROINTESTINAL PHYSIOLOGY

Lower oesophageal pH monitoring in pregnant women at term has shown an increased incidence of reflux compared to nonpregnant controls. This process is reversed by the second postpartum day. At term the pregnant woman should therefore be regarded as having an incompetent lower gastro-oesophageal sphincter (Vanner & Goodman 1989).

Studies on gastric secretion during pregnancy indicate that whilst gastric acid secretion may be decreased during the second trimester, it is essentially unchanged at term (Murray et al 1957).

Pregnancy does not significantly delay the gastric emptying of liquids or solids, but established labour may cause an unpredictable delay in gastric emptying that is markedly potentiated by the use of narcotic analgesia (Nimmo et al 1975a). By 24 h postpartum, gastric emptying is essentially normal (Whitehead et al 1993).

PROPHYLAXIS AGAINST ACID PULMONARY ASPIRATION

The use of antacids and H_2 antagonists should now be an established routine prior to both elective and emergency Caesarean section.

Antacids

The aspiration of stomach contents in late pregnancy has long been known to be associated with a high level of morbidity and mortality (Mendelson 1946, Report 1964–1966). Inhalation of solid material may lead to respiratory obstruction, whilst the pulmonary aspiration of acidic gastric contents will produce a severe pneumonitis. The severity of this acute lung injury is related to both the acidity and volume of the inhaled gastric contents. It has been suggested that if the pH of inhaled stomach contents was greater than 2.5 and the volume less than 0.4 ml kg^{-1}, then severe acid aspiration is unlikely. These values, which were extrapolated from animal studies, have been questioned (Gibbs et al 1979). In any case, general anaesthesia for the pregnant woman at term is potentially dangerous, as relaxation of both lower and upper oesophageal sphincters may lead to aspiration of stomach contents unless appropriate precautions are taken.

Mendelson (1946), in his classic paper, proposed the witholding of solid food during labour and prophylactic administration of 'warm antacid solutions' as a means of reducing the lethal consequences of inhaling acidic gastric contents. In subsequent years, as the mortality from Mendelson's syndrome was catalogued in the Confidential Reports into

Maternal Deaths, it was suggested that antacids should be administered every 2 h during labour with a further bolus before induction of anaesthesia. Initially, antacids containing magnesium were the most commonly employed because of their powerful in vitro neutralizing capacity, and because they did not interfere with gastric emptying or result in rebound gastric acid secretion. This regime, however, ignored the possibility that the repeated administration of antacid would cause an increase in intragastric volume and would thereby fail to reduce the risk of reflux and regurgitation with aspiration. Successive Maternal Mortality Reports confirmed this failure, and it was also shown that the aspiration of particulate-containing antacids was potentially as toxic as inhaling acid solutions and, in addition, did not mix quickly with gastric contents (Holdsworth et al 1980). The result was that nonparticulate antacids, such as 0.3 M sodium citrate, came into widespread clinical use. The short duration of action of nonparticulate antacids such as sodium citrate, however (median duration of action is approximately 30 min), means that they should be administered shortly before induction of general anaesthesia; they are of little value given prophylactically.

H_2 receptor antagonists

H_2 receptor antagonists are now widely used to prevent acid aspiration as they not only increase intragastric pH but also reduce the volume of gastric fluid. They have no effect on acid already present in the stomach. Both cimetidine and ranitidine are effective, but the latter is more popular as it has a longer duration of action and is devoid of effects on hepatic enzymes.

Ranitidine (150 mg orally) should be administered to all mothers presenting for elective Caesarean section on the night prior to, and the morning of, surgery. In the event of an emergency Caesarean section, ranitidine (50 mg) should be given intravenously as soon as the decision for surgery is made and, in addition, 30 ml of 0.3 M sodium citrate should be administered immediately prior to induction of anaesthesia.

Recent interest has focused on omeprazole. This drug inhibits gastric acid production by selectively blocking the proton pump in the gastric parietal cells. It is well tolerated by mother and baby, but as yet appears to offer no advantage over ranitidine.

METOCLOPRAMIDE

Several studies have attempted to reverse the delay in gastric emptying caused by opioids. Intramuscular metoclopramide (10 mg) significantly increased gastric emptying in a group of primigravidae, some of whom had received pethidine during labour (Howard & Sharp 1973). Another study could not show a reversal of the delay in gastric emptying caused by pethidine or diamorphine (Nimmo et al 1975b). In patients undergoing elective surgery intravenous but not intramuscular metoclopramide has been shown to antagonize the delay in gastric emptying caused

Table 1.
Prophylaxis against acid pulmonary aspiration

Elective Caesarean section	
Regional block	Oral ranitidine (150 mg), 8 and 2 h prior to surgery
General anaesthesia	Oral ranitidine (150 mg), 8 and 2 h prior to surgery; 0.3 M sodium citrate (30 ml) immediately prior to induction
Emergency Caesarean section	
Regional block and general anaesthesia	Intravenous ranitidine (50 mg); oral 0.3 M sodium citrate (30 ml)
	Intravenous metoclopramide (10 mg), if opiates have been administered or food has recently been ingested
	If general anaesthesia, empty stomach through nasogastric tube during the operation
Women in labour with increased risk of Caesarean section	Oral ranitidine (150 mg), every 6 h during labour; oral 0.3 M sodium citrate prior to induction

by morphine premedication (McNeill et al 1990). Thus, since metoclopramide is also known to increase gastro-oesophageal sphincter pressure (Cotton & Smith 1981), there is clearly a case for the intravenous administration of this agent before emergency Caesarean section, particularly if the mother has recently ingested semisolid food. Table 1 illustrates a prophylactic regime against Mendelson's syndrome.

BIBLIOGRAPHY

Cotton B R, Smith G. Single and combined effects of atropine and metoclopramide on the lower oesophageal sphincter pressure. British Journal of Anaesthesia 1981; 53: 869–879

Gibbs C P, Schwartz K J, Wynne J W, Hood C I, Kluck E J. Antacid pulmonary aspiration in the dog. Anesthesiology 1979; 51: 380–385

Holdsworth J D, Johnson K, Mascall G, Gywynne Roulston R, Tomlinson P A. Mixing of antacids with stomach contents. Another approach to the prevention of the acid aspiration (Mendelson's syndrome). Anaesthesia 1980; 35: 641–650

Howard G A, Sharp D S. Effect of metoclopramide on gastric emptying during labour. British Medical Journal 1973; i: 446–448

McNeill M J, Ho E T, Kenny G N C. Effect of IV metoclopramide on gastric emptying after opioid premedication. British Journal of Anaesthesia 1990; 64: 450–452

Mendelson C L. The aspiration of stomach content into the lungs during obstetric anaesthesia. American Journal of Obstetrics and Gynecology 1946; 52: 191–205

Murray F A, Erskine J P, Fielding J. Gastric secretion in pregnancy. British Journal of Obstetric Gynaecology 1957; 64: 373–381

Nimmo W S, Wilson J, Prescott L F. Narcotic analgesics and delayed gastric emptying during labour. Lancet 1975a; i: 890–893

Report on Confidential Enquires into Maternal Deaths in England and Wales 1964–1966. HMSO, London, 1969

Report on Confidential Enquiries into Maternal Deaths in England and Wales 1967–1969. HMSO, London, 1972

Report on Confidential Enquiries into Maternal Deaths in the United Kingdom 1985–1987. HMSO, London, 1991

Vanner R G, Goodman N W. Gastro-oesophageal reflux in pregnancy at term and after delivery. Anaesthesia 1989; 44: 808–811

Whitehead E M, Smith M, Dean Y, O'Sullivan G. An evaluation of gastric emptying times in pregnancy and the peripineum. Anaesthesia 1993; 48: 53–57

CAESAREAN SECTION – GENERAL ANAESTHESIA

I. Mettam

PROCEDURE

Caesarean section is usually performed by lower uterine segment incision, rarely by classical uterine incision. Urgency ranges from planned and scheduled, to life-saving emergency.

PATIENT CHARACTERISTICS

The majority are fit females with an obstetric problem. A minority have significant systemic disease.

Physiology of late pregnancy:
- Reduced respiratory reserve
- Susceptibility to acid aspiration
- Likelihood of aortocaval compression.

INDICATIONS FOR GENERAL INSTEAD OF REGIONAL ANAESTHESIA

- Extreme urgency
- Patient preference
- Existing or anticipated hypovolaemia
- Sepsis
- Clotting abnormality
- Neurological disease
- Failed regional technique.

PREOPERATIVE ASSESSMENT

The majority of women will have been

screened in the antenatal clinic. While elective patients should have a routine preoperative visit, emergencies may only have a rapid assessment. Standard history and examination is appropriate, with particular enquiry for evidence of pre-eclampsia, diabetes, anaemia, or other significant disease.

Investigations

- Recent Hb
- Scan result indicating site of placenta
- Blood grouped and screened for antibodies with sample saved. Preoperative cross-match only if excessive bleeding likely, if antibodies expected to delay cross-match, or if blood not able to be supplied within 20 min of an urgent request.

PREMEDICATION

Avoid sedatives as these will affect the neonate.

> **Acid aspiration prophylaxis:**
> *H2 antagonist*
> - Elective – give oral ranitidine (150 mg) previous night and 2–4 h preoperatively
> - Emergency – give 50 mg i.v. as soon as operative delivery is anticipated
>
> *Antacid*
> 0.3 M sodium citrate, 30 ml orally 5 min before induction

THEATRE PREPARATION

- A suitably experienced anaesthetist
- A trained anaesthetic assistant
- A full range of equipment and drugs for general anaesthesia; difficult-intubation aids should be immediately to hand
- Facilities and personnel for resuscitation of neonate
- Universal donor blood stored near theatre.

PERIOPERATIVE MANAGEMENT

Monitoring

As a minimum:

- ECG
- Noninvasive BP
- Spo_2
- Carbon dioxide and oxygen analysers.

Any additional monitoring, as indicated.

Positioning

Avoid full supine position at all times, including during transfer.

On operating table place supine with pelvic wedge (usually tilt to left but occasionally better to right).

Many units prepare and drape abdomen before induction to minimize induction–delivery interval and drug accumulation in fetus, especially for emergencies. Some units anaesthetize the patient in an anaesthetic room in a standard fashion for elective cases.

Induction

Rapid sequence induction:

- Large-bore, free-flowing intravenous infusion
- Sleep dose of thiopentone (3–4 mg kg^{-1}) giving rapid loss of consciousness but minimal placental transfer; etomidate is indicated in some cases for improved cardiovascular stability
- Suxamethonium (1–1.5 mg kg^{-1}) to allow the airway to be rapidly secured under optimal intubating conditions
- Opioids and other measures to blunt response to intubation only in mothers at risk – balance against risk to neonate.

Maintenance before delivery

Ensure maternal anaesthesia, but minimize fetal effects.

- Nitrous oxide (50%) in oxygen to ensure optimal fetal oxygenation
- Supplement with volatile agent to a total MAC of 1.0–1.5
- Maintain neuromuscular block with vecuronium or atracurium, which have an appropriate time-course, freedom from cardiovascular effects, and minimal placental transfer
- IPPV to normocapnia for pregnancy (P_aco_2 4 kPa).

Maintenance after delivery

- Syntocinon (5 units i.v.) stat plus infusion (15 units in 500 ml over 3 h)
- Give intravenous opioids in a standard dose
- Increase nitrous oxide to 70%
- Ensure that concentration of volatile agent is adequate for anaesthesia, but limited in order to avoid significant effect on uterine contractility.

Intraoperative problems

- Aortocaval compression

- Failed intubation
- Massive bleeding
- Drug reaction
- Amniotic fluid embolus.

Emergence and recovery
Airway remains at risk until full recovery of reflexes. Extubate on side when neuromuscular block is adequately reversed and tracheal tube no longer tolerated. Must be fully recovered in a suitable environment until safe to be transferred to postnatal ward.

POSTOPERATIVE PERIOD

Standard opioid and/or NSAID analgesia. Early mobilization to reduce risk to thrombo-embolism. Adequate fluid intake to replace losses and encourage lactation.

BIBLIOGRAPHY

Lussos S A, Datta S. Anesthesia for Cesarean delivery. Part III: General anesthesia. International Journal of Obstetric Anesthesia 1993; 2: 109–123

Moir D D, Thorburn J. General anaesthesia. In: Moir D D, Thorburn J (eds) Obstetric anaesthesia and analgesia, 3rd edn. Baillière Tindall, London, 1986

CROSS REFERENCES

Antacid prophylaxis
Surgical Procedures 20: 400
Difficult and failed intubation
Surgical Procedures 20: 408
Hypertensive disease of pregnancy
Surgical Procedures 20: 414
Management for the mother with coexisting medical disease
Surgical Procedures 20: 419
Obstetric haemorrhage
Surgical Procedures 20: 422
Amniotic fluid embolism
Anaesthetic Factors 33: 612
Thrombotic embolism
Anaesthetic Factors 33: 664

CAESAREAN SECTION – COMBINED SPINAL–EPIDURAL ANAESTHESIA

L. E. S. Carrie

DEFINITION

Combined spinal–epidural (CSE) techniques are those whereby local anaesthetic and/or other antinociceptive agents may be introduced into both the subarachnoid and epidural spaces to provide pain relief.

VARIETIES

- Single needle–single interspace: after epidural injection, the needle is advanced through the dura and arachnoid for subarachnoid injection.
- Double needle–double interspace: usually an epidural catheter is introduced first, before subarachnoid injection at an adjacent interspace.
- Needle through needle–single interspace: a needle placed in the epidural space acts as a guide for a spinal needle passed through it. After subarachnoid injection the spinal needle is removed and an epidural catheter introduced (currently the most popular method). A recent report describes the introduction of catheters into both subarachnoid and epidural spaces by this method.
- Needle beside needle–single interspace: a special device is required which is essentially an epidural needle with a spinal needle introducer attached to, or incorporated in, its shaft.

ADVANTAGES FOR CAESAREAN SECTION

A CSE technique offers:
- The speed of onset, the reliability and the low toxicity potential of spinal anaesthesia, combined with
- The potential of an epidural catheter to modify or prolong the blockade.

EQUIPMENT

Single needle–single interspace method
A fine-gauge or pencil-point needle is preferable to reduce the incidence of postdural puncture headache. The serious limitation is that an epidural catheter cannot be introduced.

Double needle–double interspace method
Any spinal and epidural needles favoured by the anaesthetist may be used.

Needle through needle–single interspace method
The important measurement is the distance by which the spinal needle, when fully inserted, protrudes past the tip of the epidural needle. A too short or too long a protrusion may lead to failure of the technique, and thus it is advisable to use one of the needle sets specifically designed for the technique, where the maximal protrusion is usually 10–12 mm.

Needle beside needle–single interspace method
A special device is required (see above). This makes possible the introduction of an epidural catheter before subarachnoid puncture. If the latter fails, however, either both device and catheter must be removed before another attempt, or the epidural catheter may be left in place and sub-arachnoid injection made at an adjacent interspace.

POTENTIAL PROBLEMS

Failure to obtain cerebrospinal fluid
Reasons include:

- Epidural needle not in epidural space, making it unlikely that the spinal needle will be directed towards the subarachnoid space (in case of single interspace techniques).
- Spinal needle protrusion through epidural needle is too short, or too lateral in the epidural space, the cylindrical dural sac being further from the ligamentum flavum in the lateral part of the epidural space. In the most lateral parts of the epidural space, the spinal needle may pass tangentially across the vertebral canal to strike its bony walls without ever piercing the sac. If spinal needle protrusion is too long, it may transfix the dural sac, passing out again anteriorly.
- Spinal needle may be correctly placed, but orifice occluded, e.g. by a nerve root.

Difficulty passing the epidural catheter, or reflux of blood along the catheter
With techniques in which the subarachnoid injection has already been given, it is important to control the spread of this solution. In these cases the 'Oxford' position is recommended (see below). The problem does not occur when the catheter is inserted first.

Subarachnoid placement of epidural catheter
A theoretical possibility with the needle through needle technique, it is a potential complication of any epidural technique, the catheter passing through the dura mater weakened by contact by the epidural needle. Epiduroscopic study has shown that this complication is not more likely to occur with the CSE technique as neither 18 gauge nor 16 gauge catheters will pass through the dural puncture made by a 25 gauge spinal needle.

Metallic particle contamination or needle-tip damage
Careful research has shown no evidence of such contamination or damage occurring as a result of contact between the needle tips.

'OXFORD' POSITION (FOR HYPERBARIC SOLUTIONS)

This is the left-lateral position with the left shoulder supported on an inflated 3-l bag and the head on three pillows. This causes lateral flexion of the upper thoracic spine, thus reproducing the uphill gradient from the mid to upper thoracic and cervical spines normally found in the supine position. After epidural catheter insertion has followed subarachnoid injection, the patient is turned to the same position on the right side.

Advantages
- Better control of the upper level of block than when using the supine 'wedged' position.
- The lateral position is superior to the wedged position for relieving aortocaval occlusion.

- If catheter-insertion difficulty occurs with needle through needle CSE techniques, a hyperbaric solution is trapped (mainly on the dependent side) at a level appropriate to analgesia for Caesarean section (i.e. mid to upper thoracic segments). If delay in turning is such as to reduce effective spread to the other side, the block can be augmented via the epidural catheter.

APPLICATION OF CSE TECHNIQUES TO CAESAREAN SECTION

Considerable flexibility of choice is available:

- Surgical analgesia may be attempted by the spinal block alone, only using the epidural catheter to modify the block if it is not perfect, to prolong it if surgery becomes lengthy, or to provide postoperative pain relief.
- Surgical analgesia may be achieved by using both subarachnoid and epidural routes from the outset.
- Spinal analgesia may be deliberately not extended to the highest segments necessary for a Caesarean section, these segments being secondarily blocked by epidural analgesia. This technique is intended to reduce the incidence of hypotension associated with the more rapid onset of spinal blockade.

In each variety, hyperbaric or isobaric spinal solutions of local anaesthetic may be used, although many obstetric anaesthetists consider the latter too difficult to control for Caesarean section.

BIBLIOGRAPHY

Carrie L E S. Extradural, spinal or combined block for obstetric surgical anaesthesia. British Journal of Anaesthesia 1990; 65: 225–233
Carrie L E S. Spinal and/or epidural blockade for Caesarean section. In: Reynolds F (ed) Epidural and spinal blockade in obstetrics. Baillière Tindall, London, 1990, p 139–150

CROSS REFERENCES

Caesarean section – spinal anaesthesia
Surgical Procedures 20: 406
Epidural for Caesarean section
Surgical Procedures 20: 412
Epidural and spinal anaesthesia
Anaesthetic Factors 32: 594
Local anaesthetic toxicity
Anaesthetic Factors 33: 642

CAESAREAN SECTION – SPINAL ANAESTHESIA

A. G. Davis

PROCEDURE AND INDICATIONS

Subarachnoid block (SAB) has recently become the most widely practiced method of anaesthesia for Caesarean section in the author's unit, having replaced epidural block, except where the latter has been in use in labour. General anaesthesia has thus been consigned to occasional use only.

Indications for Caesarean section in which the use of SAB has proved satisfactory, despite having been considered controversial, include:

- *Acute fetal distress.* A decision-to-delivery interval of 20–30 min can be achieved, which is usually acceptable.
- *Placenta praevia.* Circulatory stability need not be compromised if preoperative bleeding is no more than slight, an experienced obstetrician is operating, and there is adequate preparation to deal with haemorrhage. It may be advisable to exclude anterior placenta praevia in the presence of a uterine scar.
- *Severe pre-eclampsia.* An unduly rapid fall in an elevated blood pressure has not been a problem.

PATIENT CHARACTERISTICS

The presence of the gravid uterus, through its effect on the dynamics of the vertebral venous system and the dural sac, profoundly affects the response to SAB, resulting in a smaller dose being required to produce a block to a given level, especially in the small-stature obese woman with a large baby.

PREOPERATIVE PREPARATION

- Gain the woman's confidence by appropriate explanation
- Assess possible technical problems.

ANAESTHETIC TECHNIQUE

Particular requirements:

- To produce a block to a predictable segmental level
- To prevent hypotension
- To prevent postdural puncture headache.

The first two requirements have, to a large extent, been met as the technique to be described has evolved through earlier experience, while success towards achieving the third has greatly increased following the advent of atraumatic spinal needles.

Protocol for technique

This should be followed with obsessional attention to every detail so that the only variable factor is the dose of hyperbaric bupivacaine which is chosen according to height and weight, as shown in Table 1.

- Preload with 1 l of Hartmann's solution
- Position the woman sitting on the operating table
- Identify the L2–L3 intervertebral space
- Use a 25 gauge pencil-point needle, distal opening facing cephalad
- Perform spinal injection over 5 s
- Immediately change the woman's position to supine wedged
- Note the time
- Monitor in order to detect and treat hypotension
- Test sensation to pin-prick at 4 min
- Head-down tilt if block has not reached T6 (unusual).

Some problem situations

When identification of landmarks is impossible due to obesity, a useful guide is that the L2–L3 space is situated at about three-fifths of the vertical distance from the woman's shoulder level to the surface on which she is sitting.

In the case of urgent operations, the time taken for transfer to the operating room should be used for rapid preloading. A spinal dose reduction of up to one-third may be necessary in the presence of a partially effective epidural – the more nearly effective the epidural the smaller the spinal dose required. When a partially effective spinal block needs to be repeated, the dose required has been found to be approximately half of the original.

Table 1.
Dosage schedule (hyperbaric bupivacaine (ml)) for spinal anaesthesia for Caesarean section*

Pregnant weight (kg)	Height (cm)								
	140	145	150	155	160	165	170	175	180
50	**1.5**	1.7	1.8	1.9					
55	**1.5**	**1.6**	1.8	1.9	2.0				
60	1.4	**1.6**	**1.7**	1.8	2.0	2.1			
65	1.4	1.5	**1.7**	**1.8**	1.9	2.1	2.2		
70	1.3	1.5	1.6	**1.8**	**1.9**	2.0	2.2	2.3	
75		1.4	1.6	1.7	**1.9**	**2.0**	2.1	2.3	2.4
80		1.4	1.5	1.7	1.8	**2.0**	**2.1**	2.2	2.4
85			1.5	1.6	1.8	1.9	**2.1**	**2.2**	2.3
90			1.4	1.6	1.7	1.9	2.0	**2.2**	**2.3**
95				1.5	1.7	1.8	2.0	2.1	**2.3**
100				1.5	1.7	1.8	1.9	2.1	2.2
105					1.6	1.7	1.9	2.0	2.2
110						1.7	1.8	2.0	2.2

* The values shown in bold relate to the mode group of body mass index (26–29) for each height.
Diamorphine (0.4 mg in 0.4 ml 0.9% sodium chloride), or fentanyl (20 mcg = 0.4 ml) is added to the chosen volume of heavy bupivacaine.

PROBLEMS AND COMPLICATIONS

Table 2 shows an audit of 207 consecutive cases performed by, or supervised by, the author since the introduction of atraumatic needles in January 1991, up to September 1993.

Table 2.
Problems and complications in 207 consecutive cases

Problem/complication	(Incidence) No.	%
Failure to produce adequate block	11	5.3
Satisfactory after repeating	7	3.4
Converted to epidural	3	1.4
Converted to general	1	0.5
Section completed under spinal block, pain felt but tolerated*	2	1.0
Hypotension requiring ephedrine	16	7.7
'High block' (dyspnoea/dysphagia/inability to cough)	0	0.0
Postdural headache	5	2.4

* Data obtained from a questionnaire.

POSTOPERATIVE MANAGEMENT

Subarachnoid diamorphine or fentanyl provides analgesia for several hours, during which time a diclofenac suppository is administered. Later, oral diclofenac provides adequate relief in 90% of women.

Most women are ambulant later the same day, with intravenous fluids discontinued but bladder catheterization continued for 24 h.

BIBLIOGRAPHY

Kestin I G. Spinal anaesthesia in obstetrics. British Journal of Anaesthesia 1991; 66: 597–607
Lussos S A, Datta S. Anaesthesia for caesarean delivery. Part 1: General considerations and spinal anaesthesia. International Journal of Obstetric Anaesthesia 1992; 1: 79–91

CROSS REFERENCES

Pre-eclampsia
Surgical Procedures 20: 424
Epidural and spinal anaesthesia
Anaesthetic Factors 32: 594
Supine hypotensive syndrome

DIFFICULT AND FAILED INTUBATION

M. Harmer

Failed intubation
- May occur in about 1 in 300 obstetric general anaesthetics
- Is becoming less common overall (though possibly the incidence is increasing) as a result of the increased use of regional anaesthesia
- May be associated with failure of oxygenation or inhalation of stomach contents
- Incidence of difficult intubation is not known

PATIENT CHARACTERISTICS

Problems are most commonly encountered because:

- Obstetric anaesthesia is often considered an emergency or has an implied urgency
- Potentially full stomach
- Patient usually has full dentition
- Anxiety as anaesthetizing 'two' patients.

PREOPERATIVE ASSESSMENT

Clinical assessment of airway and risk of difficult intubation (can be performed in a matter of seconds):

- Mouth opening (should be greater than 5 cm or three finger breadths)
- Mallampati view (pharynx should be visible)
- Jaw slide (should be able to push the lower incisors anterior to the upper incisors)

- Neck movement (full, unhindered range of at least 90°)
- Weight (original 'booking' weight less than 90 kg)
- Evidence or possibility of laryngeal swelling (severe pre-eclampsia or URTI).

If two or more of the above are abnormal, avoid general anaesthesia and/or summon senior help.

Equipment that should be immediately available:
- Selection of laryngoscopes (long and standard blade, short-handled or polio blade)
- Selection of tracheal tubes (size 5.0 mm upwards)
- Gum elastic bougie
- Selection of oral and nasal airways
- Laryngeal mask airway (size 3)
- Cricothyrotomy kit (or equipment for transtracheal ventilation and suitable connectors).

Standard precautions at induction of anaesthesia:
- Ensure adequate preoxygenation (this 'buys' time if a problem is encountered)
- Ensure proper positioning of patient (head in best position, breasts not pushed into midline by folded-up arms)
- Ensure adequate skilled assistance
- Ensure adequate equipment (see above)
- Rapid sequence induction.

Problems that might be encountered
Insertion of the laryngoscope may be impossible (see Figure 1) because of:

- Cricoid hand in the way (adjust without releasing)
- Breasts in the way (retract breasts or use short-handled or polio blade laryngoscope)
- Relaxant has not had time to work (wait)
- Muscle rigidity (could be malignant hyperthermia or can ordinarily occur with suxamethonium)
- Undiagnosed anatomical abnormality (should have been identified in preoperative assessment).

If unable to insert the laryngoscope, abandon attempts and proceed to failed laryngoscopy/ intubation drill.

View at laryngoscopy may be restricted:

- If whole or posterior portion of the glottis is visible, intubation should be possible (may need to use gum elastic bougie to guide tube).
- If only the epiglottis is visible, use bougie.
- If epiglottis is not visible, try long-blade laryngoscope. If still not visible, abandon attempts at intubation. Even if the glottis is visible, be prepared for laryngeal/tracheal swelling and have a selection of tracheal tubes readily available.

If intubation has been achieved without full visualization of the glottis, check tube position very carefully and, if in any doubt, take it out!

If intubation is deemed impossible, proceed to failed intubation drill.

Failed intubation drill (unable to insert laryngoscope or intubate):
- Act quickly, do not waste time with further attempts
- Do not give more suxamethonium; if the first dose did not help, why should a second?
- Maintain cricoid pressure
- Do not turn – it is easier to maintain the airway and ventilate in the supine position; the cricoid pressure will protect against regurgitation
- Attempt to ventilate the lungs with 100% oxygen
- If able to ventilate, consider the urgency of the situation with regard to possible options (see later)
- If unable to ventilate, proceed to failed ventilation drill.

Failed ventilation drill
The objective is to ensure, above all else, adequate maternal oxygenation (fetal well-being must be of secondary importance).

- Carefully ease the cricoid pressure. Wrongly or too forcefully applied cricoid pressure can cause airway obstruction.
- If still unable to ventilate, insert laryngeal mask airway (cricoid pressure will need to be released to allow passage).
- If still unable to ventilate, perform a cricothyrotomy or use transtracheal ventilation. Ensure correct placement before attempting ventilation for fear of causing extensive surgical emphysema of the neck if misplaced.
- If ventilation is still impossible, consider tracheostomy as a last resort. Tracheostomy has a poor 'track record' in failed intubation, and may be associated with extensive bleeding.

Once ventilation (and oxygenation) is possible, the urgency and the need to continue with the anaesthetic should be considered.

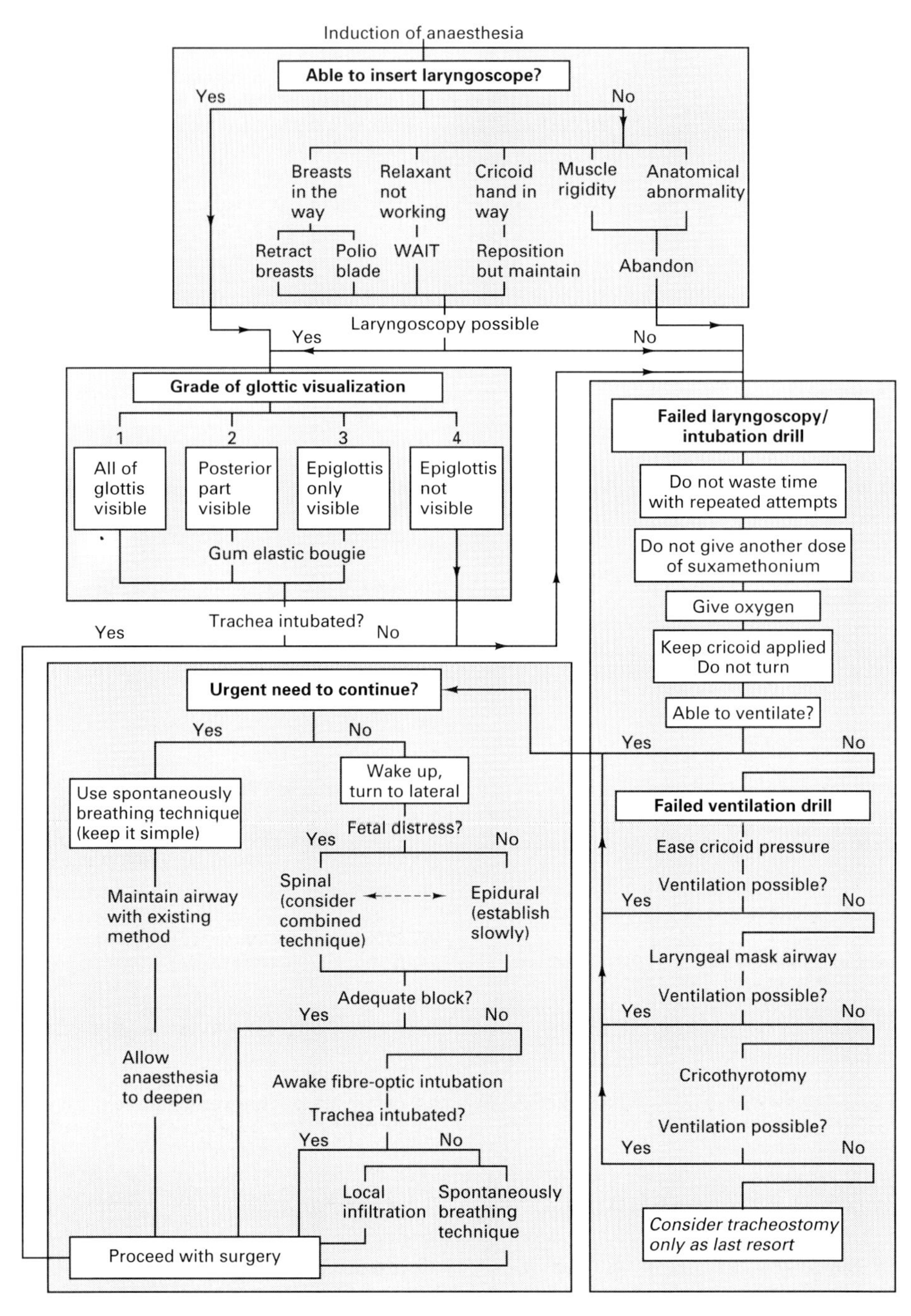

Figure 1
Difficult and failed intubation in obstetrics.

Factors indicating the need for continuing with general anaesthetic

This should ideally be assessed preoperatively and patients allocated a risk rating so that in the event of a failed intubation a line of management has been identified.

There is no option but to continue with a general anaesthetic if there is:

- Maternal cardiac arrest
- Extensive maternal bleeding

In both situations, evacuation of the uterus is fundamental to a successful outcome:

- No easy alternative to general anaesthesia, e.g. clotting disorder, cardiac valvular disease
- Severe and sudden fetal distress, whilst not an absolute indication to continue with general anaesthesia, could be considered an indication.

If the procedure is elective or for failure to progress in labour or for maternal distress, there is no urgent need to continue immediately with the anaesthetic.

Fetal distress that is not severe and sudden might not be considered a sufficient indication to continue with a general anaesthetic. The degree of fetal distress that will warrant continuation should be part of a locally decided policy.

Urgent need to continue with general anaesthetic:

- Keep cricoid pressure applied (unless already removed to allow ventilation)
- Use a simple, spontaneously breathing technique with whatever airway management was used in the initial establishment of ventilation
- Avoid further instrumentation of the pharynx unless essential to maintain the airway
- Use any available agents and deepen anaesthesia as quickly as possible
- Ensure adequate depth of anaesthesia before commencing surgery – if too light, may get laryngeal reflexes to surgical stimulation
- At end of surgery, turn to lateral position and recover in the head-down position.

No urgent need to continue with general anaesthetic

- Wake up and turn mother into lateral position
- Use a regional technique
- If no fetal distress present, may use either a spinal or an epidural anaesthetic (or a combined approach); if an epidural is used, great care must be taken to avoid an inadvertent total spinal block and the block should be established very slowly
- If there is fetal distress, a spinal block may be preferable as it will allow surgery to commence with the minimum of delay.

Failure of regional technique

Although rare, this can occur. If so:

- Repeat the technique or try the other type (if spinal used first, try epidural, and vice versa); however, watch carefully for an exaggerated block
- Consider an awake fibre-optic intubation, but only if experienced at the technique
- Consider using a spontaneously breathing technique without intubation, having taken steps to reduce gastric contents
- Consider local anaesthetic infiltration by the surgeon on an 'inject-and-cut' basis.

POSTOPERATIVE MANAGEMENT

- Ensure that the patient has full control of her airway before handing over care to a nurse
- Counsel the patient and give advice about future management.

In any event, it should be possible to ensure that there is always an alternative if one method of management has failed. Always remember that failure to intubate does not in itself cause permanent harm, but failure to oxygenate does. Maternal oxygenation must, therefore, be the main objective in managing difficult or failed intubation in obstetrics, whilst fetal well-being is a secondary consideration.

BIBLIOGRAPHY

Cobley M, Vaughan R S. Recognition and management of difficult airway problems. British Journal of Anaesthesia 1992; 68: 90–97

King T A, Adams A P. Failed intubation. British Journal of Anaesthesia 1990; 65: 400–414

Wilson M E, Speiglhalter D, Robertson J A, Lesser P. Predicting difficult intubation. British Journal of Anaesthesia 1988; 61: 211–216

CROSS REFERENCES

Difficult airway
  Anaesthetic Factors 30: 558
Malignant hyperthermia: clinical presentation
  Anaesthetic Factors 33: 644

EPIDURAL FOR CAESAREAN SECTION

J. P. Millns

PROCEDURE

For this to be successful, three parties must be considered:

- The mother must be pain free and reassured that both she and her baby are alright
- The surgeon, while gentle, requires the block to be adequate enough to allow safe delivery and haemostasis, without maternal vomiting
- The technique must not affect the neonate adversely.

PATIENT CHARACTERISTICS

Patients for Caesarean section are generally fit.

PREOPERATIVE ASSESSMENT AND INVESTIGATIONS

This must include:

- Reason for surgery and obstetric status – note conditions that may rule out use of epidural block, e.g. hypovolaemia, coagulopathy
- General health, especially conditions which may obviate use of an epidural, e.g. severe aortic stenosis, central nervous system disease
- Outcome of previous epidural anaesthetics
- Examination of spine for possible insertion difficulty
- Assessment of the upper airway for potential intubation difficulty

- BP and result of ward urine test and haemoglobin estimation; proteinuria may alert one to pre-eclampsia.

A full explanation of the procedure must be given. Possible problems to be discussed should include:

- Chances of technique failure
- Possibility of intraoperative pain despite an 'adequate' block – discuss solutions
- Effects and treatment of hypotension
- Dural tap.

Mothers must realize that it is usual to feel tugging during surgery. Pros and cons of epidural anaesthesia compared to other anaesthetic techniques are summarized in Table 1.

Table 1.
Advantages and disadvantages of epidural anaesthesia

Advantages
Avoids hazards of general anaesthesia
Allows parental participation
Catheter insertion permits repeated top-ups
Lower frequency and severity of hypotension than with spinal anaesthesia
Postoperative pain relief possible with epidural opioid or local anaesthetic
Disadvantages
Slower onset time than spinal
Possibility of dural tap
Prolonged numbness likely postoperatively
Greater likelihood of failure than with spinal anaesthesia
Shivering more likely than with spinal anaesthesia

In emergencies, the reason for operation must be noted and an estimate of available time made. Early communication of a need for surgery must be encouraged within the delivery suite, since this will allow optimal use of existing epidurals.

PREMEDICATION

Antacid prophylaxis, according to hospital policy.

TRANSFER TO THEATRE

- Never with mother supine
- Anticipate maternal nausea when moving the mother, once the block is established.

INDUCTION

Commence noninvasive BP and fetal heart monitoring. In the event that fetal status deteriorates during setting up an epidural, one must be prepared to proceed to an alternative technique if the extent of the block is not adequate for surgery at that stage.

Despite many preloading methods being practiced, none abolish hypotension reliably. If the systolic blood pressure still falls by 10% or more, treat with ephedrine.

Generally, incremental top-up methods produce less hypotension and are preferred in situations of fetal compromise, e.g. pre-eclampsia.

Freshly prepared lignocaine (2%) with 1:200 000 adrenaline produces suitable conditions quicker than 0.5% bupivacaine, although it does not last so long.

The addition of 50–100 μg of fentanyl to the epidural reduces the incidence of intraoperative pain.

Alkalinization of the local anaesthetic will speed up onset of the block.

The block must be tested and extend from T6 to S5. Note the levels on the anaesthetic chart. In the event of inadequate sacral anaesthesia, consider use of a supplementary saddle-block spinal block.

MONITORING

- ECG
- BP
- Spo_2.

THEATRE MANAGEMENT

Once the mother is positioned, wedged or tilted, on the operating table, ensure that she is comfortable, has a stable BP and a normal fetal heart rate prior to surgery commencing.

Administer supplemental oxygen up to delivery.

After delivery use syntocinon, rather than ergometrine, to lessen vomiting. Beware of hypotension with boluses of syntocinon.

COMPLICATIONS

Shivering

The incidence may be reduced by warming intravenous and local anaesthetic solutions;

alternatively, addition of epidural opioid may help.

Venous air embolism

This may cause chest pain and dyspnoea. The use of a 5° reverse Trendelenburg position may help to reduce the incidence, while also discouraging blood from tracking upwards to the diaphragm. The latter may otherwise result in annoying shoulder-tip pain.

Inadequate anaesthesia

Pain, if it occurs, is experienced usually at the stage of peritoneal suturing. If a small dose of intravenous opioid or the use of Entonox does not rectify the problem quickly, do not hesitate to offer the mother the chance of going to sleep.

POSTOPERATIVE MANAGEMENT

- Routine observations should include assessment of fundal height and vaginal blood loss
- Do not sit the mother up too quickly; hypotension and nausea may result
- Where use has been made of an epidural opioid for pain relief postoperatively, the respiratory rate will need to be monitored.

BIBLIOGRAPHY

Epidural block for Caesarean section and circulatory changes. Editorial. Lancet 1989; ii: 1076–1078

King M J, Bowden M I, Cooper G M. Epidural fentanyl and 0.5% bupivacaine for elective Caesarean section. Anaesthesia 1990; 45: 285–288

Lussos S A, Datta S. Anesthesia for cesarean delivery. Part II: Epidural anesthesia; intrathecal and epidural opioids; venous air embolism. International Journal of Obstetric Anesthesia 1992; 1: 208–221

Moir D D, Thorburn J. In: Obstetric anaesthesia and analgesia, 3rd edn. Baillière Tindall, London, 1986, p 259–261, 317–319

Norton A C, Davis A G, Spicer R J. Lignocaine 2% with adrenaline for epidural Caesarean section. Anaesthesia 1988; 43: 844–849

CROSS REFERENCES

Complications of position
Anaesthetic Factors 33: 618

Local anaesthetic toxicity
Anaesthetic Factors 33: 642

HYPERTENSIVE DISEASE OF PREGNANCY

S. C. Robson and D. Thomas

INTRODUCTION

The requirement for intensive monitoring and fluid management is mainly in women with severe pre-eclampsia (Tables 1 and 2) or eclampsia. Fluid management is particularly important in this disease because:

- The relatively low plasma volume, pulmonary artery capillary wedge pressure (PCWP) and cardiac output increase the

Table 1.
Definitions of severe pre-eclampsia

Hypertension (BP ≥140/90 mmHg) with proteinuria (≥0.5 g/24 h or ≥2+ on urinalysis) **and** one of the following:

- Epigastric pain, headache, visual disturbance
- Clonus (>3 beats)
- Platelet count <100 × 10^9, ALT >50 IU l^{-1}

Severe hypertension (systolic BP ≥170 mmHg or diastolic BP ≥110 mmHg) with proteinuria (≥0.5 g/24 h or ≥2+ on urinalysis)

Table 2.
Haemodynamic findings in severe pre-eclampsia

Low plasma volume
Low/normal cardiac output
Low/normal CVP/PCWP
Increased myocardial contractility
Low COP

likelihood of fetal distress and oliguria, particularly following vasodilation
- Endothelial damage, low colloid oncotic pressure (COP) and excessive fluid administration increase the risk of pulmonary oedema.

MONITORING

Laboratory investigations:
- Haemoglobin (with or without blood film),
  - platelets
  - clotting studies.
- Urea and electrolytes:
  - ALT
  - bilirubin
  - albumin.

Fluid balance
Hourly input/output.

Central venous pressure (CVP):
- Indications – oliguria (<100 ml/4 h), Caesarean section, haemorrhage
- Relationship with PCWP – low CVP (<4 mmHg) reasonable indicator of low PCWP; CVP >6 mmHg may be associated with PCWP of >16 mmHg
- Site – antecubital long line preferable.

PCWP/CARDIAC OUTPUT

Risks preclude routine use, but should be considered in women with pulmonary oedema or compromised myocardial function.

Blood pressure:
- Automated recording (every 15 min) – beware of underestimation of diastolic BP in severe pre-eclampsia by oscillometric devices
- Indications for treatment – sustained mean arterial pressure >125 mmHg or diastolic BP >110 mmHg
- Treatment – hydralazine (5 mg i.v. bolus; repeated every 15–20 min as necessary); alternative drugs labetolol (20 mg i.v. bolus) or nifedipine (10 mg p.o.).

Sao_2
Indicated in women at risk of pulmonary oedema (high CVP/PCWP or low COP/albumin) or respiratory depression (magnesium sulphate, diazepam, chlormethiazole or opioid infusions).

FLUID MANAGEMENT

Maintenance fluid – Ringer lactate solution 1 l/12 h (Figure 1).

Additional fluid will be required in the following circumstances:

- Prior to epidural block.
- Oliguria with a low CVP (<4 mmHg) – 5% albumin. Up to 1000 ml can be used to restore CVP to normal. If hypovolaemia is secondary to haemorrhage or haemolysis, give blood not albumin.
- Prior to antepartum vasodilation – 5% albumin. Administration of intravenous hydralazine without fluid preloading may precipitate fetal distress and oliguria. Prior administration of 500 ml albumin prevents these complications.
- Haemorrhage/haemolysis – blood. Aim to keep Hb >9 g dl^{-1}.
- Thrombocytopenia – platelets. Aim to keep platelet count $>20 \times 10^9$ in nonsurgical and $>50 \times 10^9$ in surgical patents.
- DIC with hypofibrinogenaemia – FFP. Aim to maintain fibrinogen >100 mg dl^{-1} and correct PT or PTT.

Management of oliguria with a normal CVP (4–8 mmHg):
- The adequacy of intravascular volume can be assessed by the CVP response to a 200 ml colloid challenge
- Dopamine (1 μg kg^{-1} min^{-1} increasing to a maximum dose of 5 μg kg^{-1} min^{-1}) increases urine output, provided the circulating volume is adequate.

Management of persistent oliguria with deteriorating renal function:
- Fluid restriction (normal saline; urine output during previous hour + 30 ml)
- Haemodialysis or haemofiltration may be required to reduce creatinine or potassium.

Pulmonary oedema
- >70% occur postpartum
- Risk increases as COP–PCWP gradient decreases below 4 mmHg. COP reaches a nadir at 12–16 h postpartum
- Majority of reported cases associated with excessive colloid or crystalloid infusions; risk precludes 'routine' administration of colloid in all cases of severe pre-eclampsia
- Treat with intravenous frusemide (20 mg increased to 40 mg if no response)
- Persistent hypoxaemia despite diuretic treatment is an indication for a pulmonary artery catheter.

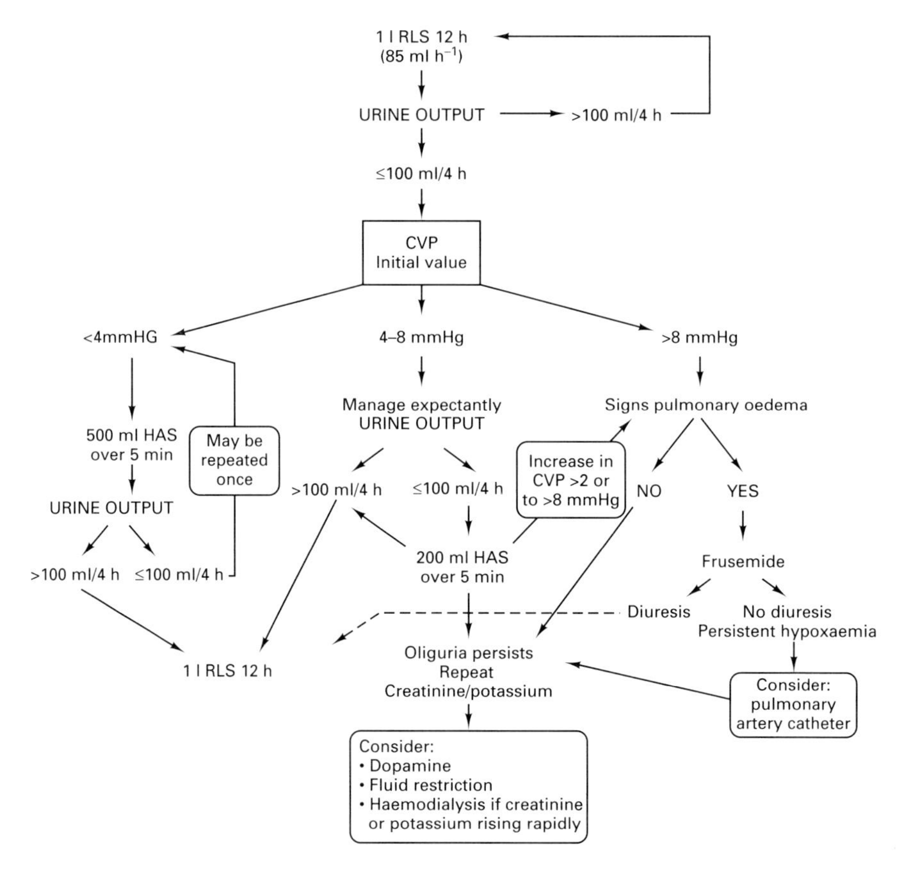

Figure 1
RLS, Ringer lactate solution; HAS, human albumin (5%) solution.

BIBLIOGRAPHY

Benedetti T J, Kates R, Williams V. Hemodynamic observations in severe pre-eclampsia complicated by pulmonary edema. American Journal of Obstetrics and Gynecology 1985; 152: 330–334

Kirshon B, Lee W, Mauer M B, Cotton D B. Effects of low dose dopamine therapy in the oliguric patient with pre-eclampsia. American Journal of Obstetrics and Gynecology 1988; 159: 604–607

Robson S C, Redfern N, Walkinshaw S. A protocol for the intrapartum management of severe pre-eclampsia. International Journal of Obstetrics and Anesthesia 1992; 1: 222–229

Wallenburg H C S. Hemodynamics in hypertensive pregnancy. In: Rubin P C (ed) Handbook of hypertension, vol 10, Hypertension in pregnancy. Elsevier, Amsterdam, 1988, p 66–101

CROSS REFERENCES

Fluid and electrolyte balance
Anaesthetic Factors 33: 626

Intraoperative hypertension
Anaesthetic Factors 33: 636

Postoperative oliguria
Anaesthetic Factors 33: 652

MANAGEMENT OF DURAL TAP AND POSTDURAL PUNCTURE HEADACHE

I. F. Russell

Dural tap may be intentional (spinal anaesthesia) or accidental (epidural analgesia). Dural tap may be recognized at the time of insertion of an epidural, but not infrequently typical postdural puncture headache (PDPH) symptoms arise in the absence of overt evidence of a dural tap.

AETIOLOGY

PDPH is believed to result from the leak of CSF through a hole in the dura at a rate faster than the brain can replace it, thus leading to a 'low pressure' headache. Early (<36 h) headaches may be related to the drug used. Late symptoms (>36 h) may be related to 'traction' on specific intra- or extra-cranial nerves and/or blood vessels, as well as to compensatory vasodilation attempting to restore intracranial volume.

Predisposing factors
- Age (young > old)
- Sex (female = male)
- Pregnant > nonpregnant
- Needle-tip design (cutting > pencil point)
- Needle size (large needles, bigger hole)
- Drug (lignocaine > bupivacaine > procaine/tetracaine mixture)
- Multiple dural punctures

SYMPTOMS

- Frontal headache (trigeminal V)
- Occipital headache (glossopharyngeal IX, vagus X)
- Neck and shoulder pain (cervical C1, C2, C3)
- Paresis of lateral gaze (abducent VI)
- Blurred/double vision, photophobia
- Hyperacute/hypoacute hearing, tinnitus (endolymph channels and semicircular canals are in communication with main CSF reservoir and may be an additional cause of these symptoms)
- Postural (worse in upright postures).

Table 1.
Summary of 15 recent studies into headache rates associated with spinal anaesthesia during pregnancy

Needle	Gauge	Incidence of PDPH (%)
Whitacre	22	0.5–3
Sprotte	24	4.2–10
Whitacre	25	0–1
Quincke	25	7–17
Quincke	26	5–20
Quincke	27	3

DIFFERENTIAL DIAGNOSIS

- Hypertension (ergometrine, PET, medical reasons, postnatal depression)
- Chronic headache syndromes (migraine, cluster headaches)
- Intracranial pathology (thrombosis, A–V malformations, extradural/intradural/subdural haematoma, tumour, infective).

PREVENTION OF PDPH

- Good epidural technique
- Nonrotation of epidural needle after entering epidural space
- Use of 26 or 27 gauge Quincke spinal needles (needles smaller than this may lead to an unacceptable spinal failure rate)
- Insertion of Quincke needles with the bevel parallel to the 'longitudinal' fibres of dura
- Use of pencil-point needles
- Insertion of spinal needles at an acute angle (e.g. lateral oblique approach).

ACCIDENTAL DURAL TAP

Initial management:
- Avoid temptation to remove epidural needle or catheter

- Insert (or leave) epidural catheter in (into) CSF:
  - May reduce incidence of headache
  - Limits trauma to patient and risk of a second dural puncture (10–15%)
  - Avoids problems of epidural in association with dural tap (erratic epidural behaviour, subdural block, total spinal block).
- Position of epidural catheter is now known
- Spinal catheter provides excellent analgesia with low-dose narcotics and/or low-dose local anaesthetic (e.g. fentanyl (25–30 mcg), bupivacaine plain (2.5–5 mg))
- Spinal catheter provides instant anaesthesia for surgical procedure (provided the hydrodynamics associated with spinal catheters are understood fully and correct technique is used).

Subsequent management:

- Clear explanation to patient of what has happened
- No restriction on mode of delivery (prophylactic forceps delivery does not reduce incidence of headache)
- Normal ambulation postdelivery (bed rest does not prevent headache, merely delays its onset)
- If headache develops, treatment depends on whether spinal or epidural catheter is in situ, and on time of onset and severity of headache
- Disagreement on value of prophylactic epidural blood patch (some claim high failure rate); since some 20–30% of women will not develop a PDPH it is probably wiser to wait before instituting invasive therapy
- Epidural injections of saline (20–40 ml) are effective; may be used during labour (before top-up with local anaesthetic), but have a short duration of effect
- Epidural infusion of saline (15–25 ml h^{-1}, postdelivery) for 24 h is effective (this treatment regimen was ceased in the author's unit after a total spinal anaesthetic ensued some 3 h after starting the infusion; IPPV was required for 3 h!)
- PDPH during labour may be treated by saline injections (up to 10 ml), injected through the 'spinal' catheter a few minutes before topping up the spinal analgesia
- Ensure adequate hydration (intravenous if appropriate, but postdelivery encourage oral fluid intake)
- Oral analgesics
- Intravenous caffeine sodium benzoate is inexpensive and has been used with some effect
- Abdominal binder (if patient will tolerate it)
- Bed rest (supine, prone position may be better)
- Epidural blood patch.

EPIDURAL BLOOD PATCH

Should be used if the headache:

- Is severe
- Interferes with mother's activity and shows no sign of diminishing over 2–3 days of conservative therapy

Effect is almost instantaneous in the majority of cases and in 90% of cases relief is permanent. Repeat blood patch (12–24 h later) may be required in a small number of cases. Occasionally some backache may ensue, lasting for 2–3 days.

Technique:

- The majority of anaesthetists in the UK do not perform blood cultures or white cell counts as a routine test
- The most experienced epiduralist available should perform the blood patch
- The epidural space should be located at or just below the site of the dural tap
- Slow injection (2 min) of the patient's own blood (taken aseptically when the epidural space has been located)
- Stop injection if pain/paraesthesia develops (down legs; in back; between shoulder blades), otherwise give 20 ml
- Place patient supine for 30 min, then mobilize
- If there are no other clinical problems and blood patch is successful, discharge patient within a few hours.

It is most important to follow-up and treat dural tap adequately. PDPH symptoms can be very debilitating and may become chronic due to inappropriate and/or ineffective therapy.

BIBLIOGRAPHY

Carrie L E S. Post dural puncture headache and extradural blood patch. British Journal of Anaesthesia 1993; 71: 179–181

Naulty J S, Hertwig R N, Hunt C O, Datta S, Ostheimer G W, Weiss J B. Influence of local anaesthetic solution on postdural puncture headache. Anesthesiology 1990; 72: 450–454

Norris M, Leighton B. Continuous spinal anaesthesia after unintentional dural puncture in parturients. Regional Anesthesia 1990; 15: 285–287

Sechzer P H, Abel L. Post spinal headache treated with caffeine. Evaluation with demand method. Current Therapeutic Research 1978; 24: 307–312

Stride P C, Cooper G M. Dural taps revisited. A 20 year survey from Birmingham Maternity Hospital. Anaesthesia 1993; 48: 247–255

CROSS REFERENCES

Local anaesthetic toxicity
Anaesthetic Factors 33: 642

Total spinal anaesthesia
Anaesthetic Factors 33: 667

MANAGEMENT OF THE MOTHER WITH COEXISTING MEDICAL DISEASE

D. Brighouse

THE PROBLEM

Improved management of chronic and congenital diseases and changing patterns of disease, coupled with improved infertility treatment and antenatal/perinatal management has led to an increase in the number of women with significant systemic disease who achieve viable pregnancies.

Coexisting disease of every system is documented in the last confidential enquiry into maternal death in the UK. The most common diseases encountered by the obstetric anaesthetist are diabetes, cardiac disease, asthma, and problems associated with neurological and orthopaedic disorders.

GENERAL PRINCIPLES

- Preconception counselling, where appropriate
- Early identification of the patient (at booking)
- Communication between obstetrician, anaesthetist and physician
- Understanding of pathophysiology of the disease, and of physiological changes of pregnancy
- Detailed preanaesthetic assessment
- Clear management plans, including place of delivery
- Involvement of senior medical staff
- Planned delivery of high-risk women.

DIABETES

Approximately 1 in 500 pregnancies.

Major maternal problems:
- Loss of diabetic control
- Polyhydramnios
- Pre-eclampsia
- Exacerbation of vascular and renal disease

Major fetal/neonatal problems:
- Macrosomia
- Fetal abnormality
- Prematurity/IRDS
- Stillbirth
- Poor glycaemic control.

Management:
- Rigorous diabetic control – insulin resistance common
- Planned delivery (usually at 38 weeks)
- Early epidural analgesia for labour; regional anaesthesia for Caesarean section
- Written protocols for intravenous insulin and glucose regime
- Beware dramatic fall in insulin requirements in recovery.

CARDIAC DISEASE

A wide range of problems, affecting approximately 1 in 350 pregnancies.

Major problems:
- Valvular disease
- Congenital heart disease – first-degree pulmonary hypertension; patients with Eisenmenger's syndrome have 50% mortality
- Dysrhythmias
- Ischaemic heart disease – incidence increasing
- Cardiomyopathies.

Antenatal assessment:
- Cardiac reserve
- ECG/echocardiography/cardiac catheterization
- Medication
- Consider delivery in unit with cardiac surgical facility.

Intrapartum monitoring:
- Consider invasive BP
- Consider central venous pressure (CVP)/ pulmonary artery pressure
- Continuous ECG.

Choice of analgesia/anaesthesia:
- Sedation reduces cardiovascular responses to stress
- Continuous conduction anaesthesia reduces stress response
- Intrathecal opioids/low-dose local anaesthetic and opioid epidural infusions provide optimal analgesia and minimize cardiovascular disturbance
- Standard obstetric general anaesthetic techniques are inappropriate – modified high-dose narcotic techniques should be used
- Continuous spinal/epidural not contra-indicated in fixed cardiac output states if appropriate invasive monitoring is used
- Senior advice essential.

Dysrhythmias:
- Supraventricular tachycardia/Wolfe–Parkinson–White syndrome common
- Consider adenosine
- Remember uterine displacement/rapid sequence induction if general anaesthesia for emergency cardioversion is needed.

ASTHMA

Approximately 1 in 100 pregnancies. One-quarter deteriorate in pregnancy.

- Treat aggressively – acute attacks may cause maternal and fetal hypoxia
- Epidural analgesia recommended for labour (avoids pain-induced bronchospasm)
- Use epidural or combined epidural and spinal anaesthesia for Caesarean section
- Beware single-shot high spinal block (reduces ability to cough).

NEUROLOGICAL AND ORTHOPAEDIC DISORDERS

Most commonly encountered:

- Multiple sclerosis:
  - Discuss antenatally
  - Document disability
  - Warn that postpartum relapse is common
  - Regional techniques not contraindicated.
- Scoliosis:
  - Assess pulmonary function
  - Consider continuous spinal block in presence of spinal instrumentation
  - Beware patchy block with epidural.
- Laminectomy: regional techniques not contraindicated.
- Spina bifida:
  - Document disability antenatally
  - Regional techniques not contraindicated.
- Epilepsy:
  - Avoid enflurane
  - May need larger doses of thiopentone
  - Regional techniques not contraindicated.

AUTOIMMUNE DISEASES

- Rheumatoid arthritis:
  - 1 in 1000 pregnancies
  - Assess antenatally
  - Look for other systemic involvement (pericardial or pleural effusions, neuropathies)
  - Early epidural
  - Anticipate major airway difficulty.
- Systemic lupus erythematosus:
  - 1 in 1600 pregnancies
  - Beware cardiomyopathy
  - Perform clotting studies.
- Idiopathic thrombocytopaenic purpura:
  - 1 in 2000–10 000 pregnancies
  - Ensure platelets >50 000 mm^{-3} for operative delivery
  - >80 000 mm^{-3} and normal bleeding time for epidural
  - Platelet transfusion produces short-term improvement (3 h)
  - Response to intravenous IgG lasts up to 4 weeks.

MORBID OBESITY

Increased risk of ischaemic heart disease, diabetes, respiratory disease (see previous sections).

Major mechanical problems:
- Bed/operating table too small
- Difficulty lifting/moving patient
- Difficult intravenous access
- Inaccuracy of noninvasive BP/fetal monitoring
- Closing volume within tidal volume when lying down.

Problems of regional analgesia/anaesthesia:
- Technical difficulty of insertion; use long needles and 22 gauge spinal needle
- Impossible to change patient position quickly
- Control of sensory block more difficult; use combined technique if possible
- Anticipate hypotension; treat aggressively
- Use supplementary oxygen.

Problems with general anaesthesia:
- Hiatus hernia invariable
- Anticipate difficult intubation
- Desaturation very rapid
- Mechanical ventilation may be difficult.

MALIGNANT HYPERPYREXIA

- Very rare in pregnancy
- No report of malignant hyperpyrexia crisis in labour
- Epidural lignocaine and bupivacaine have been used safely
- Avoid pethidine and ergometrine
- Syntocinon appears safe
- Avoid general anaesthesia unless life-saving
- Ensure that dantrolene is available in the obstetric unit.

BIBLIOGRAPHY

Maresh M. Medical complications in pregnancy. Baillière's Clinical Obstetrics and Gynaecology 1990; 1: 129–147

Ostheimer G W (ed). Manual of obstetric anesthesia, 2nd edn. Churchill Livingstone, Edinburgh, 1992, p 276–339

Ward M E, Douglas M J. Medical aspects of obstetrics: diabetes, asthma, cardiac disease. Current Opinion in Anesthesiology 1993; 3: 483–486

CROSS REFERENCES

Multiple sclerosis
Patient Conditions 1: 19
Diabetes mellitus
Patient Conditions 2: 42
Asthma
Patient Conditions 3: 68
Valvular heart disease
Patient Conditions 4: 95
Obesity
Patient Conditions 5: 148
Rheumatoid disease
Patient Conditions 8: 202
Systemic lupus erythematosus
Patient Conditions 9: 234
Pre-eclampsia
Surgical Procedures 20: 424
Malignant hyperpyrexia
Anaesthetic Factors 33: 644
Preoperative preparation of patient with respiratory disease
Anaesthetic Factors 34: 697

OBSTETRIC HAEMORRHAGE

E. A. Thornberry

20

Peripartum haemorrhage is a major cause of maternal mortality. It may be defined as follows.

Antepartum haemorrhage: bleeding from the genital tract between 28 completed weeks of pregnancy and the onset of labour.

Postpartum haemorrhage – primary: greater than 500 ml of blood loss from the genital tract after delivery of the fetus until 24 h after birth.

Postpartum haemorrhage – secondary: abnormal bleeding, between 24 h and 6 weeks postpartum.

> **Normal blood loss at parturition:**
> - 500 ml for a single vaginal delivery
> - 900 ml for a twin vaginal delivery
> - 700–1000 ml for a Caesarean section
> - Compensated by an increase in the blood volume by a factor of 0.3–0.6 (i.e. 1–2 l)

ASSESSMENT

- Obstetric history – to establish diagnosis
- Clinical signs
  - Maternal: level of consciousness; pulse; BP
  - Fetal: heart rate; CTG
- Estimate of blood loss – measured or concealed
- Obstetric examination – speculum examination; ultrasound
- General medical history and examination – to assess fitness for anaesthesia.

RESUSCITATION

- Summon extra staff:
  - Midwives
  - Obstetricians
  - Anaesthetists.
- Position patient
  - Head-down
  - Raise legs
  - (Ante- or intrapartum) left side.
- Oxygen.
- Intravenous access – two large-bore cannulae.
- Haematology:
  - Send blood for
    - (i) Full blood count
    - (ii) Clotting screen
    - (iii) Group and cross-match (at least 6 units)
  - Request group-specific blood if blood group known, whilst waiting for cross-match.
- Fluid resuscitation:
  - Crystalloid (1–2 l)
  - Colloids (gelatin solutions; hetastarch)
  - Blood (start with O Rh negative unless patient known to have anti-c antibodies)
  - Use a blood warmer
  - Use a pressure bag.
- Maternal monitoring:
  - Essential:
    - (i) Blood pressure (automatic noninvasive BP or intra-arterial monitoring helpful)
    - (ii) Pulse (via ECG or plethysmograph)
    - (iii) Central venous pressure (CVP) (continuously displayed preferable)
    - (iv) Urine output
    - (v) Pulse oximetry
  - Optional:
    - (i) Temperature
    - (ii) Blood gases
    - (iii) Acid–base status
    - (iv) Left atrial pressure (in pre-eclampsia the CVP may not accurately reflect the fluid balance and more invasive monitoring is justified).
- Fetal monitoring: Heart rate (CTG).
- Treat the cause of the bleeding.

MANAGEMENT OF PRIMARY CAUSE OF BLEEDING

See Tables 1 and 2.

Table 1.
Causes of peripartum haemorrhage

Antepartum and intrapartum
Placenta praevia
Abruptio placenta
Uterine rupture
Trauma
Advanced ectopic pregnancy
Other genital-tract bleeding
Postpartum
Uterine atony
Retained placenta
Cervical and vaginal lacerations
Placenta accreta
Uterine inversion
Coagulopathy
Cervical and uterine abnormalities

Table 2.
Aetiology of coagulopathies in obstetrics

- DIC secondary to:
  - Abruptio placentae
  - Pre-eclampsia
  - Chorioamnionitis
  - Amniotic fluid embolism
  - Prolonged intrauterine death
  - Massive transfusion
- HELLP syndrome
- Pre-existing disease
- Iatrogenic (heparin)

Indications for medical treatment:
- Atonic uterus – give oxytocin, ergot alkaloids or prostaglandins
- Coagulopathy – give fresh frozen plasma, cryoprecipitate, platelets.

Indications for surgical treatment:
- Delivery of fetus
- Delivery of placenta or retained products
- To repair local trauma or ruptured uterus
- To replace an inverted uterus
- To ligate iliac vessels or perform hysterectomy in cases of failed medical treatment.

ANAESTHETIC MANAGEMENT

If an effective epidural is in situ, cardiovascular stability can be maintained and the patient is conscious, then surgical intervention can proceed under regional block.

Except in the above circumstances, a general anaesthetic is the method of choice.

Etomidate is useful at induction because it causes minimal hypotension. Ketamine can be used, but increases uterine tone (proceed with caution if uterine tone already increased).

Use of inhalational anaesthetics before delivery allows a higher concentration of oxygen to be administered. All inhalational agents relax the uterus with progressive depression of uterine contractility above 1 MAC. Above 2 MAC inhalational agents also block the uterine response to oxytoxics. Isoflurane 0.5 MAC or less does not cause uterine depression, and therefore is the agent of choice. If the uterus is tetanically contracted (common with abruption) the relaxation induced by an inhalational agent may improve placental perfusion.

POSTOPERATIVE MANAGEMENT

Intensive monitoring should continue. The advantages of transferring the patient to an ITU or HDU should be considered. Severe cases should be transferred asleep, ventilated, with full monitoring in transit. In less severe cases the patient can be managed on a labour ward.

OUTCOME

Overall death rate from obstetric haemorrhage in England and Wales (1979–1987) is 5 per million deliveries.

Haemorrhage caused 7.2% of the maternal mortality in the UK between 1985 and 1987.

The risk is increased by age, particularly in women over 35 years.

Morbidity and mortality is reduced if efficient resuscitation is instigated. Resuscitation is more efficient if there is a prearranged protocol. Many units have a 'haemorrhage trolley' (Table 3) in addition to their resuscitation trolley, with all the necessary equipment gathered in one place.

Table 3.
Suggested items for an 'obstetric haemorrhage trolley'

Surgical gloves
A selection of intravenous cannulae
Fixing tape
Blood giving sets
Pressure bags (×2)
Crystalloid and colloid fluids
Blood sampling bottles
Blood collecting system
Syringes
Needles
Appropriate laboratory forms
Local anaesthetics
CVP lines
Dressing pack
Antiseptic
Water manometer or CVP transducer and flushing set
Scale for water manometer
Blood-warming coils
Urinary catheter and hourly measuring collecting bag
Blood gas syringes

BIBLIOGRAPHY

Suresh M S, Kinch R A. Antepartum hemorrhage. In: Datta S (ed) Anesthetic and obstetric management of high-risk pregnancy. Mosby Year Book, 1991, p 89–107
Baskett T F, Writer W D R. Postpartum hemorrhage. In: Datta S (ed) Anesthetic and obstetric management of high-risk pregnancy. Mosby Year Book, 1991, p 108–134
Report on Confidential Enquiries into Maternal Deaths in the United Kingdom 1985–87, p 28–36

CROSS REFERENCES

Inherited coagulopathies
Patient Conditions 7: 178
Blood transfusion
Anaesthetic Factors 33: 616

PRE-ECLAMPSIA

N. Redfern

PROCEDURE

Of severely pre-eclamptic mothers, 40–60% require Caesarean section (less than 32 weeks, 97%).

PATIENT CHARACTERISTICS

- 15% of mothers suffer from mild, 8% moderate, and 2% severe pre-eclampsia.
- Higher incidence in multiple pregnancy.
- Two-thirds are primiparous.
- Greater risk of complications (e.g. cerebral haemorrhage, death) in multiparous patients 25 years old and over.
- Baby may be very premature (24–40 weeks).
- Severe pre-eclamptic patients have a high systemic vascular resistance (SVR) and low colloid osmotic pressure. They are therefore particularly prone to develop pulmonary oedema from rapid infusion of relatively low volumes of fluid (500–1000 ml). Rapid vasodilation without adequate volume loading can, however, lead to sudden severe hypotension. Strict attention to fluid balance is vital.

PREOPERATIVE ASSESSMENT

Hourly fluid balance.

Investigations

- Full blood count and platelets:
  - Clotting screen in severe pre-eclampsia if platelets <100 000.

- Urea and electrolytes:
  - Albumin
  - ALT
  - AST
  - bilirubin.

It is inappropriate to wait for results in an emergency.

PERIOPERATIVE MANAGEMENT

Antihypertensive prophylaxis

Before induction of anaesthesia, maternal blood pressure should be well controlled (mean arterial pressure <125 mmHg, systolic BP <170 mmHg). Patients may present on calcium antagonists (e.g. nifedipine) or methyldopa.

For preoperative control:
- Hydralazine
  - Drug of choice
  - 5–10 mg bolus doses until effect achieved
  - Renal and uterine blood flow improved if BP maintained
  - Can cause fetal distress if patient not preloaded
  - Give 500 ml fluid prior to starting hydralazine if patient has not received intravenous fluid therapy.
- Labetalol
  - Useful if persistent tachycardia
  - 5–10 mg boluses, or infusion
  - Disadvantages:
    - (i) May further compromise myocardial function if cardiac output is low and systemic vascular resistance is very high
    - (ii) Can precipitate pulmonary oedema
    - (iii) May cause loss of baseline variability in CTG.

Anticonvulsant prophylaxis

None are of proven benefit.

- Diazepam may cause sedation and postoperative hypoxia
- Phenytoin is less effective, especially in eclamptics
- Chlormethiazole introduces a large volume load; the airway reflexes may be lost when oversedated
- Magnesium sulphate:
  - Potentiates neuromuscular blockers
  - Reduces or abolishes fasciculations with suxamethonium
  - Reduces the requirement for nondepolarizing muscle relaxants by up to 50%
  - Can cause respiratory arrest and cardiovascular collapse in large doses
  - Blood concentration should be monitored when in use.

Monitoring:
- Noninvasive BP – 1-min intervals before delivery
- Pulse oximeter
- ECG
- Urinary catheter
- $ETco_2$
- Nerve stimulator (pregnant patients may need less muscle relaxant)
- Fluid balance and blood loss
- A central venous pressure (CVP) line should be inserted for the following indications:
  - Severe pre-eclampsia
  - Oliguria unresponsive to single fluid challenge (500 ml)
  - Haemorrhage
  - HELLP (haemolysis, elevated liver enzymes, low platelets) syndrome
  - Insert via antecubital fossa if possible (coagulopathy).
- Pulmonary artery capillary wedge pressure (PCWP) risks preclude routine use but it should be considered in women with pulmonary oedema or compromised myocardial function.

Theatre and patient preparation:
- 15° left-lateral tilt
- Apprehension may further increase maternal blood pressure
- Full explanation of:
  - Anaesthetic interventions
  - Neonatal resuscitation and SCBU
- Emotional support from partner may be very useful.

ANAESTHETIC TECHNIQUE

Epidural anaesthesia

The method of choice, provided:

- Platelets >80 000, and clotting screen normal
- Patient is fully conscious
- No other contraindication exists (e.g. bacteraemia, local sepsis, severe haemorrhage, hypovolaemia, patient refusal)
- Adequate circulating blood volume
- Low-dose aspirin (75 mg day^{-1}) is not a contraindication, but should be stopped 5–7 days prior to surgery, if possible

- For Caesarean section preload with 500 ml colloid and 500–1000 ml crystalloid; if more required, insert CVP line
- If epidural block inadequate prior to surgery, it can often be improved with opioids (fentanyl 50 μg), or a careful spinal block (1 ml 0.5% heavy bupivacaine, patient in lateral position).

General anaesthesia

Indicated when:

- Patient not fully conscious following eclampsia
- Coagulopathy or low platelet count
- There is severe haemorrhage necessitating operation while patient still hypovolaemic
- Life-threatening fetal or maternal emergency.

Technique:

- Routine H_2 blockers and antacid prophylaxis, plus metoclopramide in an emergency
- Preoxygenation and rapid sequence induction mandatory
- Laryngeal oedema may make intubation very difficult.

The hypertensive response to laryngoscopy and intubation is exaggerated in pre-eclamptics, but worst in older multiparous patients. Cerebral haemorrhage causes 65% of deaths from pre-eclampsia. It is therefore vital to:

- Control BP well before induction
- Obtund the hypertensive response to intubation (try one or more of – labetalol (5–10 mg), lignocaine (1 mg kg^{-1}), alfentanil (10 μg kg^{-1}), fentanyl (2.5 μg kg^{-1})
- Remember that the danger of hypertension is as great at extubation as intubation – consider further dose of labetalol.

Spinal anaesthesia

Controversial for Caesarean section in severe pre-eclampsia, because the sudden extensive sympathetic block can result in marked hypotension and severe fetal distress, even after apparently adequate preloading of the circulation. Saddle block can be used for forceps delivery, and after delivery.

POSTOPERATIVE MANAGEMENT

Monitor:

- Urine output – if oliguric insert a CVP line
- Noninvasive BP – every 15 min
- Spo_2 – give oxygen if <90% (usual cause is opioid analgesia, but remember pulmonary oedema).

Keep patient in HDU for 24 h or longer if still in oliguric phase of disease.

Ensure good postoperative analgesia:

- Patient-controlled analgesia with an opioid is recommended
- Use of a NSAID and postoperative epidural infusions is controversial in the presence of coagulopathy.

Repeat laboratory investigations every 6–12 h (platelets lowest 24–48 h postdelivery).

COMPLICATIONS OF PRE-ECLAMPSIA

Eclampsia

If not fully conscious following eclamptic seizure, delivery should be expedited and the patient managed postdelivery on the ITU. May require period of postoperative ventilation, and neurological investigation (CT scan). Administration of sedative anticonvulsants may potentiate respiratory depressant effect of opioids. Eclampsia can occur up to 48 h postdelivery. Eclampsia can occur with minimal BP elevation. Magnesium prevents seizure recurrence.

HELLP syndrome

Haemolysis, elevated liver enzymes, low platelets (HELLP):

- Occurs in 4–12% cases of severe pre-eclampsia
- Intravascular deposition of fibrin in the liver sinusoids causes obstruction to blood flow and liver distension.

Patients present with:

- Right upper quadrant or epigastric pain
- Nausea or vomiting
- Usually mild elevation of AST, ALT, bilirubin
- Hypertension and proteinuria (often mild)
- Rarely, liver rupture, causing CVS collapse.

Before anaesthesia, the following are essential:

- Cross-matched blood
- FFP and platelets available
- Give platelets before surgery if platelet count <50 000.

Choice of anaesthetic:

- Epidural anaesthesia relatively contra-indicated unless platelet count, coagulation screen and bleeding time normal
- For general anaesthesia use drugs with minimal hepatic or renal metabolism and monitor blood glucose concentration perioperatively.

BIBLIOGRAPHY

Clark S L, Cotton D B. Clinical indications for pulmonary artery catheterisation in the patient with severe pre-eclampsia. American Journal of Obstetrics and Gynaecology 1988; 158: 453–458

Crosby E T. Obstetrical anaesthesia for patients with the syndrome of haemolysis, elevated liver enzymes and low platelets. Canadian Journal of Anaesthesia 1991; 38: 227–233

Mudie L L. Pre-eclampsia: its anaesthetic implications. British Journal of Hospital Medicine 1990; 43: 297–300

Ramanathan J. Pathophysiology and anaesthetic implications in pre-eclampsia. Clinical Obstetrics and Gynaecology 1992; 35: 414–425

CROSS REFERENCES

Epidural and spinal anaesthesia
Anaesthetic Factors 32: 594
Complications of position
Anaesthetic Factors 33: 618
Intraoperative hypertension
Anaesthetic Factors 33: 636
Postoperative oliguria
Anaesthetic Factors 33: 652
Postoperative pain management
Anaesthetic Factors 33: 655

ANAESTHESIA FOR THE PATIENT WITH A RETAINED PLACENTA

E. J. Roberts

PROCEDURE

- Manual removal of placenta with exploration of uterine cavity
- Occurs in 1% of all vaginal deliveries
- Placenta may be abnormally adherent or separated but retained by hypotonic uterus or constriction ring.

PATIENT CHARACTERISTICS

- Usually recently delivered
- May present some days after delivery, but patients are usually immediately postpartum
- May have persisting problems from pregnancy or before, e.g. anaemia, diabetes mellitus
- Previous uterine surgery increases the risk of placenta accreta.

PREOPERATIVE ASSESSMENT AND INVESTIGATIONS

Retained placenta is the third most common cause of postpartum haemorrhage and these women may be hypovolaemic and shocked. The patient's cardiovascular status should be carefully examined for signs of hypovolaemia, which may be hard to find. Look for hypotension, tachycardia or orthostatic changes. Estimates of blood loss may be unreliable. Resuscitate as necessary (Table 1).

Patients are at a high risk from the acid-aspiration syndrome. Pharmacological agents (e.g. pethidine in labour) and physiological

Table 1.
Plan of resuscitation for postpartum haemorrhage

Cross-match blood
Hb
Two 14 gauge intravenous lines
Warm intravenous fluids
Colloid or blood intravenously
Arterial line and central venous pressure, if indicated

changes of pregnancy persist for some days. Antacid prophylaxis should be given and, wherever possible, a regional technique employed.

Nonparticulate oral antacid, e.g. 30 ml sodium citrate with an H_2 receptor antagonist (cimetidine or ranitidine), is required. Retained placenta is the commonest obstetric complication requiring an anaesthetic at the place of confinement, and so may precipitate a 'flying squad' call.

PREMEDICATION

Antacid prophylaxis, as above.

PERIOPERATIVE MANAGEMENT

Monitoring:
- ECG
- Noninvasive BP
- Sao_2
- $ETco_2$.

Anaesthetic technique
If a regional block, e.g. epidural, is in situ, it is simplest and safest to extend or reinstate the block, bearing in mind that sympathetic block will exacerbate the bleeding. If bleeding is controlled and vital signs are stable, a spinal or epidural may be instituted.

Persistent bleeding which is not controlled and/or is accompanied by deteriorating vital signs is a contraindication to institution or augmentation of regional anaesthesia.

If general anaesthesia is used, then a rapid sequence induction is indicated. Intubation may be more difficult than in the nonpregnant patient. The anaesthetic drugs are a matter of personal preference, bearing in mind the following points:

- Volatile agents may contribute to bleeding due to uterine relaxation, but may be a useful tocolytic to facilitate exploration of the contracting uterus
- Ketamine should be avoided as it increases uterine tone
- Intravenous nitroglycerin has been used to induce uterine relaxation in the patient with retained placenta, but this is controversial and so is probably only of academic interest.

POSTOPERATIVE MANAGEMENT

It is desirable to have the patient awake, alert and free of pain as soon as possible, in view of the need to care for the new baby. A regional technique will favour this.

Following general anaesthesia the patient should be recovered in a recovery room with full monitoring and all the usual precautions taken to prevent aspiration of stomach contents. NSAIDs are usually adequate for analgesia.

Oxytoxics may be needed, and it is prudent to maintain intravenous access until the patient is taking fluids orally.

OUTCOME

In most cases in the UK the outcome is uncomplicated. This is in marked contrast to the Third World where there is a significant mortality and morbidity.

Previous uterine surgery increases the small risk of placenta accreta. This may lead to life-threatening postpartum haemorrhage and should be borne in mind. In the presence of intractable bleeding, the patient may need an emergency hysterectomy. Transfusions of 30–50 units of blood are not uncommon. The incidence of placenta accreta is increasing: about 1 in 3000 deliveries. It is particularly likely to occur after a Caesarean section for placenta praevia.

UNUSUAL COMPLICATIONS

There were two fatalities reported in the 1985–1987 triennial report on maternal mortality. One was caused by failure to diagnose a kinked and obstructed endotracheal tube. The second was consequent on late diagnosis compounded by refusal of a blood transfusion on religious grounds.

A preliminary report has suggested a higher than expected incidence of backache following manual removal of placenta under regional block. Numbers are so far very small.

A case report has been published describing long-term (3 days) reversible paraplegia following spinal anaesthesia for this condition. Clinical investigation suggested prolonged positioning on the operating table was the probable cause.

BIBLIOGRAPHY

Anaesthetic management of patients with placenta accreta. Canadian Journal of Anaesthesia 1979; 34: 613–617

Extradural, spinal or combined block for obstetric surgical anaesthesia. British Journal of Anaesthesia 1990; 65: 225–233

The anaesthetist and the obstetric flying squad. Anaesthesia 1986; 41: 721–725

Ostheimer G W (ed). Manual of obstetric anaesthesia, 2nd edn. Churchill Livingstone, Edinburgh

CROSS REFERENCES

Antacid prophylaxis
Surgical Procedures 20: 400

Intraoperative hypotension
Anaesthetic Factors 33: 638

21

UROLOGY

L. Bromley

OVERVIEW

L. Bromley

Patients presenting for urological operations are of all ages and degrees of fitness. Paediatric reconstructive urology is a highly specialized area where operations are performed on newborn babies and repeated operations will take place throughout childhood and adolescence. This takes place in specialist centres and is not covered in this section.

The majority of urology patients are elderly men. The increased incidence of benign hyperplasia of the prostate gland with age is largely responsible. There is an association between cigarette smoking over long periods and bladder cancer. The combination of maturity onset diabetes and incomplete bladder emptying predisposes to urinary-tract infections. These three factors act to skew the population presenting for urological investigation and operation.

As with anaesthesia for any group of elderly patients, intercurrent diseases are of the utmost importance to the anaesthetist. Where obstruction of the lower urinary tract has been longstanding, it is of great importance to ensure that kidney function is normal and urea and creatinine are not rising. Formal preoperative assessment is essential, with particular reference to smoking-related diseases. Many patients return on a regular basis for repeat examination, it is a mistake to assume that recent, e.g. 3 months ago, uneventful anaesthesia will allow the anaesthetist to omit a preoperative visit. Other important medical events are more likely in this age group, and a history should always be taken.

A number of urologists have an interest in the problems of continence in women. These problems sometimes arise after traumatic childbirth, or may be related to gynaecological surgery. There seems to be no hard-and-fast rule on who should deal with these conditions, and local practice is the deciding factor. It may therefore be the case that operations such as colposuspension, or Stamey's operation may appear in one hospital on a urology list, and in another on a gynaecology list.

Urologists were among the first surgeons to realize the potential of minimally invasive surgery. The transurethral prostatectomy was one of the first minimally invasive procedures, and although it is not without its problems, and there is some doubt as to whether the mortality is lower over a 5-year period, the technique is now universally accepted. In the last 3 years there has been a growing interest in performing other operations, particularly nephrectomy, laparoscopically, and staging of advanced prostate cancer by laparoscopic sampling of para-aortic lymph nodes. The introduction of the flexible cystoscope has allowed urologists to perform many diagnostic cystoscopies without general anaesthesia in the out-patient clinic. This has enabled them to select patients for general anaesthesia cystoscopy who need biopsy of the bladder mucosa, or more extensive examination.

The management of renal stones has been revolutionized in the last 10 years. Renal stones were formerly a major source of renal damage, and the passage of stones with associated renal colic is one of the commonest urological emergencies. Stones are now treated with a combination of minimally invasive techniques, and open operations are becoming rare. The use of ultrasonic lithotripsy, percutaneous nephrolithotomy, and ureteric lasering of stones have virtually abolished use of the Dormia basket and open removal.

Major urological surgery falls into two groups: operations performed for malignant conditions of the genitourinary tract, and operations for reconstruction of congenital malformations. A number of attempts have been made in both areas to provide the patient with as normal a function as possible postoperatively. Previously, urinary diversion into an ileal conduit was used as a replacement for bladder function, but increasingly surgery is designed to refashion and to replace the bladder with a pouch constructed from a piece of bowel (caecoplasty, ileoplasty, or gastroplasty). This pouch can be attached to the trigone, if suitable, allowing normal voiding of urine postoperatively. If the bladder neck is to be removed, a continent stoma may be fashioned with the appendix, allowing catheterization of the stoma at regular intervals (Mitroffanof procedure).

A urologist is part of the team of specialists managing spinal-injury patients, where procedures to restore continence by using artificial urinary sphincters and to restore erectile function by using penile implants, may be required. This group of patients has its own set of anaesthetic problems. Loss of erectile function is also found amongst diabetic men, and operations are performed to overcome this. Ligation of penile veins, implantation of rods or inflatable devices are undertaken. These patients are frequently long-standing diabetics and, in considering their anaesthetic management, the other sequelae of diabetes must be investigated, and blood-sugar control managed perioperatively.

The most commonly performed urological procedures are reviewed in detail in this section.

CROSS REFERENCES

Spinal chord injury (acute)
Patient Conditions 1: 23
Spinal chord injury (chronic)
Patient Conditions 1: 26
Diabetes mellitus
Patient Conditions 2: 42
The elderly patient
Patient Conditions 11: 252

CYSTOSCOPY

L. Bromley

PROCEDURE

- Examination of the urethral and bladder mucosa using a rigid fibre-optic cystoscope passed through the urethra
- Diagnostic for initial investigation of symptoms, particularly haematuria or recurrent urinary-tract infections
- Check cystoscopy is performed after treatment of bladder cancer to look for recurrence, often combined with diathermy or resection of recurrences
- Frequently performed as a day-case
- Fibre-optic cystoscopy using a flexible cystoscope is usually performed under local anaesthesia.

PATIENT CHARACTERISTICS

Patients for cystoscopy are frequently:

- Male, over 50 years of age
- Have a high incidence of chronic disease.
- ASA status II and III.

PREOPERATIVE ASSESSMENT AND INVESTIGATIONS

- Assessment of cardiovascular and respiratory systems
- Assessment of renal function
- If repeat cystoscopy, ask if there has been any change in health status since last visit
- Check previous anaesthetic records
- Assess suitability for day-case anaesthesia.

PREMEDICATION

Patients having day-case cystoscopies are frequently not premedicated. If required, a benzodiazepine is appropriate.

PERIOPERATIVE MANAGEMENT

Monitoring:
- ECG
- Noninvasive BP
- Sao_2.

Anaesthetic technique:
- *General anaesthesia*, spontaneously breathing. Induction commonly with propofol, airway management with face-mask or laryngeal mask airway. Volatile agent of choice or use a TIVA technique with propofol. Biopsy and resection of tumour will require analgesic supplementation.
- *Regional anaesthesia* may be indicated in severe respiratory disease. Caudal block may be sufficient, but filling of the bladder may cause discomfort which is not blocked by a caudal. A low spinal block is more reliable.

These anaesthetics, despite their simplicity, can be the most challenging to give smoothly. Unpremeditated patients who are elderly and frequently have respiratory disease can be very difficult to settle to spontaneous-breathing anaesthesia. The combination of propofol and the laryngeal mask has made the anaesthetist's task easier, but there is still a great deal of skill to performing this anaesthetic well.

POSTOPERATIVE MANAGEMENT

Diagnostic and check cystoscopies were no resection has taken place do not result in significant postoperative pain. In the case of a biopsy, intraoperative supplementation of the anaesthetic with an intravenous analgesic will be sufficient, and simple analgesics can be prescribed for the postoperative period.

Day-case patients are allowed to go home after they have recovered, taken a drink, and passed urine. They should be accompanied.

OUTCOME

Many patients have repeat cystoscopies at regular intervals over a long period of time.

The management of carcinoma of the bladder by radiotherapy and intravesical chemotherapy ensures a steady supply of patients for this procedure. These patients are often very knowledgeable about the procedure, and their wishes, particularly regarding premedication, should be given due consideration. A small number of patients have disease that cannot be controlled with this treatment and go on to have a cystectomy.

BIBLIOGRAPHY

Brodrick P M, Webster N R, Nunn J F. The laryngeal mask airway. A study of 100 patients during spontaneous breathing. Anaesthesia 1989; 44: 238–241

Harrison D A, Langham B T. Spinal anaesthesia for urological surgery. A survey of failure rate, postdural headache and patient satisfaction. Anaesthesia 1992; 47: 902–904

CROSS REFERENCES

Diabetes mellitus
Patient Conditions 2: 42
The elderly patient
Patient Conditions 11: 252
Day-case surgery
Anaesthetic Factors 29: 542
Preoperative assessment of pulmonary risk
Anaesthetic Factors 34: 697

CYSTECTOMY

L. Bromley

PROCEDURE

Cystectomy is the operative removal of the urinary bladder, usually undertaken for treatment of carcinoma of the transitional epithelium of the bladder, or more rarely for sarcoma of the bladder wall. Some operations of cystectomy are performed for intractable interstitial cystitis.

The operation is performed via an abdominal incision, and involves a procedure to divert the flow of urine to a different reservoir. This may entail implanting the ureters into a length of ileum which has been isolated from the gut externalized as a stoma, known as an 'ileal conduit'. Alternatively, part of the stomach, caecum, or colon may be used to fashion a pouch into which the ureters are implanted. This pouch can be drained by using the appendix as a continent stoma, which can be intermittently catheterized. This operation carries the eponymous name of 'Mitroffanof'. It is sometimes possible in benign conditions to attach the pouch to the trigone, or straight onto the bladder neck.

Patients having this operation for the removal of tumours will have received radiotherapy to the pelvis, and consequently the operative bleeding may be difficult to control.

PATIENT CHARACTERISTICS

Patients for cystectomy are generally:

- Over 50 years of age
- High incidence of smokers
- ASA grade II to IV.

These patients have commonly had a number of previous general anaesthetics for check cystoscopies. They commonly have chronic disease in other systems, particularly disease associated with smoking.

PREOPERATIVE ASSESSMENT AND INVESTIGATIONS

- Systematic review and optimization of chronic disease states is important
- Availability of blood for transfusion
- Discussion of postoperative pain relief; consent for epidural, if chosen.

PREMEDICATION

Analgesic premedication is indicated. An antisialogogue is optional; anticholinergic drugs may cause confusion in elderly people.

THEATRE PREPARATION

This is likely to be a long operation, and maintenance of body temperature is important. A warm operating theatre, warming blanket, fluid warmer and humidification of inspired gases are all necessary.

PERIOPERATIVE MANAGEMENT

Monitoring:

- ECG
- Invasive arterial pressure
- Central venous pressure (CVP)
- Sao_2
- $ETco_2$
- Blood loss
- Core temperature.

Anaesthetic technique

General anaesthesia alone or combined with epidural anaesthesia is used. A combination of general anaesthesia and epidural is particularly useful where the epidural block is to be used for postoperative analgesia. The potential for excessive blood loss combined with the inability to measure urine output during the surgery makes monitoring of CVP mandatory.

As with any long procedure, the use of thromboembolic prophylaxis should be discussed with the surgeon.

POSTOPERATIVE MANAGEMENT

The management of postoperative pain is best achieved via an epidural infusion of low-dose local anaesthetic and opioids. The local practice as to nursing and the management of epidurals containing opioids varies. It may be necessary to manage the patient on a HDU. If the latter is the case, the patient should be electively booked for the HDU before surgery. Providing that the patient is haemodynamically stable and normothermic at the end of the procedure, there is no other indication for HDU admission.

Where there is significant chest disease, postoperative physiotherapy is indicated. The combination of large abdominal incision and the use of opioids postoperatively is an indication for prescribing additional oxygen for the first three postoperative days and nights.

OUTCOME

This is a major operation and the postoperative mortality is between 3% and 5%.

BIBLIOGRAPHY

Beydon L, Hassapopoulos J, Quera M A et al. Risk factors for oxygen desaturation during sleep after abdominal surgery. British Journal of Anaesthesia 1992; 69: 137–142

Hobbs G J, Roberts F L. Epidural infusion of bupivacaine and diamorphine for post operative analgesia use on general surgical wards. Anaesthesia 1992; 47: 58–62

Morris R H. Influence of ambient temperature on patient temperature during intra abdominal surgery. Archives of Surgery 1971; 173: 230–233

CROSS REFERENCES

The elderly patient
Patient Conditions 11: 252
Blood transfusion
Anaesthetic Factors 33: 616
Postoperative pain management
Anaesthetic Factors 33: 655

NEPHRECTOMY

L. Bromley

PROCEDURE

- Removal of kidney with or without part of the ureter
- Performed with the patient positioned on the side
- Access for surgeon improved by 'breaking' the table
- Potential for considerable blood loss.

PATIENT CHARACTERISTICS

- Procedure can be undertaken at any age
- In cases of chronic infection, patient may be debilitated.
- ASA I–IV.

Common associations with nephrectomy

Nephrectomy is performed for tumour, hydronephrosis, chronic infection and, rarely, for staghorn calculi which cannot be treated by others means. Patients with renal tumours may have pulmonary metastasis. Patients who have had chronic infections may have had poor health for some time, and may be poorly nourished, with low albumin.

PREOPERATIVE ASSESSMENT

- Exclude associated conditions
- Systematic review of other medical conditions
- Discuss postoperative analgesia and obtain consent for epidural block
- Ensure availability of blood.

PREMEDICATION

Analgesic premedication, with or without an antisialogogue, is indicated.

PERIOPERATIVE MANAGEMENT

Theatre preparation

Careful positioning of patient for this operation is important. The patient is placed on the table with the side of operation uppermost, and great care must be taken to support the patient and prevent them rolling off the table. Supports which fasten to the table may be used, or alternatively a bean-bag-type of support. This latter type of support helps to reduce heat loss. Fluids should be warmed. Care must be taken that the legs are supported by pillows and that the arms are not touching any part of the metal supports.

Anaesthetic technique

The positioning of the patient on the side results in a ventilation–perfusion mismatch between the lungs; IPPV is mandatory. In addition, there is a risk of surgical disruption of the pleura during the dissection.

Epidural analgesia via a low thoracic or high lumbar catheter is the most effective form of postoperative analgesia in these cases. Thus the combination of light general anaesthesia with IPPV with an epidural is the preferred method of anaesthesia. If an epidural is not possible, intercostal nerve blocks from T9 to T12 are a useful supplement to general anaesthesia and will give some postoperative pain relief.

The potential for blood loss during this operation is an indication for invasive monitoring. A large-bore-cannula, a central venous pressure line and an intra-arterial BP line are recommended. Monitoring should also include the following:

- ECG
- Sao_2
- $ETco_2$
- Blood loss
- Temperature.

At the end of the procedure, if there is any suggestion of damage to the pleura, several large-volume breaths may be given to attempt to detect any pleural leak. If there is a pneumothorax, it must be drained.

POSTOPERATIVE MANAGEMENT

Nephrectomy is a painful operation and requires optimal postoperative pain relief. This is best provided by continuous epidural infusion of a mixture of opioids and low-dose local anaesthetics. If local policy requires patients with epidural infusions to be nursed in a HDU, then a bed should be booked preoperatively.

There is a risk of atelectasis in the dependent lung and good physiotherapy is essential, for which good pain relief is also important.

OUTCOME

Long-term outcome depends largely on the aetiology of the renal damage. Operative mortality is of the order of 1%.

BIBLIOGRAPHY

Nunn J F. The lateral position in anaesthesia. In: Nunn's applied respiratory physiology, 4th edn. Butterworth-Heinemann, Oxford, 1993

CROSS REFERENCES

Blood transfusion
Anaesthetic Factors 33: 616
Complications of position
Anaesthetic Factors 33: 618

OPEN PROSTATECTOMY

H. Owen Reece

21

PROCEDURE

Open prostatectomy is performed in one of two ways:

- *Retropubic prostatectomy* – when a benign hypertrophic prostate is too large for transurethral resection
- *Radical prostatectomy* – for clearance of a malignant prostatic tumour and lymph nodes (if they are involved on frozen section; see below).

PATIENT CHARACTERISTICS

- Over 50 years of age
- High incidence of chronic disease
- ASA grade II–IV.

PREOPERATIVE ASSESSMENT AND INVESTIGATIONS

- Identification and assessment of chronic disease.
- Deep view thrombosis prophylaxis (elasticated stockings are recommended; patients are not routinely heparinized because it is felt that, on balance, the decreased haemostasis may do more harm than good).
- Blood transfusion availability (3 units for retropubic prostatectomy, 6 units for radical prostatectomy).
- Antibiotic prophylaxis (cefuroxime and metronidazole is a popular combination).
- Assessment of the suitability for spinal or epidural analgesia. This is a particularly valuable technique to use in conjunction with general anaesthesia for radical prostatectomy because it provides excellent postoperative analgesia, reduces the perioperative blood loss and decreases the quantity of inhalational agent required.

PREMEDICATION

- An opioid premedicant, for example papaveretum or morphine, is suitable. It has the advantage of pre-empting the nociceptive stimulus, although if an epidural technique is contemplated these are not necessary.
- A benzodiazepine is a suitable alternative and will provide anxiolysis and amnesia. All elderly patients are at risk of becoming confused if anticholinergics which cross the blood–brain barrier (e.g. hyoscine) are employed.

THEATRE PREPARATION

- Patient positioning requires care, since surgery is often lengthy.
- Monitoring nasopharyngeal temperature is an easy and effective means of measuring body temperature. Body temperature should be maintained with a warming mattress, warmed intravenous fluids and a ventilator circuit humidifier.

PERIOPERATIVE MANAGEMENT

Monitoring:

- Arterial BP (via an arterial line for a radical prostatectomy)
- ECG
- Sao_2
- $ETco_2$
- Core temperature
- Fluid balance and blood loss
- Central venous pressure (for radical prostatectomy).

Anaesthetic technique

The combination of epidural and general anaesthesia with a continuous infusion of muscle relaxant and minimal volatile agent is a suitable technique. For retropubic prostatectomy, epidural analgesia is sufficient, if required.

During radical prostatectomy there will be an interval (which may be substantial) during which a frozen section of pelvic lymph node is examined histologically. If the nodes contain metastatic deposits, surgery will not proceed.

Retropubic prostatectomy leaves the prostatic capsule intact, and bleeding, though significant, is not as great (1–2 l) as in radical prostatectomy, in which the capsule is removed. In the latter case the blood loss may be as much as 4 l. It has been suggested that fibrinolysins, which exacerbate bleeding, are released by prostatic handling.

POSTOPERATIVE MANAGEMENT

If an epidural infusion is already in situ, then a combination of local analgesia and an epidural opioid will provide excellent analgesia for both procedures.

Postoperative blood loss and urine output should be monitored.

OUTCOME

With good case selection, the 5-year survival is 95%. Operative mortality is very low.

BIBLIOGRAPHY

Madsen R E, Madsen P O. Influence of anaesthesia on blood loss in transurethral resection of the prostate. Anesthesia and Analgesia 1967; 46: 330–332

Richmond C E, Bromley L M, Woolf C J. Preoperative morphine pre-empts postoperative pain. Lancet 1993; 342: 73–75

Smart R F. Endoscopic injection of the vasopressor ornithine-8-vasopressin on transurethral resection. British Journal of Urology 1984; 56: 191–197

CROSS REFERENCES

The elderly patient
Patient Conditions 11: 252
Blood transfusion
Anaesthetic Factors 33: 616
Thrombotic embolism
Anaesthetic Factors 33: 664
Preoperative assessment of pulmonary risk
Anaesthetic Factors 34: 697

PERCUTANEOUS NEPHROLITHOTOMY

J. Frossard

PROCEDURE

Percutaneous nephrolithotomy (PCNL) is a procedure whereby stones in the renal pelvis are removed with a nephroscope via a dilated percutaneous puncture made under X-ray control.

PATIENT CHARACTERISTICS

Patients for PCNL are generally:
- Any age
- ASA I–IV
- May have a compromised renal function.

PREOPERATIVE INVESTIGATIONS

- Exclusion of commonly associated medical conditions
- Review of renal function
- Blood transfusion availability
- Antibiotic prophylaxis.

PREMEDICATION

At the anaesthetist's discretion.

PERIOPERATIVE MANAGEMENT

Monitoring:
- ECG
- Noninvasive BP
- Sao_2
- $ETco_2$
- Estimation of blood loss
- Core temperature.

Anaesthetic technique:
- Intravenous cannula for access
- Muscular paralysis, because the patient will be placed prone and coughing must be avoided during renal puncture
- Use an armoured tracheal tube.

Positioning:
- The patient is placed first in the lithotomy position and a retrograde catheter is placed in the ureter to allow for opacification of the percutaneous puncture and to prevent fragments of stone passing down the ureter.
- The patient is then turned to the prone position:
  - Ensure that there is enough man-power to turn the patient
  - Protect the eyes, shoulders, knees, elbows
  - Place arm with intravenous access above the head (beware of brachial plexus strain)
  - The other arm with the BP cuff may be placed by the side
  - Place a pillow under the chest to free the abdomen for ventilation
  - Place a pad under the flank to prevent a mobile kidney from rotating anteriorly in the prone position
  - Turn the head to the side to be punctured in order to prevent neck strain
  - Drape the patient in a foil blanket (with a hole cut in it for the puncture site) because the patient often becomes wet (this will help to conserve heat; do not use a foil blanket if diathermy is to be used)
  - Warm irrigation fluid.

COMPLICATIONS

Haemorrhage

Tears in the parenchyma may occur if the rigid scope is not handled with care.

Bleeding requiring transfusion following percutaneous renal manipulation is rare. Most reports quote 3%. About 0.5% of cases may require balloon tamponade of the tract or arterial embolization. Transfusion is very rare in patients that have small stones, and bleeding is not related to the size of the track.

Extravasation

Any tear in the pelvicalyceal system will result in some extravasation of the irrigant fluid. It is important, therefore, that normal saline is used as the endoscopic irrigant. Water and glycine can cause fluid intoxication because they are absorbed from the peritoneum.

Pleural complications

If an intercostal puncture is performed to reach an upper calyceal calculus, the pleura may be entered and either a minor pleural reaction seen or following endoscopy there could be a massive collection of irrigant fluid and air within the thoracic cavity.

Infection

The most serious complication that must be guarded against is infection. Stones containing infection may be disintegrated at percutaneous nephrolithotomy, releasing bacteria into the urine and, therefore, potentially into the bloodstream. Prophylactic antibiotics should be used routinely. Bacteraemia is unavoidable, but the time of the endoscopy should be limited. If a large infected stone is being disintegrated and infection is clearly present, endoscopy should be limited to 1 h. Endoscopy for a noninfected stone should be limited to 1.5 h. If Gram-negative septicaemia is suspected, the patient should be treated aggressively immediately.

POSTOPERATIVE MANAGEMENT

Intravenous fluids should be given to increase urine output and flush out any gravel via the nephrostomy left in situ. Analgesia, as required, with opioids and/or NSAIDs if renal function is normal.

BIBLIOGRAPHY

Marberger M, Stackl W, Hruby W. Percutaneous lithopaxy of renal calculi with ultrasound. European Urology 1982; 8: 236–237

Pollack H M, Banner M P. Percutaneous extraction of renal and ureteric calculi; technical considerations. American Journal of Roentgenology 1984; 143: 778–784

Schultz P E, Hanno P M, Wein A J et al. Percutaneous ultrasonic lithotripsy: choice of irrigant. Journal of Urology 1983; 130: 858–860

CROSS REFERENCES

Blood transfusion
Anaesthetic Factors 33: 616

Complications of position
Anaesthetic Factors 33: 618

TUR syndrome
Anaesthetic Factors 33: 675

TRANSURETHRAL PROSTATECTOMY

L. Bromley

PROCEDURE

- 95% of prostatectomies are performed endoscopically
- The patient is placed in the lithotomy position
- Continuous irrigation of the bladder with a solution of 1.5% glycine occurs during the resection
- The operation may be performed as a repeat procedure.

PATIENT CHARACTERISTICS

- Over 50 years of age; male
- High incidence of chronic disease
- ASA status I–IV.

Common associations with transurethral prostatectomy

The patient may present with haematuria or may have longstanding obstruction, increasing the risk of renal failure. Urinary-tract infection can complicate large residual volumes of urine. These patients have a higher incidence of cardiopulmonary problems, hypertension, obesity and diabetes mellitus.

PREOPERATIVE ASSESSMENT AND INVESTIGATIONS

- Exclude associated conditions
- Systematic review of intercurrent illness
- Discuss anaesthetic technique and decide on suitability for regional anaesthesia.

PREMEDICATION

Anxiolysis with a benzodiazepine is suitable for patients having a regional technique. For general anaesthesia analgesic premedication may be preferred.

PERIOPERATIVE MANAGEMENT

Theatre preparation

Warm irrigating fluid should be used in order to maintain core temperature.

Anaesthetic technique

This operation can be conducted using a regional technique: either spinal or epidural anaesthesia. This method is commonly used, although a number of patients prefer to be asleep during the operation. There are advantages to a regional technique:

- These patients often have intercurrent chest disease, and benefit postoperatively from not having a general anaesthetic
- The awake patient is a better monitor of the onset of the 'transurethral (TUR) syndrome', as any confusion can be detected rapidly
- There is a reduction in the incidence of postoperative thromboembolic disease.

If a general anaesthetic is to be used, paralysis and ventilation is not specifically required for this operation which can be performed with the patient breathing spontaneously through a laryngeal mask.

Monitoring:

- ECG
- Noninvasive BP
- Sao_2
- Temperature.

The TUR syndrome

This is caused by the absorption of the irrigating fluid during resection of the prostate (see section 675). Symptoms include hypertension, visual disturbances, dyspnoea, mental changes, and circulatory collapse.

POSTOPERATIVE MANAGEMENT

The TUR syndrome can develop at any stage in the postoperative period and the nursing staff should be aware of this. The initial postoperative period is not characterized as particularly painful, the most painful period being at the time when the catheter is removed.

OUTCOME

The reported hospital mortality is 0.2–2.5% and may be as low as 0.5–1% in specialist centres. There is evidence of increased intermediate and long-term mortality and morbidity with TURP compared with open prostatectomy, and with other minimally invasive surgery in this age group. These reports can all be attributed to cardiovascular morbidity and mortality factors. Studies also suggest that haemodynamic changes relating to a drop in core temperature may be responsible.

BIBLIOGRAPHY

Evans J, Singer M, Chapple C, Macartney N, Walker M, Milroy E. Haemodynamic evidence for cardiac stress during transurethral prostatectomy. British Medical Journal 1992; 304: 666–670.

Hahn R. Prevention of TUR syndrome by detection of trace ethanol in the expired breath. Anaesthesia 1990; 45: 577–581

Roos N, Wennberg J, Malenka D et al. Mortality and re-operation after open and transurethral resection of the prostate for benign prostatic hyperplasia. The New England Journal of Medicine 320: 1120–1123

CROSS REFERENCES

The elderly patient
Patient Conditions 11: 252

Blood transfusion
Anaesthetic Factors 33: 616

Fluid and electrolyte balance
Anaesthetic Factors 33: 626

TUR syndrome
Anaesthetic Factors 33: 675

22

VASCULAR SURGERY

A. J. Mortimer

OVERVIEW

J. M. Hopkinson and A. J. Mortimer

Vascular surgery principally comprises the operations of carotid endarterectomy, infrarenal aortic reconstruction and limb salvage by revascularization or amputation procedures. The most common underlying condition requiring treatment is atherosclerotic disease of the conducting arteries causing progressive arterial occlusion. This results in ischaemic symptoms when oxygen delivery is insufficient to satisfy tissue oxygen consumption. Intermittent claudication is the commonest symptom of peripheral vascular disease, which occurs when arterial blood flow is reduced by 75% or more (approximately 50% reduction in arterial diameter). Rest pain in a limb represents advanced disease requiring urgent investigation.

MORTALITY

Elective and emergency vascular surgical procedures have a high morbidity and a mortality between 5% and 50% because of the coexistence of numerous associated conditions.

Age

The majority of patients are between 60 and 80 years old. Younger patients are associated with advanced atherosclerotic disease, as occurs in familial hyperlipidaemia and diabetes mellitus.

Sex

Males predominate, although peripheral vascular disease is increasing in females.

ASA physical status

Advanced age and the presence of coexisting disease places patients into group III (the majority), group IV, or group V (ruptured aorta).

Coexisting disease

- *Hypertension (50%).* Hypertensive disease affects the conducting arteries supplying the heart, brain and kidneys, as well as the arteriolar resistance vessels throughout the circulation. In the heart this results in left ventricular hypertrophy, reduced ventricular compliance, and the need for filling pressures higher than normal to ensure adequate cardiac output. In the brain and kidneys, autoregulation of blood flow is shifted to the right, exposing these vital organs to reduced blood flow when the perfusion pressure is reduced. The widespread increase in arteriolar resistance means that patients manifest exaggerated responses to excess induction agents (hypotension) and light anaesthesia (hypertension).
- *Coronary artery disease (angina 15%; previous myocardial infarction 50%).* Approximately two-thirds of all patients have atherosclerotic disease of the coronary arteries. This manifests as angina or previous myocardial infarction. Subendocardial infarction, as opposed to transmural infarction, is the most frequent problem, and is more likely to occur in hypertensive subjects. Perioperative myocardial infarction occurs mostly in the first postoperative week. The incidence is highest on the third postoperative day, and ranges from 3% in 8% in published series. Myocardial performance is the single most important determinant of outcome following a major vascular operation.
- *Congestive cardiac failure (15%).* Failure of one or both ventricles occurs in 15% of all patients. Left ventricular failure (pulmonary oedema) or right ventricular failure (dependent oedema) and associated symptoms must be treated prior to surgery.
- *Pulmonary disease (25–50%)* Chronic obstructive pulmonary disease (COPD) is common because of the high incidence of smokers. Preoperative lung function tests are rarely of help, as the symptoms are obvious. The most useful assessment of cardiorespiratory function is arterial blood-gas estimation. Whilst hypoxia (P_aO_2 <7.0 kPa) is occasionally found, hypercarbia

($P_{a}CO_2$ >7.0 kPa) is rare. Regular nebulizers with or without physiotherapy should be considered.

- *Renal disease (5–15%).* Chronic renal failure caused by hypertensive disease, congestive cardiac failure, and involvement of the renal arteries in atherosclerotic and/or aneurysmal disease, is detected by elevated plasma creatinine and urea concentrations preoperatively. A baseline 24-h urinary creatinine clearance estimation is useful before aortic surgery.
- *Endocrine disease – diabetes mellitus (10%).* Diabetic patients comprise a large number of those undergoing peripheral arterial reconstruction. The microvascular circulation is affected predominantly and, as a consequence, revascularization is sometimes inappropriate. Amputation of toes and limbs is commonly undertaken to control local infection which may be adversely affecting diabetic management. Optimal control of blood glucose levels, hydration and blood loss is essential in the perioperative period. Insulin-dependent patients should be managed on an intravenous fluid and a sliding-scale insulin regime. Those on oral antidiabetic agents should omit their dose on the morning of surgery. These agents sometimes have long durations of action (up to 24 h) and it is advisable to commence a glucose intravenous infusion with hourly blood glucose monitoring, in order to avoid hypoglycaemia.

CONCURRENT MEDICATION

Most patients are receiving medication from one or more of the groups listed below. Except for oral antidiabetic agents, *all* drugs should be continued on the day of surgery and thereafter, irrespective of the pharmacological group, the following especially:

- Antianginal agents
- Antihypertensive agents
- Antiarrhythmic therapy
- Antiplatelet drugs
- Bronchodilators
- Inotropes.

BIBLIOGRAPHY

Kaplan J A (ed). Vascular anaesthesia. Churchill Livingstone, New York, 1991

Roizen M F (ed). Anaesthesia for vascular surgery. Churchill Livingstone, New York, 1990

Smith G. Anaesthesia for vascular surgery. In: Bell P R F, Jamieson C C V, Ruckley C V (eds) Surgical management of vascular disease. W B Saunders, London, 1992, ch 20, p 291–307

CROSS REFERENCES

Diabetes mellitus
  Patient Conditions 2: 42
Intraoperative hypertension
  Anaesthetic Factors 33: 636
Intraoperative hypotension
  Anaesthetic Factors 33: 638
Postoperative oliguria
  Anaesthetic Factors 33: 652
Preoperative assessment of cardiovascular risk in noncardiac surgery
  Anaesthetic Factors 34: 692
Preoperative assessment of pulmonary risk
  Anaesthetic Factors 34: 697

22

ABDOMINAL AORTIC RECONSTRUCTION – ELECTIVE

J. M. Hopkinson and A. J. Mortimer

PROCEDURE

This is a major surgical procedure which is performed on a high-risk patient group, aimed at reducing the mortality from rupture (aneurysm) or the unpleasant symptoms of claudication (occlusive disease).

The procedure involves aortic cross-clamping with resultant haemodynamic and ischaemic complications. A tube (aneurysm) or a bifurcation graft (occlusive disease) is inserted below the origin of the renal arteries. The principal perioperative complication is myocardial infarction.

PREOPERATIVE ASSESSMENT AND INVESTIGATIONS

Aims:

- Correct patient selection for surgery to improve outcome. Identify a low-risk subgroup – either no coronary artery disease or mild coronary artery disease with normal investigations.
- Optimize general condition by treating coexisting problems, in particular congestive cardiac failure and hypertension.
- Defer patients with recent (less than 6 months ago) myocardial infarction.
- On the basis of surgical and anaesthetic assessment, conservative management may be indicated.

General assessment:

- Routine clinical assessment of the cardiovascular and respiratory systems
- Full anaesthetic and drug history

Investigations:
- Haemoglobin, platelets, white cell count
- Cross-match 6 units of blood
- Urea, creatinine, electrolytes, blood glucose
- Resting 12-lead ECG
- Chest X-ray
- Respiratory function tests (PEFR, FEV_1/FVC, if history of chronic obstructive pulmonary disease (COPD))
- Echocardiography (left ventricular and valvular function plus ejection fraction)
- Abdominal CT scan to define the limits of the lesion

- Further investigations may be considered to quantify the degree of coronary artery disease and myocardial dysfunction:
  - Ambulatory 24-h ECG to detect conduction abnormalities and silent myocardial ischaemia
  - Radionuclide dipyridamole–thallium scanning (MUGA scan) to detect abnormalities of coronary artery perfusion
  - Angiography and coronary revascularization prior to aortic surgery, if indicated by the presence of severe coronary artery disease or other cardiac disease
  - Carotid artery surgery prior to aneurysm repair if
    (i) asymptomatic and >90% stenosis,
    (ii) symptomatic and >70% stenosis.
- Arrange for an ICU/HDU bed for postoperative cardiorespiratory monitoring and provision of adequate analgesia.

PREMEDICATION

- Explain to patient about the procedure, anaesthetic management and postoperative care
- Anxiolytic drugs (amnesia is also useful), e.g. temazepam or lorazepam
- Continue usual cardiac medication, especially antianginal and antihypertensive drugs
- Avoid anticholinergics which may compromise the coronary circulation due to tachycardia.

PERIOPERATIVE MANAGEMENT

Anaesthetic room:

- Reassure the patient and maintain a calm environment

- Oxygen via a clear face-mask
- Establish initial monitoring as follows:
  - ECG
  - Pulse oximetry
  - Invasive arterial pressure line under local anaesthesia (radial artery)
  - Central venous pressure (CVP) catheter or pulmonary artery (PA) catheter in the right internal jugular vein
- Epidural catheter (thoracic or lumbar).

Note: the CVP line, PA catheter and epidural catheter may be inserted postinduction if preferred. A useful technique is to insert a PA catheter sheath in the right internal jugular vein of all patients. A PA catheter can then easily be inserted without delay if required perioperatively.

Induction of anaesthesia:
- Pre-oxygenate the patient
- Maintain haemodynamic stability during induction and endotracheal intubation
- Insert a nasogastric tube (postoperative ileus is common)
- Insert a urinary catheter.

Maintenance of anaesthesia

A balanced anaesthetic technique with IPPV to normocapnia is recommended. Maintain cardiovascular stability at all times – vasopressors or vasodilators may be required. Humidify inspired gases, warm intravenous fluids and use a heated mattress on the operating table to minimize heat loss.

Intraoperative monitoring:
- ECG – leads II and V5 with ST segment analysis for early warning of subendocardial ischaemia
- Sa_{O_2}
- Capnography
- $F_{I}O_2$
- Core temperature
- Invasive arterial BP
- CVP
- PA flotation catheter if left ventricular dysfunction has been identified preoperatively (ejection fraction less than 50%)
- Fluid balance – measure blood loss and urine output.

Positioning

Supine with arms out for access (take care with the brachial plexus). Table break may be requested.

Specific points
- Heparinization (5000 units) is generally requested prior to aortic cross-clamping.
- Have to hand a selection of vagodilators (e.g. glyceryl trinitrate) and vasopressors (e.g. metaraminol or methoxamine).
- Aortic cross-clamping produces a marked increase in left ventricular afterload in patients with aneurysmal disease. It is not generally a problem in patients with occlusive aortoiliac disease who have a well-developed lumbar collateral circulation. An increased left ventricular end-diastolic pressure may, however, precipitate myocardial ischaemia due to reduced coronary flow. Possible techniques of management include:
  - Add a volatile agent to produce a dose-dependent reduction in myocardial contractility
  - Use a vasodilator drug (e.g. glyceryl trinitrate infusion) following cross-clamping
  - An epidural sympathetic block reduces the response to cross-clamping.
- Aortic cross-clamp release .may cause profound hypotension. Therefore:
  - Prior to cross-clamp release, volume load the patient guided by either CVP or PA wedge; increase to 5 mmHg above baseline value
  - Request controlled cross-clamp release by the surgeon
  - Use a vasopressor if necessary.
- Blood loss may be high, requiring transfusion (average 4 units). Therefore:
  - Cross-match 6 units minimum preoperatively
  - Consider preoperative autologous donation
  - Consider normovolaemic haemodilution postinduction (2 units)
  - Intraoperative cell salvage is useful.

POSTOPERATIVE MANAGEMENT

- Transfer to a HDU or ITU is required for 24 h
- A short period of ventilation may be required in high-risk patients to enable haemodynamic stability, normothermia and adequate analgesia to be attained
- Supplementary face-mask oxygen should be administered for a minimum of 3 days postoperatively
- Physiotherapy should be commenced early to optimize lung expansion.

Analgesia

There are various suitable techniques:

- Intravenous opioid infusion together with a patient-controlled analgesia system
- Epidural local anaesthetic infusion, with or without opioids
- Bilateral intercostal nerve blocks (these need repeating at intervals and there is a risk of pneumothorax).

POSTOPERATIVE COMPLICATIONS

Surgical:

- Ischaemic limb ('trash-foot') due to embolization
- Haemorrhage from graft anastomoses
- Ischaemia of the gastrointestinal tract.

Return to theatre may be required with all the attendant risks.

Medical:

- Subendocardial ischaemia and infarction
- Renal failure – depends on preoperative renal function, site of cross-clamping and postoperative cardiac function
- Pulmonary complications – basal atelectasis, hypoxaemia, respiratory failure.

OUTCOME

- Mortality ranges from 5% to 10% (as compared with that for elective adult cardiac surgery of 1–5%)
- Outcome depends on age, coexisting disease and the nature of the surgical procedure
- Perioperative myocardial infarction is the principal cause of mortality.

BIBLIOGRAPHY

Cunningham A J. Anaesthesia for abdominal aortic surgery – a review (Part 1). Canadian Journal of Anaesthesia 1989; 36: 426–444

Cunningham A J. Anaesthesia for abdominal aortic surgery – a review (Part 2). Canadian Journal of Anaesthesia 1989; 36: 568–577

Hessell E A. Intraoperative management of abdominal aortic aneurysms: the anaesthesiologist's viewpoint. Surgical Clinics of North America 1989; 69: 775–793

CROSS REFERENCES

Blood transfusion
Anaesthetic Factors 33: 616
Complications of position
Anaesthetic Factors 33: 618
Postoperative oliguria
Anaesthetic Factors 33: 652
Preoperative assessment of cardiovascular risk in noncardiac surgery
Anaesthetic Factors 34: 692
Preoperative assessment of pulmonary risk
Anaesthetic Factors 34: 697

ABDOMINAL AORTIC RECONSTRUCTION – EMERGENCY

J. M. Hopkinson and A. J. Mortimer

PROCEDURE

Ruptured or leaking aortic aneurysms are fatal if untreated and emergency repair is the patient's only chance of survival. Patients, by definition, are ASA IV or V (E) and urgent surgery in a specialist unit is required. Rapid decisions need to be made on the value of surgery in any particular case because mortality is high, even in specialist units (50% or more).

PREOPERATIVE ASSESSMENT AND INVESTIGATIONS

- Identify patients for whom surgery is appropriate – certain criteria such as age, premorbid condition, response to initial resuscitation and urine output may be useful.
- Formal assessment and investigations are rarely possible, but attempts should be made to establish severity of any coexisting disease.
- Whilst assessing the patient, establish reliable intravenous access with two large-bore peripheral venous cannulae, and insert a percutaneous pulmonary artery catheter sheath in the right internal jugular vein. Send blood for Hb, platelets, cross-match, baseline coagulation tests and urea and electrolytes. Baseline renal function measurement is useful later for post-operative management.
- Use crystalloid or colloid solutions to maintain a systolic pressure of greater than 80 mmHg and transfer to theatre. There is little to be gained by increasing the blood pressure above 100 mmHg, as haemorrhage may increase.
- Insert an in-dwelling urinary catheter.

PERIOPERATIVE MANAGEMENT

- Notify the ITU of potential need for a bed
- Transfer to the operating theatre, with face-mask oxygen
- Try and reassure a very frightened patient and explain what you are doing
- Two anaesthetists should be in attendance
- No time should be wasted attempting to set up invasive arterial pressure monitoring or central venous lines at the beginning; it is more important for the surgeon to cross-clamp the aorta as soon as possible
- Colloid, blood, blood products and rapid infusers with warming coils should be prepared
- When the surgeons are scrubbed and ready to operate, and all anaesthetic equipment is available, the patient can be anaesthetized.

Induction:

- A standard rapid sequence induction with minimal dose of induction agent, as in any hypovolaemic patient
- As soon as the airway is secured instruct the surgeon to proceed
- Anticipate sudden hypotension as the abdominal tamponade effect is lost at laparotomy.

Maintenance:

- A balanced anaesthetic technique with IPPV and 100% oxygen is appropriate. Fentanyl and small increments of a volatile agent are suitable.
- When the aorta has been cross-clamped a degree of haemodynamic stability can usually be obtained, and this period is suitable for the insertion of the invasive monitoring lines (arterial pressure and pulmonary artery catheter).
- Humidify the anaesthetic gases, use a warming mattress and warm intravenous fluids to minimize the inevitable large heat loss.
- A nasogastric tube is required and should be inserted at a convenient moment because postoperative ileus is common.
- Position the patient supine with both arms out for access (take care with the brachial plexus).

Monitoring:
- ECG (leads II and V5 with ST segment analysis for subendocardial ischaemia)
- Sa_{O_2} (beware of problems in the hypovolaemic patient with poor peripheral perfusion)
- Capnography
- $F_{I}O_2$
- Invasive arterial pressure.
- Central venous pressure or, preferably, a pulmonary artery catheter
- Core temperature
- Fluid balance.

Specific points:
- Haemorrhage, continuing during surgery, is common and large volumes of blood may need to be administered. This may result in a dilutional coagulopathy requiring correction with FFP and platelets, depending on the results of coagulation studies.
- Cross-clamp release may cause severe hypotension despite best efforts to replace blood loss. The cross-clamp may need to be reapplied whilst further fluid is administered.
- Controlled cross-clamp release by the surgeon and the use of vasopressors may be required.

POSTOPERATIVE MANAGEMENT

- Transfer to the ITU with continued ventilatory support. Haemodynamic stability, normothermia and analgesia can be attained and coagulopathies treated.
- Extubate when the patient's condition allows. Continuous face-mask oxygen and frequent physiotherapy will then be necessary, possibly for several days.
- Close monitoring of renal function is required. Renal failure occurs commonly in this patient group.
- Recovery will depend on the success of the surgical repair, and the presence or absence of complications such as myocardial infarction, and renal and respiratory failure.

POSTOPERATIVE COMPLICATIONS

Surgical:
- Uncontrollable haemorrhage
- Limb ischaemia due to embolization ('trash-foot')
- Gastrointestinal or spinal cord ischaemia.

Medical:
- Myocardial infarction
- Pulmonary complications (basal atelectasis, hypoxaemia, adult respiratory distress syndrome)
- Renal failure.

OUTCOME

- The mortality among patients who undergo emergency surgery is 60–80%.
- It is of great importance that patients are not subjected to surgery when there is no real hope of survival. Appropriate patient selection is imperative and only suitably experienced surgeons and anaesthetists should be involved in the care of these patients.
- Adequate analgesia and nursing care should be provided for those patients where surgery is not appropriate, so they may die in peace and with dignity.

BIBLIOGRAPHY

Cunningham A J. Anaesthesia for repair of abdominal aortic aneurysms. In: Atkinson R S, Adams A P (eds) Recent advances in anaesthesia and analgesia. Churchill Livingstone, London, 1992, p 49–69

Earnshaw J J, Horrocks M. Advances in aortic aneurysm surgery. Hospital Update 1991; May: 366–374

Rutherford R B, McCroskey B L. Ruptured abdominal aortic aneurysms: special considerations. Surgical Clinics of North America 1989; 69: 859–868

CROSS REFERENCES

Coronary artery disease
Patient Conditions 4: 107

Blood transfusion
Anaesthetic Factors 33: 616

Complications of position
Anaesthetic Factors 33: 618

Intraoperative hypertension
Anaesthetic Factors 33: 636

Intraoperative hypotension
Anaesthetic Factors 33: 652

Postoperative oliguria
Anaesthetic Factors 34: 692

Preoperative assessment of cardiovascular risk in noncardiac surgery
Anaesthetic Factors 34: 697

Preoperative assessment of pulmonary risk
Anaesthetic Factors

CAROTID ENDARTERECTOMY

J. M. Hopkinson and
A. J. Mortimer

PROCEDURE

A surgical procedure on the extracranial portion of the carotid artery to improve oxygen delivery to an ischaemic brain, and prevent further strokes due to plaque or platelet embolization. Temporary occlusion of the carotid artery is required and the brain is dependent on collateral flow via the circle of Willis to maintain cerebral oxygen delivery. The anaesthetist must maintain the balance of oxygen supply and demand of brain tissue by careful attention to technique.

Careful positioning of the patient is required, with moderate cervical extension and rotation of the head away from the side of operation, avoiding obstruction of venous drainage (take care in patients with degenerative cervical disc disease).

PREOPERATIVE ASSESSMENT AND INVESTIGATIONS

Aims:

- Optimize general patient condition by treating coexisting problems, in particular control congestive cardiac failure and hypertension. It is necessary to wait until 3–6 months after a myocardial infarction if possible.
- Determine the range of blood pressure the patient normally tolerates (see ward chart).

General assessment:

- Routine clinical assessment of the cardiovascular and respiratory systems
- Full anaesthetic and drug history
- Investigations:
  - Haemoglobin, platelets
  - Urea, creatinine, electrolytes, blood glucose
  - Resting 12-lead ECG
  - Chest X-ray.

Further specific investigations may be indicated which might include echocardiography, and respiratory function tests (PEFR, FEV_1/FVC).

PREMEDICATION

- Explain the procedure and anaesthetic management to the patient
- Anxiolytic drugs (amnesia is also useful), e.g. a short-acting benzodiazepine (temazepam)
- Continue the usual cardiac medication, especially antianginal and antihypertensive drugs.

PERIOPERATIVE MANAGEMENT

- An anaesthetic technique is required that provides stable cardiovascular conditions, avoiding myocardial and cerebral ischaemia
- General anaesthesia with controlled ventilation is ideal, although if surgery is of predictably short duration general anaesthesia with spontaneous respiration following endotracheal intubation is acceptable (take care to minimize hypercapnia)
- Local infiltration and regional techniques (cervical epidurals) are rarely used in the UK. see below ->

PREPARATION

Intravenous hydration during the period of starvation will maintain normovolaemia and, therefore, lessen the hypotensive response to induction of anaesthesia.

ANAESTHETIC ROOM

- Reassure the patient; maintain a calm environment.
- Oxygen via a clear face-mask.
- Institute monitoring:
  - ECG
  - Pulse oximetry
  - Invasive arterial pressure line under local anaesthesia (radial artery).

- Secure intravenous access with a 16 gauge cannula – commence either 0.9% NaCl or Hartman's infusion. Avoid dextrose solutions because hyperglycaemia worsens any damage caused by perioperative ischaemia.

INDUCTION OF ANAESTHESIA

- Preoxygenate
- Maintain cardiovascular stability during induction and endotracheal intubation
- Thiopentone is the induction agent of choice (reduces intracranial pressure and cerebral oxygen consumption); propofol using a TIVA technique may be equally as good
- A preformed Rae cuffed oral endotracheal tube is ideal to allow easy connection to ventilator tubing and provide good access for the surgeon
- Eye protection for the patient.

OPERATING THEATRE

Maintenance of anaesthesia

A balanced anaesthetic technique with IPPV to normocapnia using air/oxygen and a volatile agent. Isoflurane is the agent of choice, but enflurane is also acceptable. Use $F_{I}O_2$ 0.5 to maintain a high SaO_2 while the carotid artery is clamped. Aim to keep the blood pressure in the previously identified normal range for the patient (normal systolic pressure + 40 mmHg). Careful use of fluids (do not overload), vasopressors and vasodilators may be necessary to maintain stability.

Monitoring:

- ECG (leads II and V5 with ST segment analysis for detection of subendocardial ischaemia)
- SaO_2
- Capnography
- $F_{I}O_2$
- Invasive arterial BP.

Specific points:

- Patient positioning – identify normal range of movements prior to induction.
- Heparinization (5000 units) required prior to clamping internal and external carotids.
- Bradyarrhythmias and hypotension may occur when the surgeon is operating around the carotid sinus nerve. If this occurs, ask the surgeon to temporarily stop dissecting and infiltrate around the carotid sinus with lignocaine. Administer ephedrine in 3-mg increments (α and β stimulation).

Heparin ~ 70 IU/kg

POSTOPERATIVE MANAGEMENT

- Light general anaesthesia should allow rapid awakening and early neurological assessment at the end of the procedure.
- Haemodynamic instability, with either hypotension (preoperative systolic BP – 40 mmHg) or hypertension (preoperative systolic BP + 40 mmHg) is common. Of these, hypotension is the more serious complication because of the risk of cerebral hypoperfusion. It should be treated if required with vasopressors (methoxamine, metaraminol or ephedrine) to restore the blood pressure to preoperative values. Hypertension should be treated with vasodilators (hydralazine, labetolol, glyceryl trinitrate) to minimize myocardial ischaemia.
- Discharge from the recovery room following 2–3 h satisfactory observation.
- Subsequent observation in a HDU for 12–24 h is ideal.

POSTOPERATIVE COMPLICATIONS

- Haemodynamic instability – hypertension may cause myocardial ischaemia or infarction which may then result in hypotension and cerebral hypoperfusion
- Airway obstruction due to tracheal compression by haematoma formation may become an acute surgical emergency
- New neurological deficit may present secondary to plaque embolization or perioperative cerebral ischaemia (approximately 3% of all patients)
- Vocal cord palsy due to recurrent laryngeal nerve damage
- Chemoreceptor dysfunction – bilateral dysfunction results in complete loss of the hypoxic response.

OUTCOME

- Depends on the severity of the cerebrovascular disease. The surgery is relatively well tolerated and, providing oxygen delivery to the brain is adequate during the cross-clamp period, is reasonably successful in preventing future stroke
- Main cause of morbidity and mortality is perioperative myocardial infarction
- Surgery on the contralateral side is often required at a later date.

BIBLIOGRAPHY

European Carotid Surgery Trialists' Collaborative Group. MRC European Carotid Surgery Trial: interim results for symptomatic patients with severe (70–99%) or with mild (0–29%) carotid stenosis. Lancet 1991; 1235–1243

Garrioch M A, Fitch W. Anaesthesia for carotid artery surgery. British Journal of Anaesthesia 1993; 71: 561–579

North American Symptomatic Carotid Endarterectomy Trial Collaborators. Beneficial effect of carotid endarterectomy in symptomatic patients with high-grade carotid stenoses. New England Journal of Medicine 1991; 325: 445–453

CROSS REFERENCES

Complications of position
Anaesthetic Factors 33: 618

Intraoperative hypertension
Anaesthetic Factors 33: 636

Intraoperative hypotension
Anaesthetic Factors 33: 638

Preoperative assessment of cardiovascular risk in noncardiac surgery
Anaesthetic Factors 34: 692

Preoperative assessment of pulmonary risk
Anaesthetic Factors 34: 697

"Deep cervical plexus block" involves separate injections on to the transverse processes of C2 to C4. Complications include injection into vertebral artery epidural space subarachnoid space and paralysis of the diaphragm. It is rarely used in the UK.

22

LEG REVASCULARIZATION AND AMPUTATIONS

J. M. Hopkinson and A. J. Mortimer

PROCEDURES

Various surgical bypass techniques are used in an attempt to revascularize lower limbs which are ischaemic due to occlusive vascular disease.

- Acute ischaemia due to embolic events is often dealt with by femoral embolectomy – local infiltration anaesthesia is generally used for this procedure.
- Chronic ischaemia due to atheromatous disease requires bypass procedures to improve the blood flow to distal regions.
- Aortoiliac disease may require an aortic bifurcation graft (see section on aortic reconstruction).
- The procedure commonly encountered is femoral–popliteal bypass, although many variations are performed. Axillofemoral bypass is generally reserved for the poor-risk patient with severe occlusive aortic disease.
- Usually prolonged procedures in a poor-risk patient group, although it is relatively noninvasive surgery.
- Patients tend to present for repeated procedures in an attempt to salvage ischaemic limbs, often culminating in progressive proximal amputation in the following sequence: (1) toes, (2) forefoot, (3), below knee, (4) above knee.
- Diabetic patients are frequently encountered in this group of procedures. Infected and necrotic tissue disturbs blood sugar control and amputation can be life-saving.

PREOPERATIVE ASSESSMENT AND INVESTIGATIONS

Aims:

- Optimize general condition by treating coexisting problems, in particular congestive cardiac failure, respiratory disease and diabetes – aim for blood glucose levels of 6–10 mmol l^{-1}.
- Formulate your anaesthetic management plan according to the findings. Routine clinical assessment of the cardiovascular and respiratory systems; full anaesthetic and drug history.

Investigations:

- Hb, platelets, white cell count
- Blood group and save serum
- Urea, creatinine, electrolytes, blood glucose
- Resting 12-lead ECG
- Chest X-ray
- Respiratory function tests (PEFR, FEV_1/FVC, if indicated).

PREMEDICATION

- Explain to the patient about the procedure and the anaesthetic management
- Anxiolytic drugs (with amnesia), e.g. the short-acting benzodiazepine, temazepam
- No premedicative drugs are indicated in some already obtunded patients
- Continue the usual cardiac and respiratory medication
- Intravenous management of diabetes, where appropriate.

PERIOPERATIVE MANAGEMENT

- The choice of anaesthetic technique will depend on expertise, the individual patient and the particular surgical procedure
- Options are:
  - General anaesthesia (spontaneously breathing or controlled ventilation)
  - Regional anaesthesia (spinal or epidural anaesthesia)
  - Combined general anaesthesia and regional anaesthesia
  - General anaesthesia together with femoral and sciatic nerve blocks.

There is probably little to choose between the above techniques. The goal is haemodynamic stability during anaesthesia. Factors to be considered will be the severity of pre-existing CVS or RS disease. Regional blockade will have advantages in certain patient groups. Regional block instituted prior to lower limb amputation (48 h) can reduce the severity of postoperative pain. Whichever technique is used, adequate oxygenation and haemodynamic stability are of paramount importance throughout.

ANAESTHETIC ROOM

- Patient reassurance, calm environment
- Institute initial monitoring: ECG, pulse oximetry and noninvasive arterial BP are adequate, unless a prolonged procedure is anticipated when invasive monitoring may be appropriate
- Intravenous access
- Induction of anaesthesia:
  - Preoxygenation
  - Maintain cardiovascular stability during induction and endotracheal intubation.

OPERATING THEATRE

Maintenance of anaesthesia:

- Balanced anaesthetic technique
- Maintain cardiovascular stability
- Humidification of gases; heated mattress to minimize heat loss
- Blood loss usually minimal.

Monitoring:

- ECG (leads II and V5 with ST segment analysis for early detection of subendocardial ischaemia)
- Sao_2
- Capnography
- $F_{I}o_2$
- Noninvasive arterial BP.

POSTOPERATIVE MANAGEMENT

- Observe in recovery until stable and adequate analgesia attained
- Oxygen via face-mask (for 3 days postoperatively in the poor-risk patient)
- Chest physiotherapy in appropriate cases
- Analgesia – either epidural local anaesthetic with opioid or parenteral opioids and NSAIDs (care with renal function) are suitable.

POSTOPERATIVE COMPLICATIONS

Surgical:

- Persistent ischaemia causing severe pain
- Progression to gangrene with localized or systemic infection

- Reoperation may be required (including amputation)
- Poor wound healing predisposing to infection
- Reperfusion injury following revascularization of the critically ischaemic limb.

systemic inflammatory response.

Medical:

- Myocardial ischaemia or infarction
- Difficult diabetic control
- Respiratory problems (atelectasis, hypoxaemia, retention of secretions).

OUTCOME

- Outcome depends on the successful bypassing of the obstructions and the severity of the arterial disease distally
- Multiple procedures and anaesthetics are often required in this high-risk patient group
- All too often the result is the requirement to amputate the limb of an ASA IV patient because of severe rest pain and gangrene
- Risk increases with the number of procedures carried out
- The patient's suffering should be minimized and analgesia should therefore be given high priority.

BIBLIOGRAPHY

Christopherson R, Beattie C, Frank S M et al. Peri-operative morbidity in patients randomised to epidural or general anaesthesia for lower extremity vascular surgery. Anesthesiology 1993; 79: 422–434

Foex P, Reeder M K. Anaesthesia for vascular surgery. Baillière's Clinical Anaesthesiology 1993; 7: 97–126

Ruckley C V. Amputations in peripheral disease. Hospital Update 1992; 1: 126–133

CROSS REFERENCES

Diabetes mellitus
Patient Conditions 2: 42

Postoperative pain management
Anaesthetic Factors 33: 655

Preoperative assessment of cardiovascular risk in noncardiac surgery
Anaesthetic Factors 34: 692

Preoperative assessment of pulmonary risk
Anaesthetic Factors 34: 697

23

TRANSPLANTATION

D. Potter

OVERVIEW

D. Potter

THE ROLE OF THE ANAESTHETIST

In relation to transplant surgery the anaesthetist has several roles to play. Preoperatively, the recipient will require selection, assessment and preparation for surgery. Intraoperative management will demand close cooperation with the surgical team, an understanding of the physiological stresses imposed by the procedure, and the supportive techniques best suited to minimize any lasting effects. Postoperative care will often involve continued support in the face of varying degrees of organ failure, with the usual anaesthetic preoccupation with sedation, analgesia, and the welfare of the whole patient.

Intensivists have an important contribution to make in the early identification and management of potential donors, before and after confirmation of brainstem death, which will involve sympathetic support of the patient's family.

Management of the donor before and during the retrieval operation will influence the function of the transplanted organs and the course and outcome for the recipient.

PATIENT SELECTION

Each transplant team has its own organ-specific criteria for listing patients for transplantation, which will depend upon the pathological diagnosis, severity of illness, technical anaesthetic and surgical factors, and an assessment of prognosis in relation to availability of organs.

PATIENT ASSESSMENT

Patient assessment depends upon the severity of organ failure, the availability and effectiveness of medical support, and the impact of the primary organ failure on other systems. The anaesthetist needs to have an understanding of the surgical procedure, and the stresses imposed by it, in assessing the chances of survival. In individual patients, as opposed to statistical groups, this remains a very inexact science.

PATIENT PREPARATION

Preparation of the patient for surgery includes:

- Medical supportive therapy for the primary organ failure
- Prompt treatment for complications as they arise
- Psychological and emotional support for the patient and their family while on the waiting list
- Anaesthetic reassessment
- Short-term measures immediately prior to surgery.

The constraints of ischaemia time do not allow much scope for immediate preoperative interventions, but dialysis, haemofiltration, or plasma exchange to correct metabolic, biochemical, or coagulation derangements are possible. Some patients with acute organ failure will be receiving intensive care and multiple forms of support prior to surgery.

The role of selective bowel decontamination prior to transplantation and immunosuppression remains controversial.

ANAESTHETIC MANAGEMENT

General principles of anaesthetic management apply:

- Appropriate premedication
- Reduction of aspiration risk
- Induction titrated to individual requirements
- Early control of the airway
- Multiple venous access of sufficient calibre to cope with anticipated transfusion requirements
- Monitoring of patient and equipment
- Maintenance with minimal depression of vital functions.

Organ-specific requirements:

- Monitoring effects of explantation

- Support during the explantation phase of surgery
- Management of the reperfusion phase
- Antibiotic and immunosuppressive therapy.

POSTOPERATIVE CARE

All transplant patients need postoperative intensive care, with varying degrees of support of respiratory and circulatory or renal function.

Monitoring includes:
- Cardiovascular system for hypovolaemia
- Clinical and microbiology for sepsis
- Graft function, for signs of rejection or impaired perfusion, sometimes requiring biopsy, and/or Doppler scans
- Secondary organ function for signs of MODS
- Drug toxicity (assays of immunosuppressive drugs and antibiotics in plasma).

Renal failure is the most common complication in all transplant patients, and may be related to poor perfusion, and/or drug toxicity.

SEDATION AND ANALGESIA

Sedation and analgesia should be titrated to individual needs using methods appropriate to the case, and which will not compromise weaning from ventilatory support. As in other forms of major surgery, intravenous infusion, under staff or patient control, and regional techniques are the commonest methods of analgesia. Intravenous infusion of propofol or a benzodiazepine is suitable for sedation.

The length of ITU stay and complication rates vary widely, but urgent exploration for bleeding, or retransplantation may be necessary, often in a very sick patient.

Later complications or unrelated surgical pathology may also necessitate anaesthesia for the transplanted patient.

DONOR MANAGEMENT

The interval between recognition, confirmation, and retrieval may extend over 48 h or more. The management of the donor during this period and during the retrieval operation has a significant effect on the subsequent function of the donated organs. The most important considerations are:

- Maintenance of adequate perfusion pressures
- Optimization of electrolyte, glucose, and acid–base status
- Maintenance of normothermia.

The retrieval operation itself may be protracted, especially if multiple organs are involved, and it is important to maintain levels of monitoring and support in the preliminary phases of the operation right up to the application of clamps and cold perfusion of the organs.

OUTCOME

The patient and graft survival rates in transplantation are steadily improving (Tables 1 and 2).

Table 1.
One-year patient survival (%) by year of operation*

	1985–86	1987–88	1989–90	1991–92
Heart	66	76	74	72
Lung(s)	–	–	58	63
Heart/lung	55	62	65	63
Liver	52	53	61	69
	1981–83	**1984–86**	**1987–89**	**1990–91**
Kidney	68	78	84	84

*Data supplied by UKTSSA.

Table 2.
Patient survival (%) after transplantation*

	1 year	3 years	5 years
Heart	73	67	62
Lung	61	42	–
Heart/lung	62	46	38
Liver	70	60	54
Kidney	84	–	64

*Figures supplied by UKTSSA.

BIBLIOGRAPHY

Davis P J, Cook D R (eds). Anesthetic principles for organ transplantation. Raven Press, New York, 1994

Fabian J (ed). Anesthesia for organ transplantation. J B Lippincott, Philadelphia, 1992

HEART TRANSPLANTATION

M. J. Boscoe

23

PROCEDURE

- Median sternotomy with cardiopulmonary bypass.
- Orthotopic heart transplant: anastomoses of left atria, right atria, donor and recipient aortas and pulmonary arteries. By far the most common operation.
- Heterotopic heart transplant: recipient and donor hearts placed in parallel with anastomoses of superior vena cavae, left atria, aortas and the pulmonary artery to right atrium. Operation of choice if only small donor heart is available in presence of severe pulmonary hypertension.

PATIENT CHARACTERISTICS

- ASA III or IV; NYHA class IV
- 83% are male in the age range 34–55 years
- 50% have ischaemic cardiomyopathy.

PREOPERATIVE ASSESSMENT AND INVESTIGATIONS

- Some will be in ITU on cardiac support (drugs, IABP, assist devices) or ventilatory support.
- Circulating volume may be low (on diuretics) or high (if in failure).
- Circulating catecholamine levels high; peripherally vasoconstricted.
- Drug therapy may include anticoagulants, heparin and coumarins, vasodilators (nitrates and ACE inhibitors) inotropes.
- Cardiac catheter study and echocardiography: ejection fraction typically <25%. Evidence of pulmonary hypertension or raised PVR >400 dyne cm s^{-5} is a relative contraindication. Reversibility of pulmonary hypertension assessed. Alternatively, a small donor heart may be placed as a heterotopic or 'piggy-back' transplant.
- Evidence of other organ dysfunction should be sought. Renal dysfunction increases risk by 50%. Hepatic congestion and dysfunction increases bleeding risks.
- Previous heart surgery indicates need for extra time to secure haemostasis in mediastinum prior to organ insertion.

PREMEDICATION

- Patients are anxious but looking forward to operation. If cardiac output reasonable, will tolerate oral benzodiazepine or intramuscular opioid, if time permitting.
- H_2 antagonist.
- Face-mask oxygen after premedication.

THEATRE PREPARATION

- Coordination with harvesting team essential. Do not anaesthetize recipient until donor heart assessed as acceptable by retrieval team.
- Strict aseptic technique for vascular access; otherwise clean anaesthetic preparation.
- History of anticoagulants, previous mediastinal surgery, complex procedures, all tend to cause a bleeding coagulopathy. Consider use of high-dose aprotinin. Clotting factors should be made available.

PERIOPERATIVE MANAGEMENT

Monitoring:

- Intra-arterial radial artery cannula and large 14 gauge peripheral venous line under local anaesthesia.
- Spo_2, ECG, $ETco_2$, urinary catheter.
- Left-sided neck lines (triple lumen). Leave right side for later cardiac biopsy. Pulmonary artery (PA) catheter or transoesophageal echo in selected cases with raised PVR. Direct PA or LA line may be preferable. Mixed venous saturation by PA oximetry may be useful.

Anaesthetic technique:

- Cardiac resuscitation drugs drawn up; preparation for emergency cardiopulmonary bypass

- Nasogastric tube for administration of cyclosporin perioperatively and for patient feeding
- Aim to maintain SVR without increasing afterload (sensitive to fall in preload and bradycardia or tachycardia as well as myocardial depression)
- Avoid sudden rise in PVR due to stress, hypoxia or hypercapnia
- Sudden removal of endogenous catecholamine drive may cause hypotension
- Most patients tolerate narcotic (fentanyl) based induction with minimal doses of benzodiazepine and sleep dose of etomidate
- Modified rapid sequence induction necessary in unfasted patient; suxamethonium followed by pancuronium, or vecuronium if tachycardia present
- Maintenance – aim to preserve perfusion of vital organs until smooth establishment of cardiopulmonary bypass
- Beware of drug interactions in perioperative period: cyclosporin and renal toxicity; anti-infective agents and hepatorenal effects; prolonged action of nondepolarizers with cyclosporin
- Immunosuppressive agent may be requested (methylprednisolone 1 g i.v.); cyclosporin and azathioprine usually already given preinduction.

POSTOPERATIVE MANAGEMENT

- Aim for post-transplant heart rate of 100–120 bpm. Atrial and ventricular pacing wires placed. Though most are in sinus rhythm, more than 50% have sinus bradycardia or A–V block.
- Most patients will have adequate cardiac output with a small dose of dopamine (5–10 μg kg^{-1} min^{-1}).
- Acute right heart dysfunction is the most common problem. It is associated with pre-existing pulmonary hypertension, a long ischaemic time (>4 h) and a small donor heart. Hyperventilation, oxygen and a small dose of isoprenaline will be inotropic and aid reduction in PVR.
- Prostaglandin E_1 or a phosphodiesterase inhibitor (e.g. enoximone or milrinone) has been useful in acute right heart failure, combined with noradrenaline.
- Rarely, IABP or left and right assist devices are necessary if vital organs are at risk of hypoperfusion.
- 90% extubated within 24 h, and can be managed similarly to routine open-heart surgery patients.

OUTCOME

- The 30-day mortality is 8.5%
- Actuarial survival figures are:
  - 79% at 1 year
  - 67.8% at 5 years
  - 55.8% at 10 years
- 86% of survivors are NYHA class I at 1 year.

BIBLIOGRAPHY

Bristow M R. The surgically denervated transplanted human heart (editorial). Circulation 1990; 82: 658–660

Camman W R, Hensley F A. Anaesthetic management for cardiac transplantation. In: Hensley F A, Martin D E (eds) The practice of cardiac anesthesia. Little Brown, Boston, 1990, ch 14

Fabian J A. Anesthesia for organ transplantation. J B Lippincott, Philadelphia, 1992

Kapoor A S, Laks H, Schroeder J S, Yacoub M H. Cardiomyopathies and heart–lung transplantation. McGraw-Hill, New York, 1991

Shaw I H, Kirk A J B, Conacher I D. Anaesthesia for patients with transplanted hearts and lungs undergoing non-cardiac surgery. British Journal of Anaesthesia 1991; 67: 772–778

CROSS REFERENCES

Preoperative assessment of cardiac patient
Patient Conditions 4: 90
Cardiomyopathy
Patient Conditions 4: 103
Cardiopulmonary bypass: principles, physiology and biochemistry
Surgical Procedures 27: 506

KIDNEY TRANSPLANTATION

J. Broadfield

PROCEDURE

Kidney transplantation may be from either a live or cadaver donor. A live donor must be fit and well (ASA I) and is subjecting him or herself to a major operation for no personal gain. If there is any query about the donor's relationship to the recipient the problem should be referred to the Unrelated Live Transplant Regulating Authority (ULTRA).

Donor tissues must be immunologically compatible. The details of the tests and their significance are changing regularly as more information emerges. They should also be free of tumour and infection (including HIV).

The graft is usually transplanted extraperitoneally to an iliac fossa because of the proximity of the bladder and suitable blood vessels (the iliac artery and vein). There is also poor viability of the distal end of the donated ureter as its blood supply is from the donor's bladder.

PATIENT CHARACTERISTICS

- Any age group (transplantation is unusual in small babies)
- The patient will suffer from the dual pathophysiology of:
  - Chronic renal failure
  - The underlying disease process (e.g. diabetes, systemic lupus, hypertension).

PREOPERATIVE ASSESSMENT AND INVESTIGATIONS

There are important aspects of the pathophysiology to note:

- The cardiovascular system:
  - Anaemia. There are many contributing factors; reversed by erythropoetin.
  - Circulating volume. Usually increased (look for CCF); may be decreased with polyuria or recent enthusiastic dialysis.
  - Hypertension. Could be either the result or the cause of the renal failure.
  - Ischaemic heart disease.
- Uraemia: pericardial effusion and tamponade (improves with good dialysis). Confirm with an echocardiogram if suspicious. Aspirate preoperatively if compromising the cardiac output.
- Water and electrolyte imbalance.
- Neuropathy (including autonomic).

Assessment of all of the above points and treatment, where appropriate, is very important.

These patients may be on large doses of a diverse selection of drugs.

Vascular access is often difficult because:

- Veins which may be needed for shunts/fistulae should not be used (especially the antecubital fossa and radial aspect of the forearm)
- Years of therapy and venesection may have taken its toll of veins.

PREMEDICATION

As appropriate, but remember that there will be problems of excreting drugs and active metabolites until the grafted kidney works. These patients are often frail.

THEATRE PREPARATION

Ensure that drugs specific to kidney transplantation are available, e.g. renal perfusion solution for live related transplantation, and immunosuppressive agents.

A sterile trolley will be required for central venous pressure (CVP) catheter insertion.

Maintenance of body temperature is important (warming blanket, warm fluids, humidification).

PERIOPERATIVE MANAGEMENT

Monitoring:

- ECG
- Noninvasive BP (avoid arms with fistulae)
- Sa_{O_2}
- ET_{CO_2}
- CVP (triple lumen helpful for drug administration)
- Fluid balance and blood loss
- Body temperature.

Anaesthetic technique

Regional techniques may be used, but there are problems:

- Duration of procedure (and hence comfort of patient)
- Occasional bleeding problems exist
- Patient apprehension.

These often make general anaesthesia the method of choice.

General anaesthesia

The modern armamentarium of anaesthetic drugs and monitoring have greatly reduced the problems of general anaesthesia in these patients.

- Hypnotics:
  - Propofol gives good postoperative recovery
  - Etomidate gives good cardiovascular stability.
- Muscle relaxants:
  - Atracurium avoids any problems of renal excretion of neuromuscular blocking drugs
  - Suxamethonium has been cited as causing problems with high serum potassium.
- Analgesia: renal excretion of opioids and metabolites needs consideration. Buprenorphine, in theory, offers the best metabolic profile.
- Volatile agents: in theory, enflurane provides the highest free fluoride levels. Isoflurane is better.

Vascularization of the graft

Maintain optimal circulating volume (CVP and peripheral temperature) with a good cardiac output at the time of revascularization. This is important:

- For the perfusion and early function of the graft
- Because this can also be a time of sudden blood loss.

Beware of excess potassium (e.g. in stored blood).

Beware of fluid overload.

N.B. The last two factors may necessitate early dialysis.

POSTOPERATIVE MANAGEMENT

- Fluids to keep graft well perfused
- Avoid haemodialysis if possible because of the problem of heparinization immediately postoperatively
- Dopamine (2–3 $\mu g\ kg^{-1}\ min^{-1}$) may help renal function, but this has been questioned.

OUTCOME

Successful transplantation improves quality of life radically.

Graft survival:

- Live related: 90% at 1 and 5 years
- Cadaver: 80–85% at 1 year and 70% at 5 years.

Other problems:

- Rejection
- Malignant disease (especially lymphoma)
- Steroid-induced cataracts.

CROSS REFERENCES

Blood transfusion
Anaesthetic Factors 33: 616
Fluid and electrolyte balance
Anaesthetic Factors 33: 626
Postoperative oliguria
Anaesthetic Factors 33: 652

23

LIVER TRANSPLANTATON

S. Cottam

23

PROCEDURE

- Laparotomy by bilateral subcostal incision with extension to xiphisternum (Mercedes' incision).
- Surgery is divided into three phases:
  - Dissection phase, with skeletonization of native liver
  - Anhepatic phase, with removal of liver and implantation of donor organ by anastomosis of vena cava (supra- and infra-hepatic) and portal vein
  - Reperfusion phase with graft reperfusion, haemostasis, completion of hepatic arterial anastomosis and biliary drainage.
- Venovenous bypass is frequently used in the anhepatic phase to maintain venous return, cardiac output, and renal perfusion when the inferior vena cava and portal vein are clamped.
- Orthotopic liver transplantation (OLT) is the common procedure (95%), although auxiliary grafting (either orthotopic or heterotopic) may be performed for patients with acute liver failure or children with isolated enzyme defects.

PATIENT CHARACTERISTICS

Patients are aged from 1 week to 70 years and fall into two distinct patient groups.

Acute liver failure (ALF)

Jaundice and encephalopathy developing in a patient with no history of chronic liver disease.

- Hyperacute liver failure – encephalopathy within 7 days of onset of jaundice
- Acute liver failure – encephalopathy in 8–28 days from onset of jaundice
- Subacute liver failure – encephalopathy in 5–12 weeks from onset of jaundice.

In the UK emergency transplantation is reserved for patients with a poor prognosis without OLT, as defined by O'Grady et al (1993) (Table 1).

Table 1. Emergency transplant criteria*

Paracetamol induced
pH <7.3 after volume repletion
(irrespective of grade of encephalopathy)

or

Prothrombin time >100 s
Creatinine >300 µmol l^{-1}
Grade 3 or 4 encephalopathy

NonParacetamol induced
Any three of the following (irrespective of the grade of encephalopathy):

- Age <10 or >40 years
- Non-A non-B hepatitis
- Halothane hepatitis
- Idiosyncratic drug reaction
- Jaundice to encephalopathy time >7 days
- Prothrombin time >50 s
- Bilirubin >300 mmol l^{-1}

*O'Grady et al (1989).

Chronic liver disease (CLD)

A wide variety of congenital and acquired disease in both adults and children may lead to end-stage liver disease. Transplantation is frequently required, as medical treatment fails to control life-threatening complications such as gastrointestinal bleeding.

COMMONLY ASSOCIATED PATHOLOGY

- Central nervous system:
  - Encephalopathy (CLD)
  - Cerebral oedema (ALF).
- Respiratory:
  - Restrictive defect due to massive ascites (50% of CLD)
  - Hypoxia due to ventilation perfusion defect (15% of CLD)
  - Pulmonary hypertension (1–2% of CLD) (relative contraindication to transplantation)

- Acute lung injury may progress to adult respiratory distress syndrome (ALF).
- Cardiovascular:
  - High cardiac output with low systemic vascular resistance (75%, CLD and ALF)
  - Pericardial effusion
  - Cardiomyopathy, especially in alcoholic liver disease or myocardial involvement in disease process, e.g. amyloid.
- Renal:
  - Pre-renal or renal failure
  - Hepatorenal syndrome both ALF and CLD.
- Gastrointestinal:
  - Portal hypertension and ascites (CLD).
- Haematology:
  - Anaemia
  - Coagulopathy
  - Abnormal fibrinolysis.

PREOPERATIVE ASSESSMENT

A multidisciplinary approach is essential to assess risk, aimed at precisely defining the multisystem involvement described above. Occult cardiovascular disease is a major cause of perioperative death; rigorous cardiac work-up, including angiography, is indicated.

PREMEDICATION

A short-acting benzodiazepine (preferably not dependent on phase-I elimination) is tolerated in the absence of hepatic encephalopathy.

PREOPERATIVE PREPARATION

- Detailed patient and relative counselling
- When an organ becomes available, liaison with donor team is essential
- Success is dependent on support services such as blood bank and laboratory services, anaesthetic technical back-up and clinical perfusionists for rapid infusion devices, cell saver and bypass equipment
- Theatre temperature is important; patient-warming devices, infusion equipment and monitoring must all be available and ready.

PERIOPERATIVE MANAGEMENT

Monitoring:
- ECG
- Invasive arterial pressure
- CVP
- Femoral venous pressure
- Pulmonary artery catheter (Svo_2 and rapid response catheter useful)
- Cardiac output computer
- Intracranial pressure (ALF)
- Core temperature
- Spo_2
- $ETco_2$
- Urine output and blood loss.

Blood samples:
- Arterial and mixed venous gases
- Full blood count
- Clotting screen
- Sodium, potassium, calcium and blood glucose
- Thromboelastography.

Intravenous access

Wide-bore venous access is mandatory for rapid infusion.

Internal jugular access is safer than subclavian in the presence of severe coagulopathy.

ANAESTHETIC TECHNIQUE

- Rapid sequence induction is advisable if patient is not fully fasted, or in the presence of massive ascites.
- Induction with narcotic (fentanyl) and sleep dose of etomidate.
- Insert a wide-bore nasogastric tube and a fine-bore enteral feeding tube for early postoperative enteral nutrition.
- Maintenance with oxygen/air/isoflurane, narcotic and relaxant infusion. IPPV with ventilator capable of minute volumes of up to $20\,l\,min^{-1}$.
- Aim to maintain renal perfusion. Low-dose dopamine or dopexamine, mannitol and the use of venovenous bypass in the anhepatic phase are all advocated.
- Maintenance of cardiac output and oxygen transport, especially in the anhepatic phase. Intraoperatively, cardiac output increases, especially on reperfusion with profound systemic vasodilation. Adequate volume loading is essential. Pressor inotropes are occasionally required, as guided by cardiac output and systemic vascular resistance. Beware of the deleterious effects of vasoconstrictors on already limited oxygen extraction.
- Intraoperative monitoring of coagulation by thromboelastography and laboratory parameters of coagulation and appropriate blood product replacement. Ionized calcium concentrations will fall due to administered citrate and will require supplementation.

- Prophylactic antibiotic administration and intraoperative doses of immunosuppression.

POSTOPERATIVE MANAGEMENT

- Continue invasive monitoring.
- 90% of patients with CLD are extubated within 24 h.
- In ALF, ITU stay may be prolonged.
- Early complications include bleeding (now <5%) and hepatic artery or portal vein thrombosis which will require early re-exploration.
- Early liver function is monitored by resolution of metabolic acidosis and resolution of coagulopathy (falling INR).
- Poor initial graft function may be treated with prostaglandins or with *N*-acetylcysteine.
- Primary nonfunction of the liver is rare in UK centres (1–2%), but will entail emergency retransplantation.
- Acute rejection is common, suggested by changes in AST and INR and confirmed by biopsy if coagulation permits. Additional steroids and/or modification of immunosuppressive regime may be required.
- Cyclosporin or FK 506 may be introduced early if renal function is satisfactory.

OUTCOME

- Patients with acute liver failure are selected for OLT if their chances of survival with medical treatment are <10%. One-year survival following emergency OLT is currently 74%.
- Patients with chronic liver disease currently have a one-year survival of 82% following OLT.
- Quality of life is improved; the majority of patients are severely incapacitated prior to transplantation.
- The majority of deaths are in the early postoperative period due to infection and multiple organ failure. Later deaths are due to complications of immunosuppression, chronic rejection or recurrence of the primary liver disease.
- Retransplantation will be required in 5–10% of patients.

BIBLIOGRAPHY

Elias E. Liver transplantation. Journal of the Royal College of Physicians of London 1993; 3: 224–232

Ginsburg R, Peachey T, Eason J, Potter D. Anaesthesia for liver transplantation. (1&2) In: Kaufmann (ed) Anaesthesia review 7. Churchill Livingstone, Edinburgh, ch 9, 10

O'Grady J, Schalm S W, Williams R. Acute liver failure: redefining the syndromes. Lancet 1993; ii: 273–275

Plevak D, Southorn P A, Narr B J, Peters S G. Intensive care unit experience in the Mayo liver transplantation program: the first 100 cases. Mayo Clinic Proceedings 1989; 64: 433–445

CROSS REFERENCES

Chronic liver disease
Patient Conditions 5: 135
The jaundiced patient
Patient Conditions 5: 142
Acute renal failure
Patient Conditions 6: 154
Chronic renal failure
Patient Conditions 6: 158
Massive transfusion
Patient Conditions 7: 180
Blood transfusion
Anaesthetic Factors 33: 616

LUNG AND HEART–LUNG TRANSPLANTATION

M. J. Boscoe

PROCEDURE

- Heart–lung transplant (HLT) with median sternotomy under cardiopulmonary bypass (CPB)
- Single lung transplant (SLT) via posterolateral thoracotomy
- Double lung transplant (DLT) either as sequential procedure via transverse sternal–bithoracic incision with bronchial anastomoses or under CPB with tracheal anastomosis via median sternotomy
- CPB may be required at any time during a SLT or sequential DLT procedure
- Lungs preserved by pulmonary artery flush with cold crystalloid with added prostacyclin PGI_2 or by donor core cooling on CPB.

PATIENT CHARACTERISTICS

- The only treatment for end-stage parenchymal lung disease and pulmonary vascular lung disease.
- HLT is the operation of choice for congenital heart disease. It is also used for primary pulmonary hypertension and some parenchymal lung disease. If the recipient heart is healthy it may be used as a 'domino heart' for another recipient.
- SLT for noninfective parenchymal lung disease, i.e. obstructive airways disease including α_1 antitrypsin deficiency and pulmonary fibrosis. Rarely for primary pulmonary hypertension.
- DLT for septic lung disease including cystic fibrosis, and for pulmonary vascular disease including primary pulmonary hypertension.

PREOPERATIVE ASSESSMENT AND INVESTIGATIONS

- Lung function tests: severely abnormal in obstructive airways disease, typical FEV_1 <30% predicted. Chest X-ray shows emphysematous bullae. CT scan may be used to select worst side to transplant.
- Baseline arterial blood gases confirm hypoxic respiratory drive in many patients with parenchymatous lung disease.
- Cardiac catheterization to measure pulmonary vascular resistance and pulmonary artery pressures. Pulmonary hypertension will make need for CPB in SLT more likely.
- Patient satisfies the criteria for donor lung selection (Table 1). Donor sputum analysis may be guide to antibiotic therapy.
- Previous intrathoracic procedures such as lung biopsy, drainage of pneumothorax or lobectomy increase risk of intraoperative bleeding due to pleural adhesions.
- Complex congenital heart disease, particularly pulmonary atresia, is associated with the presence of extensive collateral vessels. Bleeding during dissection and postoperatively is a serious cause of morbidity and mortality.
- Preoperative drugs may include: antiplatelet and anticoagulant drugs, steroids, nifedipine and prostaglandin infusions to reduce pulmonary hypertension.

PREMEDICATION

- Usually none for many patients as they already have borderline respiratory function. Premedication prevents

Table 1.
Criteria for donor selection

Criteria for donor selection
Age <50 years
No primary pulmonary disease
Chest X-rays normal
$P_{a}O_2$ >300 mmHg on $F_{I}O_2$ = 1.0 and PEEP = 5 cmH_2O
Recipient matching for ABO group and size

stress-related crises in the presence of pulmonary hypertension.
- Close cooperation with donor retrieval team is important. Ischaemic time for lungs is optimally <4–5 h.

THEATRE PREPARATION

- Clean anaesthetic equipment
- Attention to sterility with insertion of lines
- All resuscitation drugs as for heart transplantation; also aminophylline
- Preparations for emergency chest drainage and CPB
- Fibre-optic bronchoscope available for every case
- Additional padding to protect peripheral nerves in patients with poor nutrition, e.g. cystic fibrosis.

PERIOPERATIVE MANAGEMENT

Monitoring:
- Preinduction:
  - ECG
  - Sp_{O_2}
  - Intra-arterial line (radial artery cannula).
- Postinduction:
  - Central venous pressure
  - ET_{CO_2}
  - Urinary catheter
  - Mixed venous saturation oximetry
  - Pulmonary artery catheter.

Anaesthetic technique:
- A balanced technique using a benzodiazepine, narcotic and etomidate for induction is usually well tolerated.
- Aprotinin reduces blood loss, particularly from ooze. Avoid transfusion of CMV positive blood into nonimmune recipient.
- Choice of airway management. Single-lumen tube for HLT and DLT with tracheal anastomoses. Left-sided double-lumen tube for both left and right SLT (as surgeon leaves long bronchial stump in native left lung) and sequential DLT. 'Univent' tube (single lumen with integral bronchus blocker) has also been used. Always check position with fibre-optic bronchoscope.
- Sudden fall in cardiac output may occur with IPPV in patients with obstructive airways disease due to hyperexpansion of lungs or tension pneumothorax. Emergency sternotomy (to relieve tamponade), chest drainage (for pneumothorax) or CPB may be required.
- Acute pulmonary hypertensive crisis may occur in patients with previous pulmonary hypertension despite smooth induction with added oxygen. Adrenaline and fluids are the best acute therapy to increase cardiac output.
- Most patients will tolerate moderate doses of a volatile anaesthetic agent. Avoid nitrous oxide. Propofol infusion may be used. Keep narcotic dose low if early extubation is planned.
- A high I/E ratio, e.g. 1:5, may be required in obstructive airways disease. Manual ventilation allowing 'permissive hypercapnia' is often necessary and desirable during dissection.
- The need for CPB during operation is indicated by desaturation on 100% oxygen, severe pulmonary hypertension, or a severe fall in cardiac index.
- Keep crystalloid fluid infusions to a minimum as new lungs are devoid of lymphatics.
- Keep $F_{I}O_2$ <0.5 to avoid theoretical toxic lung damage to donor lungs associated with free radicals.
- Elective extubation may be desirable at the end of a SLT operation with insertion of thoracic or lumbar epidural for postoperative analgesia.
- Weaning from bypass may require inotropes, often isoprenaline (reduces PVR, and maintains rate).
- Surgeon may want to examine bronchial anastomosis with a large fibre-optic bronchoscope at the end of the operation. This will require exchange of a double- for a single-lumen tube.

POSTOPERATIVE MANAGEMENT

- There is loss of carinal reflex below tracheal anastomosis in HLT. Patients fail to cough on endobronchial suction. Physiotherapy is important.
- High $P_{a}CO_2$ should be expected post-operatively (may be due to denervation or carbon dioxide retention preoperatively). Extubation policy should regard pH as more important.
- Long ischaemic time or poor-quality organ may result in early graft dysfunction. Failure of gas exchange due to pulmonary oedema, infection or rejection.
- Early mediastinal shift in ventilated SLT patient with emphysematous native lung due to compression of new lung by

hyperexpansion of native lung is managed by independent lung ventilation using a double-lumen tube and two ventilators.
- Perioperative problems include pneumothorax and blood clot in airway.
- Global myocardial dysfunction following HLT may be due to poor preservation or long ischaemic time. Temporary right heart failure may occur following ischaemia related early lung dysfunction with elevated PVR.
- Diagnosis of cause of graft dysfunction may require transbronchial biopsy and bronchoalveolar lavage.
- Immunosuppressive regime may consist of cyclosporin, azathioprine, antithymocyte globulin and steroids. Methylprednisolone (1 g) is given intraperatively and for acute rejection episodes.
- Long-term problems affecting airway include healing and infection, and necessitate multiple anaesthetics for diagnostic bronchoscopy, bronchial dilatation, cryotherapy and, occasionally, stent insertion.
- Obliterative bronchiolitis, an obstructive disease possibly due to chronic rejection, occurs in up to 40% at 4 years with no effective cure except retransplantation.

OUTCOME

About 60–70% of both ventilation and perfusion go to the new lung following SLT. The 1-year survival for HLT is about 60% (reflects serious pathology). The 1-year survival for SLT and DLT varies in the range 70–85%. The major cause of late mortality after lung transplantation is obliterative bronchiolitis.

BIBLIOGRAPHY

Boscoe M J. Anaesthesia for lung and heart–lung transplantation. In: Prys Roberts C, Brown B R (eds) General Anaesthesia. Butterworth-Heinemann, Oxford, 1994, vol 6

Novick R J, Menkis A H, McKensie F N. New trends in lung preservation: a collective review. Journal of Heart and Lung Transplantation 1992; 11: 377–392

Smiley R, Navedo A. Postoperative independent lung ventilation in a single lung patient. Anesthesiology 1991; 74: 1144–1148

Triantafillou A N, Heerdt P M. Lung transplantation. International Anesthesiology Clinics 1991; 29: 87–109

CROSS REFERENCES

Heart transplantation
Surgical Procedures 23: 460
One-lung anaesthesia
Anaesthetic Factors 32: 602
Preoperative assessment of pulmonary risk
Anaesthetic Factors 34: 697

MANAGEMENT OF THE ORGAN DONOR

M. Rela

23

Demand for donor organs exceeds supply and patients still die on the waiting list for transplantation. Early recognition of the potential donor, and organ-oriented support after all prospect of patient survival has been lost is one important factor in redressing this imbalance.

PROCEDURE

The surgical procedure varies depending upon the number of organs to be retrieved. The salient features of multiple organ retrieval, in which at least two teams are usually involved, are as follows:

- Chest and abdomen are opened through a midline incision
- The organs are examined for suitability
- The liver is mobilized first, and the anatomy of the hilar structures determined
- Distal abdominal aorta and superior mesenteric vein (SMV) are prepared for cannulation
- Descending thoracic aorta prepared for cross clamping.
- Cardiac team prepare superior and inferior vena cavae (SVC and IVC)
- Ascending aorta is cannulated for infusion of cardioplegia
- Heparin (300 units per kg body weight) is given
- Antibiotics and steroids may be requested
- Cannulation of abdominal aorta and SMV
- IVC is incised within the pericardium
- Heart and liver are allowed to empty
- Thoracic aorta is cross-clamped at the arch and above the diaphragm
- Cold perfusion of abdominal and thoracic organs is started simultaneously, using cardioplegia for the heart, UW solution via the portal system for the liver, and Marshall's solution via the distal aorta for the kidneys
- Pericardium and peritoneum are irrigated with chilled saline
- Organs are removed in the order: heart (with lungs en bloc if required), liver, pancreas and then kidneys
- Spleen and lymph nodes are removed for tissue typing, and iliac artery and vein for possible use in vascular reconstruction.

This sequence may be modified in an unstable donor or according to individual team protocols. When heart and lungs are being retrieved, full cardiopulmonary bypass and whole-body cooling may be used.

DONOR SELECTION

Following identification of a potential organ donor, cardiovascular and respiratory support should be maintained while the viability of the brainstem is being assessed.

General donor assessment:

- History
- Physical examination
- Laboratory investigations.

General exclusion criteria for organ donation:

- Age >65 years (variable, depending on individual unit policies)
- Untreated sepsis
- Acquired immunodeficiency syndrome (AIDS)
- Viral hepatitis B or C
- Viral encephalitis
- Active tuberculosis
- Malignancy excluding primary brain tumours
- Risk of rare viral disease such as Jakob–Creutzfeldt disease and recipients of human pituitary growth hormone.

High-risk groups such as prostitutes or intravenous drug abusers, who are HIV antibody negative should be considered on an individual basis with the status of the potential recipient. Cardiac arrest and prolonged hypotension do not necessarily contraindicate organ donation and the suitability of individual organs depends upon postresuscitation function.

ASSESSMENT FOR INDIVIDUAL ORGANS

Heart-donor selection

Exclusions:

- History of hypertension, ischaemic heart disease, cardiomyopathy or valvular disease.
- Excessive inotrope requirement.

Exogenous and endogenous catecholamines have a deleterious effect on myocardial energy stores and post-transplant function.

Inclusions:

- Age <50 years
- Normal chest X-ray
- Normal 12-lead ECG
- Inotrope requirement <10 μg kg min^{-1} of dopamine to maintain systolic pressure >90 mmHg after correction of hypovolaemia
- Echocardiogram for evaluation of myocardial function if dopamine requirement >10 μg kg min^{-1} to maintain systolic pressure >90 mmHg after resuscitation from cardiac arrest, prolonged hypotension or chest trauma.

Pulmonary-donor selection

Exclusions:

- Chronic lung disease, heavy smoking, pulmonary aspiration and parenchymal trauma
- High alveolar–arterial oxygen gradient (P_aO_2 <300 mHg, F_IO_2 1.0, PEEP ≤+5 cmH_2O)
- Respiratory sepsis – tracheal colonization with fungus or bacteria adversely affect the outcome by increasing the morbidity and mortality.

Inclusions:

- Age <50 years
- Normal chest X-ray (minor chest X-ray abnormalities are noted in 27% of donors and do not contraindicate the possibility of lung donation)
- Normal bronchoscopy.

Liver-donor selection

Exclusions:

- Age >60 years
- History of chronic liver disease and/or viral hepatitis. Alcohol abuse with potential liver disease is more difficult to assess from history and liver function tests, unless the latter are widely deranged. Marked elevations in serum transaminase levels can occur in donors subjected to short periods of hypotension or asystole. If the levels of transaminase decrease in the subsequent 48 h the liver can be used.

Kidney-donor selection

Exclusions:

- History of chronic renal insufficiency or recurrent urinary tract infection
- Serum creatinine >170 μmol^{-1} is associated with decreased graft survival.

MEDICAL MANAGEMENT

The principal goals include early recognition and treatment of haemodynamic instability, maintenance of a systemic perfusion pressure to maximize post-transplantation allograft function, and the prevention and treatment of complications related to brainstem death and supportive care.

General ITU care plus:

- Pulmonary artery catheterization may be necessary to minimize inotrope requirement
- Warming blankets to maintain a temperature above 35°C (hypothermia impairs cardiac, renal and hepatic function).

Laboratory investigations

- Haematology:
  - ABO and Rhesus blood group
  - Full blood count
  - Prothrombin time.
- Biochemistry:
  - Electrolytes
  - Glucose
  - Urea
  - Creatinine
  - Liver function tests
  - Arterial blood gases.
- Microbiology:
  - Blood cultures
  - Urine cultures
  - Sputum cultures.
- Serology:
  - HBsAg
  - Anti-HCV
  - CMV
  - HIV
  - HLA tissue typing.

Cardiovascular system

The predominant haemodynamic abnormality seen in brain-dead patients is hypotension due to the destruction of pontine and medullary vasomotor centres. A systolic pressure of less than 80 mmHg is inadequate for optimal liver function. Maintaining a minimum systolic pressure of 90–100 mmHg is necessary to ensure adequate perfusion to all vital organs.

Hypovolaemia should be corrected and inotropic support added judiciously, using a pulmonary artery (PA) catheter if necessary. Dopamine is the preferred vasopressor because of its potential for maintaining renal and mesenteric blood flow. Although dopamine at a greater dose than 10 $\mu g\ kg^{-1}\ min^{-1}$ does not seem to affect early cardiac allograft survival, doses above this range can increase the risk of acute tubular necrosis and reduce renal allograft survival. If additional inotropic support is required, dobutamine is preferred to minimize any increase in myocardial oxygen demand. Exogenous and endogenous catecholamines have a deleterious effect on myocardial energy stores and post-transplant function, and inotropic dosage should be kept to the minimum compatible with adequate perfusion pressures by optimizing volume status using a PA catheter if necessary.

Respiratory system

Adequate oxygenation should be maintained by controlled ventilation, with PEEP $\leq$5 cmH_2O and $F_IO_2 \leq 0.5$. Excessive PEEP impairs liver perfusion, and increases the risk of pulmonary barotrauma.

Acid–base status should be optimized as far as possible.

Renal/metabolic systems

A urine output of at least 100 ml h^{-1}, especially in the hour preceding retrieval, has been shown to be one of the most important factors determining renal allograft function in the recipient. If urine output is inadequate after volume expansion at a systolic pressure of 90–120 mmHg, mannitol or frusemide should be administered to establish a diuresis.

Avoid hypernatraemia and maintain adequate stores of intrahepatic glycogen by using hypotonic saline with dextrose as maintenance fluid. Destruction of the hypothalamic–pituitary axis results in central diabetes insipidus. Desmopressin is the preferred vasopressin analogue because of its long duration of action and low pressor activity. The high pressor activity of other vasopressin preparations can cause reduced blood flow to the liver and cause post-transplant acute tubular necrosis and nonfunction of kidneys.

INTRAOPERATIVE MANAGEMENT

- Anaesthetic agents are not required
- Full cardiovascular and respiratory support should be maintained up to the time of clamping vessels
- Full neuromuscular blockade
- Full systemic heparinization
- Avoid premature cooling.

BIBLIOGRAPHY

Darby J M, Stein K, Grenvik A, Stuart S. Approach to the management of the heart beating 'brain-dead' organ donor. Journal of the American Medical Association 1989; 261: 2222–2228

Harjula A, Starnes V A, Oyer P E, Jamieson S W, Shumway N E. Proper donor selection for heart–lung transplantation. Journal of Thoracic and Cardiovascular Surgery 1987; 94: 874–880

Jordan C A, Snyder J. Intensive care and intra-operative management of the brain-dead organ donor. Transplantation Proceedings 1987; 19: 21–25

Pruim J, Klompmaker I J, Haagsma E B, Bijleveld C M A, Sloof M J H. Selection criteria for liver donation: a review. Transplant International 1993; 6: 226–235

CROSS REFERENCES

Diagnosis of brain death
Anaesthetic Factors 34: 695

24

ORTHOPAEDICS

A. Loach

OVERVIEW

A. Loach

Orthopaedic surgery is a successful and expanding specialty concerned with elective surgery of bones and connective tissue. Success is based chiefly upon the replacement of diseased or worn joints in elderly patients with synthetic prostheses.

JOINT REPLACEMENT

One-fifth of the population is aged 65 years or over, and this proportion is increasing alarmingly: last year over 50 000 joint replacements were performed and there remains a backlog of cases for surgery. Increasing numbers of cases are also presenting for revision surgery due to loosening of the original prosthesis, infection of the prosthesis or, more rarely, fracture. Hip replacement is now rivalled by knee replacement, where recent improvements have concentrated on using resurfacing procedures, which conserve bone stock for future revision, rather than elaborate hinge prostheses. Replacement arthroplasty is available for all large joints plus the small joints of the hand; interest is growing rapidly in elbow and shoulder replacement.

ARTHROSCOPY

Arthroscopy of all major joints is undertaken and machine tools are being developed for arthroscopic surgery to permit many procedures, meniscectomy or condylar drilling, for example, to be undertaken as day-cases – an area where orthopaedic surgery has trailed behind other fields of surgery.

SPINAL SURGERY

Surgery to the spine may involve decompressive laminectomy or discectomy (although percutaneous injection of the disc under X-ray control, with a proteolytic enzyme, chymopapain, is gaining popularity), whilst more extensive surgery is undertaken to improve scoliosis and correct congenital deformity. Monitoring of cord function by detection of evoked responses has become mandatory during these procedures to avoid ischaemic injury or traction injury to the cord.

INTERNAL FIXATION

Internal fixation of fractures of long bones soon after trauma has been shown to improve recovery and reduce the requirement for ITU care. Such cases, therefore, increasingly appear on daily elective accident service lists. Patients are commonly young and fit and pose few problems for anaesthesia during internal fixation by either plating or intramedullary nailing procedures. However, manipulation of long-bone fractures is now known to liberate fat from marrow cavities into the circulation and reaming of the medullary cavity for nailing may be followed by fat embolism syndrome of varying severity.

OTHER SURGERY

These procedures may include: resection of tumours of bone or connective tissue (sometimes involving huge fore- or hind-quarter amputation); debridement and removal of sequestra for the treatment of osteomyelitis; reconstructive repair of trauma with tendon transplantation; limb straightening, lengthening or shortening with a variety of external fixators.

PROBLEMS IN ORTHOPAEDIC ANAESTHESIA

Bleeding

It is the commonest error in orthopaedic anaesthesia to underestimate blood loss. Cut bone surfaces ooze steadily and control is difficult, so that bleeding persists throughout an operation and may reach major proportions: it is essential to keep a running total of loss from the weighing of swabs and sucker contents (then add one-third). Long operations involve high blood loss, as does resection of tumours which may be very vascular, and operations on patients with Paget's disease. Procedures such as excision arthroplasty (Girdlestone's procedure) which leave an unfilled space, may be followed by severe occult bleeding.

Infection

Infection of bone is difficult to eradicate even over many years, so surgeons take every possible precaution to avoid it. Arthroplasties may be carried out in a sterile (Charnley) enclosure, which tends to isolate the anaesthetist and makes monitoring of surgical progress and blood loss more difficult. Comprehensive patient monitoring is vital. Prophylactic antibiotics are employed when metal is implanted and must be given before a limb tourniquet is applied. If deep-seated infection is suspected, antibiotics are generally withheld until samples have been collected for bacteriological examination.

Venous thromboembolism

Orthopaedic patients are particularly at risk of venous thromboembolism because of their age, their immobility and sluggish circulation in the legs during surgery, especially if the legs are placed in awkward positions which might kink vessels. Needless mortality continues to be incurred by ignoring this hazard (NCEPOD 1993). Prophylaxis should be used: graduated compression stockings, anticoagulants, warfarin or, probably better, low-molecular-weight heparin, intravenous dextran and/or early mobilization. Epidural anaesthesia improves leg blood flow.

Age

Many patients are elderly: two-thirds of joint replacements are in patients over 65 years of age. These are elective operations to improve the quality of life and preoperative selection is vital to avoid death or damaging morbidity due principally to cardiovascular events, strokes and renal failure. Some patients have already undergone heart-valve replacement, coronary-artery surgery or renal transplantation, and require careful assessment.

Splints

The effect of splints must be anticipated. On the legs they make turning a patient difficult and may contribute to deep vein thrombosis; on the trunk they may provide a restrictive ventilatory defect, particularly during anaesthesia; halotraction from chest to head may make intubation difficult.

Cooling

Loss of 1°C body temperature per hour of surgery is common and caused by:

- Laminar down-draught in a Charnley enclosure
- Exposure of large areas of the patient
- Evaporation from large wounds
- Ventilation with unhumidified gases
- The endothermic effect of curing plasters
- The use of regional blocks and resulting vasodilatation
- The use of hypotensive agents such as sodium nitroprusside.

Elderly patients and very young patients compensate poorly for heat loss. Body temperature should be monitored, inspired gases should be humidified and intravenous infusions warmed. Active body warming may be needed using a hot-air blower.

BIBLIOGRAPHY

Loach A. Orthopaedic anaesthesia. Edward Arnold, London, 1993

CROSS REFERENCES

Metabolic & degenerative bone disease
Patient Conditions 8: 200
Rheumatoid disease
Patient Conditions 8: 202
Spinal surgery
The elderly patient
Patient Condition 11: 252
Blood transfusion
Anaesthetic Factors 33: 616
Fat embolism
Anaesthetic Factors 33: 625
Thrombotic embolism
Anaesthetic Factors 33: 664

ARTHROSCOPY

A. Loach

24

PROCEDURE

Arthroscopy is the percutaneous internal examination of a joint using a fine-bore telescope similar to a laparoscope. The joint may be viewed directly by the surgeon through the telescope or, more likely, a video camera is attached to the arthroscope and the magnified image displayed on a television screen.

Miniature power tools can be introduced through separate ports and therapeutic procedures performed under visual control without opening the joint.

This surgery is easily possible as day-surgery.

All of the larger joints may be examined.

PATIENT CHARACTERISTICS

Most patients are fit young sportsmen for assessment of injury. Older patients undergo arthroscopy for assessment of distribution and severity of joint damage prior to total joint arthroplasty.

PREOPERATIVE ASSESSMENT AND INVESTIGATIONS

Fit sportsmen present few problems. Anabolic steroid intake may be by injection with the remote risk of HIV.

In older patients, undertake a systematic review for likely chronic diseases.

Day-surgery preparation when booked as day-cases.

PREMEDICATION

Seldom required and may prejudice recovery of day-cases.

THEATRE PREPARATION

Arthroscopy of hip, knee and elbow is performed with the patient supine.

Shoulder arthroscopy is performed in the 'deckchair' position.

PERIOPERATIVE MANAGEMENT

Monitoring:
- ECG
- Sa_{O_2}
- Noninvasive BP.

Regional anaesthesia

Regional anaesthesia is suitable for knee, elbow and shoulder. It is particularly good for day-cases. Postoperative analgesia is good and postoperative vomiting rare. It permits demonstration to a patient of any pathology (or its absence) on the television monitor.

Regional anaesthesia is ineffective in the presence of synovitis.

Techniques of regional anaesthesia for arthroscopy

Knee:
- Marcain (0.5%) with adrenaline (20 ml) into joint
- Infiltrate portals of entry of instruments with lignocaine and adrenaline
- Surgeon must be prepared to work without a tourniquet (not necessary if adrenaline-containing solution is used) and accept poor relaxation of the joint.

Shoulder:
Interscalene brachial plexus block.

Elbow:
- Interscalene or axillary brachial plexus block.
- Sedation is seldom required.

General anaesthesia

Standard techniques suitable for day surgery are adequate.

POSTOPERATIVE MANAGEMENT

If the joint is filled with bupivacaine at the end of surgery then rectal diclofenac and simple analgesics are adequate for analgesia, and patients may go home that day.

OUTCOME

Arthroscopic surgery will increase as financial pressures militate against in-patient treatment, and also as hardware improves with technical development.

BIBLIOGRAPHY

Allum R L, Ribbans W J. Day case arthroscopy and arthroscopic surgery of the knee. Annals of the Royal College of Surgeons of England 1987; 69: 225

CROSS REFERENCES

HIV and Aids
Patient Conditions 7: 174
Metabolic & degenerative bone disease
Patient Conditions 8: 200
Rheumatoid disease
Patient Conditions 8: 202
Overview
Surgical Procedures 24: 474
Day-case surgery
Anaesthetic Factors 29: 542
Local anaesthetic techniques
Anaesthetic Factors 32: 600
Local anaesthetic toxicity
Anaesthetic Factors 33: 642
Thrombotic embolism
Anaesthetic Factors 33: 664

MANIPULATION UNDER ANAESTHESIA

A. Loach

PROCEDURE

Manipulation under anaesthesia (MUA) is performed;

- To correct deformity due to a fracture before plastering
- To overcome stiffness in a total joint replacement caused by postoperative adhesions
- To improve movement after patellectomy
- To improve position after an osteotomy, before replastering.

PATIENT CHARACTERISTICS

Patients may be any age: on the whole, fractures occur in the young and active; joint replacements in the elderly.

MUA for fracture is semi-urgent to reduce pain; it is urgent if there is any vascular impairment. These patients may therefore be unprepared.

MUA is required after joint replacement and patellectomy in the elderly.

PREOPERATIVE ASSESSMENT AND INVESTIGATIONS

For elective procedures after joint replacement, patients are fasted. Other considerations are as for total hip arthroplasty.

For fractures, ascertain:
- Time since last meal and relation to accident

- Brief medical history (sportsmen may be asthmatic)
- Drug intake and allergy.

For large-bone fracture, establish an intravenous infusion.

PREMEDICATION

Not required.

THEATRE PREPARATION

MUA is often performed in the anaesthetic room.

PERIOPERATIVE MANAGEMENT

Monitoring:
- Sao_2
- ECG
- Noninvasive BP.

Anaesthetic technique
Regional or general anaesthesia is suitable.

For the arm, regional anaesthesia is often preferred because it is simple and saves an out-patient from having a general anaesthetic. Axillary brachial plexus block or intravenous regional anaesthesia (IVRA) are both acceptable (Table 1).

Table 1.
IVRA technique

- Establish i.v. line in both hands/forearms
- Check cuff connections and place cuff around upper arm
- Exsanguinate limb as thoroughly as possible
- Inflate cuff to systolic BP plus 100 mmHg
- *Slowly* inject 40 ml prilocaine (0.5%)
- Do not release cuff until 30 min has elapsed from injection of prilocaine, and then monitor pulse
- Someone must monitor cuff pressure throughout

For the leg a general or regional anaesthetic is suitable. General anaesthesia is carried out as for day-cases. Use an epidural and a catheter if the patient is to receive continuous passive motion.

POSTOPERATIVE MANAGEMENT

MUA after joint replacement or after patellectomy gives rise to great pain. Therefore, consider:

- A suitable regional block
- Patient-controlled analgesia.

MUA for fracture usually relieves pain, and simple analgesics only are required.

BIBLIOGRAPHY

Davis A H, Hall I D, Wilkey A D, Smith J E, Walford A J, Kale V R. Intravenous regional anaesthesia. The dangers of the congested arm and the value of occlusion pressure. Anaesthesia 1984; 39: 416

Grice S C, Norell R C, Balestrieri F J, Stump D A, Howard G. Intravenous regional anaesthesia, evaluation and prevention of leakage under the tourniquet. Anesthesiology 1986; 65: 316

CROSS REFERENCES

Metabolic & degenerative bone disease
Patient Conditions 8: 200
Total hip arthroplasty
Surgical Procedures 24: 481
Local anaesthetic techniques
Anaesthetic Factors 32: 600
Blood transfusion
Anaesthetic Factors 33: 616
Fat embolism
Anaesthetic Factors 33: 625
Local anaesthetic toxicity
Anaesthetic Factors 33: 642
Thrombotic embolism
Anaesthetic Factors 33: 664

REPAIR OF FRACTURED NECK OF FEMUR

P. McKenzie

PROCEDURE

Repair of fractured neck of femur is performed via the supine, lateral or intermediate position.

(A)
- Screws to femoral head
- Screw and femoral plate
- Other 'pin-and-plate' methods.

(B)
- Cemented or uncemented primary femoral prosthesis
- Total hip replacement (rarely).

PATIENT CHARACTERISTICS

- 65–95+ years old
- Female/male ratio 2:1
- Very high incidence of chronic disease
- Dementia and confusional states common
- Multiple medication common
- Dehydration common: extent often difficult to assess accurately
- Fracture may be pathological.

PREOPERATIVE ASSESSMENT

- Assess the state of hydration; rehydrate intravenously if required
- Full history, examination and routine investigations
- Blood cross-match
- Antibiotic prophylaxis and allergy history.

PREMEDICATION

Analgesia and acid aspiration prophylaxis, if necessary. Sedative and anticholinergic drugs should be avoided.

PERIOPERATIVE MANAGEMENT

Monitoring:

- ECG
- Noninvasive BP
- Spo_2
- $ETco_2$
- Fluid balance.

Anaesthetic technique

Operative blood loss moderate (200–300 ml); unaffected by choice of regional or general anaesthesia.

Regional anaesthesia is most commonly by the subarachnoid route. Spinal anaesthesia can be technically difficult in the elderly. Analgesia for positioning the block can be provided by a small dose of intravenous ketamine (20–30 mg). Profound falls in arterial pressure may occur, as patients are often more hypovolaemic than they appear and this is best treated with a vasopressor such as methoxamine in 2 mg increments. This can cause bradycardia, and pretreatment with glycopyrrolate is wise.

Supplemental oxygen should be given to all patients, despite the fact that there is no change in blood gases except when a prosthesis is inserted.

Advantages of regional anaesthesia are:
- Reduction in deep venous thrombosis rate
- Useful in the presence of severe respiratory disease
- Avoids postoperative deterioration of Spo_2 if patients breathe air.

For general anaesthesia, any careful technique is suitable, and there is no difference in outcome between controlled and spontaneous ventilation. Avoidance of hypoxia and hypocarbia and use of short-acting muscle relaxant drugs (if required), e.g. atracurium, are important.

Problems associated with prosthesis insertion

The insertion of a prosthesis may be associated with a fall in blood pressure and oxygen saturation, which may be severe. Treatment with vasopressors and high $F_{I}O_2$ are most appropriate. Causes are embolism of one or more of: fat, air, thromboplastins and acrylic monomer.

Deep venous thrombosis

The incidence measured by objective methods is extremely high (75% approximately). If spinal anaesthesia is used this is reduced to around 40%.

General anaesthesia increases the risk of deep venous thrombosis (DVT) by

- Reducing venous return
- Increasing blood viscosity by reduction in red cell deformability (flexibility).

Spinal anaesthesia reduces the risk of DVT by:

- Increasing venous flow
- Reducing blood viscosity by decreased haematocrit and increased deformability.

POSTOPERATIVE MANAGEMENT

Severe hypoxaemia can occur after general anaesthesia if patients do not receive added oxygen. This is most severe in the period between 5 and 10 min after the end of anaesthesia. The aetiology is unclear.

Postoperative confusional states have been now shown not to relate to the type of anaesthesia but to episodes of hypoxaemia. It is thus essential that all patients breathe added oxygen continuously for at least 6 h and preferably 24 h after surgery. Patients are usually in less pain after operation than before. Judicious use of opioids or appropriate nerve blocks are satisfactory in control of pain. The use of NSAIDs is potentially hazardous in this type of patient.

OUTCOME

There is no significant difference in long-term outcome whether spinal or general anaesthesia is used.

Mortality rates at 1 month are variously reported from 32% in older studies to 5.2% in recent studies. At 6 months, mortality is around 15%. After 6 months, death rates have returned to that predicted by actuarial data.

BIBLIOGRAPHY

Coleman S A, Boyce W J, Cosh P H, McKenzie P J. Outcome after general anaesthesia for repair of fractured neck of femur: a randomised trial of spontaneous versus controlled ventilation. British Journal of Anaesthesia 1988; 60: 43–47

McKenzie P J. Anaesthesia and the prophylaxis of thromboembolic diseases. Current Anaesthesia and Critical Care 1993; 4: 26–30

McKenzie P J. Anaesthesia for orthopaedic surgery. In: Smith, Nimmo, Robotham (eds) Anaesthesia, 2nd edn. Blackwell, Oxford, 1993

McKenzie P J. Anaesthesia and the accident service. In: Loach (ed) Anaesthesia for orthopaedic patients. ABL Longman, Edinburgh, 1993

McKenzie P J, Wishart H Y, Smith G. Long-term outcome after repair of fractured neck of femur. Comprising of subarachnoid and general anaesthesia. British Journal of Anaesthesia 1984; 56: 581–585

CROSS REFERENCES

Metabolic and degenerative bone disease
Patient Conditions 8: 200

Rheumatoid disease
Patient Conditions 8: 202

The elderly patient
Patient Conditions 11: 252

Total hip arthroplasty
Surgical Procedures 24: 481

Blood transfusion
Anaesthetic Factors 33: 616

Fat embolism
Anaesthetic Factors 33: 625

Local anaesthetic toxicity
Anaesthetic Factors 33: 642

Thrombotic embolism
Anaesthetic Factors 33: 664

TOTAL HIP ARTHROPLASTY

A. Loach

PROCEDURE

Total hip arthroplasty (THA):

- Requires the lateral, semilateral (most commonly) or supine position
- Uses a posterior or anterolateral incision (L4–S3)
- Uses a cemented or screw-in acetabular prosthesis followed by a cemented, or in younger patients an uncemented, femoral prosthesis
- Is increasingly performed as a revision procedure following loosening, infection or fracture of an earlier prosthesis.

PATIENT CHARACTERISTICS

- Age group 50–90+ years
- May have unsuspected accompanying disease (Table 1)
- ASA status I–IV
- Many are extremely active old people; farmers have a particularly high incidence.

Table 1.
Incidence of chronic disease in the elderly

Medical condition	Incidence (%)
Systemic hypertension	45
Previous myocardial infarction	21
Rhythm other than sinus	18
Angina	13
COAD	20
Renal disease	5

COMMON ASSOCIATIONS WITH THA

- Primary osteoarthritis or secondary to fractured neck of femur
- Rheumatoid arthritis and ankylosing spondylitis (to give upright posture)
- Avascular necrosis after fractured neck of femur or steroid therapy, e.g. for immunosuppression after transplantation, or NSAIDs.

PREOPERATIVE ASSESSMENT AND INVESTIGATIONS

- Exclude commonly associated medical conditions, e.g. anaemia from analgesic gastropathy
- Systematic review of likely chronic diseases, especially myocardial ischaemia (angina often masked by inactivity), hypertension, renal failure from analgesics, possible carcinoma, e.g. bronchus
- Blood transfusion availability
- Plan deep venous thrombosis (DVT) prophylaxis (compression stockings, regional block, anticoagulant, dextran)
- Antibiotic prophylaxis.

PREMEDICATION

Seldom necessary in the elderly, and likely to cause confusion. If essential, give a minimal dose of a benzodiazepine.

THEATRE PREPARATION

Care with positioning; elderly patients are particularly fragile. Ample padding; evacuated beanbag ensures good support. Do not forget items, e.g. diathermy plate. If using a Charnley enclosure, patients are subsequently inaccessible.

Maintain body temperature with warm fluids or a hot-air blower (blankets burn); humidification if intubated.

Blood loss measured during THA ranges from 300 to 1500 ml, and is doubled in the first 24 h postoperatively. Blood loss during THA is strongly related to anaesthetic technique and is reduced by regional anaesthesia and induced hypotension. This reduction may be cancelled by increased postoperative loss.

PERIOPERATIVE MANAGEMENT

Monitoring:

- Sa_{O_2}

- Direct BP if history of cardiovascular disease, otherwise noninvasive BP is adequate
- Blood loss and fluid balance
- ECG
- Core temperature
- $ETCO_2$.

Anaesthetic technique

Regional anaesthesia is the method of choice (Table 2) because the risk of venous thromboembolism is reduced due to increased leg blood flow and better venous drainage. There is excellent postoperative analgesia, decreased blood loss and attenuation of the stress response. Cementing may be improved because of reduced bleeding from bone.

Spinal and epidural techniques may be difficult in the elderly (look at hip X-rays for the lower spine); positioning may be impeded by pain.

Sedation during surgery may be needed. Use a light general anaesthetic or an infusion of propofol in low dosage (1–2 mg kg^{-1} h^{-1}). Added oxygen should be provided throughout.

General anaesthesia may be necessary if the patient rejects regional anaesthesia or block is impossible (ankylosing spondylitis, previous spinal fusion, gross scoliosis). Venous and arterial bleeding may be reduced with the modest hypotension from a volatile anaesthetic agent. Intravenous antibiotics may produce severe hypotension if given in bolus.

Cement-induced hypotension

Hypotension, occasionally severe, may occur during cement and prosthesis insertion, particularly into the femoral shaft. This is probably due to air embolism during impaction of the prosthesis. It does not occur if the surgeon uses a cement gun to layer the cement from the bottom of the cavity. Absorption of liquid polymer cellular debris, and fat also occurs marked by lasting hypoxaemia, and a rise in pulmonary vascular resistance. Hypotension is amplified by hypovolaemia and undertransfusion. Fat embolism syndrome has been reported when press-fit prostheses have been cemented. Intravenous fluid therapy must be adequate at this stage and the F_{IO_2} increased to 0.5 at least.

Table 2.
Regional anaesthesia used for THA

Spinal or epidural	Sole agent or with sedation. One-shot, limited postoperative analgesia; catheter technique continuous
Lumbar plexus block	With general anaesthesia. Less autonomic block
Paravascular inguinal block	With general anaesthesia. Poor analgesia

Thromboembolism

This is common after THA, principally due to femoral vein thrombosis (80%), possibly caused by extreme flexion and adduction during surgery kinking vessels, or by the heat of cement curing. Apart from cardiac causes, venous thromboembolism is the commonest cause of death following THA; prophylaxis is mandatory. Spinal and epidural anaesthesia reduce DVT significantly.

POSTOPERATIVE MANAGEMENT

Pain relief may be provided by continuous epidural analgesia with epidural opioids or slow infusion of local anaesthetics. Patient-controlled analgesia is effective and usually small doses only are required.

Rewarming may cause a fall in blood pressure but beware severe bleeding into operation site.

Urinary output should be monitored and added fluids given, if necessary, to maintain urinary output.

OUTCOME

The overall mortality from THA is 1–2%, rising with age to 5% at 90 years. Few studies include mortality at home. No reduction in mortality at 6 months has been demonstrated with regional anaesthesia and studies to date have been unable to show any difference in postoperative confusion.

BIBLIOGRAPHY

Evans R D, Palazzo M G A, Ackers J W L. Air embolism during total hip replacement: comparison of two surgical techniques. British Journal of Anaesthesia 1989; 62: 243

Michel R. Air embolism in hip surgery. Anaesthesia 1980; 35: 858

Seagroatt V, Tan H S, Goldacre M, Bulstrode C, Nugent I, Gill L. Elective total hip replacement: incidence, fatality and short-term readmission rates in a defined population. British Medical Journal 1991; 303: 1431

Watson J T, Stulberg B N. Fat embolism associated with cementing of femoral stems designed for press-fit application. Journal of Arthroplasty 1989; 4: 133

CROSS REFERENCES

Ankylosing spondylitis
  Patient Conditions 8: 194
Metabolic and degenerative bone disease
  Patient Conditions 8: 200
Rheumatoid disease
  Patient Conditions 8: 202
The elderly patient
  Patient Conditions 11: 252
Blood transfusion
  Anaesthetic Factors 33: 616
Complications of position
  Anaesthetic Factors 33: 618
Fat embolism
  Anaesthetic Factors 33: 625
Local anaesthetic toxicity
  Anaesthetic Factors 33: 642
Postoperative pain management
  Anaesthetic Factors 33: 655
Thrombotic embolism
  Anaesthetic Factors 33: 664

25

ENDOCRINE SURGERY

C. J. Hull

GENERAL CONSIDERATIONS

A. Batchelor and C. J. Hull

Some endocrine disorders are amenable to surgical correction. Such patients are exposed to several hazards in addition to those associated with the general surgical process.

- The patient suffers from an endocrine disorder which may, in itself, make anaesthesia and surgery especially hazardous. Uncorrected hyperthyroidism is a good example. Such patients are likely to develop dangerous tachydysrhythmias regardless of the type of surgical intervention.
- The surgical procedure may provoke the release of hormones and their precursors into the general circulation. This is a particular problem in the case of phaeochromocytoma, where massive quantities of catecholamines may be released causing life-threatening hypertension and/or tachycardia.
- When a hormone-excreting tumour has been removed the patient may be faced with the consequences of acute withdrawal. Thus removal of a large phaeochromocytoma may amount to sudden cessation of a high-dose catecholamine infusion, leading to severe hypotension and hypoglycaemia.
- Removal of functioning endocrine tissue may leave the patient with a secretory mass which is smaller than that required to maintain normal health. Thus total adrenalectomy, thyroidectomy or parathyroidectomy will lead to the development of typical hyposecretory syndromes which threaten survival unless corrected by immediate replacement therapy.

TOTAL ADRENALECTOMY

Every effort is made to conserve adrenal tissue, so that in many cases the patient is left with at least some adrenal function. While a single adrenal gland may be removed with almost no impact on global adrenal function, many patients lose at least part of their single remaining gland. Such patients must be supported with steroid cover through the postoperative period and until a formal assessment can be made of adrenocortical potential. In adult patients hydrocortisone (25 mg) is administered at the commencement of surgery followed by 100 mg in divided doses during the first 24 h, reducing to approximately 25 mg daily by day 5. Some patients, however, finally face the prospect of total adrenalectomy. They require normal hydrocortisone cover through the peri-operative period and may require mineralocorticoid supplementation (fludrocortisone, up to 0.3 mg daily) from day 3 onwards. Finally, they must be stabilized on life-long replacement therapy with both glucocorticoid and mineralocorticoid drugs.

BIBLIOGRAPHY

Wheeler M H. The adrenal glands. In: Burnand K G, Young A E (eds) The new Airds companion in surgical studies. Churchill Livingstone, Edinburgh, 1992

CROSS REFERENCES

Iatrogenic adrenocortical insufficiency
Patient Conditions 2: 54
Multiple endocrine neoplasia
Patient Conditions 2: 59
Hypertension
Patient Conditions 4: 111

PARATHYROID SURGERY

A. Batchelor and C. J. Hull

Parathyroidectomy is usually undertaken for removal of a parathyroid adenoma.

DIAGNOSIS

The clinical picture is due to hypercalcaemia. The commonest presentation is caused by deposition of insoluble calcium salts in the kidney, leading to stone formation. Renal or ureteric colic are the inevitable consequences.

Such patients often are hypertensive and develop progressive renal impairment with increased serum urea and creatinine concentrations. In more advanced cases patients suffer severe skeletal pain and even pathological fractures as a result of calcium mobilization.

Parathyroid tumours may be visualized using CT or scintigraphy, but the distinction between normal and abnormal glands often rests finally on surgical exposure and frozen-section microscopy.

Associated conditions

- Peptic ulceration
- Anaemia
- Myopathy.

In multiple endocrine neoplasia type I, parathyroid adenoma is associated with pancreatic islet cell tumour and adenoma or hyperplasia of the anterior pituitary.

LABORATORY FINDINGS

- Raised serum urea
- Raised serum creatinine
- Raised serum calcium
- Raised serum parathormone levels
- Reduced serum phosphate
- Raised urinary calcium
- Reduced urinary phosphate.

PREOPERATIVE PREPARATION

Some patients present with severe hypercalcaemia which should be corrected before surgery is considered. Such patients often suffer from fluid and electrolyte depletion as a consequence of intractable vomiting. In patients with adequate renal function these disturbances may be corrected using intravenous fluid therapy with a loop diuretic to promote calcium clearance. Hypocalcaemic drugs such as sodium clodronate, calcitonin and plicamicin also may be used. Of these, plicamicin is the most rapidly effective, but its use is limited to a few days due to marrow toxicity.

Steroids have been used, but are of very limited value. Rarely, life-saving surgery may be required when these measures fail to abate severe hyperparathyroidism.

SURGICAL PROCEDURE

Exploration of all four parathyroid glands is essential, since both adenomas and simple hyperplasias may be solitary or multiple. Rarely, parathyroid adenomas appear at ectopic sites and can be localized only by scintigraphy.

PREMEDICATION AND ANAESTHESIA

The surgeon requires a quiet, bloodless field if he is to identify the tiny glands.

This does not necessitate hypotensive anaesthesia, but does place a high premium on good technique. Avoidance of coughing and straining during the induction sequence are high priorities. A variety of techniques may serve, but the authors favour benzodiazepine premedication, induction of anaesthesia with small initial doses of alfentanil (0.25–0.5 mg) and midazolam (1–4 mg), followed by etomidate titrated to moderately deep anaesthesia, vecuronium (6–8 mg), endotracheal intubation and controlled ventilation with oxygen, nitrous oxide and a volatile anaesthetic agent. Supplemental doses of alfentanil and vecuronium are administered as required.

The procedure may be prolonged, and so effective heat conservation and fluid replacement should be maintained from the outset. In patients with major preoperative electrolyte disturbances, serum potassium should be monitored throughout surgery. Blood loss usually is minimal.

Patients should be positioned with great care in order to avoid pathological fractures.

Monitoring

- ECG
- Sao_2
- $ETco_2$
- Noninvasive BP
- Core temperature
- Ulnar nerve stimulation with evoked twitch responses.

POSTOPERATIVE COMPLICATIONS

- Accidental division of the recurrent laryngeal nerve.
- Acute hypocalcaemia may follow total parathyroidectomy.

CROSS REFERENCES

Hyperpara thyroidism
Patient Conditions 2: 46
Multiple endocrine neoplasia
Patient Conditions 2: 59
Prolonged anaesthesia
Anaesthetic Factors 32: 604

PHAEOCHROMOCYTOMA

A. Batchelor and
C. J. Hull

Phaeochromocytoma is a tumour of chromaffin tissue. It may be benign (usually) or malignant, solitary or multiple, and may occur within the adrenal gland, or at a wide variety of paraganglionic sites ranging from the base of the bladder to the base of the skull. Of the tumours, 10% are associated with genetic problems such as multiple endocrine neoplasia (MEN) type II, where phaeochromocytoma is associated with thyroid carcinoma and parathyroid hyperplasia. It also is associated with neurofibromatosis, cerebellar haemangioblastoma and Lindau von Hippel disease. Some 10% are extra-adrenal, multiple, bilateral, or malignant.

Occasionally, phaeochromocytoma develops in childhood, where the prevalence of nonadrenal sites is greater than in adults.

DIAGNOSIS

Patients commonly present with the following:

- Hypertension – this may be paroxysmal (50%) or continuous, and may have been treated for some years before phaeochromocytoma is suspected
- Headache
- Sweating
- Cardiovascular problems ranging from arrhythmias to catecholamine cardiomyopathy
- Hyperglycaemia and glycosuria; some patients may even require insulin therapy.

Ectopic tumours in the neck may be provoked by head movement, and those at the base of the bladder by micturition.

The presentation depends upon the relative proportion of adrenaline and noradrenaline secreted into the bloodstream. Predominantly noradrenaline-secreting tumours present with hypertension, headache and pallor, while adrenaline-secreting tumours tend to present with tachycardia and arrhythmias. Some patients develop a hypermetabolic state similar to that seen in severe hyperthyroidism.

INVESTIGATIONS

Confirmation of diagnosis is achieved by estimation of:

- Urinary hydroxymethylmandelic acid (HMMA)
- Urinary metadrenalines
- Plasma catecholamines.

In equivocal cases, the pentolinium test may be useful. Administration of intravenous pentolinium suppresses neurally mediated noradrenaline release, and so reduces plasma catecholamine concentrations in nonphaeochromocytoma patients.

Tumour localization depends on CT and ^{131}I *m*-iodobenzylguanidine (MIGB) scintigraphy.

SURGICAL PROCEDURE

Of the tumours, 90% occur in the adrenal medulla. The lateral position gives best access to the adrenal gland, but in the event of any doubt regarding the contralateral gland or ectopic sites, the surgeon will usually elect for laparotomy in the supine position. Some surgeons, taking a very aggressive approach and arguing that the incidence of recurrence in the remaining gland is unacceptably high, perform bilateral adrenalectomy, even when the tumour is solitary. However, the accepted approach in the UK is more conservative. Since recurrences may occur at a great variety of sites, it is considered more rational to preserve as much normal adrenal tissue as possible and then to monitor the patient over a prolonged period.

Since extra-adrenal tumours may be found anywhere from the base of skull to the pelvis, usually along the paraganglionic line, their removal may require a variety of surgical approaches.

PREOPERATIVE MANAGEMENT

Multisystem preoperative assessment is necessary, with special emphasis on the cardiovascular system. All patients should have echocardiography, since cardiomyopathy is often symptomless and unsuspected.

PREOPERATIVE BLOCKADE

Published recommendations range from nothing to many weeks of alpha with or without beta adrenergic blockade. No adequate trials of preoperative preparation exist in the literature, but a reduction in mortality from 50% to 0–3% was coincident with the introduction of preoperative blockade. The authors place great emphasis on proper preoperative blockade managed by the anaesthetic team.

Adrenergic blockade does not prevent the release of catecholamines, but does obtund the physiological response, producing unimpaired myocardial performance and tissue oxygen delivery.

Recommendations for preoperative blockade

Alpha blockade using phenoxybenzamine (10 mg orally twice daily) increased as tolerated.

- *Aim*: stabilization of BP. Increase dosage until a postural BP drop develops, with reduction of symptoms such as sweating. The object is to allow restoration of normal circulating volume, and in patients with cardiomyopathy a period of cardiac rest which may allow some recovery.
- *Side-effects:*
  - Stuffy nose
  - Dizziness on standing (initial treatment should be as an in-patient)
  - Drowsiness and blurred vision (the patient should not drive)
  - Tachycardia, which can be controlled with a beta blocker (propranolol or atenolol) introduced after alpha blockade is established.

At least 7–10 days of established blockade is required, but many patients benefit from a longer period of treatment, particularly those with cardiomyopathy or ST–T wave changes. Plasma volume increases during blockade, thus preventing severe hypotension after tumour removal. In patients with cardio-myopathy, blockade must be continued for several weeks, so as to maximize recovery before operation.

PREMEDICATION

- An anxiolytic such as temazepam. Avoid atropine because of tachycardia. Phenoxybenzamine decreases sweating.
- Deep venous thrombosis prophylaxis.

THEATRE PREPARATION

Drugs:
- Phentolamine may be useful during the induction of general anaesthesia if this provokes a hypertensive surge.
- Sodium nitroprusside infusion for control of hypertensive surges during surgery. This is best administered through a central line in order to achieve the fastest possible response.
- Noradrenaline ready in case of post–resection hypotension.
- Propranolol ready for control of tachycardia. Large doses (>50 mg) may be required.

Maintenance of temperature in a vasodilated patient:
- Warm all intravenous fluids
- Use a warming blanket on the operating table
- Warm and humidify inspired gases.

ANAESTHESIA

Aim
To avoid provocation of catecholamine release by anaesthetic drugs or manoeuvres, to suppress the adrenergic response to surgical stimulation, and to minimize haemodynamic responses to tumour handling and devascularization.

Monitoring:
- ECG (CM5 lead preferred)
- Arterial line for continuous BP measurement
- Central venous pressure (triple-lumen catheter)
- A pulmonary artery flotation (Swan–Ganz) catheter is essential because:
  - Rises in pulmonary artery capillary wedge pressure (PCWP) indicate left ventricular strain
  - There are great changes in systemic vascular resistance; changes in blood pressure have no correlation with changes in cardiac output
  - Right and left filling pressures may differ in patients with phaeochromocytoma.
- Spo_2
- Core temperature.

ANAESTHETIC TECHNIQUE

High lumbar epidural block plus general anaesthesia. Combined opioid + LA regional blockade augments preoperative alpha blockade and provides postoperative analgesia. Since these patients already have extensive peripheral vasodilation, it is most unusual for the epidural to cause hypotension.

Avoid histamine-releasing drugs such as morphine and atracurium. Most anaesthetic drugs have been reported as being used successfully, but the most rational combination is alfentanil, etomidate, vecuronium and isoflurane.

Control of arterial pressure and heart rate during surgery
Despite preoperative preparation, marked swings in blood pressure may be seen during manipulation of the tumour. These should be controlled with short-acting agents such as nitroprusside and propranolol. Esmolol would seem to be an even more suitable beta blocker, but in practice has proved disappointing in the face of extreme tachycardias.

Alpha blockade leads to increased plasma volume, but even then it is usually necessary to administer additional intravenous fluids during the dissection phase if hypotension following tumour devascularization is to be prevented.

After ligation of all venous drainage from the tumour, arterial pressure commonly declines. This may be associated with a high cardiac output and very low systemic vascular resistance, requiring noradrenaline treatment, low cardiac output requiring inotropic support, or both. The Swan–Ganz catheter simplifies decision-making during this phase. An adequate period of preoperative blockade, combined with generous intraoperative fluid loading monitored by PCWP may obviate the need for post–resection catecholamines.

POSTOPERATIVE CARE

The patient should be managed in an ITU or

HDU by nursing staff familiar with the special problems posed by these patients.

Blood pressure
Despite persisting alpha and beta blockade, arterial pressure usually stabilizes remarkably quickly, and vasoactive medication can be withdrawn within a few hours. In some cases, hypertension persists for several days before settling down, but in a small minority hypertension may persist, raising the possibilities of residual tumour or underlying essential hypertension.

Blood glucose
High catecholamine levels increase blood glucose and block the secretion of insulin. Tumour removal and loss of catecholamines may result in hypoglycaemia, either via a rebound increase in insulin secretion and/or via a decrease in lipolysis and glycogenolysis. Persisting beta blockade will mask the signs of hypoglycaemia. Failure to detect severe hypoglycaemia has led to disastrous outcomes in several reported cases. Blood glucose should be monitored every half hour for the first 24 h, and corrected promptly if subnormal.

Steroids
If bilateral adrenalectomy has been carried out, steroid replacement will be required.

Analgesia
Abrupt withdrawal of catecholamines and residual concentrations of blocking drugs may cause marked somnolence. Such patients are very sensitive to the sedative actions of opioids, such that conventional doses may result in dangerously deep sedation. Continuous or, even better, patient-controlled epidural analgesia avoids this problem and provides superior pain control.

UNEXPECTEDLY ENCOUNTERED PHAEOCHROMOCYTOMA

Very occasionally, a patient will exhibit severe hypertension with a tachycardia and possibly arrhythmias and hyperpyrexia during surgery for an unrelated condition. Once the possibility of an undiagnosed phaeochromocytoma has been raised alpha blockade with phentolamine must be instituted immediately. Surgery should be completed as rapidly as possible and no attempt made to resect the tumour unless this is essential to the patient's immediate survival. Then, diagnosis, localization and preparation may be undertaken as usual.

OUTCOME

In adequately prepared patients mortality is 0–3% in reported series. Mortality is high (of the order of 50%) in patients diagnosed during operation. In a series of 40 000 postmortems, phaeochromocytoma was found in 0.13%. In those patients whose tumours were identified at autopsy, 27% died in the perioperative period from a cardiovascular collapse of unknown cause.

25

BIBLIOGRAPHY

Hull C J. Phaeochromocytoma. British Journal of Anaesthesia 1986; 58: 1453–1468
Mihm F G. Pulmonary artery monitoring in patient with phaeochromocytoma. Anesthesiology 1982; 57: A42
Roizen M F, Hung T K, Beaupre P N et al. The effect of alpha-adrenergic blockade on cardiac performance and tissue oxygen delivery during excision of phaeochromocytoma. Surgery 1983; 946: 941–945
Stenstrom G, Kutti J. The blood volume in phaeochromocytoma patients before and during treatment with phenoxybenzamine. Acta Medica Scandinavica 1985; 218: 381–387
Sutton M G, Sheps S G, Lie J T. Prevalence of clinically unsuspected phaeochromocytoma: Review of a 50 year autopsy series. Mayo Clinic Proceedings 1981; 56: 354–360

CROSS REFERENCES

Iatrogenic adrenocortical insufficiency
Patient Conditions 2: 54
Multiple endocrine neoplasia
Patient Conditions 2: 59
Hypertension
Patient Conditions 4: 111
Prolonged anaesthesia
Anaesthetic Factors 32: 607
Intraoperative hypertension
Anaesthestic Factors 33: 636

26

PAEDIATRICS

G. Meakin

OVERVIEW

G. Meakin

The fundamental differences between paediatric patients and adults concerning anaesthesia have been discussed earlier (p. 255). This section deals with the practical aspects of anaesthetic management.

PREOPERATIVE PREPARATION

The child should be admitted to a suitably decorated children's ward, in which a selection of toys is available. In addition, the child should be encouraged to bring a favourite toy from home. The child's nickname, if one is used, should be entered in the nursing notes and used by the carers. At the preoperative visit, the anaesthetist should explain the proposed procedure in simple terms, avoiding words which may cause alarm. For example, if intravenous induction of anaesthesia is planned, it is more tactful to describe this as a 'scratch on the hand' rather than a 'prick from a needle'. A parent may be invited to accompany the child at induction of anaesthesia.

Anaesthetic assessment

The case notes should be reviewed with particular attention to:

- Age and weight (is the weight appropriate?)
- History of prematurity
- Previous illnesses and medications
- Allergy and any unusual syndrome
- Previous anaesthetics
- History of upper respiratory tract infection.

Children with a history of upper respiratory tract infection within 4 weeks of operation are at an increased risk of respiratory complications during or after anaesthesia. Ideally, elective surgery should be postponed for 4–6 weeks, but this is not always practical as symptoms tend to recur. Moreover, many children with recurrent symptoms will be suffering from allergy. If a decision is made to proceed, a drying agent should be administered preoperatively and the patient intubated to minimize the risk of coughing or laryngospasm during anaesthesia. Careful monitoring and supplemental oxygen will be required during recovery.

Physical examination should be carried out with particular attention to:

- Loose deciduous teeth
- Signs of difficult intubation (limited mouth opening, micrognathia, large tongue, noisy breathing)
- Pyrexia (38°C), cough, malaise and audible signs of lower respiratory tract infection
- Possible venepuncture sites.

When signs of lower respiratory tract infection are present, elective surgery must be postponed for 4–6 weeks to allow hyperactive airways to return to normal.

Investigations are not required routinely in healthy children undergoing relatively minor surgery. Haemoglobin estimation is required in patients at increased risk of anaemia. The significance of anaemia should be judged by its clinical effects. Because of compensatory mechanisms, symptoms rarely appear until the haemoglobin falls below 6 g/100 ml.

A formal assessment of the risk of anaesthesia should be made using the ASA classification and entered into the patient's notes.

Fasting and premedication

Clear fluids should be withheld for 3 h and solid food and milk for 6 h preoperatively to ensure minimum volume of gastric contents at induction of anaesthesia.

Infants do not require sedative premedication, but they may be given atropine (20 μg kg^{-1} i.m.) preoperatively, or preferably intravenously at induction of anaesthesia to prevent reflex bradycardia. Older children will benefit from sedative premedication and the application of EMLA cream to possible venepuncture sites.

MANAGEMENT OF ANAESTHESIA

Induction

Induction of anaesthesia may be accomplished by intravenous injection of a short-acting hypnotic or inhalation of a volatile anaesthetic agent. Intravenous induction of anaesthesia is quicker, creates less operating-room pollution, and may be less disturbing to the child than inhalational methods.

Tracheal intubation

Infants and children are intubated with the head in a neutral position. Raising the head on a low pillow does not improve the view of the larynx in these patients because there are fewer intervertebral joints above the larynx that can be flexed. The most effective manoeuvre is the application of external pressure at the level of the cricoid cartilage to push the larynx into view.

In infants a flat-blade laryngoscope such as the infant Magill which passes posterior to the epiglottis may be more suitable than a curved one, since it flattens out the curvature of the epiglottis and can be used to lift it forwards to expose the larynx. In children aged over 1 year, laryngoscopy can usually be accomplished using a medium-sized Macintosh blade with the tip placed in the vallecula.

Since the narrowest part of the larynx before puberty is the cricoid ring, cuffed tracheal tubes are not usually required in infants and children. The correct sized tube is one that passes easily through the cricoid ring and allows a slight leak at 20–25 cmH_2O pressure. The following formula may be used as a guide in children aged 2 years and over:

$$\text{Tube size (internal diameter in mm)} = \frac{\text{Age (years)}}{4} + 4.5$$

Using this formula any quarter sizes should be rounded down. Tube sizes in infants and children aged less than 2 years have to be memorized. A normal neonate weighing 3 kg requires a 3 mm tracheal tube; premature and low-weight babies may require a 2.5 mm tube. Other tube sizes can be interpolated.

Tracheal tubes should be cut to a length which allows the tip of the tube to be placed in the midtrachea, while 2–3 cm protrudes from the month for fixation. The following formula may be used to estimate orotracheal tube length in children aged over 2 years:

$$\text{Orotracheal tube length (cm)} = \frac{\text{Age (years)}}{2} + 13$$

Orotracheal tube lengths for patients aged less than 2 years have to be memorized. The length for neonate is 10 cm, and for a 1-year old is 12 cm; other tube lengths can be interpolated. The position of the tracheal tube should be checked by auscultation of the lung fields.

Maintenance of anaesthesia

In general, infants are poor candidates for anaesthesia with spontaneous ventilation because of poor pulmonary mechanics (p. 255). In these patients, the combination of tracheal intubation and balanced anaesthesia with full doses of muscle relaxants, controlled ventilation, minimum concentrations of volatile anaesthetics and reduced doses of opioids is recommended. This regimen provides ideal surgical conditions with minimal cardiovascular depression and rapid return of laryngeal reflexes at the conclusion of anaesthesia.

Children aged over 1 year undergoing long operations will also benefit from balanced anaesthesia. However, for many children undergoing operations lasting less than 30–40 min, simple inhalation anaesthesia with 66% nitrous oxide in oxygen and halothane (1–2%) may be adequate. This may be combined with an opioid analgesic (e.g. morphine 0.1 mg kg^{-1} i.m.), local infiltration, or a regional block to provide analgesia in the postoperative period.

Anaesthetic breathing systems

Most modern breathing systems incorporating low resistance valves can be adapted for paediatric use. Nonabsorber systems are favoured by paediatric anaesthetists as they are more compact, and the inspired concentration of anaesthetic is essentially the same as that set at the vaporizer. An adequate fresh gas flow is required to eliminate carbon dioxide (Table 1).

Monitoring

The published guidelines for minimum standards of monitoring during anaesthesia apply equally well to children as to adults. A range of paediatric cuffs must be available for measurement of blood pressure; the correct sized cuff is one which covers two-thirds of

Table 1.
Fresh gas flow requirements of anaesthetic circuits

Enclosed Mapleson A (e.g. Carden A mode)
Controlled or spontaneous ventilation:
Fresh gas flow ($1\ min^{-1}$) = Alveolar ventilation $\approx 0.6 \times \sqrt{}$ Weight (kg)

T-pieces (e.g. Bain and Jackson Rees)
Controlled ventilation:
Fresh gas flow ($1\ min^{-1}$) = Minute ventilation $\approx 0.8 \times \sqrt{}$ Weight (kg)
Spontaneous ventilation:
In theory, Fresh gas flow ($1\ min^{-1}$) > 2 × Minute ventilation
In practice, Fresh gas flow ($1\ min^{-1}$) = $\sqrt{}$ Weight (kg)

the upper arm. Temperature measurement is mandatory in children, and neuromuscular transmission monitoring is useful in view of the marked variation in response to muscle relaxants.

Intraoperative fluid therapy

An intravenous infusion should be established for all but minor procedures. A 22 gauge cannula can generally be sited in a peripheral vein in an infant, while a 20 gauge cannula is suitable for children. Maintenance fluid and electrolyte requirements can be calculated from the equation given on p. 256. A balanced salt solution, such as Ringer lactate, should be given to replace third-space losses.

Blood loss should be measured by swab weighing or colorimetry. In general, losses less than 10% of the blood volume (estimated at 80 ml kg^{-1}) either require no replacement or can be replaced by crystalloid solution. Losses of 10–20% can be replaced by colloids or blood, but losses over 20% must be replaced by blood.

POSTOPERATIVE MANAGEMENT

At the conclusion of anaesthesia the child should be turned into the lateral position and transported, breathing oxygen, to a fully equipped recovery room. Details of the operative procedure and any special instructions should be given to the recovery nurse assuming care of the child. Recovery-room protocol should include airway maintenance, provision of oxygen therapy, monitoring of oxygen saturation, pulse, respiration and blood pressure, and the completion of a postanaesthetic recovery chart. The anaesthetist should ensure that the child is fully awake and that postoperative fluids and analgesics have been ordered before the child is returned to the surgical ward.

BIBLIOGRAPHY

Meakin G. Anaesthesia for infants and children. In: Healy T E J, Cohen P J (eds). A practice of anaesthesia, 6th edn. London: Edward Arnold 1995

Meakin G, Jennings A D, Beatty P C W, Healy T E J. Fresh gas requirements of an enclosed afferent reservoir breathing system during controlled ventilation of children. British Journal of Anaesthesia 1992; 68: 43–47

Steward D J. Screening tests before surgery in children. Canadian Journal of Anaesthesia 1991; 38: 693–695

Westhorpe R N. The position of the larynx in children and its relationship to the ease of intubation. Anaesthesia and Intensive Care 1987; 15: 384–388

CROSS REFERENCES

Infants and children
Patient Conditions 11: 255

CIRCUMCISION

S. Stainthorpe

PROCEDURE

Usually performed as a day-case procedure.

PATIENT CHARACTERISTICS

Patients for circumcision are usually:
- Aged over 1 month
- ASA status grade I–III.

PREOPERATIVE ASSESSMENT

- Exclude of active upper respiratory tract infections
- Exclude of contact with childhood infections
- Exclude of hypospadias abnormality
- No family history of bleeding diathesis or anaesthetic problems.

PREOPERATIVE INVESTIGATIONS

None necessary unless there is a positive medical indication.

PREOPERATIVE PREPARATION

- Abstinence from food and food drinks (e.g. milk, soup) for 6 h
- Total starvation for 3 h
- Explanation to parents and child, including explanation of local procedure and how long its effect may last.

PREMEDICATION

- Application of topical local anaesthetic preparation (e.g. EMLA cream) over possible venepuncture sites
- If anxiolytic required, oral midazolam (0.5 mg kg^{-1}) may be given 30–45 min preoperatively.

THEATRE PREPARATION

Escort for accompanying parent leaving anaesthetic room when child is asleep.

PERIOPERATIVE MANAGEMENT

Monitoring:
- Pulse oximetry
- $ETCO_2$.
- ECG
- BP.

General anaesthesia:
- Intravenous or inhalation induction
- Spontaneous ventilation via laryngeal mask for children over 1 year; IPPV via endotracheal tube for children under 1 year
- If local anaesthesia is not performed before the procedure, the general anaesthetic should be deep when the foreskin is clamped, to prevent laryngospasm.

Local anaesthesia

Penile block using 0.5% bupivacaine (1–3 ml) *without* adrenaline (Table 1); or caudal block, single shot using 0.25% bupivacaine (0.5 ml kg^{-1}) (Table 2). Both are performed after induction as supplement to general anaesthesia and for postoperative pain relief.

POSTOPERATIVE MANAGEMENT

Good analgesia is essential during the early postoperative period. Be prepared to supplement the local block with an intravenous narcotic if local block is not adequate when the child wakes.

OUTCOME

Discharge may be delayed by:
- Over sedation
- Failure to micturate (more likely with inadequate analgesia; penile block has a higher failure rate than caudal)
- Large haematoma can be caused by penile block or manipulation of the surgical site by a restless child in pain
- Difficulty walking (more likely if caudal block used)
- Vomiting.

Table 1.
Complete penile block

- The nerves lie deep and superficial to Buck's fascia and may be separated by a midline septum
- Supine position
- Routine skin preparation
- Use the smallest size of needle with which the operator is familiar
- Palpate the lower border of the symphysis pubis with the left index finger and retract the penis
- Insert the needle between finger and arch of pubis until there is a slight 'give' or bone is struck; if bone is struck, 'walk' the needle inferiorly till it is free
- Bupivacaine should be injected either side of the midline by two sperate needle punctures or by directing the needle from a single puncture
- Aspirate before injection
- Inject half the dose either side, 2/3 deep and 1/3 superficial to Buck's fascia
- Minimal swelling should be seen
- Analgesia should last about 6 h, during which period the child is able to micturate without pain

Table 2.
Caudal block of the sacral nerves

- The sacral hiatus appears higher in children than adults. It may be located by placing the child on his side with the legs flexed to a right angle at hips and knees
- The smallest needle with which the operator is familiar should be used
- When the caudal space has been identified, the needle should not be advanced in small children. The dura mater extends more caudally in children and there is increased chance of piercing it or an anterior blood vessel
- Children's circulation is stable after caudal extradural block

BIBLIOGRAPHY

Goulding F J. Penile block for postoperative pain relief in penile surgery. Journal of Urology 1981; 126: 337

White J, Harrison B, Richmond P, Proctor A, Curran J. Postoperative analgesia for circumcision. British Medical Journal 1983; 286: 1934

CROSS REFERENCES

Infants and children
Patient Conditions 11: 255
Local anaesthetic toxicity
Anaesthetic Factors 33: 642

CONGENITAL DIAPHRAGMATIC HERNIA

A. J. Charlton

26

PRESENTATION

Incidence is 1 in 4000 live births. Right-sided hernia (20%) is associated with higher mortality, as is detection by antenatal ultrasonography (increasingly common).

Presents with respiratory failure at or shortly after birth. Patients have bilateral pulmonary hypoplasia and tend to revert to fetal pattern of circulation with severe right–left shunting.

Death occurs due to:

- Inadequate gas exchange surface
- Fixed high pulmonary vascular resistance (decreased vascular cross-sectional area, but normal cardiac output)
- Reversible pulmonary hypertension (abnormal muscularity of pulmonary vessels)
- Additional anomalies (in about 5%).

RESUSCITATION

Immediate tracheal intubation when diagnosis is known. Avoid inflations by mask, which distends the herniated viscera, worsening mediastinal shift.

Pass nasogastric tube to deflate gut and keep on free drainage. Use muscle relaxants to facilitate IPPV for transport.

PREOPERATIVE PREPARATION

No longer considered an emergency; surgery worsens lung mechanics.

Time (days) should be taken to stabilize gas exchange by meticulous intensive medical management aimed at avoidance of trigger factors for pulmonary vasoconstriction (hypoxia, hypercarbia, acidosis).

Monitoring

Peripheral arterial cannulation allows blood pressure monitoring and blood gas sampling with minimal disturbance. Most published predictive indices require postductal oxygen values. Transcutaneous oxygen and carbon dioxide transducers aid continuous monitoring. Pulse oximeters placed pre- and post-ductally may demonstrate the variability of shunting.

Ventilation

- Muscle relaxants (e.g. tubocurarine infusion) give optimal control of ventilation and decrease oxygen consumption
- Conventional or high frequency IPPV can be used
- Risk of pneumothorax from high inflation pressures
- PEEP rarely of benefit until weaning.

Acid–base status

Acidosis should be corrected with buffers. Alkalosis may enhance pulmonary circulation, achieved either by systemic alkalinization (to pH 7.5–7.6) or hyperventilation ($P_{a}CO_2$ 25–30 mmHg).

Pulmonary circulation

Refractory hypoxaemia may respond to vasodilating agents, such as tolazoline (1 mg kg^{-1} bolus followed by up to 1 mg kg^{-1} h^{-1} if effective and urine output is normal), prostacyclin or nitric oxide inhalation.

Fluid balance

Preoperative restriction (6 ml kg^{-1} per 24 h) avoids fluid retention. Circulating volume should be maintained with plasma or blood (maintain Hb above 14 g dl^{-1}).

Sedation

If oxygenation is shown to be labile in response to handling (unusual), a narcotic (e.g. morphine infusion) may be helpful.

SURGERY

Usually undertaken via an upper abdominal incision, which permits correction of the gut malrotation. In about 5% of cases closure can only be achieved with a prosthetic patch.

ANAESTHESIA

- Surgery causes little disturbance if delayed to permit inspired oxygen requirement to stabilize below 50%
- The exact pattern of preoperative ventilation should be continued
- Volatile agents should be avoided (cardiovascular depression)
- Fentanyl in large doses (up to 25 μg kg^{-1}) obtunds all response to surgery (even with 100% oxygen) and has negligible cardiovascular effect
- Monitoring should include ECG, direct or indirect arterial pressure, pulse oximetry, capnography and body temperature.

POSTOPERATIVE CARE

General intensive care with attention to fluid and nutritional requirements (enteral or parenteral) must continue. Weaning from IPPV in severe cases may take months. After tracheal extubation a period of CPAP (e.g. via nasopharyngeal tube) may be required. The most severely affected survivors have little respiratory reserve and may succumb to respiratory infection.

EXTRACORPOREAL MEMBRANE OXYGENATION (ECMO)

Although its place in congenital diaphragmatic hernia management is still not clear, ECMO has been used pre-, intra- and post-operatively. If available it should be considered in the presence of deterioration to an oxygenation index (OI) of greater than 0.4 ($OI = F_IO_2 \times$ Mean airway pressure$/P_aO_2$). Patients who do not achieve a best postductal PO_2 of 100 mmHg on conventional treatment do not usually survive with ECMO.

OUTCOME

Mortality in large series ranges from 29% to 55%. Survivors may exhibit chronic lung disease and developmental impairment.

BIBLIOGRAPHY

Charlton A J. The management of congenital diaphragmatic hernia without ECMO. Paediatric Anaesthesia 1993; 3: 201–204

Charlton A J, Bruce J, Davenport M. Timing of surgery in congenital diaphragmatic hernia. Anaesthesia 1991; 46: 820–823

Rice L J, Baker S B. Congenital diaphragmatic hernia. Does extracorporeal membrane oxygenation (ECMO) improve survival? Paediatric Anaesthesia 1993; 3: 205–208

Sakai H, Tamura M, Hosokawa Y, Bryan A C, Barker G A, Bohn D J. Effect of surgical repair on respiratory mechanics in congenital diaphragmatic hernia. Journal of Pediatrics 1987; 111: 432–438

Wilson J M, Lund D P, Lillehei C W, O'Rourke P P, Vacanti J P. Delayed repair and preoperative ECMO does not improve survival in high-risk congenital diaphragmatic hernia. Journal of Pediatric Surgery 1992; 27: 368–375

CROSS REFERENCES

Infants and children
Patient Conditions 11: 255

CONGENITAL HYPERTROPHIC PYLORIC STENOSIS

R. Walker

PROCEDURE

Repair of congenital hypertrophic pyloric stenosis (Ramstedt's procedure) is performed:

- Either via a transverse incision in the right upper quadrant, or a hemicircumferential supraumbilical incision (both in a skin crease)
- By a longitudinal serosal and muscular incision down to the mucosa of the pylorus
- Patency is checked by passage of air through the pylorus injected via a nasogastric tube at operation.

PATIENT CHARACTERISTICS

- Typically first-born male children (male > female)
- Age 3–8 weeks old
- Incidence 1:300 live births, but considerable regional variation
- Symptoms and signs are shown in Table 1.

Common associations:
- Renal anomalies
- Increased unconjugated bilirubinaemia (17%).

Table 1.
Clinical features

- Bile-free vomiting after every feed, becoming projectile
- Hungry
- Dehydrated (may vary from mild to severe hypovolaemia)
- Visible peristalsis in left upper quadrant from left to right
- Palpable tumour

Diagnosis confirmed by palpation of tumour (with or without test feed); if in doubt, confirm by abdominal ultrasound

PREOPERATIVE ASSESSMENT, INVESTIGATIONS AND RESUSCITATION

The operation is never urgent and full resuscitation is imperative. This may take several days.

Preoperative management involves the cessation of oral feeding, passage of a nasogastric tube and correction of the fluid and electrolyte status.

There are two main problems:
- Dehydration: assessment of volume status (N.B. 1 l water is approximately equal to 1 kg weight) (Table 2).
- Biochemical defect: hypochloraemic metabolic alkalosis; hypokalaemia.

Loss of hydrochloric acid in the vomitus results in metabolic alkalosis. Correction of this defect depends on retention of hydrogen ion by the kidney. Since hydrogen and potassium ions are exchanged for sodium in the distal renal tubule, retention of hydrogen ions results in increased potassium excretion and hypokalaemia. If dehydration becomes severe, increased reabsorption of sodium ions

Table 2.
Assessment of hydration in the infant

	Mild	Moderate	Severe
Loss of body weight (%)	5	10	15
Clinical signs	Dry skin and mucous membranes	Mottled cold periphery. Loss of skin turgor. Sunken fontanelle. Oliguria, low BP	Shocked. Moribund
Replacement (ml kg^{-1})	50	100	150

increases excretion of both hydrogen and potassium, exacerbating hypokalaemic alkalosis.

Treatment requires replacement of the calculated fluid deficit with 0.9% saline with potassium (40 mmol l^{-1}).

In severe dehydration up to half of the calculated fluid deficit may be required in the first hour, and 20 ml kg^{-1} may be given as salt-poor albumin. Once the circulation is restored and urine output of at least 1 ml kg^{-1} h^{-1} is established, the remaining deficit can be replaced over 24–48 h. Maintenance fluid requirements should also be given as 0.18% saline in 5% dextrose.

The serum electrolytes and acid–base status must be normal before surgery takes place.

PREMEDICATION

Intramuscular atropine (20 μg kg^{-1}) if preferred 1 h preoperatively. Nil else.

THEATRE PREPARATION

Increase ambient temperature in theatre to 24–26°C. Warming blanket, warm gamgee padding, fluid warmer and warm-air blower should be available.

PERIOPERATIVE MANAGEMENT

Monitoring:
- ECG
- Noninvasive BP
- Spo_2
- $ETco_2$
- Core temperature
- Peripheral nerve stimulator
- Fluid balance and blood loss.

ANAESTHETIC TECHNIQUE

General anaesthesia should be induced in the operating theatre with all efforts made to maintain the infant's body temperature. All precautions protecting against a full stomach should be employed. The nasogastric tube should be aspirated prior to induction. Two techniques are commonly used:

- A rapid sequence induction with pre-oxygenation, cricoid pressure, thiopentone (5–7 mg kg^{-1}), suxamethonium (1.5–2 mg kg^{-1}).
- An inhalational induction with oxygen and halothane followed by tracheal intubation.

Both techniques of induction should be followed by muscle paralysis (atracurium 0.5 mg kg^{-1}) and IPPV.

Following the relatively short procedure, the infant should be extubated awake, and vigorous in the left lateral position.

POSTOPERATIVE MANAGEMENT

Postoperative pain relief can be provided by wound infiltration with local anaesthetics and oral or rectal paracetamol. Only rarely are more potent analgesics required.

The infant can be fed 8 h postoperatively and 70% of infants tolerate this. Graduated feeding regimens are of no proven benefit.

OUTCOME

Recurrence of the disease reflects inadequate surgery. Morbidity in other areas is associated with related disease pathology.

BIBLIOGRAPHY

Atwell J D, Levick P. Congenital hypertrophic pyloric stenosis and associated anomalies in the genitourinary tract. Journal of Paediatric Surgery 1982; 16: 1029

Daley A M, Conn A W. Anaesthesia for pyloromyotomy: a review. Canadian Anaesthetic Society Journal 1979; 16: 316

Dawson K D, Graham D. The assessment of dehydration in congenital pyloric stenosis. New Zealand Medical Journal 1991; 104: 162–163

Steven I M, Allen T H, Sweeney D B. Congenital hypertrophic pyloric stenosis. The anaesthetists' view. Anaesthesia and Intensive Care 1973; 1: 544

Vivori E, Bush G H. Modern aspects of the management of the newborn undergoing operation. British Journal of Anaesthesia 1977; 49: 51

Winters R W. Metabolic alkalosis of pyloric stenosis. In: Winters R W (ed) The body fluids in paediatrics. Little & Brown, Boston, 1973, p 402

Wooley M M, Felsher B F, Asch M J et al. Jaundice, hypertrophic pyloric stenosis and glucoronyl transferase. Journal of Paediatric Surgery 1974; 9: 359

CROSS REFERENCES

Infants and children
Patient Conditions 11: 255

TRACHEO-OESOPHAGEAL FISTULA AND OESOPHAGEAL ATRESIA

S. G. Greenhough

PROCEDURE

Tracheo-oesophageal fistula (TOF) and oesophageal atresia repair is performed as follows:

- Left lateral position (right side up)
- Axillary skin crease or axillary longitudinal incision
- Extrapleural approach, if possible
- Requires compression collapse of right lung
- In the presence of oesophageal atresia, closure of TOF and either primary oesophageal anastomosis or oesophagostomy and gastrostomy is required.

PATIENT CHARACTERISTICS

- Generally less than 1-week old
- Incidence of 1 in 3500 live births
- 30% of babies are premature.

There are several different combinations of fistula and atresia. The three most common are: oesophageal atresia and lower pouch fistula (80%), oesophageal atresia with no fistula (10%), and tracheo-oesophageal fistula with no oesophageal atresia (2%). (Figure 1).

COMMON ASSOCIATIONS WITH TOF

- 20–25% have associated major cardiac anomalies
- Polyhydramnios in the mother is common
- Increasing antenatal diagnosis
- 10% incidence of VACTERL syndrome.

PREOPERATIVE ASSESSMENT AND INVESTIGATIONS

Routine:

- Haemoglobin
- Urea and electrolytes
- Cranial ultrasound
- Single X-ray of chest and abdomen
- Cross-match blood.

Specific:

- Rectal examination
- Renal ultrasound
- Echocardiogram
- Blood gases if indicated, especially if premature.

PREOPERATIVE MANAGEMENT

- Replogle tube to prevent aspiration of saliva.
- Small number of premature babies may require positive pressure ventilation. If lung compliance is low and the fistula large, immediate surgery may be the only method of achieving adequate ventilation.

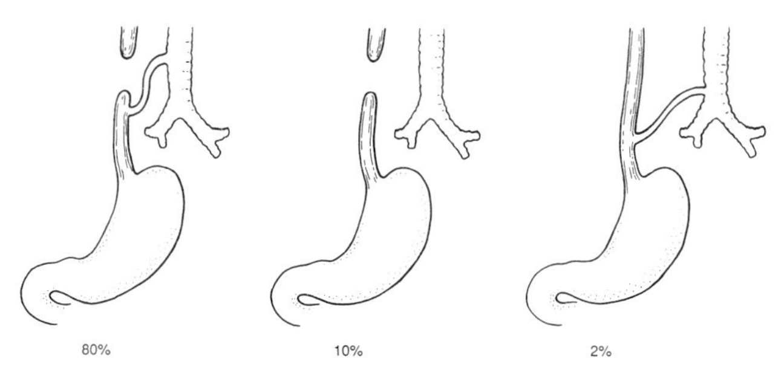

Figure 1
Common presentations of oesophageal atresia.

THEATRE PREPARATION

- High theatre temperature
- Warming blanket
- Humidification of inspired gases.

PERIOPERATIVE MANAGEMENT

Induction:
- In the operating theatre
- Awake intubation or thiopentone and atracurium.

Tracheoscopy:
- Requires ventilating bronchoscope to identify the fistula position
- A small percentage of cases will have upper and lower pouch fistulas.

Monitoring:
- ECG
- Sao_2
- Noninvasive BP
- $ETco_2$
- Core temperature.

Care should be taken with siting the monitoring. The axillary artery in the uppermost arm may be compressed by surgical traction.

Maintenance
Oxygen and nitrous oxide with 0.2–0.5% halothane. Inspired oxygen may occasionally require to be increased during lung collapse.

SPECIAL CONSIDERATIONS

Many authors stress the importance of endotracheal tube placement relative to the fistula in order to prevent excessive quantities of gas being forced into the stomach. In our unit we believe this risk to be overstated, and site normal length endotracheal tubes irrespective of fistula position. Gastric distension is much more commonly the result of overvigorous ventilation with high airway pressures. Gentle hand ventilation is the best way of avoiding this. Lung collapse is produced by surgical retraction, which has the advantage of compressing both alveoli and blood supply together, making ventilation–perfusion mismatch uncommon. This method of collapsing the lung does, however, commonly result in intermittent tracheal obstruction caused by overenthusiastic retraction by the assistant. Hand ventilation using a Jackson Rees modified T-piece allows obstruction to be detected instantly and also allows reinflation of the compressed lung periodically during periods of surgical inactivity.

IMMEDIATE POSTOPERATIVE PERIOD

Although TOF repairs can be managed without elective postoperative ventilation, we have found it difficult to predict which patients will require ventilation and which will not. In order to decrease the risk of collapse requiring emergency ventilation, often during the hours of darkness, we now electively ventilate TOF repairs overnight. A small number, particularly the preterm babies, may require longer periods of ventilation. It is common surgical practice to request ventilation for difficult TOF repairs for periods of between 5 and 10 days postoperatively. If the baby is ventilated care should be taken with both tracheal suction and physiotherapy to avoid the risk of disruption of the repair.

OUTCOME

- Good in TOF with no other abnormalities
- Overall survival is about 90%
- If there are associated anomalies, mortality is much higher
- A small number have tracheal weakening at the site of the fistula and may require aortopexy, tracheopexy or, in severe cases, tracheoplasty before extubation is possible.

BIBLIOGRAPHY

Goh D W, Brereton R J. Success and failure with neonatal tracheo-oesophageal anomalies. British Journal of Surgery 1991; 78: 834–837

Waterston D J et al. Oesophageal atresia: tracheo-oesophageal fistula. A study of survival in 218 infants. Lancet 1962; i: 819–822

CROSS REFERENCES

Infants and children
Patient Conditions 11: 255

27

CARDIAC SURGERY

P. Hutton

27

CARDIOPULMONARY BYPASS: PRINCIPLES, PHYSIOLOGY AND BIOCHEMISTRY

J. P. Benson and P. Hutton

The objective of cardiopulmonary bypass (CPB), is to allow surgery on the heart and great vessels whilst the rest of the body is perfused with oxygenated blood and the products of metabolism are removed. Bypass necessitates anticoagulation with heparin (usually 3 mg kg^{-1}), and haemodilution. Abnormal surface interactions between blood, air and plastics damage cells and denature proteins. Air and particulate microemboli may enter the bypass circuit via suction, so blood filters are essential.

THE CPB CIRCUIT

This is shown diagrammatically in Figure 1. Venous cannulae are inserted into either the right atrium, the venae cavae, or (more rarely) the femoral vein. The large-bore venous return line drains blood, under gravity, from the patient on the table to the bypass machine on the floor. In the oxygenator, the blood is oxygenated and carbon dioxide is removed and the heat exchanger allows heating and cooling of the blood. Roller pumps return the blood to the body via an aortic or (more rarely) a femoral cannula.

There are usually two additional auxiliary roller pumps which feed blood into the circuit. One (sometimes called the 'coronary sucker' or 'cardiotomy sucker'), acts as a sucker to return blood in the operative field to the bypass circuit. The other (sometimes called the 'vent') aspirates gently from the left ventricle or pulmonary artery to prevent ventricular distension. During bypass when the heart is arrested and there is no effective ejection, blood draining from the bronchial and thesebian veins and retrogradely across the aortic valve collects in the left ventricle. Ventricular distension causes mechanical damage, impairs subendocardial perfusion and can result in fatal sub-endocardial infarction.

Poor venous return is occasionally a problem and can result from kinks, air locks, drainage

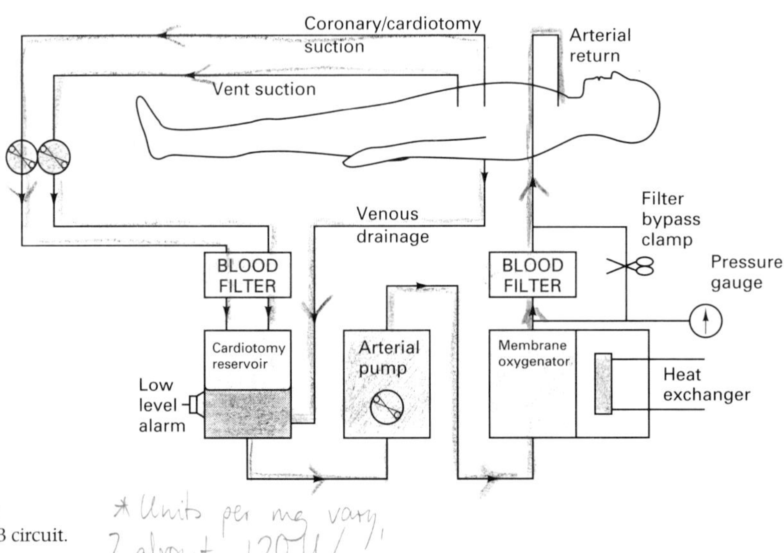

Figure 1
The CPB circuit.

tube malposition, decreased circulating blood volume, sequestration of blood into body cavities or into the tissues or from vasodilator therapy. When the heart is rotated by the surgeons operating on the circumflex arteries, not only can venous return be impaired, but also venous drainage from the brain may be sufficiently obstructed to cause jugular venous hypertension with an acute rise in central venous pressure. This obviously needs immediate correction. Complications of aortic cannulation are embolization (from air and wall debris), haemorrhage, dissection and malposition. The most common form of malposition is for the cannula to abut the aortic wall, and this can be detected by high arterial supply line pressures in the presence of normal flow rates. It is usually amenable to repositioning. Sometimes the cannula can feed directly into one of the carotid arteries. This situation can be avoided by checking for carotid pulses after insertion of the arterial return cannula before the commencement of perfusion.

MANAGEMENT OF ANTICOAGULATION

The activated clotting time (ACT), should be kept three times greater than the baseline, or over 450 s, by the use of heparin. The patient must be anticoagulated adequately before the arterial return cannula is inserted, or a clot will form on its tip and within its lumen. At the end of bypass the action of the heparin is reversed with protamine. Protamine is a potent vasodilator and falls in blood pressure should be anticipated and treated. No blood must be returned to the pump via suction after this. If it is, clot formation can occur in the pump making an emergency return to bypass impossible and preventing the blood being used later for autotransfusion.

TEMPERATURE, FLOW AND PRESSURE ON CPB

There are many controversies surrounding the management of CPB. For instance, some centres routinely use normothermic bypass whenever possible, whilst others invariably use hypothermic bypass. The advantages claimed for normothermic bypass are reduced bypass time (no cooling or warming needed), and reduced postoperative cooling and shivering with its increased metabolic demand and tissue hypoxia. For normothermic bypass, flow rates of greater than 2.2 l min^{-1} m^{-2} are usually used.

Hypothermic bypass reduces metabolism and oxygen consumption falls by a factor of 2.5 (known as the QIO), for every 10°C fall in temperature. Moderate hypothermia (25–28°C) is commonly used for adult coronary and valve work, with an associated reduction in flow rate. For some operations (e.g. on the aortic arch), circulatory arrest is needed. The brain will tolerate approximately 1 h of arrest during deep hypothermia at 15–18°C. Even moderate hypothermia permits a brief (approximately 12 min) period of circulatory arrest, which may be life-saving if there is a catastrophic mechanical failure or circuit disruption.

Management protocols vary considerably in relation to the perfusion pressure to be maintained on bypass. When the aorta is clamped and the heart protected by cardioplegia as far as the heart is concerned myocardial perfusion pressure is irrelevant. If the aorta is not cross-clamped the heart is least likely to suffer ischaemic damage if it is kept empty, beating and well perfused. During intermittent cross-clamping techniques, the fibrillating ventricle consumes more oxygen than the beating but unloaded heart. At normothermia, with autoregulation, cerebral blood flow is maintained at 50 mmHg mean perfusion pressure. Under hypothermia, with reduced metabolic demand, lower perfusion pressures can be tolerated and some workers regard 30 mmHg as satisfactory. Certainly there are a number of retrospective studies which indicate no relationship between hypotension during bypass and postoperative neurological dysfunction. Typical UK practice is to fix the flow rate and then keep the mean perfusion pressure above 50 mmHg and below 80 mmHg. Pharmacological management of BP centres around the use of alpha agonists (metaraminol, phenylephrine, noradrenaline) and smooth-muscle relaxants (sodium nitroprusside, glyceryl trinitrate).

The use of pulsatile flow is controversial and outcome data on its benefits are lacking. Physiological models would suggest that such flow improves perfusion and oxygen uptake; achieving it requires intermittent roller pump action or external reservoir compression, both of which add complexity to the circuit.

BIOCHEMICAL AND HAEMATOLOGICAL CONTROL OF CPB

For adult patients the CPB is primed with

Table 1. (from Hindman et al, 1993)
Alpha stat versus pH stat blood gas management

In vivo temperature (°C)	Measured and reported at 37°C				Corrected to in vivo temperature			
	pH_a		P_aCO_2 (mmHg)		pH_a		P_aCO_2 (mmHg)	
	Alpha stat	pH stat	Alpha stat	pH stat	Alpha stat	pH stat	Alpha stat	pH stat
37	7.40	7.40	40	40	7.40	7.40	40	40
33	7.40	7.34	40	47	7.44	7.40	35	40
30	7.40	7.30	40	54	7.50	7.40	29	40
27	7.40	7.26	40	62	7.55	7.40	26	40
23	7.40	7.21	40	74	7.60	7.40	22	40
20	7.40	7.18	40	84	7.65	7.40	19	40

1.5–2 l of balanced asanguinous salt solution (e.g. Hartman's solution), to which heparin is added. This causes significant haemodilution with a reduction in the total oxygen carrying capacity per millilitre. On the other hand, by reducing viscosity, haemodilution improves blood rheology and prevents microcirculatory sludging during hypothermia. Most anaesthetists consider a haematocrit of 20% to be satisfactory on bypass.

Oxygen flow into the oxygenator should be sufficient to maintain an arterial P_aO_2 of over 100 mmHg. If this produces unacceptable hypocapnia then carbon dioxide will need to be added to the oxygenator gas flow to reduce carbon dioxide washout. Some centres now use in-line electrodes to monitor both arterial and venous blood gas status, the oxygen saturation in the venous line being used to confirm acceptable blood flow rates, with the A–V difference across the pump confirming satisfactory oxygenator function.

There is controversy over the optimum method of blood gas management during hypothermic CPB. The alpha stat method aims to achieve a pH of 7.4 and a P_aCO_2 of 40 mmHg when blood drawn from the hypothermic patient is measured at 37°C: the pH stat method aims to achieve a pH of 7.4 and a P_aCO_2 of 40 mmHg when blood drawn from the hypothermic patient is measured at the in vivo temperature. A comparison between the two methods is shown in Table 1. Alpha stat management is thought to preserve autoregulation and coupling of flow and metabolism in the brain better than pH stat, and therefore is currently gaining favour.

The most important electrolyte to monitor on CPB is potassium, because correct levels optimize contractility and suppress dysrhythmias. High levels can be reduced by haemofiltration, diuresis, and insulin and dextrose and countered by calcium. Low levels can be corrected by giving incremental doses of 10–20 mmol of potassium chloride.

TEMPERATURE MEASUREMENTS ON BYPASS

It is vital to measure the body temperature on bypass. The temperature of the nasopharynx is generally used to approximate to that of the brain. Thorough rewarming is essential. Normal central blood temperatures at the end of bypass after the patient has been rewarmed do not, however, represent the temperature in peripheral, poorly perfused tissues. After the discontinuation of CPB an 'afterdrop' is usually seen, which is caused by the opening up of cold, vasoconstricted tissue beds. This can lead to postbypass shivering with its high metabolic load.

REFERENCES

Hindman B J, Lillehaug S L, Tinker J H. Cardiopulmonary bypass and the anesthesiologist. In: Cardiac Anesthesia 3rd Edn, Ed by Kaplan J A, Saunders, Philadelphia, 1993, pp 919–950

THE SEQUELAE OF CARDIOPULMONARY BYPASS

C. Lorenzini and
P. Hutton

During cardiopulmonary bypass (CPB), normal physiology and biochemistry are significantly altered by changes in blood pressure and flow, temperature and haemodilution. The blood is in contact with abnormal surfaces in the oxygenator, heat exchanger, reservoir, tubing, cannulae and filters. These factors can lead to systemic and cerebral complications. Fortunately, the incidence of serious morbidity from them is sufficiently low for CPB to be regarded as a safe procedure in the majority of patients. There is, however, a much higher incidence of more minor and subtle effects which are usually temporary and which the patient may not notice.

Blood flow, pressure and temperature are abnormal during CPB. At the onset of CPB using a crystalloid prime there is usually a sharp drop in the blood pressure to unacceptably low levels which gradually recovers. This is caused by the lower systemic flow and the sudden fall in blood viscosity as the crystalloid is pumped into the circulation. Subsequently during bypass the systemic vascular resistance usually gradually increases to above normal levels.

Although the endocrine response cannot be separated from that due to anaesthesia and surgery, during CPB there is a generalized increase in serum catecholamine levels in excess of those seen in operations not utilizing CPB. There is no pulmonary metabolism of noradrenaline; renin secretion is increased, and with this follows angiotensin activation and aldosterone secretion. Vasopressin levels increase considerably during CPB and remain elevated for up to 48 h following surgery. These increased levels of catecholamines, angiotensin and vasopressin, together with local tissue vasoconstrictor agents, lead to arteriolar constriction. A mild hyperglycaemia is usually seen following CPB, due to increased gluconeogenesis, peripheral insulin resistance, a decrease in serum insulin and raised ACTH and cortisol levels.

Total body water is increased at the end of CPB, the extra water being contained in the extracellular and extravascular spaces. Haemodilution and the increased capillary permeability resulting from activation of inflammatory mediators are the major factors causing this fluid shift.

DAMAGING EFFECTS OF THE CPB CIRCUIT

The exposure of blood to abnormal surfaces during CPB causes platelet activation and aggregation, the net effect being a reduction in platelet numbers and an impairment in function of those which remain. Platelet damage is probably the most important factor in the bleeding diathesis associated with CPB. Proteins are denatured by contact with foreign surfaces, and this can lead to activation of various clotting and fibrinolytic cascades with consumption of clotting factors, microcoagulation, fibrin generation and complement activation. The complement cascade results in the production of powerful anaphylotoxins which increase capillary leakage, mediate leucocyte chemotaxis and facilitate leucocyte aggregation and enzyme release. There is mechanical damage to leucocytes and erythrocytes from the shear stresses caused by turbulence from the pumps, suckers, abrupt changes in velocity of blood flow and cavitation around the cannula tip. Damage to blood produces fibrin microemboli, aggregates of denatured protein and lipoproteins and platelet and leucocyte aggregates. Particulate emboli in spilt blood are aspirated by suckers and returned to the bypass circuit. There can be significant air emboli during aortic cannulation, during filling of the beating heart after removal of the aortic cross-clamp and during discontinuation of CPB despite meticulous de-airing techniques. In about 1 in 1000 procedures a critical incident will occur from malfunction of the extracorporeal circuit.

SPECIFIC ORGAN DAMAGE ASSOCIATED WITH CPB

Heart

CPB, per se, has only a minor effect on cardiac dysfunction unless there has been inadequate myocardial protection or perfusion. Post-bypass cardiac function is more closely related to the preoperative condition of the heart and the success of surgery.

Lungs

Abnormalities of lung function following CPB are frequent, with clinical manifestations of atelectasis and pulmonary oedema. Acute lung injury leading to adult respiratory distress syndrome (ARDS) occurs in 1–2% of patients. A reduction in FRC with an increased A–a difference may persist for up to 10 days. Sputum retention and ineffective coughing, which contribute to pulmonary morbidity, are consequences of the surgery and post-operative care rather than the CPB.

Kidneys

Renal dysfunction occurs to some degree in 1–4% of patients following CPB. It is usually due to acute tubular necrosis and, although potentially reversible, is associated with a high mortality. Factors associated with an increased risk of renal failure are pre-existing renal impairment, long bypass times and low cardiac output. Drugs such as aminoglycoside antibiotics and NSAIDs may be contributory.

Gastrointestinal tract

Gastrointestinal tract complications develop in less than 2% of patients following CPB, but the associated mortality is high. The commonest problem is upper gastrointestinal bleeding and is maximal on the 10th postoperative day. Hyperbilirubinaemia has been reported in up to 20% of patients. Rare complications are ischaemic bowel and ischaemic pancreatitis.

Neurological

These can be divided into global, focal or neuropsychological complications. Global damage often presents as a prolonged depression of conscious level unrelated to sedation and is seen in up to 3% of patients. In serious cases there are frequently signs of widespread neurological dysfunction present. Patients in coma for over 24 h have a high mortality, and poor prognostic signs include extensor posturing, the absence of motor responses, and seizures. Choreoathetosis is a rare but serious complication occurring almost exclusively in paediatric patients who have had total circulatory arrest. Sensori-neural hearing loss is often missed clinically, but up to 13% of patients have been reported to have a hearing loss of greater than 10 dB following CPB.

Focal events or strokes (defined as a focal CNS deficit of relatively sudden origin that lasts for more than 24 h), are the major cause of persisting neurological disability following cardiac surgery. They are usually seen as an acute hemiparesis or visual field defect and have been reported as occurring in 1–6% of patients after coronary artery bypass grafting. Approximately 70% of cardiac related strokes occur intraoperatively and 30% in the early postoperative period. Acute focal deficits due to air emboli usually resolve steadily over the first 24 h. Membrane oxygenators have been shown to produce fewer microemboli than bubble oxygenators, and there are fewer microvascular occlusions seen in the retinal microcirculation when using a membrane oxygenator as compared with a bubble oxygenator.

Neuropsychological testing provides a sensitive technique to quantify the effects of cerebral damage, but is difficult to undertake and not all workers agree on the clinical relevance of the results. The deficits found are mainly related to concentration, memory, learning and speed of visual motor response. In addition, depressed patients perform worse and complain of difficulties more often. In one study of 298 patients who were subjected to 10 different neuropsychological tests, a significant deterioration occurred in one test for over three-quarters of the subjects, but over half of them were unaware of any problem themselves. It is not clear what relevance, if any, this has on their future life.

The most important risk factors for cerebral damage during CPB are increasing age, a previous cerebrovascular event, pre-existing carotid or cerebrovascular disease, aortic atherosclerosis, valve surgery, left ventricular thrombus, poor preoperative cardiac function, the occurrence of microemboli and long bypass times. Current evidence suggests that the best way to reduce the sequelae of CPB is to perform the surgery meticulously and expeditiously, with minimum suction of shed blood, using a membrane oxygenator and a 40 μm main arterial filter.

CROSS REFERENCES

Cardiopulmonary bypass: principles, physiology and biochemistry
Surgical Procedures 27: 506

CORONARY ARTERY BYPASS GRAFTING

J. M. Freeman and P. Hutton

PHYSIOLOGICAL CONSIDERATIONS

Coronary artery disease (CAD) is the leading cause of death in Western societies and coronary artery bypass graft (CABG) surgery comprises 50–60% of most cardiac surgical programmes. The heart extracts oxygen to a greater extent than any other organ with only minimal increases in oxygen extraction possible; therefore, any increase in oxygen demand must be met by increasing flow. In health this is done by autoregulation and in the absence of CAD maximal flow is four to five times as great as at rest. The coronary arteries arborize on the surface of the heart to form a mass of smaller epicardial arteries from which 'B' branches perforate directly through the myocardium to reach the endocardium (Figure 1). These vessels are subject to torsion and pressure during muscular contraction which in the left ventricle results in the majority of useful myocardial perfusion occurring during diastole. The only collateral circulation exists at subendocardial level and becomes of importance if there is a blockage in an epicardial vessel. Patients with classic CAD are asymptomatic at rest. As the severity of the stenosis increases, coronary flow reserve declines, resting CBF is preserved by progressive vasodilation of the micro-circulation, and the onset of angina of effort occurs with increased demand. Coronary artery bypass grafting aims to bypass epicardial blockages with the internal mammary artery or with vein grafts taken from the leg and so increase myocardial blood flow and oxygen delivery.

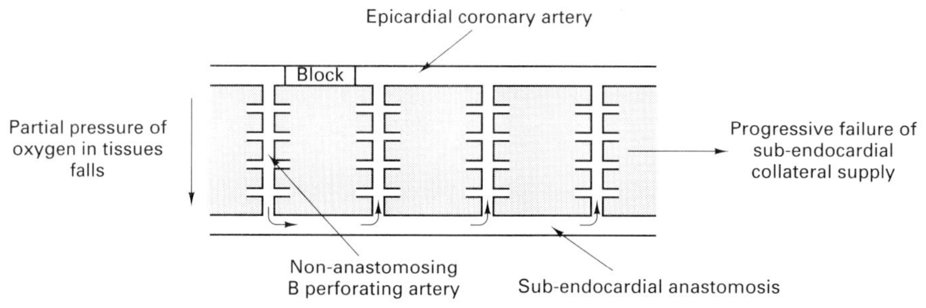

Figure 1
Perfusion of the left ventricular wall.

GENERAL ANAESTHETIC CONSIDERATIONS

Preoperative assessment

This comprises history, examination and investigations. The history should concentrate on the symptoms of ischaemic heart disease, i.e. degree of angina pectoris and, when it occurs, previous infarction, exercise tolerance, shortness of breath and orthopnoea. Look also for a history of diabetes mellitus, renal disease, hypertension, vascular disease and pulmonary disease. These are all added risk factors for CABG patients. A knowledge of perioperative medication is essential with antianginal agents and anticoagulant or platelet-inhibiting drugs being of particular importance. While the patient should continue with the usual antihypertensive and/or antidysrhythmic medication, platelet-inhibiting drugs, such as aspirin, should be stopped 2 weeks prior to surgery to avoid antiplatelet effects at operation.

On examination, physical findings are often few in this group of patients, but look for signs of right and left ventricular failure and check the arterial pulses. If there is a marked difference in right- and left-sided pulses one should monitor from the strongest, as this will be the better reflection of aortic root pressure. If there are carotid bruits or stenoses make a note to avoid jugular lines on that side.

Investigations involve routine preoperative tests which include urea and electrolytes, haemoglobin, chest X-ray, ECG, as well as more invasive procedures, e.g. cardiac catheterization. The latter can give information on left ventricular function and ejection fraction. A low ejection fraction, the presence of ventricular dyssynergy, high left ventricular end diastolic pressure (LVEDP) or pulmonary hypertension suggest a strong possibility of post-CABG myocardial dysfunction. All patients *must* have a baseline 12-lead ECG for postoperative comparison.

Premedication

The purpose of premedication is to pharmacologically reduce apprehension, fear, and the stress of painful events, e.g. insertion of intra-arterial catheter prior to induction. Commonly used drugs include benzodiazepines (e.g. oral diazepam or temazepam) and intramuscular opiates (e.g. morphine or papaveretum). Metoclopramide and ranitidine may be used to reduce the volume and acidity of the gastric contents. Heavy premedication should be supplemented with face-mask oxygen in a safe clinical environment.

Intraoperative management

Remember antibiotic prophylaxis.

Monitoring

Commence by establishing good peripheral venous access, an arterial line and a multilead ECG (leads II and V5). Following induction, additional monitoring will involve insertion of a central venous catheter, using the internal jugular or subclavian routes, temperature probes and urinary catheter. The use of a pulmonary artery catheter (PAC) varies from centre to centre, but one would be indicated in patients with abnormal left ventricular function, recent myocardial infarction or postinfarction sequelae, e.g. ventricular septal defect, left ventricular aneurysm, mitral regurgitation. In some patients who may or may not need a PAC it is sensible to insert a PAC sheath to facilitate easy insertion of a PAC postoperatively if required.

Anaesthesia

The fundamental principle of any anaesthetic technique is to minimize myocardial ischaemia and prevent awareness. It is probably the experience of use of the available drugs which is of greater importance than the particular agent itself. Prior to induction of anaesthesia the patient should be preoxygenated. Induction of anaesthesia needs to be smooth with cardiovascular stability, but simultaneously adequate to prevent the sympathetic response to laryngoscopy and intubation. Agents which have been used successfully for induction with or without opioid supplementation include: thiopentone, ketamine, etomidate and propofol. Some centres use high-dose opioid techniques (fentanyl 50 mcg kg^{-1}) for the whole procedure, with very modest benzodiazepine supplementation.

Probably the most commonly used induction technique in UK practice is a slow bolus of opioid (fentanyl 10–15 mcg kg^{-1}) followed by a small dose of induction agent. Maintenance is usually provided by an opioid infusion (e.g. alfentanil 50 mcg kg^{-1} h^{-1}), combined with a low dose of either a volatile or an intravenous agent. Propofol by infusion can be used for maintenance at a rate of 5–6 mg kg^{-1} h^{-1} to achieve adequate serum levels during cardiopulmonary bypass (CPB). Of the volatile agents, isoflurane has received much attention because its known vasodilator properties have been implicated in causing myocardial ischaemia through the coronary steal mechanism. However, this has been shown not to be of relevance at concentrations less than 1.5%. Both enflurane and halothane have been and are still used for maintenance in CABG anaesthesia. Many anaesthetists run a 'renal' dose of dopamine at 2–3 μg kg^{-1} min^{-1} and if there is poor urine flow in the presence of an adequate circulating fluid volume and blood pressure commence a frusemide infusion. All the currently available muscle relaxants have been used to produce adequate intubating and maintenance conditions during anaesthesia for CABG. The cardiovascular side-effects of pancuronium are sometimes used therapeutically to counter the bradycardias caused by the fentanyl group of drugs.

During dissection of the internal mammary artery one should observe the blood pressure during insertion of the Chevalier retractor. There can be a genuine fall due to right ventricular compression or (if the arterial cannula is in the ipsilateral arm) an artefactual fall due to stretching of the subclavian artery.

The management and sequelae of bypass are described in other sections. Adjust serum potassium to between 4.5 and 5.5 mmol l^{-1} prior to cessation of bypass.

In addition to the goals of providing anaesthesia and muscle relaxation, in the pre- and post-bypass periods myocardial ischaemia must be minimized by the anaesthetist, and this requires constant observation of the ECG. If ischaemic changes do occur (which can be manifested by dysrhythmias and low cardiac output as well as by ST segment changes), always make sure immediately that the patient is ventilating well with a satisfactory $F_{I}O_2$ and SpO_2. The mainstays of good cardiovascular management are meticulous attention to fluid balance (using information from direct visual inspection of the heart, central venous pressure (CVP), PAC (if present), left atrial catheter (if present) and surgical palpation of the pulmonary artery), and tight control of the cardiac output and blood pressure. The latter can best be achieved by the appropriate combination of vasodilators (e.g. sodium nitroprusside, glyceryl trinitrate), inotropes (e.g. dobutamine, adrenaline), and a volatile anaesthetic agent. In the absence of severe hypotension or tachycardia causing poor coronary perfusion, glyceryl trinitrate infusion can be used to treat ischaemic changes. Rapid elevations in diastolic coronary perfusion pressure are easy to achieve with short-acting alpha agonists (e.g. metaraminol), but these do of course also increase systolic work and may constrict vital microvasculature. The key to postbypass care is to optimize the intravascular volume by transfusion from the pump and then, if the cardiac output and blood pressure are still poor, to introduce an inotropic agent.

Following the cessation of CPB and the heart taking over the circulation the true cardiac performance is usually not seen for several minutes because it often has energy stores within the myocardium which accumulated whilst it was perfused and beating but with no load on full bypass. A heart which had good initial ventricular performance and was satisfactorily grafted can be expected to continue to beat well. The heart can, however, be disadvantaged by poor myocardial protection during CPB and/or by reperfusion injury. This can result in the 'stunned myocardium' which functions badly and needs a period of hours to days to recover fully. Perioperative infarcts may also occur. In both these situations inotropes are usually necessary. If drug therapy shows no alleviation of the ischaemic picture (from continued ST segment change, reduced cardiac output, elevation of pulmonary artery wedge pressure (PAWP), increasing acidosis), it is usually an indication for a balloon pump. This is the only treatment modality that simultaneously increases myocardial oxygen supply whilst decreasing demand. In the immediate postbypass period calcium antagonists and beta blockers are relatively contraindicated and must be used with extreme caution since their negative inotropic effects are both magnified and unpredictable.

Postoperative care

Postoperative management of the adult patient on the ITU is dealt with in the relevant section. In brief, the principles of management prior to extubation are to maintain stable haemodynamics (MAP 65–85 mmHg; CVP 8–12 mmHg; heart rate 80–110 beats min^{-1}; Hb 9–10 g dl^{-1}), good blood gases and adequate urine output, together with good analgesia.

CROSS REFERENCES

Coronary artery disease
Patient Conditions 4: 107
Cardiopulmonary bypass: principles, physiology and biochemistry
Surgical Procedures 27: 506
Premedication
Anaesthetic Factors 29: 549

POSTOPERATIVE CARE OF ADULT PATIENTS AFTER CARDIOPULMONARY BYPASS

V. Patla and T. H. Clutton-Brock

The increase in demand for cardiac surgery, caused mainly by coronary artery disease has led to a marked rise in the number of patients presenting to postoperative ITUs. The trend has been towards the development of specialized postcardiac surgery units with protocol-based care becoming the norm. The protocols used and the duration of post-operative ventilation, etc., vary considerably from one unit to another, and frequently derive more from tradition than proven clinical outcome. Nevertheless, the basic principles of postoperative care are common to all patients and are summarized below. For convenience the postoperative period has been divided into transfer, early and late phases.

TRANSFER PERIOD

Following the completion of surgery, patients are usually transferred to their intensive care bed and theatre and transported on it to the ITU. The distances involved vary enormously from one hospital to another. This is a period of great potential instability and, unless the transfer distance is very short indeed, at the very least ECG and intra-arterial pressure monitoring should be continued. The development of modern transport monitors has made this a much easier task.

THE EARLY POSTOPERATIVE PERIOD (0–6 h)

The essentials of the early postoperative care of these patients are summarized in Table 1.

Table 1.
Care in the early postoperative period

Analgesia and sedation
Assisted ventilation ± PEEP
Measurement of arterial blood gases, potassium, haemoglobin, etc.
Adjustment of inspired oxygen concentration
Maintenance of cardiac rhythm; treatment of arrhythmias
Control of postoperative hypertension
Haemodynamic monitoring
Manipulation of cardiac filling pressures
Maintenance of adequate cardiac output
Maintenance of adequate renal perfusion and urine output
Fluid management; colloid replacement, crystalloids
Monitoring and treatment of clotting/platelet abnormalities
Reduction of heat loss; assisted rewarming

Analgesia and sedation

Adequate opioid analgesia is essential, but there is wide variability in the drugs and routes of administration used; fentanyl, alfentanil and morphine are all popular. The use of high doses of fentanyl (40–60 μg kg^{-1}) intraoperatively provides analgesia well into the postoperative period; alfentanil is a potent short-acting agent and is given by continuous infusion. Morphine is widely available, cheap and has useful additional sedative properties, but care should be taken in patients with poor renal function due to the accumulation of active metabolites. The NSAIDs are now widely used after general surgery, but they all inhibit the renal protective actions of prostaglandins during hypotension and should be used with great caution in the early postoperative period. In some patients, despite adequate analgesia, additional sedation may be required; midazolam, propofol and isoflurane (0.4–0.6%) are popular and combine a short duration of action with acceptable haemodynamic stability. Shivering is an important complication in the early postoperative period as it markedly increases oxygen consumption and must be suppressed by adequate analgesia and sedation.

Assisted ventilation

The duration of mechanical ventilation after cardiac surgery is very variable even in routine patients, varying from none (extubation on the operating table) to several hours. Improvements in surgical and anaesthetic techniques with a reduction in cardiopulmonary bypass times, less hypothermia, etc., have led to a trend towards earlier extubation in many centres. Safety is an important consideration and it seems prudent to continue mechanical ventilation until adequate rewarming (at the least to central normothermia), adequate analgesia, haemostasis and haemodynamic stability have been achieved.

A degree of atelectasis is common after cardiac surgery, especially if the pleura has been breached during internal mammary dissection. Low levels of PEEP (2.5–5 cmH_2O) are widely used after cardiac surgery; they improve oxygenation in the presence of pulmonary oedema and may play a role in reversing atelectasis. The adverse haemodynamic effects of PEEP are exacerbated by hypovolaemia.

Most modern intensive care ventilators incorporate the facilities for weaning in the form of synchronized intermittent mandatory ventilation (SIMV) with inspiratory assist. Mandatory breaths are gradually reduced to zero and, if adequate ventilation is maintained, then the patient is extubated. Many factors may precipitate more prolonged periods of mechanical ventilation. These include: previous lung pathology, haemodynamic instability, persistent pulmonary oedema, delayed neurological recovery, and pulmonary infection.

Monitoring

Table 2 lists the basic monitoring required in the postoperative period.

Table 2.
Basic monitoring after cardiopulmonary bypass

ECG (rate, rhythm, ST changes)
Intra-arterial blood pressure
Central venous pressure
$F_{I}O_2$, respiratory rate, airway pressures, tidal and minute volumes
Arterial blood gases
Pulse oximetry
Serum potassium
Blood loss
Haemoglobin, clotting screen, platelet count
Blood sugar
Core and peripheral temperatures
Chest X-ray
Urine output

Haemodynamic manipulation

Skilled haemodynamic monitoring and manipulation are essential after cardiopulmonary bypass. In UK practice most routine patients do not have pulmonary artery catheters inserted and the adequacy of cardiac output has to be estimated from a combination of arterial blood pressure, urine output, peripheral rewarming and the absence of a metabolic acidosis. Early hypotension is most commonly due to hypovolaemia exacerbated by the vasodilatation that occurs during the rewarming phase. Central venous pressures should be maintained by the infusion of colloids, including blood, if indicated. The pressure required is variable, but in the absence of significant ventricular dysfunction, pulmonary hypertension, etc., a level of 5–8 mmHg is a reasonable starting point. Hypertension after cardiopulmonary bypass is also common and should be treated to avoid excessive left ventricular workloads, suture-line disruption and bleeding. *Having ensured adequate analgesia* and sedation, nitrodilators (glyceryl trinitrate, sodium nitroprusside) form the mainstay of treatment.

Arrhythmias are common after cardiac surgery and require aggressive treatment because of their effects on cardiac output and blood pressure. When they occur, *always* quickly ensure that the patient has not become acutely hypoxic from a simple cause such as ventilator disconnection. Hypokalaemia is a common contributing factor and serum potassium should be maintained at 4.5–5.0 mmol l^{-1}. Following cardiopulmonary bypass, ventricular function is often impaired and many patients have relatively fixed stroke volumes. Persistent bradycardias should be avoided by making use of isoprenaline infusions, pacing, etc., to maintain the heart rate; rates of 90–100 beats min^{-1} are usually considered optimal.

The absolute indications for the instigation of more complex haemodynamic monitoring in the form of pulmonary artery wedge pressure measurements and thermodilution cardiac output measurements are difficult to define. Failure to rewarm, oliguria, worsening metabolic acidosis and persistent hypotension despite apparently adequate filling pressures are all good indications. Pericardial tamponade should be high on the list of suspected causes if these conditions develop in the postoperative period.

Inotropic agents such as adrenaline and dobutamine are indicated if the cardiac index is low despite adequate filling. A low systemic vascular resistance occurring after prolonged bypass may require the use of noradrenaline.

Renal function

Although acute renal failure requiring dialysis is rare after uncomplicated cardiac surgery, degrees of oliguria are common. Although there is little scientific evidence, dopamine at 'renal' doses (e.g. 3 μg kg^{-1} h^{-1}) is widely used both intra- and post-operatively. It is important to maintain a diuresis in the postoperative period so as to reverse the anaemia from haemodilution caused by the bypass prime and the cardioplegia. If oliguria persists despite an adequate cardiac output and blood pressure, small doses of a loop diuretic are indicated.

Fluid management

Cardiac filling pressures should be maintained by the infusion of colloid solutions, including the modified gelatins, albumin solutions and blood. Free water is required for the formation of urine, and in the absence of pulmonary oedema our routine practice is to give all patients 1 ml kg^{-1} h^{-1} of 5% dextrose in water. Although circulating hypovolaemia is common, tissue dehydration is rare in the immediate postoperative period, the usual problem being an increase in total body water.

THE LATE POSTOPERATIVE PERIOD (after 6 h)

In a routine case, following extubation, the activities described above are continued, but the emphasis shifts towards preparing the patient for return to the HDU or ward. Most patients require oxygen to be administered by face-mask to maintain arterial saturations above 95%. Oral or rectally administered analgesics may be prescribed and the patient undergoes regular chest physiotherapy. Where postoperative complications develop, or if the patient's progress is slow, the intensive care administered during the first few hours is continued. In these circumstances every effort must be made to look for correctable causes of the failure to progress. Observing the deterioration closely but without intervention achieves nothing.

CROSS REFERENCES

Cardiopulmonary bypass
Surgical Procedures 27: 506
Postoperative oliguria
Anaesthetic Factors 33: 652
Postoperative pain management
Anaesthetic Factors 33: 655

AORTIC VALVE SURGERY

D. W. Riddington and P. Hutton

AORTIC STENOSIS

Physiological considerations

Aortic stenosis can be either congenital (in which case the valve is abnormal and bicuspid in over 50% of cases), or acquired (usually from rheumatic involvement of a previously normal valve). In the absence of other valvular disease, AS is almost always congenital in origin: if it is of rheumatic aetiology there is usually involvement of the mitral valve as well. The normal aortic valve area (AVA), is 2.5–3.5 cm^2. 'Severe' aortic stenosis has an AVA of <0.7 cm^2, and 'moderate' aortic stenosis has an AVA of 0.7–1.2 cm^2.

As aortic stenosis develops there is a progressive increase in outflow obstruction to the left ventricle. Systolic pressures within the left ventricle rise and a pressure gradient develops between the left ventricle and the aorta. Increased systolic chamber pressure stimulates parallel replication of sarcomeres with consequent wall thickening and concentric ventricular hypertrophy. The consequences of this are two-fold. Firstly, the ventricle relaxes poorly during diastole, so left ventricular end diastolic pressure (LVEDP) rises and higher filling pressures are needed to maintain cardiac output. The ventricle becomes increasingly dependent on atrial contraction to ensure diastolic filling and the atrium (in sinus rhythm), contributes up to 40% of LVEDV in AS compared to 10–15% in normals. The sudden onset of atrial fibrillation (which suggests a rheumatic aetiology), can precipitate a major fall in cardiac output. Secondly, the balance between myocardial oxygen supply and demand becomes precarious. This is because increased myocardial bulk and high cavity pressures increase myocardial oxygen demand, whilst increased wall thickness and raised LVEDP predispose to subendocardial ischaemia. The relationship between diastolic time (determined by HR), LVEDP, and the systemic diastolic pressure available for coronary perfusion (determined by cardiac output and systemic vascular resistance) is therefore critical. Coincident coronary artery disease is a serious added risk factor for these patients.

With aortic stenosis there is usually a long (can be up to 50 years or more) asymptomatic period, and sudden death may be the first presenting feature. The most common symptoms are angina, syncope, dyspnoea and dysrhythmias. When symptoms finally occur the stenosis is severe, their significance is ominous and if the stenosis is not surgically corrected death occurs within a few years.

The ECG will show LVH if aortic stenosis is significant, often with ST segment changes of left ventricular strain. Unless there is LVF the chest X-ray will show a normal transverse diameter of the heart. If LVF has supervened there will be cardiomegaly and lung field changes. Specialist investigation is by coronary angiography and ultrasound.

GENERAL ANAESTHETIC PRINCIPLES

Anaesthetic technique is similar to that described for coronary artery bypass grafting (CABG). The physiological objective is to maintain the basic haemodynamic state by carefully managing heart rate, filling pressure and systemic blood pressure. Give antibiotic prophylaxis.

Hypotension

Very dangerous. Caused by low cardiac output, hypovolaemia or vasodilatation. It implies that a ventricle generating high intracavity pressures is being perfused by a low pressure arterial system. Needs immediate correction with an alpha agonist, whilst the underlying cause is remedied.

Tachycardia

Dangerous. Produces myocardial ischaemia (sometimes acute LVF), and reduces cardiac output by increasing dynamic impedance of stenosis. Treat cause (light anaesthesia, hypovolaemia, etc.). *Do not* give beta blockers. Persistent dysrhythmias affecting cardiac output may need d.c. countershock.

Bradycardia

Moderate degrees tolerated. Reduces dynamic impedance of stenosis. If severe with very low diastolic pressures, use tiny doses of glycopyrrolate and avoid overcorrection at all costs.

Preload on left ventricle

Must be maintained to ensure filling of hypertrophied ventricle.

Afterload on left ventricle

Changes have little effect on valve pressure gradient and hence LV load, but the effect on systemic blood pressure in the aortic root significantly changes coronary perfusion.

MONITORING

Invasive arterial monitoring is mandatory prior to induction. ECG monitoring must be able to detect left ventricular ischaemia and diagnose dysrhythmias; use V_5 and standard lead 2 leads. In practice, it may be difficult to interpret 'ischaemic' changes due to pre-existing ST abnormalities caused by LVH (strain pattern).

The central venous pressure (CVP) is a poor indicator of left ventricular filling when left ventricular compliance is reduced. A flotation catheter, however, may cause severe and persistent dysrhythmias as it passes through the right ventricle. Their use is controversial and there is little published work on which to base an informed decision.

Persistent ischaemia in the face of appropriate corrective measures necessitates early institution of cardiopulmonary bypass. In the event of cardiac arrest, defibrillate immediately. Only internal massage is effective because of valve stenosis, and emergency bypass may be required. Do not commence anaesthesia unless a theatre and bypass facilities are immediately available.

Intraoperative care, management of bypass and postoperative care are as described elsewhere for CABG and ITU.

AORTIC REGURGITATION

Physiological considerations

Aortic regurgitation may be acute or chronic. Chronic causes are rheumatic valve disease, connective-tissue disorders or a congenital bicuspid valve. Acute aortic regurgitation is most commonly caused by infective endocarditis or trauma. The basic problem is volume overload of the left ventricle caused by blood leaking through the incompetent aortic valve during diastole. The degree of regurgitation is determined by the size of the regurgitant orifice and the diastolic time interval. Systemic vasodilatation, increased inotropy and tachycardia all contribute to increased forward flow in patients with aortic regurgitation and may explain the phenomenon of mild exercise tolerance with symptoms at rest. Over a period of time, eccentric left ventricular hypertrophy, gross cardiomegaly and impaired oxygen supply result.

Mild to moderate degrees of chronic regurgitation are well tolerated and there is a long asymptomatic period. Symptoms, when they arise, are usually those of LVF or angina. The life expectancy of patients with significant aortic regurgitation is about 9 years. Sudden death is rare. In acute aortic regurgitation there is a sudden volume overload of the left ventricle with a dramatic rise in the LVEDP. Ventricular dilatation enlarges the mitral valve annulus resulting in functional mitral regurgitation. Pulmonary oedema is marked and refractory. Very severe aortic regurgitation with gross distortion of the valve ring can result in dissection, which may involve the coronary arteries.

GENERAL ANAESTHETIC PRINCIPLES

Anaesthetic technique is as for CABG. Only severe aortic regurgitation is a major anaesthetic risk. If there is an associated dissection, refer to the appropriate section. Remember antibiotic prophylaxis.

Bradycardia

Allows time for back flow into the ventricle and increases regurgitant fraction. Treat carefully with glycopyrrolate or very small dose of adrenaline or isoprenaline.

Tachycardia

If mild, it is well tolerated, because it increases dynamic impedance of reverse flow through valve.

Preload

This needs to be maintained to keep the dilated ventricle full.

Afterload

This needs to be kept low to enhance forward flow. A balance has to be found between good cardiac output and an aortic perfusion pressure adequate to perfuse the coronary arteries of the dilated ventricle.

Monitoring

As for aortic stenosis. In severe cases, use of a pulmonary artery flotation catheter allows one to maximize cardiac output by afterload reduction, whilst maintaining preload by titrating fluid replacement to pulmonary artery capillary wedge pressure (PCWP).

Principles of intra- and post-operative management are as for CABG and ITU care.

CROSS REFERENCES

Aortic valve disease
Patient Conditions 4: 95
Elective surgery
Anaesthetic Factors 29: 545
Premedication
Anaesthetic Factors 29: 549

MITRAL VALVE SURGERY

M. P. Wilkes and
T. H. Clutton-Brock

27

MITRAL STENOSIS

Physiological considerations

Mitral stenosis continues to present regularly to specialist units, despite the success of antibiotic therapy against acute rheumatic fever. The history of the condition is a gradual deterioration over many years. By the time surgical intervention is required these patients are classically dyspnoeic and exhibit a relatively fixed, low cardiac output, often in association with atrial fibrillation. The area of the normal adult mitral orifice is 4–6 cm^2 and the severity of mitral stenosis is graded by reduction in this area into mild (1.5–2.5 cm^2), moderate (1.1–1.5 cm^2) and severe (0.6–1.0 cm^2). The narrowed mitral valve restricts flow between the left atrium and ventricle and the degree of stenosis thus limits both early diastolic ventricular filling and the contribution of atrial contraction to late diastolic ventricular filling. Increased left atrial work inevitably causes dilatation of the thin-walled left atrium. In the normal heart the two phases of diastole are clearly distinguishable using echocardiography, but in mitral stenosis the echocardiographic pattern shows a plateau and loss of late diastolic filling because the dilated left atrium generates less force than normal. In the presence of atrial fibrillation the uncoordinated movements of the left atrium no longer contribute to this second diastolic phase, reducing end diastolic ventricular volume by up to 30%. Duration of diastole is therefore of great importance in mitral stenosis, and excessive tachycardia compromises cardiac output, especially in the presence of atrial fibrillation. Many of these patients will be on long-standing digitalis therapy and this should be continued into the perioperative period, along with appropriate potassium supplementation. The primary purpose of this therapy is to control ventricular rate, rather than to enhance myocardial contractility. Mean left atrial pressure (LAP) is usually greater than 15 mmHg, and factors causing increased filling of the left atrium are liable to precipitate pulmonary oedema. The natural history of the condition is progression to pulmonary hypertension and, eventually, to cor pulmonale as a response to left- and then right-sided heart failure.

General anaesthetic principles

The main areas of anaesthetic consideration for this group are heart rate, rhythm and preload. Anaesthetic technique is similar to that described for coronary artery bypass grafting (CABG) and must include antibiotic prophylaxis.

- Bradycardia:
  - Causes a decrease in cardiac output due to a fixed stroke volume.
- Tachycardia:
  - Decreases ventricular filling time and thus cardiac output
  - Increases LAP and may result in pulmonary oedema.
- Atrial fibrillation:
  - Will further decrease ventricular filling by up to 30%
  - Is often long standing and, if so, will be highly resistant to cardioversion
  - May be induced by anaesthesia
  - Digitalis toxicity may be induced by intraoperative hypokalaemia.
- Preload:
  - Hypovolaemia may result in reduced LAP, and thus a further reduction in left ventricular filling
  - Excessive fluid load may result in pulmonary oedema.
- Afterload:
  - A large decrease in systemic vascular resistance (SVR) may cause severe hypotension due to a relatively fixed cardiac output.

Monitoring considerations

The pressure gradient across the mitral valve means that pulmonary artery wedge pressure (PAWP) overestimates the left ventricular end-diastolic pressure (LVEDP). However, in the absence of significant changes in heart rate, PAWP trend measurements reliably track left-sided filling pressure. A reflex tachycardia following excessive blood loss will make this technique inaccurate, and in some cases it may be more appropriate to place a left atrial pressure catheter at operation for postoperative monitoring.

Summary

Cardiac anaesthesia for mitral stenosis is guided by the principles of any good anaesthetic, but requires greater care in preventing extremes of heart rate and changes in circulating volume. It is often complicated by the presence of, or a tendency to develop, atrial fibrillation. This may precipitate sudden, rapid drops in cardiac output. This dysrhythmia is often extremely resistant to both external and internal cardioversion, and inotropic support may be required to support systemic blood pressure. Inotropes may in turn cause tachycardia, thus worsening the situation, and should be administered with caution. These patients also have a relatively fixed cardiac output and severe reductions in SVR may be associated with a severe reduction in systemic blood pressure. Potent vasodilators including the nitrovasodilators should be used with extreme caution in this group.

MITRAL INCOMPETENCE

Physiological considerations

Mitral incompetence results in dilatation of both the left atrium and the left ventricle. During systole the regurgitant flow causes high pressure to be transmitted to the left atrium and increases left ventricular work. In contrast to mitral stenosis, there is no obstruction to forward flow through the valve, with the exception of a combined stenotic and regurgitative lesion. Any increase in systemic vascular resistance will limit left ventricular forward ejection and thus encourage retrograde flow into the more compliant atrium. An increased afterload causes decreased forward flow and increased regurgitant flow, and in this respect these patients are sensitive to peripheral vasoconstrictors. The magnitude of regurgitant flow is determined by the size of the regurgitant orifice and the pressure gradient across it; the orifice size tends to parallel ventricular size. Increased preload causes left atrial dilatation and further stretching of the mitral valve orifice which may result in a decrease in ventricular forward flow due to an increased regurgitant flow into the atrium. In common with mitral stenosis these patients may progress to pulmonary hypertension and cor pulmonale. It is important to realize that acute mitral incompetence may be due to posterior left ventricular papillary muscle damage induced by myocardial infarction. In this case the left atrium may be small, making replacement of the valve technically difficult. This group are especially sensitive to increases in SVR. Patients with mitral regurgitation caused by coronary artery disease, including those with recent myocardial infarction, require extremely careful anaesthesia.

General anaesthetic principles

Anaesthetic technique is similar to that described for CABG and must include antibiotic prophylaxis. The anaesthetic aims for these patients are centred around the maintenance of forward flow through the left ventricle:

- Systemic vascular resistance:
  - An increased SVR increases the tendency for regurgitative flow, and vasoconstrictors should be avoided.
- Preload:
  - A large increase in preload causes atrial distension and the relatively rapid onset of pulmonary oedema.
- Heart rate:
  - Bradycardia reduces ventricular filling and increases the degree of regurgitation; however, a moderate tachycardia increases forward flow, and is thus preferable.

Monitoring considerations

It has been suggested that faster, fuller and vasodilated are the principles on which forward flow in mitral regurgitation may be maintained. In these circumstances (especially when using potent vasodilators and with the dangers of vascular overfilling) a pulmonary artery catheter allows assessment of intravascular filling, measurement of cardiac output and evaluation of therapeutic intervention. In patients with high pulmonary artery pressures, evidence of tricuspid regurgitation should be looked for in the central venous pressure trace. Passive tricuspid regurgitation results from right ventricle dilatation in the face of increased afterload from pulmonary hypertension (PHT). There are few attractive therapies for this combination of PHT and right ventricular failure, and attention should be paid to basic principles, including the avoidance of hypoxia, hypercarbia and acidosis. One promising therapeutic strategy for the treatment of PHT is the use of prostaglandin E_1 (prostacyclin), a potent dilatator of pulmonary arterial smooth muscle. It has been noted that prostacyclin is also a systemic vasodilator. However, it has the theoretical advantage of having pulmonary endothelial first-pass metabolism, and may be considered as a 'pulmonary-specific' vasodilator when given via the right atrium.

Summary

Anaesthesia for replacement of an incompetent mitral valve is dominated by the need for a relatively low SVR allowing the left ventricle to eject the majority of its output into the systemic circulation and reducing regurgitant flow into the left atrium. A high end-systolic LAP increases the incidence of pulmonary oedema and inhibits diastolic left atrial filling.

BIBLIOGRAPHY

Braunwald E. Valvular heart disease. In: Braunwald E (ed) Heart disease. W B Saunders, Piladelphia, 1992

Chaffin J S, Dagget W M. Mitral valve replacement: a nine year follow up of risks and survivals. Annals of Thoracic Surgery 1979; 27: 3–12

CROSS REFERENCES

Mitral valve disease
Patient Conditions 4: 114
Cardiopulmonary bypass: principles, physiology and biochemistry
Surgical Procedures 27: 506
Premedication
Anaesthetic Factors 29: 549

THORACIC AORTA SURGERY

T. McLeod and P. Hutton

PHYSIOLOGICAL AND PATHOLOGICAL CONSIDERATIONS

Aortic dissection

Aortic dissections are characterized by an intimal tear followed by a longitudinal separation within the media of the wall which extends parallel with the lumen. It usually presents acutely with severe anterior or posterior chest pain. Depending upon position and progression, dissections can cause aortic valve incompetence, interruption of the coronary, cerebral, spinal, subclavian, mesenteric, renal or femoral arteries. Clinical presentation may be related to these secondary effects. Young patients can have an associated connective tissue disorder such as Marfan's syndrome. The major classification is into types A (involving the ascending aorta), and B (distal to the origin of the left subclavian), as shown in Figure 1. The characteristics of type A and B dissections are shown in Table 1.

Aneurysmal dilatations

These are usually asymptomatic until they leak or produce symptoms due to compression on surrounding structures such as the superior vena cava, left main bronchus or lung. Intimal deterioration can occlude smaller arteries; paraplegia, for example, may be the presenting symptom. There is often a history of hypertension and diabetes together with aneurysmal dilatation of the abdominal vessels.

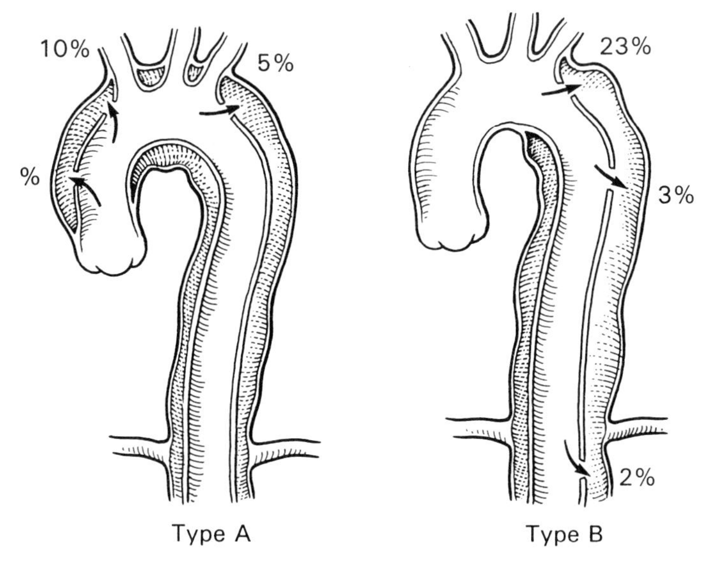

Figure 1
Type A and type B aortic dissections. (Reproduced from Elgin et al, 1985)

Table 1.
Characteristics of type A and type B aortic dissections*

	Type A	Type B
Frequency (%)	65–70	30–35
Male/female ratio	2:1	3:1
Average age	50–55	60–70
Associated hypertension (%)	50	80
Hypertension on admission	±	++
Associated atherosclerosis	±	++
Aortic regurgitation (%)	50	10
Intimal tear	Always present	Absent in 5–10%
Acute mortality (%)	90–95	40

*Reproduced with permission from Ergin et al 1985.

Although clinical presentation and plain chest X-rays may suggest a diagnosis, accurate diagnosis depends upon special investigations such as aortography, CT scan, MRI scan and echocardiography.

ANAESTHETIC CONSIDERATIONS

Preoperative

Perform a full neurological assessment and record any deficits. Reduce hypertension with the use of vasodilators (e.g. sodium nitroprusside). Catheterize and check renal function.

Insert two large-bore cannulae and an arterial line in the arm least affected by the lesion. Order at least 10 units of blood. Accompany patient to scan room, etc., and be prepared to resuscitate. Continued or suddenly increasing pain may indicate further dissection and the need for immediate surgery.

Perioperative

Antibiotic prophylaxis is essential. Provide renal protection with dopamine, mannitol and frusemide. The anaesthetic technique is as for coronary artery bypass grafting. Insert a femoral arterial line for pressure monitoring on bypass and to ensure major vessel continuity after clamp removal.

- *Type A with involvement of ascending aorta only.*
  Full cardiopulmonary bypass (CPB) is necessary with cardioplegia for myocardial protection. Replacement of the aortic valve and reimplantation of the coronary arteries may be required in addition to grafting of the ascending aorta.
- *Type A with involvement of aortic arch.*
  As above, but in addition the operation on the cerebral vessels requires total circulatory arrest at <18°C.

- *Type B with involvement of the descending aorta.*
  Does not require CPB and is approached via a left thoracotomy. A double-lumen tube is preferred, to allow deflation of the left lung.

All of these operations necessitate cross-clamping of the aorta. When the clamp goes on there may be proximal hypertension, requiring the use of vasodilators. Unclamping produces a sudden fall in left ventricular afterload and systemic BP. Fluid loading and/ or vasoconstrictor agents will be required.

Postoperative
Ensure stable haemodynamics. Monitor and preserve renal function wherever possible. The incidence of renal failure is 5% and is related to preoperative renal function and the cross clamp ischaemic time. Central and peripheral neurological function need careful observation, although there is little that can be done to affect the course of intraoperative damage from ischaemia or embolization. The incidence of paraplegia is 5–10%. Postoperative hypotension should be avoided since it may contribute to the incidence of late-onset paraplegia.

BIBLIOGRAPHY

Ergin M A, Galla J D, Lansman S et al. Acute dissections of the aorta; current surgical treatment. Surgical Clinics of North America 1985; 63: 721

CROSS REFERENCES

Diabetes mellitus
Patient Conditions 2: 42
Hypertension
Patient Conditions 4: 111
One-lung anaesthesia
Anaesthetic Factors 32: 602
Blood transfusion
Anaesthetic Factors 33: 616

SPINAL OPIOIDS AND CARDIAC SURGERY

N. M. Turner and A. P. Jackson

The clinical use of spinal opioids originated in the late 1970s when, following the description of opioid receptors in the spinal cord, various opioid drugs were administered both intrathecally and epidurally. The application of these techniques to cardiac surgery followed soon afterwards and, although the majority of the clinical experience to date in cardiac anaesthesia has been with intrathecal morphine, epidural opioids have also been used.

The advantages claimed for intrathecal morphine in cardiac surgery are:

- Excellent analgesia, which can persist well into the postoperative period following ITU discharge
- Reduced vasodilator use in the ITU
- less respiratory depression when compared to intravenous opioid use
- Reduced hormonal stress response to surgery
- Reduction in the need for infusion pumps and related equipment, with the consequent advantages of simplicity and cheapness.

It should be noted that, although intrathecal morphine results in a reduction in the patient's demand for analgesia, there have been few controlled studies comparing this technique with other methods of analgesia and no studies have conclusively proven that intrathecal morphine provides better analgesia. Furthermore, although intrathecal morphine is associated with a modest improvement in respiratory parameters such as peak expiratory flow rate and postoperative arterial carbon dioxide tension, it has not been shown to reduce time to extubation or ITU stay.

Unfortunately, The technique is, however, associated with some of disadvantages, ranging from the undesirable to the life-threatening. Spinal puncture is a procedure which requires a significant amount of skill and is associated with a small failure rate, particularly in the elderly, as well as the rare complications of infection and neurological sequelae. Postspinal headache does not appear to be a problem in the cardiac surgical patient, urinary retention is not an issue owing to the necessity for catheterization, and backache attributable to dural puncture has not been reported. In common with IV opioids, up to 20% of patients will suffer from nausea and/or vomiting, and a much smaller number experience pruritus which is often confined to the facial dermatomes and which may be severe.

The two most important problems associated with the use of spinal opioids in cardiac surgery are respiratory depression and the potential for spinal haematoma formation. Respiratory depression is characteristically delayed following the use of hydrophillic drugs such as morphine. It is believed to be due to slow rostral spread of the drug by bulk flow in the cerebrospinal fluid which acts on the respiratory centre in the floor of the fourth ventricle many hours after administration. Several papers have attested to the fact that the phenomenon does not occur after the first 24 h, during which time close respiratory monitoring is clearly required. This prerequisite is easily provided in the post-cardiac surgery patient as it is usual practice to nurse these patients either in an ITU, HDU or step-down unit during this time. The respiratory depression associated with intrathecal morphine may be precipitated by the concomitant use of opioids by other routes (including premedicant drugs) which should be given with caution, if at all. It is easily reversed with a carefully titrated dose of intravenous naloxone which is insufficient to antagonize analgesia.

The controversy surrounding the use of spinal and epidural blocks in patients with abnormalities of coagulation reaches its zenith in cardiac surgery, as the patient is required to be fully anticoagulated. Spontaneous epidural haematomata in the presence of a coagulopathy, and haematomata following axial blocks, although rare, have been reported in the literature, and can lead to irreversible neurological damage. However, several large series from the 1980s have demonstrated the safety of axial blockade in patients who have subsequently been heparinized for vascular surgery, provided that the procedure is abandoned if a 'bloody tap' is obtained. Indeed, there have been no reports of epidural haematoma following intrathecal morphine for cardiac surgery.

Notwithstanding the above argument, it is generally accepted that the pre-existence of an iatrogenic or other coagulopathy is an absolute contraindication to spinal puncture, although, if there were very strong indications, some anaesthetists might proceed in a patient receiving low-dose heparin or anti-platelet drugs. The other contraindications to spinal puncture – local infection, spinal deformity, neurological disease, raised intracranial pressure and patient refusal – also apply to the administration of intrathecal morphine.

In our institution we use 0.03 mg kg^{-1} morphine diluted with 10 ml normal saline administered to the lumbar CSF using a 25 gauge trocar pointed or a 24 gauge Sprotte needle. Asepsis must of course be meticulous and the use of bacterial filters is recommended. The dose of morphine is reduced by 20% for each decade of life over 60 years and the dose is adjusted for the very tall or very short patient. Patients with a history of postoperative nausea and vomiting are given a pre-emptive antiemetic. Following successful intrathecal injection, additional postoperative analgesia is rarely required; propofol is useful should additional sedation be necessary.

BIBLIOGRAPHY

Aun C, Thomas D, St John-Jones L, Colvin M P, Savage T M, Lewis C T. Intrathecal morphine in cardiac surgery. European Journal of Anaesthesiology 1985; 2: 426–429

El-Baz N, Goldin M. Continuous epidural infusion of morphine for pain relief after cardiac operations. Journal of Thoracic and Cardiovascular Surgery 1987; 93: 878–883

Mathews E T, Abrams L D. Intrathecal morphine in open heart surgery. Lancet, 1980, 2: 543

Odoom J A, Sih I L. Epidural analgesia and anticoagulant therapy: experience with one thousand cases of continuous epidurals. Anaesthesia 1983; 38: 254–259

Twycross R G, McQuay H J. Opioids. In: Wall P D, Melzack R (eds) Textbook of pain, 2nd edn. Churchill Livingstone, Edinburgh, 1989

CROSS REFERENCES

Epidural and spinal anaesthesia
Anaesthetic Factors 32: 594

Postoperative pain management
Anaesthetic Factors 33: 655

CONGENITAL HEART DISEASE: GENERAL PRINCIPLES AND PREOPERATIVE ASSESSMENT

C. Jerwood and M. A. Stokes

CONGENITAL HEART DISEASE (CHD)

- Incidence 6–8 per 1000 live births
- 2–3 times more common in premature infants
- Often associated with other abnormalities (diaphragmatic hernia, gastroschisis, tracheo-oesophageal fistula, imperforate anus)
- Often accompanies specific genetic disorders or known teratogens: Down's syndrome (40%), maternal alcohol (25%), rubella (35%), diabetes (3–5%).

SIMPLE PATHOPHYSIOLOGICAL CLASSIFICATION OF CHD

- Is there obstruction to blood flow (e.g. coarctation of the aorta, valvular stenoses)? Increased work needed to overcome obstruction; flow decreased distal to obstruction
- Is there shunting between pulmonary and systemic circulations and, if so, in which direction?
  - Shunting left to right (L–R) with increased pulmonary blood flow. Acyanotic (e.g. atrial septal defect (ASD), ventricular septal defect (VSD), PDA). Risk of volume or pressure overload to pulmonary circulation.
  - Shunting right to left (R–L) with decreased pulmonary blood flow. Cyanosis occurs because of anatomical reduction in flow (e.g. tetralogy of Fallot), or physiological mixing of saturated and desaturated blood (e.g. single ventricle).

PRESENTATION

Depending on the defect, may present in neonatal period, infancy, or childhood. Some defects have little effect on function and are picked up on routine medical checks.

- Cardiac failure presents as breathlessness on feeding and exertion, failure to thrive, pallor, sweating and hepatomegaly
- Cyanosis may be intermittent (crying, exercise) or continuous (at rest).

AIMS OF SURGERY

- Total correction
- Palliation
- Preparation for future palliative or definitive repair.

PREOPERATIVE ASSESSMENT

Anatomy and function are very variable and individual assessment is essential.

History and examination:
- Level of activity (cardiac reserve) and symptoms
- Murmurs, peripheral pulses and skin temperature.

Investigations:
- Chest X-ray (heart position, size and shape; increased or decreased pulmonary vascular markings)
- ECG (R axis deviation normal in infancy)
- Echocardiography (anatomy, function, cardiac output)
- Catheterization (site and magnitude of shunts, pressures, saturations)
- Haematocrit (increased in lesions with decreased pulmonary flow; significant risk of thrombosis if >60%).

Medications:
- Diuretics, digoxin, captopril
- Warfarin, aspirin
- Antibiotics (see endocarditis prophylaxis)

Previous surgery:
Review records. Note airway problems, dental hygiene.

INDUCTION

The aim is for a smooth induction, with impeccable airway control and balanced systemic and pulmonary vascular resistances. Consider sedative and antisialogogue premedication, EMLA cream. Intravenous induction is generally preferred although children with mild functional impairment (e.g. ASD, small VSD) will tolerate inhalational induction.

L–R shunts:
- An increase in SVR increases L–R shunting. An increase in PVR reduces L–R shunting.
- Intravenous induction may be prolonged because of recirculation in the lung.
- Inhalational uptake is minimally influenced by L–R shunt unless there is poor cardiac output. An agent with low blood gas solubility coefficient will then show increased speed of uptake. Pulmonary congestion increases incidence of atelectasis.

R–L shunts:
- Avoid prolonged starvation times. Polycythaemia and increased blood viscosity increase risk of thrombosis.
- Scrupulous attention to avoiding air and particulate embolization.
- Aim is to avoid worsening the shunt (hypoxia, hypotension).
- Raised intrathoracic pressure decreases pulmonary blood flow.
- Cyanotic patients have a blunted ventilatory response to hypoxia which may persist after lesion is corrected.
- Intravenous induction is rapid, but reduce dose to avoid precipitous drop in systemic vascular resistance.
- Volatile anaesthetic uptake is slow.

Obstructive lesions:
- Avoid dehydration, as reduced heart volume may worsen functional stenosis
- Similarly, avoid tachycardia.

MONITORING

- ECG
- Pulse oximetry: consider pre- and post-ductal sites (see coarctation of aorta).
- Temperature: multiple sites for cardiopulmonary bypass – heart (oesophageal), brain (nasopharyngeal or tympanic), and peripheral skin. Monitors cooling and rewarming of specific organs and helps assess perfusion.
- Invasive pressures, arterial and venous: in small children pulmonary artery and left atrial pressure lines can be brought out directly through the surgical field.

- Capnography: note increased arterial to $ETCO_2$ gradient with R–L shunting and reduced pulmonary blood flow.
- Urine output.
- Arterial blood gases, electrolytes, glucose, and ionized calcium (especially for neonates).
- Activated clotting times.
- Ventilation (F_IO_2, airway pressure, PEEP, tidal volume).

CROSS REFERENCES

Adult congenital heart disease
Patient Conditions 4: 92
Atrial septal defect
Patient Conditions 4: 96
Congenital heart disease in adult life
Patient Conditions 4: 121
Tetralogy of fallot
Patient Conditions 4: 127
Infants and children
Patient Conditions 11: 255
Cardiopulmonary bypass: principles, physiology and biochemistry
Surgical Procedures 27: 506

MANAGEMENT OF SPECIFIC CONGENITAL CARDIAC CONDITIONS

J. Payne and M. A. Stokes

PATENT DUCTUS ARTERIOSUS

Failure of the duct to close can cause a significant left–right (L–R) shunt. Symptoms include recurrent chest infections. Medical management involves treating heart failure (diuretics) and pharmacological closure of the duct (prostaglandin inhibitor, e.g. indomethacin). Interventional management includes surgical ligation or 'umbrella' device closure (via cardiac catheterization).

Anaesthetic considerations:

- Relatively quick operation via left thoracotomy
- Postoperative ventilation may be necessary (especially if heart failure is present)
- Avoid hypothermia (many infants small and premature)
- Cross-match blood (vessels may be damaged during ligation).

Postcorrection

May be assumed to have normal cardiovascular systems and do not require routine endocarditis prophylaxis for subsequent surgery.

COARCTATION OF THE AORTA

The presentation depends on the age of the child and degree and site of stenosis. There are often other cardiac anomalies. Neonates may present acutely with heart failure and absent femoral pulses. In this group the lesion is proximal to the ductus, so blood flow to the lower body is dependent on flow through the ductus arteriosus. Prostaglandin E infusion is required preoperatively to keep the duct open. Repair involves left thoracotomy, resection of the stenosed segment and end-to-end anastomosis, or a subclavian 'flap' to increase the aortic size. More complicated lesions (e.g. interrupted aortic arch) are repaired on bypass.

Anaesthetic considerations:

- Arterial line and Spo_2 probe sited preductally (right arm). Additional postductal (lower limb) BP cuff or arterial line and Spo_2 probe useful for comparison.
- Aorta is cross-clamped. In infants and older children, vasodilators (e.g. sodium nitroprusside) may be required to control upper body hypertension.
- Hypotension can occur on release of the clamps, requiring volume or inotrope (e.g. calcium) administration.
- Document cross-clamp times (risk of spinal cord ischaemia).

ATRIAL SEPTAL DEFECT

Generally well tolerated in children, most having mild or no symptoms. Atrial pressures are low, hence degree of L–R shunting is small. However, if the defect is large, or remains unrepaired, increased pulmonary blood flow causes vascular damage, increased PVR, and risk of shunt reversal. Most common defect is the secundum atrial septal defect (ASD), lying at the fossa ovalis. An ostium primum ASD occurs lower down in the atrial septum and may be associated with abnormal atrioventricular valve function (particularly mitral regurgitation).

Anaesthetic considerations:

- Surgery is generally straightforward, with a short bypass time; hence early awakening and extubation is appropriate
- Rhythm problems occur if atrioventricular node compromised
- Risk of paradoxical embolus.

Postcorrection:

- Most children will have normal function.
- Atrioventricular valve malfunction can persist.
- Simple secundum defects (repaired without use of prosthetic material) do not require endocarditis prophylaxis for subsequent surgery. Prophylaxis is required following repair of ostium primum defects.

VENTRICULAR SEPTAL DEFECT

The effect of a ventricular septal defect (VSD) on cardiovascular function depends on its size. Small lesions (many of which close spontaneously during the first year) may cause few symptoms, with only moderate amounts of L–R shunting. More severe shunting occurs with larger defects, depending on the ratio of systemic to pulmonary vascular resistances. If left uncorrected, increased pulmonary blood flow eventually leads to obstructive vascular disease, right–left (R–L) shunting (Eisenmenger's syndrome), and systemic desaturation.

Anaesthetic considerations:

- The aim is to minimize shunting by balancing systemic and pulmonary vascular resistances.
- Good airway control during induction is very important. Hypoxia increases PVR and may cause reversal of shunt (systemic desaturation).
- Risk of air and particulate embolization.
- Impaired left ventricular function may persist.
- Endocarditis prophylaxis is required.

TETRALOGY OF FALLOT (TOF)

The tetralogy of Fallot (TOF) is the association of a VSD with an obstruction to the right ventricular outflow tract (usually infundibular stenosis), together with right ventricular hypertrophy and a malaligned aorta 'overriding' the VSD. Pulmonary blood flow is reduced by a variable amount (some children have few symptoms unless stressed, whereas others present in early infancy with cyanosis, particularly if the pulmonary arteries are also small). Cyanotic 'spells' are due to infundibular spasm and cause an increased shunt across the VSD to the systemic circulation. Such cyanotic spells are precipitated by catecholamines (fear, anxiety, exercise) and handling of the heart at operation. Preoperative treatment includes beta blockade. In infants with small pulmonary arteries, a systemic to pulmonary shunt (e.g. Blalock–Taussig, subclavian to pulmonary artery) is inserted via a thoracotomy in the neonatal period, to ensure pulmonary blood flow while the vasculature develops. Definitive correction is usually performed towards the end of the first year of life. Correction consists of patch repair of the VSD and relief of the obstruction to the right ventricular outflow tract.

Anaesthetic considerations:

- Preoperative hydration (see R–L shunts, above)
- Sedative premedication (helps reduce cyanotic spells)
- As in VSD repair, avoid hypotension and hypoxia on induction, which tend to increase R–L shunting
- N.B. Intraoperative desaturation and reduced $ETco_2$ values also occur in other acute situations such as hypovolaemia and air embolus
- Treatment of infundibular spasm:
  - Increased F_Io_2
  - Analgesia
  - Beta blockade (propranolol 0.1 mg kg^{-1} i.v.)
  - Volume ± alpha agonist (noradrenaline) to increase systemic vascular resistance
- Risk of embolization.

Postcorrection:

- Usually totally corrected, but risk of residual VSD and outflow tract obstruction; rhythm disturbance
- Impaired left and right ventricular function may persist
- Endocarditis prophylaxis.

TRANSPOSITION OF THE GREAT ARTERIES

In transposition of the great arteries (TGA) the aorta arises from the right ventricle and the pulmonary trunk from the left. To be compatible with life, mixing must occur through a septal defect or patent ductus. If the neonate has an intact septum, an atrial communication (Rashkind balloon septostomy) is performed. Physiological correction involves septating the atria such that systemic venous return preferentially flows into the left ventricle, then into the pulmonary trunk (Senning or Mustard operation). Anatomical correction involves switching the aorta and pulmonary trunk (with reimplantation of the coronary arteries). Longer term, the right ventricle is unable to power the systemic circulation indefinitely and right ventricular failure may occur. Cardiovascular function is usually good following anatomical correction, although the long-term outcome is yet to be determined.

CROSS REFERENCES

Atrial septal defect
Patient Conditions 4: 96
Tetralogy of fallot
Patient Conditions 4: 127
Infants and children
Patient Conditions 11: 255
Cardiopulmonary bypass: principles, physiology and biochemistry
Surgical Procedures 27: 506
Premedication
Anaesthetic Factors 29: 549
Intraoperative cyanosis
Anaesthetic Factors 33: 634
Intraoperative hypertension
Anaesthetic Factors 33: 636
Intraoperative hypotension
Anaesthetic Factors 33: 638

POSTOPERATIVE CARE OF PAEDIATRIC PATIENTS AFTER CARDIOPULMONARY BYPASS

P. Hall and M. Stokes

GENERAL PRACTICE POINTS

- Analgesia (an opioid infusion is recommended)
- Sedation.

CARDIOVASCULAR

- Contractility is reduced with a long bypass time or ventriculotomy. Consider early use of inotropes (dobutamine, dopamine) ± vasodilator (nitroprusside) to reduce afterload. Use right and left atrial pressures and heart rate as a guide to volume loading.
- Dysrhythmias may be the result of surgical damage. Exclude a metabolic cause (pyrexia, potassium) or irritation by invasive monitoring. Treat by cardioversion (d.c. shock, adenosine), antidysrhythmics, or pacing.
- Cardiac tamponade is usually secondary to blocked chest drains. Look for pulsus paradoxus, rising right atrial pressure and systemic hypotension. Treatment is urgent surgical evacuation.
- Adequacy of cardiac output assessed by peripheral perfusion, core–skin temperature gradient, urine output, acid–base balance.

RESPIRATORY

- Mechanical ventilation until fully rewarmed and haemodynamically stable.
- Ensure endotracheal tube is correctly positioned (chest X-ray) and secure (nasotracheal route in small children).
- Use PEEP and regular physiotherapy to prevent atelectasis.
- Ventilatory requirements may alter because of pulmonary oedema (capillary leakage if bypass time long) or altered pulmonary flow (V/Q mismatch).
- Limit peak inspiratory times and PEEP to minimize risk of barotrauma.

RENAL

- Postoperative fluid and electrolyte disturbances are more likely if the child was previously hypoxic, hypertensive, or receiving diuretic therapy.
- Hypovolaemia is unmasked by vasodilatation on rewarming.
- Hormonal responses cause sodium and water retention.
- Potassium and calcium losses increase, so monitor carefully.
- Maintenance fluids are initially restricted (50–60 ml kg day^{-1}), increasing to normal (120 ml kg day^{-1}) by 3 days.
- If oliguric (<0.5 ml kg h^{-1}), check patency of catheter, review volume replacement and systemic pressures. Consider frusemide and dopamine. A few children may require peritoneal (cross-flow) dialysis.

NEUROLOGICAL

- Complications are infrequent but may be secondary to periods of hypoxia, electrolyte disturbance, hypoglycaemia, embolization.
- Phrenic nerve damage (surgical trauma, or from ice used for topical cooling).

GASTROINTESTINAL

- Opioids, nitrates and hypokalaemia all reduce smooth-muscle tone and increase risk of abdominal distension.
- Hepatic failure is uncommon, but may occur secondary to congestion or hypoxia. Monitor liver function.
- Start enteral nutrition on first postoperative day and parenteral nutrition within 3 days if absorption poor.

BIBLIOGRAPHY

Cote, Ryan, Todres, Goudsouzian (eds). A practice of anaesthesia for infants and children, 2nd edn. W B Saunders, Philadelphia, 1993

Katz, Steward (eds). Anaesthesia and uncommon pediatric diseases, 2nd edn. W B Saunders, Philadelphia, 1993

Lake C. Pediatric cardiac anesthesia. Appleton & Lange, New York 1988

CROSS REFERENCES

Infants and children
Patient Conditions 11: 255
Fluid and electrolyte balance
Anaesthetic Factors 33: 626
Postoperative oliguria
Anaesthetic Factors 33: 652
Postoperative pain management
Anaesthetic Factors 33: 655

28

NON-THEATRE PROCEDURES

B. J. Pollard

DENTAL CHAIR

J. Eddleston

HISTORY

The first recorded anaesthetic for a dental chair procedure was in 1844. Horace Wells was given nitrous oxide by Gardner Quincy Colton for the extraction of a tooth.

The number of general anaesthetics administered in dental practice in the UK is declining:

- 1.5 million in 1965
- Approximately 275 000 in 1992.

Why the reduction?

- There has been a substantial overall reduction in dental caries over the last 20 years:
  - in 1973, 7% of 12-year olds were caries-free
  - in 1993, 50% were caries-free.
- There has been a transition from general anaesthesia to 'relative analgesia' or sedation.

INDICATIONS

- Children
- Mentally or physically handicapped patients
- Local infection (local anaesthetics are ineffective)
- Allergy to local anaesthesia.

PATIENT SELECTION

- Out-patient anaesthesia
- Usually children aged 2–15 years old
- ASA status grade I–II
- Procedures should be of short duration; usually simple extractions
- Standard instructions and stipulations for day-case anaesthesia apply.

EQUIPMENT

All dental surgeries or clinics where general anaesthesia is administered must be equipped with:

- Dental chair capable of head-down tilt
- Facilities for intubation and positive pressure ventilation
- Resuscitation drugs
- Defibrillator
- Electrocardiogram, noninvasive BP measuring device, pulse oximeter
- A capnograph must be used where tracheal intubation is performed
- A Boyle's-type anaesthetic machine is strongly advised in preference to intermittent-flow machines.

PERIOPERATIVE MANAGEMENT

Posture (supine or semirecumbent):

- Mortality not related to posture
- Sa_{O_2} not influenced by posture (supine versus semirecumbent)
- Supine position associated with reduced incidence of fainting
- Supine position easier for anaesthetist.

Induction:

- Intravenous or inhalation.
- Intravenous more common now after introduction of EMLA cream.
- Insertion of intravenous cannula mandatory.
- Intravenous induction agents used are methohexitone or propofol:
  - Methohexitone 2 mg kg^{-1} for children <40 kg and 1.5 mg kg^{-1} for >40 kg
  - Propofol 3.5 mg kg^{-1}.
- Inhalational agents: halothane is still the agent of choice. Isoflurane is associated with more respiratory problems and desaturation compared to halothane and enflurane.

Maintenance:

- Nitrous oxide/oxygen/volatile agent using a nasal mask of Goldman type

or, alternatively,

- Incremental doses of induction agent, e.g. propofol.

Intraoperative monitoring:
- ECG
- BP
- Sa_{O_2}
- ET_{CO_2}, if tracheal intubation performed.

Airway control

Airway obstruction can be due to:

- Foreign body:
  - Mouth pack
  - Mouth prop insertion
  - Blood clot
  - Tooth.
- Downward pressure on mandible during lower-teeth extraction.
- Large tonsils or adenoids.
- Dislocation of temporomandibular joint.

Airway patency aided by use of:
- Nasopharyngeal airway
- Nasal CPAP
- Brain laryngeal mask
- Nasotracheal intubation.

Cardiac dysrhythmias:
- Patients are anxious and unpremedicated, with high circulating catecholamine levels.
- Hypoxia and hypercapnia (obstruction/hypoventilation) have an additive effect.
- Halothane sensitizes the myocardium to catecholamines; enflurane and isoflurane are less arrhythmogenic.
- Inhalational induction is associated with an increased incidence of dysrhythmias compared with intravenous induction.
- Stimulation of the trigeminal nerve during dental extraction may trigger dysrhythmias via the sympathoadrenal system. The incidence is reduced if periodontal injection of local anaesthetic is performed.

Scavenging:
- Difficult because of leakage of gas through open mouth
- Inhalation induction increases pollution in dental surgeries.

Emergence and recovery:
- In the dental chair or transferred to trolley and placed in lateral position
- Supervision of patient is mandatory until full recovery
- Discharge instructions as for day-case anaesthesia.

Analgesia:
- Oral NSAIDs (e.g. paracetamol, diclofenac)
- Periodontal injection of local anaesthetic.

OUTCOME

Mortality 1 in 248 000 dental anaesthetics.

BIBLIOGRAPHY

Evans C S, Dawson A D G. O_2 saturation during general anaesthesia in the dental chair: a comparison of the effect of position on saturation. British Dental Journal 1990; 168: 157–160

Reilly C S. Anaesthesia in the dental chair. Current Anaesthesia and Critical Care 1992; 3: 6–10

Report of an Expert Working Party. Department of Health. General anaesthesia, sedation and resuscitation in dentistry. 1991

Simmons M, Miller C D, Cummings G C, Todd J G. Outpatient paediatric dental anaesthesia. Anaesthesia 1989; 44: 735–738

CROSS REFERENCES

Infants and children
Patient Conditions 11: 255
Day care surgery
Anaesthetic Factors 29: 542
Complications of position 33: 618

ELECTROCONVULSIVE THERAPY

B. Holt

PROCEDURE

Seizure therapy was first introduced for the treatment of schizophrenia in 1934. The early ECTs were unmodified, i.e. no sedation, anaesthesia, relaxation, ventilation, or supplemental oxygen. Amnesia and cyanosis were believed to be beneficial and were encouraged. In 1963 the treatment was modified by the use of intravenous anaesthetic agents, neuromuscular blockade and ventilation with oxygen. With the advent of more potent neuropharmacological agents, ECT fell into disuse, but has recently undergone a revival.

Despite 50 years of use, the mechanism of action is still in dispute, but recent research suggests that biochemical changes occur at the cellular and subcellular level. What is not in doubt is the efficacy and dramatic improvement in the treatment of depression, schizophrenia, mania, and other conditions.

PATIENT CHARACTERISTICS

Patients for ECT are all adult and, with the growth of psychogeriatrics, many are in the older age group. In the elderly many cases of depression are brought on by the patient's poor general health. Patients can therefore be suffering from many chronic conditions and are often on many different medications for respiratory, cardiac, and musculoskeletal disorders. In addition, they will almost certainly be on drugs for their psychiatric condition.

PREOPERATIVE ASSESSMENT

History taking can often be difficult, in psychiatric patients and is often unreliable in relation to the physical condition. One of the major effects of ECT is on the parasympathetic and sympathetic nervous system. There is first stimulation of the parasympathetic system followed by stimulation of the sympathetic system. This can give rise to bradycardia followed by tachycardia with concomitant changes in BP that place a considerable stress on the whole cardiovascular system. These changes are, however, transient, and although the observed changes can be alarming they seldom require treatment.

ECT raises intracranial pressure (ICP) and any indication of raised ICP due to any cause is an absolute contraindication to treatment by ECT.

Drug interactions are not normally a problem, and even mono-aminoxidase inhibitors can be continued provided due cognisance is taken of potential problems. The only drug likely to cause problems is lithium, which should be discontinued prior to treatment.

PREMEDICATION

- Anxiolysis (if required) with benzodiazepines
- Anticholinergics are not now generally given prior to ECT, but should be readily available in case of an exaggerated vagal response.

THEATRE PREPARATION

ECT should only be undertaken where full anaesthetic and resuscitation back-up is available, and preferably in a specially designated room with a fully monitored recovery area.

PERIOPERATIVE MANAGEMENT

Monitoring:

- ECG
- Noninvasive BP
- Sa_{O_2}.

INDUCTION

Methohexitone and thiopentone are the agents of choice. Propofol is not approved for use in ECT. Etomidate causes increased muscle tone and is not recommended for ECT.

Muscle relaxation is used to reduce the incidence of fractures related to ECT. Succinylcholine (0.5 mg kg^{-1}) is the drug of choice. Following modified ECT only 2% of patients suffer muscle pain.

Intubation is not normally necessary and the airway can be maintained by correct head position. Assisted ventilation with 100% oxygen is mandatory until spontaneous respiration returns. Because of the seizure and clamping of jaws that occurs with ECT, it is advisable to insert an oral airway or mouth gag to prevent the tongue being bitten.

Following administration of ECT, bradycardia and even asystole may occur, and many anaesthetists still administer atropine or glycopyrrolate routinely. These drugs may accentuate the sympathetic response that invariably follows, putting undue stress on the myocardium and recent studies have suggested a greater degree of morbidity from this. The use of a short-acting beta blocker such as Esmolol has been advocated to attenuate the sympathetic response to ECT, and should be available to treat arrhythmias and hypertension that persist into the recovery period.

POSTOPERATIVE MANAGEMENT

Patients having had ECT should be closely monitored until fully recovered.

OUTCOME

Mortality following ECT is 0.03%.

Arrhythmias, myocardial infarction, congestive cardiac failure and sudden cardiac arrest are the commonest causes of death, nearly always occurring during the recovery period.

BIBLIOGRAPHY

O'Flaherty D, Giesecke A H. Electroconvulsive therapy and anaesthesia. Current Opinions in Anaesthesiology 1991; 4: 436–440

Selvin B L. Electroconvulsive therapy – 1987. Anesthesiology 1987; 47: 367–385

Varassi B et al. Circulatory responses during electroconvulsive therapy. The comparative effect of placebo, esmolol, and nitroglycerine. Anaesthesia 1992; 47: 563–567

CROSS REFERENCES

The elderly patient
Patient Conditions 11: 252
Intraoperative hypertension
Anaesthetic Factors 33: 636
ICP/CBF Control 33: 662

PART 3

ANAESTHETIC FACTORS

29

PREOPERATIVE ASSESSMENT

B. J. Pollard

DAY-CASE SURGERY

B. J. Pollard

29

Table 1.
Guidelines for patient selection for general anaesthesia

Age greater than 6 months
Age less than 70 years
ASA status I or II
ASA III may be acceptable (should be discussed on an individual basis between surgeon and anaesthetist)
Patient should live within 1 h drive of the unit
There must be a responsible adult to escort the patient home
Avoid procedures which are likely to last for longer than about 60 min
Avoid procedures where severe postoperative pain is likely
Avoid procedures where significant postoperative bleeding is likely.

A day-case (ambulatory) patient is one who is an in-patient for several hours for purposes of investigation or minor surgery and does not stay overnight in hospital. There are a number of advantages for the patient:

- Less disruption of family life
- More pleasant for the patient and the family
- Usually able to return to work or school earlier
- Waiting time is reduced
- Less risk of hospital-acquired infections in susceptible individuals
- Incidence of postoperative respiratory complications is decreased.

The principal advantages to the hospital are that waiting lists are reduced for many minor operations and day-case activity is generally cheaper per patient.

PATIENT SELECTION

This is very important. Inappropriate selection of patients will hamper the smooth working of the unit and lead to operations being cancelled or deferred. It is useful for the day-case unit to draw up a series of guidelines for the surgeon (Table 1). If there is any doubt (e.g. diabetes, obesity), the surgeon and anaesthetist should discuss the case individually. The potential suitability for a local or regional block must also be remembered.

Suitable procedures

These are too numerous to list, but include most minor gynaecological, urological, general, dental, plastic and ENT procedures.

TIMING OF THE PREOPERATIVE ASSESSMENT

All day-case patients should preferably be seen by an anaesthetist in advance of the day of surgery. This is not always possible and various alternatives have been developed.

Clinic assessment

An anaesthetic assessment clinic approach is used in some centres. This should not be more than about 4 weeks before admission, otherwise the patient's condition might have changed. Patients should be advised to telephone and defer their surgery if they develop an acute upper respiratory tract infection.

Questionnaire assessment

A questionnaire is sent to the patient in advance of their admission date and they are requested to complete it and return it to the day-case unit. This works well, provided the questions are relevant and well worded. The range of topics which can be covered is wide (Table 2), and each day-case unit has its own individual version of this sort of questionnaire.

Computer assessment

Interactive assessment by computer may be the method of the future. This could take place in the GP's surgery, for example. It may be particularly good for patients who live some distance from the day-case unit.

Table 2.
Example questionnaire topics

Have you ever had previous in-patient treatment; general anaesthesia; surgery?
Do you take any medicines on a regular basis (including the contraceptive pill)?
Any allergies?
Any bleeding problems?
Breathlessness or chest pain?
Previous or present serious illnesses, e.g. diabetes, epilepsy, asthma, hypertension, heart disease?
Risk of pregnancy?
Family problems with anaesthesia?
Smoking habits, drinking habits?

ASSESSMENT OF THE PATIENT

Age

Most day-case units accept patients between the ages of 6 months and 70 years. Some will go down to 1 month, provided the infant was not a preterm delivery.

Personal circumstances

There must be a responsible adult to accompany the patient home. If the patient lives a long distance from the facility, they should stay overnight within about 30 miles of the facility.

Preoperative starvation

The normal rules apply. It is important to emphasize the importance of preoperative starvation to the patient because it is less easy to be certain that the patient has not had a meal than when the patient is already in hospital.

Review of systems

A routine history and examination should be undertaken, with particular emphasis on:

- Past medical and surgical history
- Drugs and allergies
- Cardiovascular system
- Respiratory system and airway
- Smoking, alcohol, social drugs
- Liver and kidneys
- Endocrine and metabolic disorders.

Investigations

The surgeon should have organized these at the original booking clinic. With respect to anaesthesia, there are no routine investigations which are always indicated. There should be a valid reason for each. The normal rules apply.

It may be necessary to repeat certain investigations on the morning of surgery, and the day-case unit should have this facility available.

PATIENT INFORMATION

It is sensible practice for each patient to receive an information sheet at the booking clinic giving important information about the procedure. This is also an opportune time to list those important points which the patient needs to know about the postoperative period (Table 3).

Table 3.
Example patient information sheet

Date, time, place of admission
Nature of procedure and anaesthetic
Preoperative starvation rules and surgical preparation requirements
What to do about taking any preoperative medication
Must arrange for a responsible adult
No driving, alcohol, machinery, etc., for 24 h
Postoperative analgesic advice
Day-case-unit phone numbers (routine and emergency)
What to do if the patient develops a cold, thinks she might be pregnant, or has any acute change in health
Advice on time off work, follow-up appointments, etc.

The patient should also receive another information sheet on discharge, re-emphasizing the essential points.

CONDUCT OF THE ANAESTHETIC

Premedication

Often unnecessary. Use an agent with a relatively short duration of action.

Induction

Propofol is presently the induction agent of choice. Methohexitone is also suitable.

Maintenance

There appears to be little to choose between the three volatile agents halothane, enflurane and isoflurane. A total intravenous technique using propofol is also suitable. The new volatile agents sevoflurane and desflurane may prove to be superior.

Analgesia

Alfentanil or fentanyl are popular because of their potency and short duration of action. The newer nonsteroidal agents, e.g. ketorolac, are being used increasingly for day-case patients.

Muscle relaxants

A short or intermediate duration non-depolarizing agent is recommended. Mivacurium, atracurium and vecuronium are all suitable. Rocuronium may also be suitable. The incidence of muscle pains following suxamethonium is very high in ambulatory patients and this drug should be avoided if possible. Mivacurium does not usually need to be reversed with an anticholinesterase agent, which avoids the potential adverse effects of this family of drugs.

DISCHARGE FROM THE DAY-CASE UNIT

Whereas early recovery is important, return to 'street fitness' is the most important factor. Batteries of complex psychomotor and cognitive performance tests have been undertaken in a number of centres. These are not possible in the routine day-case unit. Each day-case unit should have a list of guidelines for safe discharge of patients (Table 4). In general, most patients are fit enough to go home after about 3–4 h.

Table 4.
Discharge guidelines

Vital signs stable for at least 1 h
No respiratory depression or undue drowsiness
Able to eat and drink and to pass urine
Able to walk unaided
No significant pain, bleeding, nausea or vomiting
Written instructions have been given to the patient and read by either patient or escort or both
Responsible adult present

COMMON POSTOPERATIVE PROBLEMS IN DAY-CASES

The facility should always exist for admission of a patient from a day-case unit for overnight stay in a hospital bed if necessary. Such reasons might include:

- Extended surgery or surgical complications, e.g. bleeding, perforation of viscus
- Perioperative complications, e.g. arrhythmias
- Problems with control of a pre-existing disease, e.g. diabetes
- Persistent nausea and vomiting
- Difficulty with pain control
- Prolonged drowsiness
- Patient request, or lack of suitable escort.

BIBLIOGRAPHY

Healy T E J. Anaesthesia for day case surgery. Baillière's Clinical Anaesthesiology 1990; 4

CROSS REFERENCES

The elderly patient
Patient Conditions 11: 252
Infants and children
Patient Conditions 11: 255
Dental chair
Surgical Procedures 28: 534
Elective surgery
Anaesthetic Factors 29: 545
Premedication
Anaesthetic Factors 29: 549
Postoperative pain management
Anaesthetic Factors 33: 655
Thrombotic embolism
Anaesthetic Factors 33: 664

ELECTIVE SURGERY

B. J. Pollard

Every patient should be assessed by an anaesthetist before anaesthesia. This should ideally be the same anaesthetist who is going to administer the anaesthetic. Performing a full history and examination on every patient is time-consuming and difficult in the context of a busy operating list. Time may be saved by confining attention to those systems of direct relevance to anaesthesia and gaining additional information from the notes of the surgical house officer.

PREVIOUS HISTORY

Anaesthetic:

- Problems with previous anaesthetics must be identified
- Difficulty with intubation or sensitivity to drugs are the commonest problems encountered
- Knowledge of the approximate dates of previous anaesthetics will allow certain agents to be avoided if necessary, e.g. halothane.

Surgical:

- May indicate the existence of previous pathology, e.g. lung resection
- If this may be a repeat operation for a recurrent problem, a more prolonged procedure may be expected.

Medical:

- Seek information on all old or ongoing disease processes
- Severity, treatment and complications should be determined.

CARDIOVASCULAR SYSTEM

Particular factors include:

- Hypertension
- Ischaemic heart disease
- Valvular heart disease
- Recent or previous myocardial infarction
- Cardiac failure
- Arrhythmias
- Exercise tolerance
- Dyspnoea and orthopnoea
- Presence of a pacemaker.

RESPIRATORY SYSTEM AND AIRWAY

Particular attention should be paid to:

- Chronic obstructive airways disease
- Productive cough
- Exercise tolerance
- Dyspnoea (grade it)
- Any tendency to bronchospasm
- Acute upper respiratory tract infection
- Mouth opening and jaw mobility
- Presence of any dental crowns, dentures or loose teeth
- Any previous surgery or trauma to the airway.

DRUG AND ALLERGY HISTORY

- What drugs the patient is taking (prescribed or proprietary) and their doses
- This gives a clue to the presence of other accidentally forgotten or concealed medical problems.
- The severity of a known disease process may be related to the strength and number of drugs being taken
- Potential drug interactions may be avoided or allowed for
- Potential allergic reactions can be avoided.

SOCIAL AND FAMILY HISTORY

- Smoking habits.
- Consumption of alcohol (units per week or day).
- Use of addictive drugs:
  - What drugs are being used?
  - By what route are they being taken?
  - How often?
- Any family history of anaesthetic problems (e.g. malignant hyperpyrexia).
- Might the patient be pregnant? Elective surgery should be postponed until after delivery if possible.

- Assess nutritional status. The obese patient and the thin cachectic patient have a number of particular problems.
- Might the patient have any ongoing infections? Elective procedures may need to be postponed while these are treated. Remember the potential hazard to theatre staff.

NEUROLOGICAL, MUSCULAR AND PSYCHIATRIC DISEASES

- Level of consciousness (chart it if necessary).
- Patients with neuromuscular disorders (e.g. myasthenia) are likely to respond in an unusual way to muscle relaxants.
- Patients with myopathies and dystrophies may have an associated cardiomyopathy.
- Psychiatric disorders do not usually themselves pose any particular problem. The drugs used to treat them are usually of more importance.
- Some patients are incapable of giving consent to surgery and this needs to be taken instead from a legally competent person, e.g. parent or guardian.

GASTROINTESTINAL DISORDERS

- These do not usually have an important effect on anaesthesia
- In patients with a hiatus hernia, or otherwise at risk from gastric reflux, appropriate precautions should be taken to prevent pulmonary aspiration of gastric contents
- When there has been a period of diarrhoea or vomiting, or continuous drainage from a fistula or nasogastric tube, fluid and electrolyte imbalances are common
- Care should be taken with the use of nitrous oxide in the presence of gas-filled loops of bowel.

LIVER DISEASE

- Many drugs used in anaesthesia are at least partly metabolized in the liver; pre-existing liver disease is therefore of profound importance in anaesthesia
- A reduction in serum albumin concentration will alter the protein binding of many drugs
- Coagulopathies are common in liver disease
- There is likely to be a reduced plasma cholinesterase level
- Look for jaundice and take appropriate precautions if present
- Consider the possibility of one of the infectious forms of hepatitis.

RENAL DISEASE

- Many of the drugs used in anaesthesia are excreted via the kidney; avoid those which are exclusively renally excreted
- The patient may be hypertensive
- The patient may be chronically anaemic
- The patient may be on dialysis
- Measure the preoperative plasma electrolytes.

ENDOCRINE AND METABOLIC DISORDERS

- Diabetic patients should be managed in one of the standard ways
- Patients with adrenocorticoid dysfunction may require steroid cover
- Look for a goitre (and remember the possibility of difficult intubation) in patients with thyroid disease.

INVESTIGATIONS

Blood tests, ECG, X-rays, pulmonary function tests, etc., should not be routinely performed without good reason, e.g. the anaemic patient should have a preoperative haemoglobin estimation, and patients taking a diuretic should have the plasma electrolytes measured. Patients of African origin or with a suspicious family history should have a Sickledex test performed. Remember to cross-match blood if need is anticipated.

A concentration of 10 g dl^{-1} is generally accepted as the lower limit for haemoglobin below which elective surgery should be postponed. In certain cases of chronic anaemia, e.g. renal failure, lower levels are acceptable.

PREOPERATIVE STARVATION

The normally accepted period of starvation is 6 h for food and 4 h for drinks alone. Recent evidence suggests that drinks are cleared more rapidly from the stomach and that 2 h may be a short enough time. A prolonged period of starvation is unpleasant and may be hazardous in infants and babies. It should be avoided.

PREOPERATIVE PREPARATION

- The correct patient should arrive in theatre with the correct notes and X-rays

- Dentures, contact lenses, prosthetic limbs, etc., should have been left on the ward
- Patients who are deaf or with impaired vision may benefit from retaining their hearing aid or glasses until the moment of induction of anaesthesia
- All lipstick and cosmetics should have been removed
- All jewellery should have been removed, or should be taped securely to the patient
- Never remove the patient's identity badge unless absolutely essential, whereupon it must be immediately reattached to a different part of the patient
- If there could be any confusion as to the site or side of the operation, the patient should have been marked with an indelible ink marker by the surgeon before leaving the ward.

BIBLIOGRAPHY

Maltby J R, Lewis P, Marbin A, Sutherland C R. Gastric fluid volume and pH: in elective patients following unrestricted oral fluid until three hours before surgery. Can. J. Anaesth. 1991, 38: 425–429

CROSS REFERENCES

Diabetes mellitus
Patient Conditions 2: 42
Malignant hypoaxaemia
Patient Conditions 2: 57
Smoking and anaesthesia
Patient Conditions 3: 85
Chronic liver disease
Patient Conditions 5: 135
Obesity
Patient Conditions 5: 148
Acute renal failure
Patient Conditions 6: 154
Sickle cell syndrome
Patient Conditions 7: 188
Pregnancy
Surgical Procedures 20: 391
Difficult airway
Anaesthetic Factors 30: 558
Preoperative assessment of cardiovascular risk in noncardiac surgery
Anaesthetic Factors 34: 692
Preoperative assessment of pulmonary risk
Anaesthetic Factors 34: 697
Scoring systems in anaesthesia
Anaesthetic Factors 34: 700

EMERGENCY SURGERY

B. J. Pollard

An emergency anaesthetic is one that is required as soon as possible. The implication is that there is not enough time available for the patient to be fully prepared for surgery. It is likely therefore that the patient's condition has not been optimized, there may be existing homeostatic disturbances, and not all of the laboratory or other tests may be available before beginning.

ASSESSMENT

In the initial assessment of the patient, the first decision which must be taken is the urgency of the procedure. If the nature of the surgery is compelling and immediate, no time should be wasted. If it is possible to introduce some delay, however short, this should be done in order to allow the patient to be more fully assessed and for the patient's condition to be optimized.

Assessment should be along the same lines as for elective procedures if time permits. Assess as fully as possible within the constraints of the degree of urgency.

If the patient cannot give any history look for warning cards and 'Medic-Alert' tags, or bracelets. Look at any previous hospital notes and emergency department records. Ask friends or relatives if present.

Perform appropriate investigations, depending upon available time. Obtain the results for those already instituted.

Look for the presence of alcohol intoxication, particularly in cases of trauma.

Remember that in urgent procedures there is an increased chance of cardiac-related death in the presence of pre-existing cardiovascular disease.

If the patient is of an ethnic origin where sickle disease is prevalent, treat as positive until proven to the contrary.

Starvation

Assume that the patient has a full stomach. Even if the last food intake was over 6 h ago the stomach may not be empty. In cases of trauma, in particular, the stomach ceases to empty at the time of injury and may still contain partly digested food 12 or more hours later.

Attempts at emptying the stomach using a nasogastric tube are not usually completely successful and should not be relied upon.

PREPARATION

Trained assistance must be available in the operating theatre. Make sure everything is prepared and ready before starting, including drawing up any drugs which you might want. If possible, check that blood has been cross-matched and is immediately available in theatre.

Consider anaesthetizing the patient in the theatre and not in the anaesthetic room to minimize delays between induction and incision. Test all equipment before starting.

Insert at least one intravenous line (minimum size 16 gauge; preferably 14 gauge). If major blood loss is expected, or if the patient is markedly hypovolaemic, insert a central venous pressure (CVP) line.

MONITORING

Attach all monitors before starting and get baseline readings. Standard minimum monitoring should consist of:

- Spo_2
- ECG
- Noninvasive BP
- $ETco_2$.

Other monitors, e.g. NMT, should be added as necessary. Core-temperature monitoring is advisable in all but the most minor emergencies. An arterial line should be considered for invasive arterial pressure monitoring. In general, time should not be wasted in securing additional monitoring lines (e.g. CVP, PAFC) unless this is deemed essential before starting. It is usually acceptable to establish these when the patient is asleep, while preparation for surgery is progressing. A urinary catheter should be inserted in major cases.

INDUCTION

Secure the airway as rapidly as possible. Use a rapid sequence induction technique with preoxygenation and cricoid pressure. Take a further blood sample if necessary for more tests, blood gases, cross-match, etc.

Give drugs slowly, particularly in the hypotensive patient. Etomidate is a good choice in hypotensive, hypovolaemic patients; it should not, however, be used as an alternative to preoperative fluid replacement if there is time for the latter.

MAINTENANCE

Almost any technique is suitable depending upon the fitness of the patient. Remember that volatile agents tend to produce vasodilatation and/or a fall in cardiac output. This may further reduce an already low blood pressure.

Do not waste time waiting for blood but give any available fluid if required, particularly colloids. All intravenous fluids should be warmed. Remember to order fresh frozen plasma, platelets, etc., if giving more than about 4 units of blood or if coagulation problems are suspected.

The condition of most patients who require emergency surgery is dynamic, and close observation is essential because rapid changes do occur.

Autotransfusion using a cell saver should be considered if blood loss is likely to be considerable or if there is any reason to avoid blood transfusion.

It must be remembered that the patient may have one or more disease processes which have not been discovered preoperatively. Keep an open mind at all times whatever happens – the patient could have almost anything wrong with them.

If the patient has suffered from trauma, remember that there may be additional unknown fractures or injuries, e.g. neck injuries, thoracic trauma. Continuing hypotension may mean continuing bleeding somewhere other than the operating site. Additional precautions apply if the patient has suffered a head injury.

RECOVERY

Reverse any residual block and discontinue anaesthesia in a routine manner. The patient should be extubated in the lateral position if possible. Administer face-mask oxygen for at least the early recovery period and consider its use for the first 24–48 h in high-risk patients.

If the surgery has been extensive, the patient has received a large transfusion, perioperative complications have occurred, or there are other concerns, it is wise to transfer the patient to a HDU or ITU for the early postoperative period. Overnight controlled ventilation may be advisable in certain cases.

CROSS REFERENCES

Sickle cell syndrome
Patient Conditions 7: 188
Elective surgery
Anaesthetic Factors 29: 545
Difficult airway – aspiration risk
Anaesthetic Factors 30: 553
Blood transfusion
Anaesthetic Factors 33: 616
Failure to breathe or wake up postoperatively
Anaesthetic Factors 33: 623
Intraoperative hypotension
Anaesthetic Factors 33: 638
Thrombotic embolism
Anaesthetic Factors 33: 664
Trauma
Anaesthetic Factors 33: 672
Preoperative assessment of cardiovascular risk in noncardiac surgery
Anaesthetic Factors 34: 692

PREMEDICATION

B. J. Pollard

Premedication is short for 'preoperative medication' or 'preliminary medication'. A drug, or a combination of drugs (the premed), is administered to the patient before anaesthesia and surgery.

There are a number of reasons for administering a premed, the commonest of which is anxiolysis. Reasons vary from patient to patient and also within the same patient at different times. It must always be remembered that not every patient needs pharmacological premedication on every occasion. A visit from the anaesthetist and an explanation of the procedure may be all that is required.

Sedative premedication may be inadvisable in the old or frail patient. Profound sedation, confusion or disorientation may result.

The administration of a sedative premed will lead to a reduction in the requirements for anaesthetic agents, reduce the potential for awareness during tracheal intubation, assist in maintaining anaesthesia, and reduce any unwanted side-effects from certain of the anaesthetic agents.

Children require a premed more often than adults. Remember to scale the dose down. Diazepam, temazepam and trimeprazine are prepared in a flavoured liquid formulation for children. Infants and neonates are special cases (see p. 255).

The factors which it is necessary to consider in premedication are listed in Table 1. Common premedicant drugs and combinations are listed in Table 2.

Table 1.
Factors to consider for premedication

Anxiolysis
Amnesia
Antiemesis
Analgesia
Antibiosis
Antithrombosis
Antisialogogue action
Antacid action
Antihistamine action
Antivagal action

Table 2.
Common premed drugs and combinations*

	Dose	Route
Adults		
Diazepam	5–15 mg	Oral
Temazepam	10–30 mg	Oral
Lorazepam	1–3 mg	Oral
Papaveretum with hyoscine	5, 10, 15 or 20 mg with 0.1, 0.2, 0.3 or 0.4 mg	Intramuscular
Children		
Diazepam	0.2 mg kg^{-1}	Oral
Trimeprazine	2–3 mg kg^{-1}	Oral

*All are given approximately 1 h preoperatively. Metoclopramide may be added as an antiemetic. There are many other combinations which are favoured by individual anaesthetists. Antacids and/or antibiotics may need to be added if needed.

ANXIOLYSIS

- Most patients are apprehensive of forthcoming surgery and anxiolysis is welcome
- Anxiety is a subjective sensation and it may be difficult to determine whether a patient is anxious or not
- The patient who has had several previous anaesthetics may be more, not less, anxious
- The severity and site of the surgery are poor indicators of potential for anxiety
- An anxiolytic premed will lessen the normal stress response to surgery and anaesthesia
- The benzodiazepines and the opioids are the agents most commonly used to secure anxiolysis in the preoperative period.

AMNESIA

- Amnesia may be appropriate for a particularly traumatic occasion, especially if further procedures are planned
- Amnesia is disliked by a number of patients who are disturbed by the removal of part of a day of their life
- Amnesic drugs will assist in reducing the incidence of awareness under general anaesthesia
- Amnesia may not be sensible if it has been necessary to go to lengths to gain the patient's confidence for a procedure; the patient may also forget all of the positive points which have been emphasized on this occasion
- The benzodiazepines are commonly used amnesics (lorazepam is the most potent); hyoscine is also a potent amnesic, although it may cause confusion in the elderly.

ANTIEMESIS

- Useful for the patient who complains of previous sickness following surgery
- The effect of an antiemetic in the premed may be waning by the end of the procedure, requiring an additional dose
- Advisable if an opioid is used for premedication
- Droperidol, prochlorperazine, metoclopramide, cyclizine and hyoscine are those most commonly used; the 5-HT_3 antagonists are usually reserved for situations when the simpler drugs do not work.

ANALGESIA

- Desirable if the patient has pain preoperatively
- Reduces the intraoperative requirements for anaesthetic agents and analgesics
- Improves comfort in the early postoperative period, but is likely to need supplementing at that time
- The opioids remain the most commonly used analgesics
- The newer nonsteroidal analgesics (NSAIDs) are enjoying an increased following, but they lack the mild sedative and euphoric effect of the opioids which is useful as a part of the premed.

Table 3.
Common antibiotic regimens for the prevention of subacute bacterial endocarditis in susceptible individuals*

Drug regimen	Dose	Route	
Amoxycillin	3 g	Oral	1 h preoperatively
Amoxycillin	1 g 0.5 g	i.m./i.v. i.m./oral	At induction, then 6 h postoperatively
Amoxycillin Gentamicin Amoxycillin	1 g 120 mg 0.5 g	i.m./i.v. i.m./i.v. Oral	At induction At induction 6 h postoperatively
Vancomycin Gentamicin	1 g 120 mg	i.v. i.v.	Infusion over 100 min, then at induction
Clindamycin	0.6 g	Oral	1 h preoperatively

**Note*: Doses should be reduced proportionately in children.
Reduce the dose of gentamicin in renal impairment.
Choice of antibiotics depends upon patient tolerance (e.g. allergies) and on expected contaminants.
For further details see *British National Formulary*, ch. 5.

29

ANTIBIOSIS

- Used principally for prophylaxis against subacute bacterial endocarditis in susceptible individuals
- The accepted regimens are given in the *British National Formulary*; the commonest are listed in Table 3
- May also be given as a part of local surgical practice for prophylaxis against postoperative infection; particularly recommended where foreign material is to be implanted.

ANTITHROMBOSIS

- Consider in patients at risk from deep venous thrombosis
- Heparin (5000 units, s.c., 12 hourly) is the commonest regime.

ANTISIALOGOGUE ACTION

- Essential for premeds in infants
- Useful when intraoral surgery is to be undertaken
- Some anaesthetists recommend this when fibre-optic intubation is planned
- The principal disadvantage is the unpleasant dry mouth experienced by the patient
- Atropine, hyoscine and glycopyrrolate are all potent drying agents.

ANTACID ACTION

- Should be used if there is an increased risk of regurgitation of gastric contents
- Particular risk factors are pregnancy, hiatus hernia with reflux, obesity
- Sodium citrate is preferable to magnesium trisilicate mixture because it is not particulate
- Ranitidine or cimetidine needs to be given 1–2 h preoperatively.

ANTIHISTAMINE ACTION

- A relatively unimportant consideration
- May offer partial protection against endogenously released histamine
- Promethazine is a suitable agent.

ANTIVAGAL ACTION

- Important in ophthalmic surgery
- Indicated if repeated doses of suxamethonium are to be administered
- Counteracts the otherwise potent vagal effects of surgery
- Not necessary in all cases; however, if not used, remember the potential for a profound bradycardia during surgery and have atropine ready to hand at all times
- Atropine and glycopyrrolate are the most effective antivagal agents for general use.

CROSS REFERENCES

Paediatric anaesthesia
Surgical Procedures 26: 494
Dental chair
Surgical Procedures 28: 534
Thrombotic embolism
Anaesthetic Factors 33: 664

30

AIRWAY

I. Calder
R. Vanner
R. Bingham

HYPOXAEMIA UNDER ANAESTHESIA

I. Calder

HYPOXAEMIA AND CIRCULATORY ARREST

Acute hypoxaemia will eventually cause circulatory arrest due to myocardial hypoxia. At some time around the point of arrest, irreversible cerebral damage occurs. The *period of anoxia* necessary to produce circulatory arrest will depend on cardiac health, the oxygen content of the body prior to the anoxic episode and the oxygen consumption. Anecdotal accounts suggest that complete airway obstruction for about 10 min will cause circulatory arrest in healthy patients.

Bradycardia and hypoxaemic cardiac arrest

Hypoxaemic cardiac arrest is invariably preceded by bradycardia. Hypoxaemia must be excluded before treating bradycardia with atropine.

CEREBRAL DAMAGE AND HYPOXAEMIA

For ethical reasons this topic is not well researched. The evidence is largely anecdotal.

Acute hypoxaemia

This causes cerebral dysfunction (confusion), particularly in the elderly, but structural damage seems to be unusual, unless hypoxaemic circulatory arrest occurs. In one report, a volunteer was confused but still conscious, despite an oximeter reading of 37%.

Cerebral damage and hypoxaemic circulatory arrest

Severe cerebral damage is invariable, but it is sometimes possible to restore circulatory function. Many survivors die later of the complications of coma.

Prolonged hypoxaemia

This has been shown to cause structural cerebral damage (diminished finger tapping ability) in mountain climbers. The subjects had saturations of about 60% for many hours.

CAUSES OF HYPOXAEMIA UNDER ANAESTHESIA

- Equipment failure
- Hypoventilation
- 'Shunt'.

Equipment failure

A rapid check of the equipment is always the first step. In particular, the $F_{I}O_2$ and the patency and correct connection of the anaesthetic circuit, and any artificial airway.

Hypoventilation

Hypoventilation results from central or peripheral depression of ventilation, and/or an obstructed airway.

The effect of hypoventilation on oxygen saturation is complex. Oxygen absorption depends more on the $F_{I}O_2$ than on alveolar ventilation. At a given inspired oxygen concentration, reducing alveolar ventilation makes little difference to oxygenation, until a 'critical' level is reached (Figure 1).

Apnoeic oxygenation

Provided the airway is at least partially open, passive entrainment of high oxygen concentrations can prevent desaturation during lengthy periods of apnoea, since the $P_{a}O_2$ only rises by about 0.5 kPa min^{-1} (see alveolar air equation in Figure 1 legend below). Insufflation of oxygen into the mouths of apnoeic, anaesthetized patients has been shown to prevent desaturation for 10 min (the study was terminated after 10 min for ethical reasons). Apnoeic oxygenation in one (brainstem dead) patient prevented circulatory arrest for 3 h and 20 min.

Practical points

- Hypoxaemia due to hypoventilation will respond rapidly to an increase in $F_{I}O_2$
- SPO_2 readings are not a reliable guide to the adequacy of ventilation, when the $F_{I}O_2$ is high – *oximeters measure saturation not ventilation.*

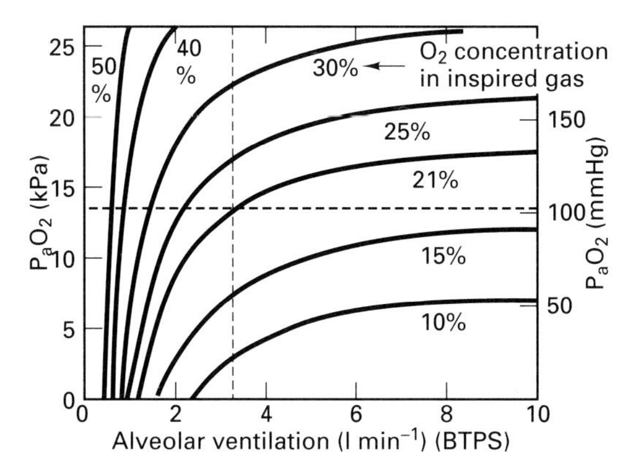

Figure 1
Effect of ventilation on alveolar gas tensions (P_aO_2, F_IO_2 and alveolar ventilation). (Reproduced with permission from Benumof 1990.)
Note that at high levels of F_IO_2 the critical level of ventilation is reduced, but when reached the P_aO_2 may fall suddenly. P_aO_2 depends upon F_IO_2 and P_aCO_2. The relationship is described by the 'alveolar air equation', which in its simplest form (applicable only to a patient breathing 100% oxygen) is:

$$P_{alv}O_2 = P_IO_2 - P_aCO_2$$

Corrections have to be introduced if there are other components to the inspired gas.

'Shunt'
The term 'shunt' is used here to mean failure of oxygenation of blood during passage through the pulmonary circulation ('venous admixture'). In most cases this is due to ventilation/perfusion mismatch.

Some causes of 'shunt':
- General anaesthesia
- IPPV
- Bronchial intubation
- Aspiration
- Embolus
- Oesophageal intubation
- Pulmonary oedema
- Malignant hyperthermia.

Reduced cardiac output and shunt:
A reduced cardiac output may result in a low mixed venous oxygen content, because more oxygen is extracted in the tissues. In many circumstances increased venous admixture causes a decrease in shunt fraction, so that P_aO_2 is not decreased. However, anaesthesia may interfere with this useful adaptation, and desaturation results. In any case, a fall in cardiac output will decrease the oxygen flux to the tissues (Oxygen flux = Oxygen content × Cardiac output) (Figure 2). It is therefore necessary to ensure that cardiac ouput is adequate, particularly when the patient has pulmonary pathology.

Practical points
- Hypoxaemia due to shunt may not respond to small increases in F_IO_2
- Hypoxaemia due to shunt will often respond to intravenous fluids, inotropes or PEEP.

PREOXYGENATION

Desaturation (SPO_2 less than 90%) is common during induction of (and emergence from) anaesthesia. This can be prevented by allowing the patient to breathe high concentrations of oxygen before induction. The patient will then remain well saturated for about 3 min, even if the airway is obstructed. The time taken to wash out the nitrogen in the lungs and a small amount in the blood and tissues depends on the alveolar ventilation. A nonrebreathing circuit must be used for this purpose, such as a Mapleson A circuit with an 8 l min^{-1} fresh gas flow.

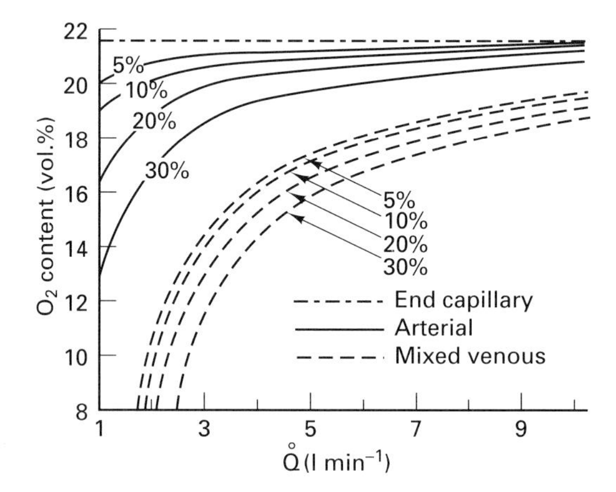

Figure 2
Oxygen content, cardiac output and 'shunt'. At higher levels of shunt a drop in cardiac output can be associated with a substantial fall in saturation. (Reproduced with permission from Kelman et al 1967.)

Less complete, but clinically valuable preoxygenation can be conveniently accomplished by applying a standard oxygen mask to all patients on arrival in the anaesthetic room.

PERIOPERATIVE HYPOXAEMIA

Desaturation (SPo_2 less than 90%) is common both before and for even a week after surgery, particularly at night. The significance of minor hypoxaemia is unknown and treatment is difficult, since oxygen delivery systems are uncomfortable and patient compliance is poor.

MONITORING OXYGEN SATURATION

- Cyanosis is a difficult sign, especially in coloured people. The surgical wound is the best site to observe.
- Pulse oximetry is regarded by most as a massive contribution to patient safety, despite the fact that it may never be possible to prove that patient outcome (in terms of death and cerebral damage) is improved.
- The accuracy of pulse oximeters is reduced by black and purple nail varnish and poor peripheral perfusion. Falsely high readings are seen in carbon monoxide poisoning.
- For ethical reasons, instrument calibration at low saturations is impossible.

BIBLIOGRAPHY

Benumof J L. Respiratory physiology and respiratory function during anaesthesia. In: Millar R D (ed) Anesthesia, 3rd edn. Churchill Livingstone, New York, 1990, p 504–549

Eichorn J E. Pulse oximetry as a standard of practice in anesthesia. Anesthesiology 1993; 78: 423–427

Hanning C D. Prolonged postoperative oxygen therapy. British Journal of Anaesthesia 1992; 69: 115–116

John R E, Peacock J E. Limitations of pulse oximetry. Lancet 1993; 341: 1092–1093

Keenan R L, Boyan C P. Cardiac arrest due to anesthesia: a study of incidence and causes. Journal of the American Medical Association 1985; 253: 2373–2377

Kelman G F, Nunn J F, Prys Roberts C et al. The influence of cardiac output on arterial oxygenation: a theoretical study. British Journal of Anaesthesia 1967; 39: 450

Moller J T, Johannessen N W, Espersen K et al. Randomized evaluation of pulse oximetry in 20,802 patients. Anesthesiology 1993; 78: 436–445

DEATH OR BRAIN DAMAGE DUE TO UPPER AIRWAY PROBLEMS

I. Calder

The true incidence of death or brain damage due to airway problems is not known. Statistics are hard to assemble; death due to airway problems may occur years after the event. Many incidents are followed by legal proceedings, usually civil but sometimes criminal. Airway problems cause the majority of deaths associated with anaesthesia.

Causes:
- Equipment
- Failed intubation/ventilation
- Oesophageal intubation
- Hypoventilation
- Aspiration

The mechanism is *hypoxaemia*, but hypercarbia and acidosis often contribute.

EQUIPMENT

Faulty equipment

Leaks and misconnections in the anaesthetic equipment must be detected by rigorous preanaesthetic checks. *Carbon dioxide cylinders* should be removed from the machine, unless specifically required. (Deaths have occurred from the rotameter's fully open position going unnoticed.)

Unavailable equipment

Never (except in bizarre, exceptional circumstances) induce general anaesthesia without access to:

- A source of oxygen
- A means of inflating the lungs
- Suction apparatus
- Muscle relaxant drugs
- Laryngoscope and tracheal tubes.

Extremely desirable equipment:
- Laryngeal mask airway
- Gum elastic bougie
- Oesophageal detector device
- Capnometer
- Oximeter
- Disconnection alarm.

FAILED INTUBATION/VENTILATION (PRIMARY AND SECONDARY)

Primary failure to ventilate the lungs with a mask and airway despite adequate relaxation and anaesthesia is, fortunately, very rare (0.01–1:10,000 patients).

Secondary failure is caused by glottic swelling after persistent attempts to intubate. *Failed intubation should not, but can, cause failed ventilation.*

OESOPHAGEAL INTUBATION

Death from oesophageal intubation nearly always follows *easy* laryngoscopy, because checks of tube position are not performed. Oesophageal intubation can be identified by:

- Auscultation of chest *and* abdomen
- Oesophageal detector device (ODD)
- Expired air carbon dioxide monitoring.

If no capnometer is available at the time when the patient is intubated then another method of confirmation must be used. The 1993 NCEPOD report (Campling et al 1993) found that capnography was only applied in the anaesthetic room in 6.7% of cases.

Detection of oesophageal intubation using the detector device is instantaneous and completely reliable. The bulb of the ODD may refill slowly in about 15% of cases, despite the tube being in the trachea. The total failure to refill associated with oesophageal intubation is unmistakeable.

If auscultation of the chest is used alone, about 25% of cases are missed, possibly because inflation of the stomach may cause quiet expiratory breath sounds. Auscultation becomes reliable if the upper abdomen is also auscultated.

Oesophageal intubation:
- Follows *easy* laryngoscopy
- Check every case

HYPOVENTILATION

An understanding of the relationships between tissue oxygen saturation, $F_{I}O_2$ and alveolar ventilation is helpful. Adequate pulse oximeter readings can give a false sense of security.

ASPIRATION

The incidence of aspiration pneumonitis is low (0.05% overall, 0.1% in emergencies); About 5% of cases die, and 17% require mechanical ventilation. Patients without symptoms 2 h after apparent aspiration are unlikely to develop pulmonary sequelae.

The stomach contains more than 25 ml of fluid with a pH of less than 2.5 in *half* of patients prepared for elective surgery. It is probably safe to allow clear fluids to within 2 h of induction.

BIBLIOGRAPHY

Andersen K H, Hald A. Assessing the position of the tracheal tube: the reliability of different methods. Anaesthesia 1989; 44: 984–989

Campling E A, Devlin H B, Hoile R W, Lunn J N. The Report of the National Confidential Enquiry into Perioperative Deaths 1993.

Caplan R A, Posner K L, Ward R J, Cheney F W. Adverse respiratory events in anaesthesia: a closed claims analysis. Anesthesiology 1990; 72: 828–833

King T A, Adams A P. Failed tracheal intubation. British Journal of Anaesthesia 1990; 65: 400–414

Olsson G L, Hallen B, Hambraeus-Jonzon K. Aspiration during anaesthesia: a computer-aided study of 185 358 anaesthetics. Acta Anaesthesiologica Scandinavica 1986; 30: 84–92

Strunin L. How long should patients fast before surgery? Time for new guidelines. British Journal of Anaesthesia 1993; 70: 1–4

Warner M A, Warner M E, Weber J G. Clinical significance of pulmonary aspiration during the perioperative period. Anesthesiology 1993; 78: 56–62

Zaleski L, Abello D, Gold M I. The esophageal detector device – does it work? Anesthesiology 1993; 79: 244–247

EFFECT OF GENERAL ANAESTHESIA ON THE AIRWAY/UPPER ALIMENTARY CANAL

I. Calder and R. Vanner

EFFECT ON OROPHARYNGEAL AND GLOTTIC STRUCTURES – THE 'NANDI EFFECT'

Induction of anaesthesia usually causes obstruction of the upper airway. Alterations in the tone of the skeletal muscles of the pharynx and neck are thought to be responsible. It has been shown that the soft palate, tongue and glottic opening may all impinge on the posterior pharyngeal wall when anaesthesia is induced. The glottic opening is similar to the tip of a Tuohy needle. This can be appreciated by examining a lateral cervical radiograph or MR scan. It is easy to see how the glottis can obstruct against the posterior pharyngeal wall. The term 'swallowing the tongue' is an oversimplification.

The obstruction is often relieved by stretching the anterior neck tissues, which is achieved by extending the head on the neck. This may need to be combined with protrusion of the mandible (the combination is the *Esmarch–Heiberg manoeuvre*).

It is sometimes easier to maintain a clear airway in the supine position, as opposed to the lateral 'coma' position usually recommended for unconscious patients. It seems that a surface under the occiput allows more effective application of the Esmarch–Heiberg manoeuvre.

RECOGNITION OF AN OBSTRUCTED AIRWAY

A *conscious patient* may be dysphonic, aphonic, anxious and, ultimately, exhausted.

A *spontaneously breathing patient* will generate large negative intrathoracic pressures (but not if there is also respiratory depression), which will cause:

- Noisy inspiration, due to turbulent gas flow (a completely obstructed airway is silent)
- Tracheal tug, intercostal recession
- Paradoxical respiratory movements.

Airway obstruction encourages gastro-oesophageal reflux.

A *ventilated patient* will have high inflation pressures.

In both spontaneous and artificial ventilation:

- Carbon dioxide excretion will be impaired – capnometer traces will be flattened or absent; arterial blood gases will reveal a respiratory acidosis
- Desaturation may be late and sudden, if the $F_{I}O_2$ is high
- Oximetry is not a good monitor of airway patency.

Signs of obstruction:
- Noise
- Tracheal tug
- Paradoxical movements
- Inflation pressure high
- Abnormal carbon dioxide trace

PULMONARY OEDEMA FOLLOWING RELIEF OF AIRWAY OBSTRUCTION

The large transpulmonary pressure gradients during obstruction may cause alveolar fluid collection. This presents as pulmonary oedema when the obstruction is relieved. Positive pressure ventilation may be required. An ARDS picture may result.

GLOTTIC REFLEXES

The MAC for glottic stimulation is 30% higher than for surgical incision. Tachycardia and hypertension follow laryngoscopy and intubation, unless adequate anaesthesia is given.

'LARYNGOSPASM'

Glottic closure reflexes are uninhibited during light anaesthesia. Laryngospasm may complicate induction of anaesthesia, surgical stimulation, extubation and recovery. It is probably the most frequent serious airway complication.

Desaturation can often be avoided by giving 100% oxygen. Deepening the level of anaesthesia (propofol or diazepam) is usually effective, but muscle relaxants may be required to relieve the spasm. As little as 5 mg of suxamethonium may be effective.

OESOPHAGEAL SPHINCTER FUNCTION AND ANAESTHESIA

The lower oesophageal sphincter

The intraluminal pressure at the gastro-oesophageal junction is 15–25 mmHg above gastric pressure, which normally prevents gastro-oesophageal reflux. The pressure is produced by smooth muscle cells of the lower oesophageal sphincter. Contraction of the surrounding skeletal muscle of the diaphragmatic crura increases the intraluminal pressure during inspiration, and also during straining. Straining does not cause gastro-oesophageal reflux in normal conscious patients. Reflux may occur spontaneously after a meal.

Reflux does not occur spontaneously during anaesthesia, but diaphragmatic tone decreases and thus its protective effect may be lost. Reflux is associated with hiccup, straining, deep inspiration with surgical stimulus, and bucking on the tracheal tube, all features of light anaesthesia.

A sudden, brief rise in lower oesophageal sphincter pressure is seen at the same time as the onset of fasciculation after suxamethonium, probably as a result of diaphragmatic contraction.

Intravenous atropine and other cholinergics can cause a decrease in lower oesophageal sphincter pressure sufficient to permit free reflux. Sphincter pressure is unaffected when atropine is combined with neostigmine.

Very small, and probably clinically insignificant, decreases in sphincter pressure are caused by intravenous and inhalational anaesthetic agents, the laryngeal mask airway and the lithotomy position.

The steep Trendelenburg position used during pelvic laparoscopy does not cause gastro-oesophageal reflux.

The oesophagus

The oesophagus is a muscular tube about 25 cm in length, which begins at the caudal border of the cricoid cartilage and ends at the cardiac orifice of the stomach, usually about 1.5 cm below the diaphragm. The upper quarter is composed of skeletal muscle only, the lower third of smooth muscle only and the middle is a mixture of the two types. The oesophagus can contain large volumes of fluid (up to 200 ml).

Refluxed gastric contents are cleared by oesophageal peristalsis, which is initiated by swallowing or local reflex.

Both general anaesthesia and intravenous atropine inhibit oesophageal motility. Oesophageal clearance may not occur despite gastro-oesophageal reflux during general anaesthesia. The refluxed contents will remain in the oesophagus, increasing the risk of regurgitation into the pharynx, until swallowing recommences as the patient awakes.

The upper oesophageal sphincter

The upper sphincter is formed by the lamina of the cricoid cartilage anteriorly and the striated muscle cricopharyngeus posteriorly. Resting upper oesophageal sphincter pressure is about 40 mmHg.

Both intravenous thiopentone and suxamethonium decrease upper oesophageal sphincter pressure to less than 10 mmHg, a pressure low enough to allow regurgitation of oesophageal contents. The low upper oesophageal sphincter pressure caused by suxamethonium is not further reduced by laryngoscopy. With thiopentone, the fall in sphincter pressure starts *before* loss of consciousness.

Intravenous induction with ketamine or inhalational induction with halothane maintains upper oesophageal sphincter pressure, in the absence of neuromuscular blockade. Upper oesophageal sphincter pressure may rise to over 100 mmHg during coughing and straining under light anaesthesia, and prevent regurgitation.

Intravenous benzodiazepines, such as midazolam, reduce upper sphincter pressure. They also depress laryngeal reflexes. Heavy sedation may allow aspiration.

There have been case reports of regurgitation during anaesthesia when a laryngeal mask has been in use. Whether regurgitation and aspiration is more frequent using this airway instead of an oral Guedel airway and face-mask remains to be seen.

BIBLIOGRAPHY

Chung D C, Rowbotham S J. A very small dose of suxamethonium relieves laryngospasm. Anaesthesia 1993; 48: 229–230

Drummond G B. Keep a clear airway (Editorial). British Journal of Anaesthesia 1991; 66: 153–156

Herrick I A, Mahendran B, Penny F J. Postobstructive pulmonary edema following anesthesia. Journal of Clinical Anesthesia 1990; 2: 116–120

Nandi P R, Charlesworth C H, Taylor S J, Nunn J F, Dore C J. Effect of general anaesthesia on the pharynx. British Journal of Anasthesia 1991; 66: 157–162

Swann D G, Drummond G B. Effect of supine and lateral positions on airway patency in anaesthetised patients. British Journal of Anaesthesia 1991; 67: 644P

Vanner R G. Mechanisms of regurgitation and its prevention with cricoid pressure. International Journal of Obstetric Anaesthesia 1993; 2: 207–215

ARTIFICIAL AIRWAYS

I. Calder

Artificial airways:
- Face-mask
- Oral/nasal airways
- Laryngeal mask
- Tracheal tube
- Cricothyroid cannula
- Tracheostomy

FACE-MASK

Designed to fit the face; many practitioners believe that edentulous patients should be encouraged to wear their dentures during anaesthesia, as a good fit is difficult if they are removed.

ORAL/NASAL AIRWAYS

The timing of airway insertion calls for judgement. An airway will often relieve an obstruction, but if the patient is too 'light', it may provoke coughing, breath holding and laryngospasm.

A nasal airway should be used in patients with fragile teeth, crowns or bridges. Nasal airways should be avoided in patients with bleeding disorders.

LARYNGEAL MASK

For easy insertion of a laryngeal-mask airway (LMA) the patient must be deeply anaesthetized or paralysed. Propofol provides the best conditions for insertion. There is a small insertion failure rate. The oesophageal detector device (ODD) can be used to check position. A bite block must be used; the device should be left in until the patient is awake. The LMA can be used as an aid to fibre-optic guided intubation (6.0 mm Mallinkrodt metal reinforced tubes).

TRACHEAL TUBE

Intubation

The glottic closure reflexes must be obtunded before a tracheal tube can be placed. This can be achieved with topical anaesthesia, deep general anaesthesia, or muscle relaxant drugs.

The tracheal tube can be placed under direct vision, over a flexible fibre-optic endoscope or retrogradely over a guide passed from the trachea, either blind or by observation of transillumination from a lighted tip (Lightwand).

Direct laryngoscopy

A 'line of vision' must be established from eye to glottis. This requires:

- Artificial *protrusion* of the mandible and tongue with the blade of the laryngoscope
- *Flexion* of the neck and *extension* at the craniocervical junction – the 'sniffing the morning air' position, described by Magill.

Size of tube

The cross-sectional area of the narrowest point of the glottic opening (true cords) corresponds to that of an 8.0 mm tracheal tube in men, and a 7.0 mm tube in women. Smaller sizes can be used, since resistance to gas flow is only clinically significant below 6.0 mm. There is little to be gained and a price to be paid (insertion is more difficult and the incidence of sore throat is higher), if larger sizes are used.

Tissue damage and orotracheal intubation

Sore throat and hoarseness are common, but should settle within 48 h. Persisting or severe symptoms require laryngological advice. Haematoma of the cords is the commonest complication; dislocation of the arytenoid (usually left) cartilage is rare, but requires immediate treatment. Arytenoid dislocation has been reported after easy intubation. Reports of recurrent laryngeal nerve palsy caused by intubation may have been describing dislocation.

Perforation of the pharyngeal mucosa by stilettes or bougies can cause mediastinitis.

Oral or nasal tube?

Nasal tube – against:

- Mucosal damage is common, both in the nasal cavity and to the posterior pharyngeal wall. Mortality from pharyngeal abscess has been reported. Damage to, or even avulsion of, the turbinates occurs. Much damage can be avoided by using a suction catheter or fibre-optic endoscope as a 'Seldinger' guide.
- Severe bleeding can occur – bleeding disorders and infected blood represent contraindications. Mucosal engorgement in pregnant women at term is a relative contraindication.
- Closed base-of-skull fractures can be converted to open fractures by nasal intubation.
- Bacteraemia is common after nasal intubation (but not after insertion of nasal airways). Half of nasally intubated patients develop bacterial sinusitis if intubated for more than 4 days; nasogastric tubes are also associated with an increased incidence of sinusitis.

Nasal tubes – for

- The nasal route is often necessary when direct laryngoscopy is difficult.
- Intraoral surgery.
- A nasal tube is easier to fix and the patient cannot bite it. There are fewer episodes of accidental extubation and main bronchus intubation with a nasal tube. It is often claimed that a nasal tube is more comfortable for the patient.

Conclusion

Nasal tubes can cause serious morbidity and occasional mortality. The popularity of long-term nasal intubation is decreasing, but it may be justified in situations in which accidental decannulation might have serious consequences.

Extubation

Desaturation is probably commoner at extubation than at any other time. Preoxygenation is recommended.

Direct laryngoscopy and suction should be performed prior to extubation, if possible. Blind suction of the pharynx may be traumatic, mucosal perforation and mediastinitis has been reported.

Laryngospasm, breath holding and severe coughing can complicate extubation, unless the patient is wide awake (patient takes his own tube out) or deeply anaesthetized (no reaction to laryngoscopy and suction). Problems arise when the level of anaesthesia is somewhere between the two extremes. It may be necessary to deepen anaesthesia and/ or reparalyse the patient.

Deep anaesthesia extubation

The airway is inevitably unprotected and must be supported. However, recovery is usually smoother in terms of coughing and laryngospasm. Desaturation is less frequent than is the case with extubation at light levels of anaesthesia.

Awake extubation

This is preferable if the patient has a difficult airway (see below). Consider *delaying* extubation during unsocial hours in difficult cases.

CRICOTHYROID CANNULAE/TRACHEOSTOMY

Percutaneous cricothyroid membrane puncture

This can be life-saving in total airway obstruction. Unfortunately the procedure is associated with considerable morbidity (29% complication rate). It should probably be reserved for 'dire emergencies or well thought out elective situations'. This means that few anaesthetists will have experience of the technique.

Anaesthetists should familiarize themselves with the anatomy and be able to construct a system capable of delivering oxygen, e.g. a tracheal tube inserted into the barrel of a syringe inserted into a 14 gauge cannula. A metal needle (such as a Tuohy epidural) may be preferred, being less likely to kink. Pulmonary barotrauma is a major problem if expiration is obstructed. A high-pressure gas source is required if ventilation is to be achieved.

Larger percutaneous cannulas, such as the Minitrach (Portex) or Quicktrach (Dulker) with 4.0 mm internal diameter have the advantage that expiration should be relatively un-obstructed and capnography can be used. They may also have a lower incidence of misplacement.

The condition(s) that made the intervention necessary may well make the insertion of a percutaneous device difficult, especially in an emergency.

Tracheostomy

Tracheostomies should be stitched in place as well as taped until a track has formed. Recannulation after accidental decannulation before a track has formed (about 10 days) is often unsuccessful.

The place of percutaneous dilatational (Ciaglia) tracheostomy is under review. The complication rate may be less than with conventional tracheostomy in the short term, but long-term follow-up is awaited.

BIBLIOGRAPHY

Bach A, Boehrer H, Schmidt H, Geiss H K. Nosocomial sinusitis in ventilated patients. Nasotracheal versus orotracheal intubation. Anaesthesia 1992; 47: 335–339

Benumof J L, Scheller M S. The importance of transtracheal jet ventilation in the management of the difficult airway. Anesthesiology 1989; 72: 828–833

Hartley M, Vaughan R S. Problems associated with tracheal extubation. British Journal of Anaesthesia 1993; 71: 561–568

Kambic V, Radsel L. Intubation injuries of the larynx. British Journal of Anaesthesia 1978; 50: 587–590

Pennant J H, White P F. The laryngeal mask airway: its uses in anesthesiology. Anesthesiology 1993; 79: 144–164

Stout D M, Bishop M J, Dwersteg J F, Cullen B F. Correlation of endotracheal tube size with sore throat and hoarseness following general anaesthesia. Anesthesiology 1987; 67: 419–421

30

DIFFICULT AIRWAY – OVERVIEW

I. Calder

A totally satisfactory definition is difficult. The clinical situation is often a mixture of the problems described below.

- *The anaesthetist must consider whether the induction of anaesthesia will result in inability to maintain the airway.*
- *If in doubt, ask for help.* Additional assistance was found to be 'the most desired aid' in a recent survey of reports of difficult intubation. This includes surgical assistance, in case an elective or emergency tracheotomy is required.
- The difficult airway comprises one or more of the following problems:
  - Difficult mask anaesthesia/ventilation
  - Difficult direct laryngoscopy
  - Difficult intubation
  - Aspiration risk
  - Uncooperative patient.

DIFFICULT AIRWAY – ASPIRATION RISK

R. Vanner

Patients at risk include those with:

- Full stomach
- Gastro-oesophageal reflux
- Oesophageal pathology
- Last half of pregnancy
- Hiccups, straining or coughing during light anaesthesia.

PROPHYLACTIC DRUGS

Decreasing the volume of gastric contents reduces the chance of regurgitation. Raising the gastric pH may limit lung damage if aspiration does occur. Oral ranitidine and sodium citrate are commonly used. Soluble paracetomol (Panadol) is also an effective antacid.

OPTIONS FOR ANAESTHESIA

- Regional anaesthesia with an awake patient
- Awake fibre-optic intubation before induction of general anaesthesia
- Intubation after rapid sequence intravenous induction with preoxygenation and cricoid pressure
- Intubation after induction in the left lateral head-down position.

Pulmonary aspiration has been reported with all the options mentioned above.

STOMACH TUBES

Patients with bowel obstruction, peritonitis, or diabetic ketoacidosis should always have nasogastric tube drainage preoperatively, which should be aspirated before induction of anaesthesia. A Salem sump tube with two lumens is the most efficient.

A recent meal may be difficult to aspirate through a tube, and inducing emesis is probably the only way to empty the stomach, albeit unreliably. It is unwise to induce emesis in a patient with a reduced conscious level.

The nasogastric tube, open to the atmosphere, should left in place during induction of anaesthesia. A nasogastric tube does not interfere with oesophageal sphincter function or cricoid pressure.

The stomach should be decompressed with a large-bore orogastric tube before extubation.

CRICOID PRESSURE

- A pillow should be placed under the occiput, not the shoulders.
- A properly trained assistant is mandatory.
- A bimanual technique is preferred by some (the neck support prevents the head from flexing on the neck); however, others prefer the single-handed technique that leaves the assistant's other hand free to help with intubation. If the bimanual technique is used another assistant is needed.
- The nasogastric tube should be left in place, but it must be open to vent gas or liquid.
- Cricoid pressure should be applied to the awake patient with a force of 10 N (1 kg), after preoxygenation but before intravenous induction.
- If retching occurs after intravenous induction, the cricoid pressure should not be released, as oesophageal rupture is unlikely at this level of cricoid force.
- Cricoid pressure should be increased to a force of 30 N (3 kg) after loss of consciousness and before the onset of suxamethonium fasciculations.
- The assistant should practice the correct application of force on a weighing scale.
- Sellick originally described a three-fingered technique, with the main force applied by the index finger; others have recommended two fingers.
- The assistant should try to keep the larynx in the midline.
- Cricoid pressure should not be released until tracheal intubation is confirmed.

BIBLIOGRAPHY

Vanner R G. Mechanisms of regurgitation and its prevention with cricoid pressure. International Journal of Obstetric Anesthesia 1993; 2: 207–215

DIFFICULT AIRWAY – DIFFICULT DIRECT LARYNGOSCOPY

I. Calder

Definition:
'Difficult' direct laryngoscopy is generally regarded as Cormack and Lehane grades 3 and 4 (see Figure 1.)

Incidence

Grade 3 glottic visibility occurs in only 1.5% of unselected patients. Grade 4 is rare; severe rheumatoid arthritis is the commonest cause.

CAUSES

Difficult laryngoscopy is caused by poor mouth opening and stiffness of the cervical spine, particularly the craniocervical junction. Swelling of the oropharyngeal tissues can also prevent vision.

Difficulty is rare in the young and healthy, whose joints are mobile.

Diseases regularly associated with difficulty include arthritis (particularly rheumatoid arthritis), oropharyngeal infections and tumours, ankylosing spondylitis, acromegaly and the Klippel–Feil abnormalities of the cervical spine. Iatrogenic causes include interdental wiring and cervical fixators.

PREDICTION

It is rare for a patient without a cause, such as the diseases already mentioned, to present severe problems. Various tests have been described (Mallampati, Patil), which appear to

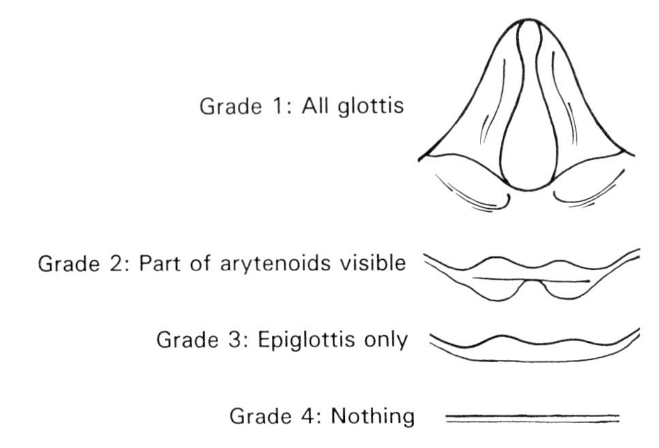

Figure 1
Cormack and Lehane's classification of glottic visibility.

perform well when applied retrospectively to difficult patients. However, prospective trials have shown that the false-positive rate associated with prediction in a general population may be as high as 96%. It is also unfortunately the case that the available tests have sensitivities of about 50% (i.e. half the cases are missed).

It is more important to be aware of the various methods of dealing with difficult laryngoscopy than to expect to be able to accurately identify the rare difficult patients without predisposing cause.

It is nevertheless good policy to routinely examine all patients, mouth opening ability, if only to confirm that laryngoscopy will be easy.

Tests of mouth opening

Tests of cervical movement appear to be difficult to apply successfully. In patients with cervical disease, radiographic evidence of poor separation of the occiput, atlas and axis on a flexion film does reliably indicate difficulty.

Difficult laryngoscopy should be expected if mandibular protrusion is impaired (grade B – edge to edge'), or pharyngeal visibility is Mallampati grade 3, *and* there is disease of the cervical spine affecting the upper three vertebrae (Figure 2). There will still be false-positive results. In patients with grade C protrusion (lower incisors cannot be protruded to touch the upper incisors), direct laryngoscopy is *always* difficult.

It is much easier to predict *easy laryngoscopy* (the arithmetic of incidence, sensitivity and specificity guarantees a low false-positive rate). A Mallampati grade 1 or mandibular protrusion grade A (lower incisors in front of upper incisors) virtually excludes difficult laryngoscopy.

The 'anterior larynx'

Poor mouth opening is usually due to temporomandibular joint dysfunction causing failure of mandibular protrusion. If the mandible cannot be held forward with the laryngoscope, the glottis cannot be properly displayed. The term 'anterior larynx' has been used to describe this situation, but is misleading since it is not the larynx which is anterior but the mandible that is posterior.

MANAGEMENT OF DIFFICULT LARYNGOSCOPY

Severe difficulty expected

Some difficulty in mask ventilation is not uncommon in difficult laryngoscopy. The Esmarch–Heiberg manoeuvre is made difficult if the cervical spine is rigid and mandibular protrusion limited.

Awake fibre-optic intubation is the method of choice, and is acceptable to most patients. Fibre-optic laryngoscopy can be regarded as part of preoperative examination and should be presented to the patient in that manner. The cardiovascular stability associated with fibre-optic intubation under topical anaesthesia is an attractive feature of the technique.

Nasal intubation is frequently easier in this

Mallampati (Pharyngeal visibility)

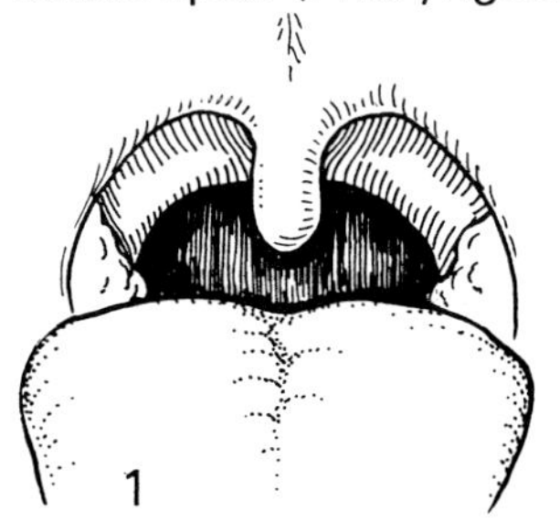

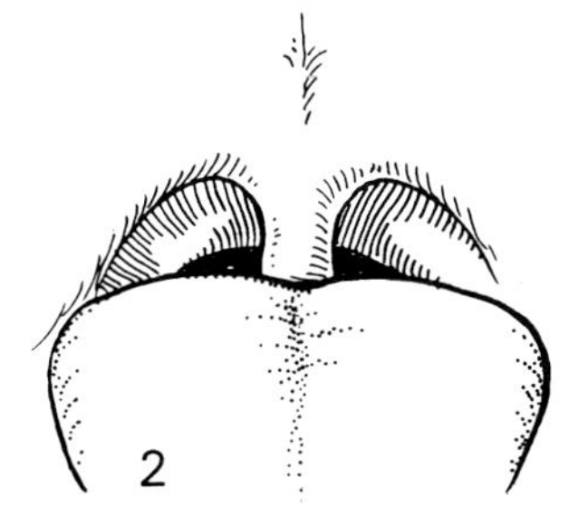

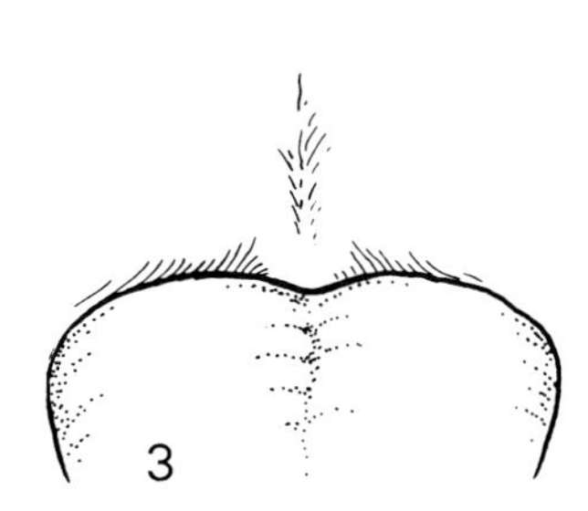

Figure 2
Tests of mouth opening.

group of patients, because of limited mouth opening, and the poor 'angle of attack' with the oral route. The nasal mucosa should be shrunk with xylometazoline (Otrivine) before endoscopy. Lignocaine is poorly absorbed from the nasopharynx; toxic reactions are unlikely. The reverse is true of cocaine. Topical anaesthesia is more effective if glycopyrrolate is given to cut down secretions. Lignocaine is irritant to the nasal mucosa; initial application should be with a warm 1% solution or 2% gel; 10% lignocaine can then be applied to nasal and pharyngeal mucosa. The glottis is liberally sprayed with 4% lignocaine through the endoscope (about 6 ml). An alternative is to inject 4% lignocaine through the cricothyroid membrane. Coughing can be very vigorous, but will result in satisfactory anaesthesia. The glottis will not be anaesthetized if the patient does not cough.

It is foolish to attempt to pass a tube of greater than 7.0 mm internal diameter over a fibre-optic endoscope. Metal-reinforced tubes (Mallinkrodt) are best, and *rotation of the tube as it is passed* is helpful. It is sensible to administer some sedation as the tube is passed, as the passage of the tube through the nose is unpleasant.

Retrogade intubation is an alternative when fibre-optic technology and skill is not available. An epidural catheter or J-tipped wire is passed through a Tuohy needle into the pharynx, recovered in the pharynx and an introducer (a fibre-optic laryngoscope is ideal) or tracheal tube passed over it. The crico-tracheal membrane may be a better entrance site than the cricothyroid membrane (reduced incidence of bleeding and deeper penetration of the glottis by the tube).

Uncooperative, unconscious or lesser degree of expected difficulty

Such patients can be managed fibre-optically under general anaesthesia, or with a gum elastic bougie or laryngeal mask airway, as described below. Preoxygenation of the patient is a sensible precaution.

Unexpected difficulty

Gum elastic bougie

This outstandingly useful item should *always* be ready for use.

Technique:

- Continue exposure of the glottis with laryngoscope throughout.
- Lubricate *only* the tip of the bougie. Pass the bougie, suitably bent, before loading a *small (6.0–7.0 mm) tube.*
- Lubricate the tip of the tube, and the bougie, as the tube enters the mouth.
- Rotate the tube 90° *anticlockwise* as it approaches the glottis.
- Remove bougie and laryngoscope. Apply oesophageal detector device.

Laryngeal mask airway

In some cases successful positioning of a laryngeal mask airway (LMA) may be all that is required. If intubation is required, a 6.0 mm tube can be passed blindly in over half of cases. Alternatively a gum elastic bougie can be passed through the LMA, which is removed and a tube passed over the bougie.

A fibre-optic laryngoscope is usually easy to pass into the trachea via a LMA. A 6.0 mm tube is then *rotated* into the trachea. The only 6.0 mm tube of adequate length is the metal-reinforced tube manufactured by Mallinkrodt. This is a very successful technique.

Specially made split LMAs have been constructed to allow larger sizes of tube to be passed and the removal of the LMA.

Blind nasal intubation

Skilful practitioners can achieve a remarkable degree of success. A combination of direct laryngoscopy and guiding a nasal tube towards the glottis with Magill's forceps is easier for most anaesthetists.

Repeated attempts are to be deprecated, as laryngeal damage and airway obstruction may result.

'Taking over ventilation before paralysis' in suspected difficult laryngoscopy

This practice is often recommended to trainees, the rationale being that the 'failure to intubate/ventilate syndrome' may be identified before the patient is rendered apnoeic by muscle relaxants.

If the airway becomes obstructed after induction, muscle relaxants are often (in practice) required to allow ventilation. The 'failure to intubate/ventilate' syndrome is very rare, although some difficulty in mask ventilation has been reported has been repeated in 1:7 cases of difficult intubation. Relying on a return of consciousness to clear the airway may not always be in the patient's interest. Relaxants should be given if the anaesthetist believes that the patient will benefit.

If difficult mask ventilation is expected, a tracheal tube or tracheostomy should be placed before induction.

Direct laryngoscopy and the unstable cervical spine

There is no evidence that direct laryngoscopy (and cricoid pressure) is more dangerous than any other method of intubation. Many patients with severe instability are in cervical fixation devices, which restrict mouth opening and cervical movements. In these circumstances, awake fibre-optic intubation is probably the method of choice.

Failed intubation in the patient with a full stomach

Repeated unsuccessful attempts at intubation can cause airway obstruction; a mature anaesthetist will admit failure early. If a gum elastic bougie cannot be passed within 1 min, serious consideration should be given to abandoning intubation attempts.

Failure occurs most commonly in obstetric practice (1:200–300 obstetrics, 1:2000 general surgery). The drill below refers to obstetric patients, but is applicable to all. The patient has already had preoxygenation, cricoid pressure followed by intravenous induction and suxamethonium.

'Failed intubation' drill:

- Inform surgeon and call for senior anaesthetic help
- Maintain cricoid pressure and keep patient in supine wedged position
- Insert an oral airway and ventilate with 100% oxygen
- Continue to mask ventilate until spontaneous ventilation starts, *then* turn the patient into the left lateral position, remove the pillow and *then* release cricoid pressure
- If mask ventilation is not possible, try the following:
  - Reduce (*not release*) cricoid pressure by half
  - Insert a laryngeal mask, continue cricoid pressure; remove laryngeal mask if no success.
  - Cricothyroid puncture.

BIBLIOGRAPHY

Calder I. Anaesthesia for spinal surgery. In: Walters J M, Ingram G S, Jenkinson J L (eds). Anaesthesia and intensive care for the neurosurgical patient. Blackwell, Oxford, 1994, p 274–317 [Detailed description of fibre-optic intubation, with photographs]

Nolan J P, Wilson M E. An evaluation of the gum elastic bougie. Intubation times and incidence of sore throat. Anaesthesia 1992; 47: 878–881

Shantha T R. Retrograde intubation using the subcricoid region. British Journal of Anaesthesia 1992; 68: 109–112

Sidhu V S, Whitehead E M, Ainsworth Q P, Smith M, Calder I. A technique of awake fibreoptic intubation. Experience in patients with cervical spine disease. Anaesthesia 1993; 48: 910–913

Silk J M, Hill H M, Calder I. Difficult intubation and the laryngeal mask airway. European Journal of Anaesthesiology 1991; supl 4: 47–51

Wilson M E. Predicting difficult intubation. British Journal of Anaesthesia 1993; 71: 333–334

Wood P R, Lawler P G P. Managing the airway in cervical spine injury. A review of the advanced trauma life support protocol. Anaesthesia 1992; 47: 798–801

DIFFICULT AIRWAY – DIFFICULT TRACHEAL INTUBATION

I. Calder

Conditions that narrow the glottis or trachea include adult epiglottitis, tumours, airway burns, and oedema due to cervical haematomas or anaphylaxis.

Stridor is the principal sign, which is said to occur at rest when the airway diameter is reduced to 4.0 mm. The diameter of the airway can be seriously reduced without stridor being present. The combination of sore throat, hoarseness and dysphagia is very suggestive of adult epiglottitis. Antibiotic therapy should be started immediately. It should be appreciated that the condition of such patients can deteriorate rapidly.

Cervical haematomas (thyroid or anterior cervical surgery) produce oedema of the glottis. *Evacuation of the haematoma does not relieve airway obstruction immediately*, and is therefore secondary to the establishment of an airway in an emergency.

Inhalation of nebulized adrenaline (1 ml of 1:1000, in 10 ml of saline) may buy some time. In anaphylactic cases adrenaline (0.5–1.0 ml of 1:10 000) should be given intravenously.

MANAGEMENT

This will depend entirely on the severity of the condition.

Patients in extremis (deteriorating conscious level)

Emergency tracheotomy or cricothyrotomy

will be required if direct laryngoscopy fails. In many cases a gum elastic bougie can be passed and a 6.0 mm tube introduced over it.

Both emergency tracheotomy and direct laryngoscopy will be facilitated by sedation and muscle paralysis, there is nothing to lose.

Less urgent cases

In such cases decision-making is more complex.

Tracheostomy under local anaesthesia is often sensible, particularly if the condition is likely to persist.

Flexible fibre-optic laryngoscopy and intubation under topical anaesthesia will be appropriate, and part of the diagnostic process, in some cases. In patients with very swollen necks it may be the only sensible option.

Inhalational induction with halothane is the traditional method. Inhalational induction can only succeed if the airway is at least partially patent. Problems can arise with a prolonged excitement phase. Complete obstruction can occur. Judicious use of an intravenous agent, such as propofol, and application of CPAP can be helpful. Intravenous glycopyrrolate may reduce troublesome secretions.

Surgical assistance

It is prudent to obtain surgical assistance if an emergency tracheostomy might be necessary.

ANTERIOR MEDIASTINAL MASSES

Obstruction of the trachea or main bronchus can occur during anaesthesia in symptomless patients. General anaesthesia should be avoided if possible. Flow/volume loops may predict airway obstruction – obstruction has occurred during both spontaneous and positive pressure ventilation.

EXTUBATION AFTER INTUBATION FOR AIRWAY OBSTRUCTION

The minimum period of intubation should probably be 24 h. Adequate sedation must be prescribed, to prevent accidental extubation. A small tube should have been passed, so that deflation of the cuff and blocking the tube can demonstrate a satisfactory airway.

BIBLIOGRAPHY

Crosby E, Reid D. Acute epiglottitis in the adult: is intubation mandatory? Canadian Journal of Anaesthesia 1991; 38: 914–919

Neuman G G, Weingarten A E, Abramowitz R M, Kushins L G, Abramson A L, Ladner W. The anesthetic management of a patient with an anterior mediastinal mass. Anesthesiology 1984; 60: 144–147

Sparks C J. Ludwig's angina causing respiratory arrest in the Solomon Islands. Anaesthesia and Intensive Care 1993; 21: 460–463

DIFFICULT AIRWAY – DIFFICULT MASK ANAESTHESIA/ VENTILATION

I. Calder

Any patient whose airway cannot be maintained under anaesthesia or whose lungs cannot be inflated with the aid of a mask, is in immediate danger of death, unless a laryngeal mask, tracheal tube or cannula can be promptly inserted.

CAUSES

- *No seal between face and mask.* Facial abnormalities. Reasons range from absence of teeth and beards to massive facial trauma.
- *Reduced cross-sectional area of airway.* Tissue swelling from infection, trauma, burns, tumour or oedoema (cervical haematoma, anaphylaxis). Laryngospasm is the commonest cause.
- *Standard airway-clearing manoeuvres not possible.* If the Esmarch–Heiberg manoeuvre cannot be performed because of cervical rigidity or poor mandibular protrusion, it may be impossible to counteract the 'Nandi effect'. Patients in halo-body frames or with interdental wiring are extreme examples of this problem. These factors are also responsible for difficult direct laryngoscopy. Difficulty with mask ventilation has been reported to occur in 1:7 difficult laryngoscopies, but complete failure is very rare (0.01–1:10 000).

PREDICTING DIFFICULT MASK VENTILATION

Cases with readily identifiable problems, such as facial injuries, can be predicted. However, serious difficulty is, fortunately, very rare in apparently normal people. It is therefore unlikely that a predictive method will be successful (see difficult direct laryngoscopy)

In general, a tracheal airway should be placed before induction of anaesthesia in patients in whom it might be difficult to perform positive pressure ventilation with a mask. In practice, this means awake fibre-optic intubation or tracheostomy under local anaesthesia.

BIBLIOGRAPHY

American Society of Anesthesiologists Task Force. Practice guidelines for management of the difficult airway. Anesthesiology 1993; 78: 597–602

Benumof J L. Management of the difficult adult airway. Anesthesiology 1991; 75: 1087–1110

Ovassapian A. Fiberoptic airway endoscopy in anesthesia and critical care. Raven, New York, 1990

Williamson J A, Webb R K, Szekely S, Gillies E R N, Dreosti A V. Difficult incubation: an analysis of 2000 incident reports. Anaesthesia and Intensive Care 1993; 21: 602–667

PAEDIATRIC AIRWAY

R. Bingham

The child's airway is smaller and anatomically distinct from that of the adult. The tongue is relatively large and forms a seal with the palate. Infants are obligatory nose breathers when breathing quietly, and airway obstruction at oropharyngeal level is likely when pharyngeal muscle tone is reduced.

The external nares are the narrowest part of the airway and contribute up to 30% of the total airway resistance. Any additional obstruction at this point (e.g. nasogastric tube) may significantly increase the work of breathing.

The larynx is more cephalad and anterior than in adulthood; the epiglottis is long, floppy and U-shaped in cross-section. Intubation with a curved blade laryngoscope is difficult as the epiglottis cannot easily be lifted from above. It is easier to view the vocal cords with a straight blade used to lift the epiglottis from underneath.

The larynx itself is cone shaped. The narrowest part is at the level of the cricoid cartilage (the cricoid ring) and is circular in cross-section. A plain, uncuffed tube will form an effective seal at this point to facilitate IPPV.

The resistance to gas flow through a tube is inversely related to the fourth power of the radius. As a result, mucosal oedema results in large changes in airway resistance. Partial airway obstruction is therefore common in infants with upper airway inflammation (e.g. following extubation or in laryngotracheobronchitis). Stridor occurs because of turbulent flow during inspiration. Wheezing occurs when the intrathoracic airways expand during inspiration, and intrathoracic airway obstruction results in an expiratory noise.

Oxygen consumption in the infant is approximately double that of an adult and there is a reduced reserve of oxygen within the lungs. Should a problem with oxygenation occur, the onset of hypoxaemia is far more rapid.

AIRWAY MAINTENANCE

During induction, children are predisposed to upper airway obstruction. Simple airway manoeuvres may be used to overcome this:

Head tilt/chin lift:

- No pillow (a protuberant occiput generates cervical spine flexion)
- Gentle extension of the head at the atlanto-occipital joint
- Do not lift the chin under the jaw (this may push the tongue base upwards and backwards and further obstruct the airway)
- Pressure is exerted on the bony mandible only.

If this fails to clear the airway there are several further options (see below).

Jaw thrust manoeuvre

This is more efficient than the head tilt/chin lift, but requires two hands.

Oropharyngeal or nasopharyngeal airway

- Oral airway may cause laryngospasm or retching
- Sizes range from 000 to 4 (estimate size by comparison to child's face; it should extend from the lips to the angle of the jaw)
- Nasal airways are better tolerated; the correct diameter is the same as that for an orotracheal tube.

Constant positive airway pressure (CPAP):

- CPAP provides a pneumatic splint which distends the structures of the oropharynx
- CPAP is best provided with a T-piece circuit and partial obstruction of the reservoir bag.

Laryngeal mask airway (LMA):

- Particularly useful in anatomical deformities associated with an anterior larynx (e.g. Pierre–Robin syndrome)

- Insertion more difficult than in adults, as the angle between the palate and posterior pharynx is more acute. Solutions include:
  - Inserting the device upside down initially and then rotating it
  - Partial inflation
  - Guiding it round the posterior pharynx with a finger.

INTUBATION

One of two techniques are employed:

- The epiglottis is visualized; the laryngoscope is then slid underneath it and the tip of the blade lifted so that the glottis is exposed
- The laryngoscope blade is deliberately advanced into the oesophagus and then, with the tip lifted anteriorly, withdrawn slowly until the larynx drops into view.

Both techniques bring the blade in contact with the epiglottis. There is therefore intense vagal stimulation, and atropine premedication is advantageous.

In order to avoid damage to the cricoid region, it is essential to choose an uncuffed tube of the correct diameter. Tubes a half-size smaller and larger than the estimated correct size should also be available. Once the tube is in place there should be a small air leak at an inflation pressure of 29–30 cmH_2O, but none during normal ventilation. If the correct size of tube is chosen (Table 1) there is no danger from aspiration of gastric contents, and a pharyngeal pack is unnecessary.

Table 1.
Paediatric tracheal tube sizes

Age	Tube size (i.d.) (mm)
Newborn	3.0
6 months	3.5
1 year	4.0
> 1 year	Age/4 + 4

The length of the tube is crucial in small infants. Problems with calculating this can be avoided by:

- The use of uncut tubes
- Passing 3 cm of through the glottis
- Careful checking for air entry into both lungs.

This system has the additional advantage that connectors for the breathing circuit, capnograph, humidifier, etc., are distanced from the child's face.

Firm fixation of the tube is vital. Most people use a system based on adhesive tape fixed to the face and then wrapped around the tube. Extra security can be obtained by the application of a sticky substance such as tincture of benzoin or nobecutaine.

For long-term intubation nasal intubation is more secure than oral. It also reduces movement of the tube in the larynx and simplifies mouth care. The incidence of complications of this method in children is low.

Regular saline instillation and suction is important, as small tubes easily become obstructed by inspissated mucus.

DIFFICULT PAEDIATRIC LARYNGOSCOPY AND INTUBATION

This problem is less common than in adults. It is usually associated with

- Obvious deformity of the child's head or neck
- Mandibular hypoplasia (e.g. Pierre–Robin or Treacher–Collins syndrome) or space occupying lesions within the oropharynx (e.g. cystic hygroma, haemangioma).

The technique used will depend on the presence or absence of airway obstruction, the site of the anatomical problem and the age of the child.

Difficult laryngoscopy without airway obstruction

Intubation is usually performed under general anaesthesia as:

- Awake intubation is physically only possible in neonates in the first few days of life
- Fibre-optic laryngoscopy under topical anaesthesia may be possible, but it may be difficult to obtain full cooperation.

The anaesthetic technique usually involves spontaneous respiration although, in the absence of obstruction, a muscle relaxant may be used. It is prudent to check that manual ventilation is possible before instituting paralysis.

A variety of options may be used for the intubation itself.

Gum elastic bougie

Most difficult paediatric intubation can be accomplished by conventional laryngoscopy using this device. Occasionally, a two-operator technique may be useful; one operator manipulates the laryngoscope and brings the larynx into view by pressing on the neck, whilst the second performs the intubation itself.

Fibre-optic laryngoscope

A 2.5 mm internal diameter tracheal tube can pass over the smallest fibre-optic laryngoscope (although difficult to control). Larger sizes (3.8 mm outer diameter) can be used in the same way as in adults.

The technique is as follows:

- Anaesthesia is maintained via the nasal airway
- A two-person technique can be used:
  - First operator guides the tip as close to the larynx as possible using a conventional laryngoscope and Magill's forceps
  - The second operator monitors the advance into the larynx through the fibre-scope itself.

Laryngeal mask airway (LMA)

A plain 5.0 mm internal diameter tracheal tube can be passed through the size 2 mask or a 6.0 mm one through the size 2.5 mask. The tube can be advanced blindly, but as the epiglottis may be down-folded in children, it is better to pass the tube under direct vision over a fibre-optic laryngoscope. The LMA can then either be left in place or removed carefully. A further alternative is to advance a Seldinger wire into the larynx through the fibre-optic scope and thread a stiff catheter/dilator over this. The LMA can then be removed and the tube railroaded in. In all these manoeuvres it is important to practise them in advance so that the sequence of events is familiar to all the participants.

Difficult laryngoscopy accompanied by upper airway obstruction

The management of this difficult problem will depend on the site and nature of the obstruction and the age of the child.

Supraglotic obstruction

Awake intubation may be possible. This may be achieved with either a conventional laryngoscope in the newborn or with a fibre-optic scope under topical anaesthesia in the cooperative older child.

GENERAL ANAESTHESIA

General anaesthesia may be preferable because coughing or straining associated with laryngeal stimulation in an awake patient may precipitate complete airway obstruction (particularly likely in infective conditions such as acute epiglottitis):

- Spontaneous respiration must be maintained, usually with halothane in oxygen.
- The delivery of CPAP with a T-piece circuit and a well-fitting mask is an essential part of the technique.
- If airway obstruction is severe it can take a long time to reach a depth of anaesthesia sufficient to permit laryngoscopy.
- In laryngeal or tracheal obstruction, the intubation itself is usually accomplished with a conventional laryngoscope and a bougie.

For the initial control of the airway, intubation is usually oral. If long-term intubation is required this may be changed electively for a nasal tube. To prevent accidental extubation, meticulous sedation is required. This is usually accomplished with a combination of a continuous intravenous morphine infusion and either intravenous benzodiazepines or, if possible, nasogastric chloral hydrate. Neuromuscular paralysis should be avoided, if at all possible, as, although accidental extubation is less likely, the consequences should it occur would be catastrophic.

BIBLIOGRAPHY

Biack A E, Hatch D J, Nauth-Misir N. Complications of nasotracheal intubation in neonates, infants and children: a review of 4 years experience in a children's hospital. British Journal of Anaesthesia 1990; 65: 461–467

Chadd G D, Crane D L, Phillips R M, Tunell W P. Extubation and reintubation guided by the laryngeal mask in a child with the Pierre–Robin syndrome. Anesthesiology 1992; 76: 640–641

Debreuil M, Ecoffey C. Laryngeal mask guided tracheal intubation in paediatric anaesthesia. Paediatric Anaesthesia 1992; 2: 344

Markakis D A, Sayson S C, Schreiner M S. Insertion of the laryngeal mask airway in awake infants with the Robin sequence. Anesthesia and Analgesia 1992; 75: 822–824

Russell S H, Hirsch N P. Simultaneous use of two laryngoscopes. Anaesthesia 1993; 48: 918

Ward C F. Pediatric head and neck syndromes In: Katz, Steward (eds) Anaesthesia and uncommon pediatric conditions. W B Saunders, Philadelphia, 1987, p 238–271

White A P, Billingham I M. Laryngeal mask guided tracheal intubation in paediatric anaesthesia. Paediatric Anaesthesia 1992; 2: 265

Wilson I G. The laryngeal mask airway in paediatric practice. British Journal of Anaesthesia 1993; 70: 124–125

Zideman D, Bingham R, Beattie T et al. Guidelines for paediatric life support. A statement by the Paediatric Life Support Working Party of the European Resuscitation Council. Resuscitation 1994; 27: 91–105

31

EQUIPMENT AND MONITORING

N. Newton

31

THE BOYLE'S MACHINE

N. Newton

Prior to the introduction of the continuous flow anaesthetic machine (the 'Boyle's machine') the concentration of anaesthetic inhaled by a patient was dependent on many factors which were variable and difficult to quantify. Observation of the patient's response to the anaesthetic was often the only means by which the concentration of anaesthetic being administered was assessed.

The essential element of the Boyle's machine is that it enables known concentrations of anaesthetic gases and vapours to be delivered accurately. This is achieved by controlling the way in which the supplies of oxygen and nitrous oxide are mixed; the resultant carrier gas is then passed through calibrated vapourizers where an accurate percentage of volatile anaesthetic agent is taken up, and subsequently delivered to the patient.

The anaesthetic machine comprises several elements, as described below.

CYLINDERS

See Table 1.

- Cylinders should be cautiously 'cracked open' before use, to blow dust away from the valve. Open valves slowly. Never use grease.
- The pin index system ensures that the correct cylinder is fitted.
- Cylinders are connected at their respective yokes via Bodok seals.

Table 1.
Gas cylinders used with the Boyle's machine

Gas	Cylinder pressure (×100 kPa)	Critical temperature (°C)
Oxygen	135	−119
Nitrous oxide*	44	36.5
Medical air	137	−141
Carbon dioxide*	49	31
(Cyclopropane*	5	125)

*These gases liquefy under pressure at room temperature; the cylinder pressure does not therefore reflect the state of filling.

PIPELINES

- Each 'complete hose assembly' is permanently attached via a noninterchangeable (NIST) connector at the machine end, and has a Schraeder probe at the distal end
- Pipeline gases are supplied at the anaesthetic machine working pressure of 400 kPa via flow restrictors
- Blackflow check valves on the anaesthetic machine prevent gases escaping from the empty cylinder yoke when a cylinder is changed or from the pipelines when these are not plugged into the gas terminal outlets.

PRESSURE GAUGES

- Aneroid 'Bourdon gauges' monitor high gas pressures in cylinders and pipelines
- Pressures are displayed as kPa × 100.

PRESSURE REGULATORS

- Reduce cylinder pressures to safe working levels (just below 400 kPa)
- Maintain a constant flow despite changes in supply pressure
- Are required for all gases where the supply pressure exceeds 1000 kPa (i.e. not needed for cyclopropane cylinders or pipeline supplies).

FLOW CONTROL VALVES

- Manually operated fine adjustment needle valves that control total flow rate and oxygen composition of carrier gas
- Oxygen control knob has distinctive shape

to avoid confusion, and is always on the left (in the UK).

FLOW METERS

- Enable flows of individual gases to be visualized and measured.
- Rotameter bobbins rotate to avoid sticking. Tubes must be vertical.

VAPORIZERS

- Plenum vaporizers have a vapourizing chamber and bypass channel
- Vapourizers are compensated for temperature and flow rate
- Control knob alters the 'splitting ratio', thereby determining the percentage of carrier gas that becomes fully saturated
- Modern vapourizers can be removed from the machine by means of the 'Selectatec mechanism' on the backbar.

PRESSURE RELIEF VALVE

- Protects the machine from high pressure due to obstruction at common gas outlet or breathing system
- Opens when the pressure exceeds 35–80 kPa.

OXYGEN FAILURE

Alarms:
- Primary audible oxygen alarm powered by oxygen as it fails. Alarms sounds when the oxygen supply pressure falls below 200 kPa (half normal pressure), giving a whistle lasting a minimum of 7 s
- Secondary alarms may operate to give a more persistent warning, e.g. a siren driven by nitrous oxide being vented.

Protection devices:
- Ensures other gases are cut off when oxygen fails
- May open the breathing system to atmosphere, allowing a nonparalysed patient to breathe air.

OXYGEN FLUSH

- Bypasses all vaporizers
- Supplies 35–75 l of oxygen per minute
- Ideally self-closing, but may have facility to be locked on (risk of awareness/barotrauma if unnoticed).

COMMON GAS OUTLET

- Final pathway for gases to leave anaesthetic machine
- Male 22 mm taper/female 15 mm taper
- Cardiff swivel allows breathing system to swing into best position – beware possible interaction between breathing system and oxygen flush.

BREATHING SYSTEM

- Connects the patient to the common gas outlet (see p. 580)
- Integral pressure-limiting valve protects the patient (opens at 60–80 cmH_2O).

VENTILATOR

Most anaesthetic machines are equipped with an automatic ventilator (see p. 587).

ANAESTHETIC GAS SCAVENGING SYSTEM

- Normally an active system using assisted flow
- Levels of nitrous oxide in operating theatre can be kept below 100 ppm with effective scavenging
- Such levels are achievable by:
  - Scavenging at all times
  - Avoiding leaving gases flowing when the patient is not connected to machine
  - Care in filling vapourizers will reduce contamination from volatile agents.

BIBLIOGRAPHY

British Standards Institution. BS 4272: Part 3: 1989 British standard specification for anaesthetic and analgesia machines. British Standards Institution, Milton Keynes

British Standards Institution. BS 6834: 1987 British standard specification for active anaesthetic gas scavenging systems. British Standards Institution, Milton Keynes

Davey A, Moyle J, Ward C (eds). Ward's anaesthetic equipment, 3rd edn. W B Saunders, Philadelphia 1992

BREATHING SYSTEMS

U. Hodges

31

Breathing systems deliver the anaesthetic mixture from a gas source to the patient (Table 1), and may be classified into systems as shown.

Table 1. Classification of breathing systems

Classification	System
Carbon dioxide absorption	Waters' canister Circle system
Rebreathing	Mapleson A Mapleson B/C Mapleson D, E and F
Nonrebreathing	Ambu E Ruben valves Nonrebreathing valves in a bag mount

CARBON DIOXIDE ABSORPTION SYSTEMS

- Soda lime (94% calcium hydroxide, 5% sodium hydroxide, 1% potassium hydroxide, with silicates to make granules)
- Baralyme (80% calcium hydroxide, 20% barium hydroxide)
- Moisture required, for efficient absorption:
  - From the patient's expired gases
  - From soda lime/Baralyme reacting with carbon dioxide (Baralyme is better in a dry climate)
- Indicators which change colour when absorbent is 'exhausted'.

Waters' canister

- 'To-and fro' system, canister between the patient and a closed bag
- Cumbersome
- Deadspace increases as granules nearest the patient become exhausted
- 'Channelling' can occur
- Not used in current practice.

Circle system

- Expired gases circulate in a direction determined by two unidirectional valves
- The fresh gas flow determines how much of exhaled gases vent through the adjustable pressure limiting (APL) valve
- Carbon dioxide absorption prevents rebreathing (Table 2)
- Low flow (<3 l min^{-1}):
  - Exhaled gases including nitrogen dilute fresh gases; oxygen concentration from machine needs to be increased
  - Nitrous oxide inflow needs to be reduced continuously as uptake declines
  - Oxygen monitoring is mandatory
  - Vapour concentration within the system must be monitored
- With mechanical ventilator:
  - For bellow-in-bottle the bellows should be of the 'rising bellows' type (collapse under gravity if leak occurs)
  - For constant-flow generator (e.g. Penlon Nuffield series 200) either interpose bellows-in-bottle or use sufficient length of tubing so that the breathing system is not contaminated by oxygen from the ventilator (risk of awareness increases of flow loss).

REBREATHING SYSTEMS

- Carbon dioxide removed by washout with adequate fresh gas flow
- In the absence of fresh gas flow, total rebreathing occurs
- Rebreathing depends on fresh gas flow (Table 3) and carbon dioxide production, which is affected by:
  - Body temperature
  - Age
  - Metabolic disturbances
  - Pregnancy
  - Sepsis
  - Stress.

Magill attachment (Mapleson A)

- Most efficient breathing system for spontaneously breathing patient

Table 2.
Advantages and disadvantages of the circle system

Advantages	Disadvantages
Economical use of fresh gas flows	Hypoxic mixture at low flows possible
Economical use of volatile agents	Unpredictable concentration of anaesthetic possible
Reduction in pollution	Nitrogen concentration increases with time
Reduction of explosion risk	Complex system (disconnections and leaks)
Maintenance of heat and moisture	Soda lime absorbs volatile anaesthetics
Spontaneous or controlled ventilation	Carbon monoxide will accumulate with time
Can use low flows	Long time constants at low flows (<3 l min^{-1}) Sevoflurane (toxic byproducts) Valves (can stick open or closed) Bulky (less portable than Mapleson systems)

Table 3.
Recommended fresh gas flows for rebreathing systems during spontaneous and controlled ventilation to achieve normocarbia

System	Fresh gas flow*	
	Spontaneous ventilation	Controlled ventilation
Mapleson A = Magill/Lack (coaxial)	70 ml kg^{-1} min^{-1}	>20 l min^{-1}
Mapleson B/C (Waters' without absorber)	$2 \times V_{min}$	$2 \times V_{min}$
Mapleson D/E/F (all geometrically T-pieces)	$3 \times V_{min}$	70 ml kg^{-1} min^{-1}
Humphrey ADE	70 ml kg^{-1} min^{-1}	70 ml kg^{-1} min^{-1}
Ohmeda enclosed afferent reservoir system	70 ml kg^{-1} min^{-1}	70 ml kg^{-1} min^{-1}

*V_{min}, minute volume.

- Minimal fresh gas flow can in theory be reduced to the same value as alveolar minute volume due to preferential venting of alveolar gas during expiration
- Inefficient for prolonged controlled ventilation.

Lack system (Mapleson A)
- Effectively the same configuration as the Magill attachment
- Relatively economical
- Accessible exhaust valve
- Easy scavenging
- Satisfactory humidity
- Unlike the Bain system, the Lack system cannot be used with a ventilator.

Bain system (Mapleson D/E)
Advantages:
- Can be used for both children and adults
- Useful where access to patient limited
- Minimal drag on endotracheal tube or mask
- Facilitates scavenging
- Easy interchange between spontaneous and controlled ventilation
- Satisfactory humidity
- Can be used with a ventilator; large tidal volumes can be used without hypocapnia.

Disadvantages:
- Inner tube can disconnect or double back causing obstruction
- Inner tube has a high resistance, e.g. can lose some of emergency oxygen flush if

Table 4.
Monitoring breathing systems

Potential hazard	Monitoring
Disconnection (leading cause of critical incidents), may be partial or complete	Clinical observation Pressure/respiratory volume/carbon dioxide monitors
Misconnections	Clinical observation Standards committees set different diameters for connections
Occlusion (obstruction)	High pressure alarm Carbon dioxide monitor
Barotrauma (excess inflow into breathing system)	High pressure alarm

pressure relief valve on the backbar is set at a low value
- Cannot use with an intermittent flow machine.

Humphrey ADE
- Combines Mapleson A, D and E principles
- Allows spontaneous or controlled ventilation by changing valve levers, without the need to change the circuit configuration
- May be coaxial, or use twin (inspiratory/ expiratory) hoses.

Enclosed afferent reservoir system
- Integrated with the anaesthetic machine
- Double expiratory valve – vents in late expiration (controlled and spontaneous ventilation).

NONREBREATHING SYSTEMS

More commonly used outside operating theatres.

Advantages:
- No rebreathing
- Spontaneous or controlled ventilation
- Fresh gas flow (FGF) = Minute volume (V_{min}).

Disadvantages:
- Wasteful
- FGF > V_{min}, valve can jam in inspiration potentially causing barotrauma
- FGF < V_{min}, reservoir bag becomes depleted
- Valves may stick or be sluggish
- Some valves are noisy.

MONITORING BREATHING SYSTEMS

See Table 4.
- Expired rather than inspired oxygen detects problems with the delivery system of Bain
- Set lower oxygen limit to detect oxygen failure, and upper oxygen limit for nitrous oxide failure
- Rigorous preanaesthetic check is essential, especially with circle and coaxial systems.

BIBLIOGRAPHY

Adams A P, Henville J D. Anaesthetic circuits and flexible pipelines for medical gases. In: Langton Hewer C, Atkinson R S (eds) Recent advances in anaesthesia and analgesia Vol 13. Churchill Livingstone, London, 1979, p 23–55

Andrews J J. Inhaled anesthetic delivery systems. In: Miller R D (ed) Anesthesia. Churchill Livingstone, London, 1990, p 171–223

Mushin W W, Jones P L. Physics for the anaesthetist, 4th edn. Blackwell, Oxford, 1987

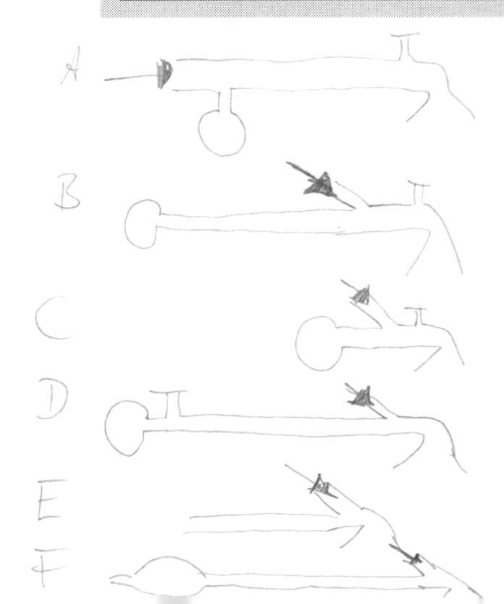

MONITORING

M. Jordan and
R. Langford

MONITORING STANDARDS

ASA Standards 1986 (amended 1990):
- Continuous presence of anaesthetist
- Monitoring of $F_{I}O_2$
- Blood oxygenation, e.g. by SpO_2
- Capnography/spirometry encouraged
- Confirmation of endotracheal tube position by $F_{E}CO_2$
- Ventilator disconnection alarm
- Continuous display of ECG
- Arterial BP, pulse at least every 5 min
- Continual monitoring of circulation, e.g. by pulse or arterial trace
- Temperature measurement available.

AAGBI Standards 1988: (revised 1994)
- Continuous presence of anaesthetist
- $F_{I}O_2$, leak/disconnection, rebreathing and overpressure alarms
- *Continuous* monitoring of ventilation and circulation by, e.g. capnography, SpO_2
- Appropriate frequency of BP and heart rate measurement
- Peripheral nerve stimulator available
- Adequate monitoring for brief cases, complicated cases and transport
- Clear handover to recovery staff.

GAS MONITORING

$F_{I}O_2$
- Simple oxygen analysers should be placed in the inspiratory limb of breathing system
- Pressurization of analyser (e.g. by minute volume divider ventilators) will cause overreading
- Multigas analysers using slow-response technology for oxygen analysis (e.g. fuel cell) may give value intermediate between $F_{I}O_2$ and $F_{E}O_2$ when sampling at tracheal tube.

$F_{E}O_2$
- Persisting $F_{I}O_2 - F_{E}O_2$ difference greater than 5% may be indicator of hypoventilation or low cardiac output state
- $F_{E}O_2$ is useful in monitoring nitrogen and nitrous oxide washout.

$F_{E}CO_2$
Sudden falls in $F_{E}CO_2$ are suggestive of disconnection, air embolism or fall in cardiac output

$P_{E}CO_2$ will also underestimate $P_{a}CO_2$ in:
- Significant intra- or extra-pulmonary shunting
- Respiratory rates too high for accurate analysis
- Tidal volumes too low for accurate sampling
- Dilution of sample by fresh gas, e.g. in Bain circuit.

Nitrous oxide and volatile agents:
- Analysers requiring selection of agent in use introduce serious errors if this is incorrect, if nitrous oxide compensation is not appropriate or if mixtures of volatile agents are used
- End-tidal volatile agent concentrations will *overestimate* arterial concentrations in presence of high A–a gradients.

Nitrogen

Sudden rises in $F_{E}N_2$ in absence of inspired nitrogen are indicative of air embolism.

RESPIRATORY MECHANICS

Pulmonary compliance monitoring, e.g. with pressure/volume or flow/volume loops is useful in:

- Patients prone to bronchospasm
- Laparoscopic or thoracoscopic surgery
- Surgery in proximity of tracheal tube.

BODY TEMPERATURE

- Oesophageal temperature correlates best with blood (core) temperature

- Nasopharyngeal or tympanic membrane temperature reflects brain temperature
- Rectal temperature lags core temperature in the adult.

OXYGEN SATURATION BY PULSE OXIMETRY (Spo_2)

In vivo, spectrophotometric measurement of haemoglobin oxygen saturation by a probe, usually located on a finger or the ear lobes (less reliable).

- Fails in low perfusion states (cold, hypovolaemia, low cardiac output) or with movement/shivering
- Erroneous results if incorrectly positioned, nail varnish not removed, or in presence of carboxyhaemoglobin or methaemoglobin
- Ideally, pulse waveform should be displayed/discernible to confirm signal strength
- Peripheral Spo_2 may lag 30–45 s behind central Spo_2
- Administration of high inspired oxygen may initially maintain oxygen saturation, even when ventilation is inadequate.

ELECTROCARDIOGRAPHY

Continuous observation of:

- Rate, rhythm (including ectopics) and conduction
- Myocardial ischaemia identified from single lead (e.g. CM_5) ST segment depression, or with greater sensitivity by computer-analysed multilead system
- Electrolyte status:
  - peaked T waves (hyperkalaemia)
  - prolonged QT (hypocalcaemia).

SYSTEMIC BLOOD PRESSURE

Noninvasive BP

The automated oscillometric technique is now the commonest.

Accuracy is mainly dependent on:
- Correct cuff size – width 20% greater than arm diameter, or 1/3 of arm circumference
- Correct application – loose wrapping results in falsely high readings.

Regular calibration of aneroid sphygmomanometers is required.

Invasive BP

A mechanoelectrical transducer produces small changes in voltage or resistance proportional to pressure waves transmitted from a vessel though fluid-filled tubing.

To obtain an optimally damped, accurate waveform:

- The connecting tubing should be of 60–120 cm length, 1.5–3.0 mm internal diameter, and made with rigid walls
- Eliminate any air bubbles in the system
- Use 4 ml h^{-1} continuous flush to prevent thrombotic occlusion.

Precautions:
- Use a small cannula to avoid arterial occlusion or damage
- Avoid accidental intra-arterial injection by using colour-coded taps
- Display waveform to prevent blood loss from disconnection.

CENTRAL VENOUS PRESSURE

Central venous pressure (CVP) is measured via a jugular, subclavian or long brachial venous cannula to indicate right atrial pressure (Table 1).

Table 1.
Complications in measuring CVP and their avoidance

Complication	Avoidance
• Air embolism	Head-down tilt during insertion Use luer-lock connections
• Sepsis	Aseptic insertion; minimize number of injections into tubing
• Pneumothorax/ haemothorax	

PULMONARY ARTERY AND CAPILLARY WEDGE PRESSURES

Measured via balloon-tipped floatation-directed catheter. Facilitates measurement of cardiac output and (by balloon occlusion of pulmonary artery (PA)) left atrial pressure.

Indications:
- Ejection fraction <40%
- Left ventricular failure/hypertrophy
- Cardiac output studies.

Complications:
- Dysrhythmias
- Sepsis
- Pulmonary infarction
- Haemorrhage.

NEUROMUSCULAR FUNCTION

The muscular response to a supramaximal electrical stimulation of a peripheral motor nerve is measured by an eye, feel, force transducer or an electromyogram.

A train-of-four (TOF) stimuli (at 2 Hz, 10 s apart) indicate the degree of neuromuscular blockade.

- TOF count (number of twitches seen):
  - satisfactory blockade if 0–2 twitches detectable
  - TOF ratio (fourth twitch force as a fraction of the first) is useful for monitoring recovery from blockade.
- Tetanic stimulation (50 or 100 Hz for 5 s) in the presence of partial nondepolarizing blockade results in 'fade' (failure to sustain muscular contraction) and 'post-tetanic facilitation' of force from a single stimulus.

BIBLIOGRAPHY

Saidman L J, Smith N Ty. Monitoring in anesthesia. Butterworth, Boston, MA, 1984

Sykes M K, Vickers M D, Hull C J. Principles of measurement and monitoring in anaesthesia and intensive care. Blackwell Scientific, London, 1991

PREOPERATIVE ANAESTHETIC MACHINE CHECKLIST

P. Bickford-Smith

31

- All anaesthetic gas machines must be checked systematically before use. A check should be performed by the anaesthetist at the beginning of each list.
- If there is a change of anaesthetist during the list, the checked status of the machine must be agreed at handover.

PERFORMING A CHECK PROCEDURE

The most serious deficiency in an anaesthetic machine is the failure to deliver adequate supplies of oxygen. Modern machines are fitted with at least two safety devices to prevent the delivery of a hypoxic gas mixture:

- A primary oxygen-supply-failure protection device (with an audible alarm)
- A secondary gas cut-off device, to prevent the common gas outlet (CGO) delivering a hypoxic gas mixture.

Some machines have a minimum ratio device which actively reduces the proportion of nonrespirable gases to guarantee adequate oxygen delivery. On machines without an integral oxygen analyser, these safety devices cannot identify a crossed pipeline or a misfilled cylinder, since they simply detect differential gas pressures. The correct function of these safety devices must be tested with an oxygen analyser, calibrated in room air (21%) and 100% oxygen (from a separate source, e.g. a wall flowmeter). Integral oxygen analysers can be used if the sampling point can be placed at the CGO.

A systematic check procedure ensures the provision and correct function of:

- The supply of medical gases, primarily oxygen
- Vaporizers for volatile anaesthetic agents
- Breathing system (tubing, bags, valves)
- Ventilator
- Suction apparatus
- Sundry apparatus (e.g. airway maintenance and intubation equipment).

MEDICAL GAS CHECK

Step 1:

- Disconnect all gas pipelines, turn off all cylinders and vaporizers
- Remove unwanted cylinders, and blank off empty yokes with blanking plugs
- Connect oxygen analyser to CGO
- Turn on electrical supply to machine
- Turn on gas supply master switch (if fitted – see note in step 6)
- Open all gas-flow-control valves.

Step 2:

- Turn oxygen cylinder *on*, check that the pressure rises on the relevant gauge to above half full; bobbin rises in oxygen flowmeter *only*, adjust to 5 l min^{-1}
- Watch analyser concentration rise towards 100%
- Turn nitrous oxide cylinder *on*, check the relevant gauge pressure shows full; check that nitrous oxide bobbin rises, adjust to 5 l min^{-1} (check that the oxygen bobbin has remained at 5 l min^{-1}).

Step 3:

- Turn oxygen cylinder *off*, press emergency oxygen button
- Watch the cylinder pressure fall, the oxygen bobbin fall, and the audible oxygen failure alarm sound (± visual indicator green to red); gas flow from CGO ceases.

Step 4:

- Connect the oxygen pipeline and perform a 'tug' test. The audible alarm should stop, and gas flow recommence at the CGO.
- Watch the oxygen bobbin *rise* to 5 l min^{-1}, and the pipeline pressure gauge rise to 400 kPa.

Step 5:

- Turn the nitrous oxide cylinder *off*, connect the nitrous oxide pipeline and perform a 'tug' test
- Watch the nitrous oxide bobbin rise to 5 l min^{-1}; the pipeline pressure gauge rises to 400 kPa.

Step 6:

- *Attempt* to turn off the oxygen flow control valve, and see if the oxygen bobbin falls to zero, or remains at around 250 ml min^{-1}.
- N.B. If the nitrous oxide bobbin also falls, and the oxygen analyser reading remains above 21%, the machine is fitted with a minimum ratio antihypoxic device. Operate the gas control master switch to turn off the basal oxygen flow.

Step 7:

- Repeat steps 2–4 for any other cylinders of gas which may be employed
- If there is no gas control master switch, turn off *all* flowmeter control valves individually.

VAPORIZER CHECK

- Detachable vaporisers must be locked correctly onto the backbar and be level
- Check the orientation of any flexible in/outflow pipes
- Check the fluid level (between full and empty)
- Turn oxygen flow *on* to 5 l min^{-1}, switch vaporizer to full scale, briefly occlude the CGO, and look for any fluid leakage
- Turn vaporizer *off*, then oxygen *off*.

VENTILATOR CHECK

- Check configuation and correct operation
- Equipment (e.g. self-inflating bag) for manual assistance of ventilation
- Presence and function of a disconnection alarm
- Set controls.

BREATHING SYSTEM CHECK

- Correct configuration, especially coaxial tubes and circle absorber systems.
- Reservoir bag and expiratory valve.
- Connector tightness (push and twist).
- Leak test: occlude patient-end, close expiratory valve, fit a manometer into the circuit with a T-piece adjacent to the bag. Distend bag to 20–35 mmHg using the oxygen flush button. Pressure should remain unchanged after 1 min.

SUCTION

- Adequate = <–60 kPa achieved in <5 s when the patient end is occluded
- All components securely assembled.

SUNDRIES

- Two laryngoscopes (check bulbs)
- Appropriate size of airways
- Face-masks.

FAULTS DETECTED DURING CHECK – ACTION

- Correct fault if possible (e.g. calibrate monitor).
- Note minor faults in the logbook.
- Major fault (e.g. persistent gas leak): *remove equipment from service* and attach label indicating type of fault, stating that machine must not be used.
- Inform theatre staff/service engineer.

BIBLIOGRAPHY

Adams A P, Morgan M. Checking the anaesthetic machine – checklists or visual aids? Anaesthesia 1993; 48: 183–186

Association of Anaesthetists of Great Britain and Ireland. Checklist for anaesthetic machines. Association of Anaesthetists of Great Britain and Ireland, 9 Bedford Square, London WC1B 3RA, 1990

Page J. Testing for leaks. Anaesthesia 1977; 32: 673

VENTILATORS

A. Pearce

The correct term is 'ventilatory breathing system'. This comprises:

- Ventilator
- Breathing system attached to patient.

FUNCTIONAL CLASSIFICATION

Inspiratory phase gas control:
- Volume – a preset volume is delivered
- Pressure – a preset pressure is not exceeded.

Cycling (inspiration/expiration):
- Time
- Pressure
- Volume
- Flow.

Inspiratory flow characteristics:
- Flow generator – the inspiratory flow pattern predetermined by ventilator settings
- Pressure generator – the inspiratory pressure applied to the patient's airway is determined by ventilator settings.

THREE COMMON TYPES OF VENTILATOR

Volume preset, time cycled, flow generator
- Includes virtually all adult ITU machines and many adult anaesthetic ventilators
- Delivery of a preset tidal volume is maintained despite changes in lung compliance
- Inflation pressure depends on lung compliance and is limited by a safety blow-off valve (usually 60 cmH_2O)
- Cycles from inspiration to expiration at the end of a preset time

- Powerful machines powered by a high pressure driving gas (400 kPa) or substantial electric motors
- Examples include Servovent, Cape, Oxford, Nuffield 200 with adult valve.

Pressure pre-set, time cycled, flow generator
- Common arrangement in paediatric ventilators
- Set airway pressure (usually 15–20 cmH_2O) not exceeded during inspiration
- Cycles to expiration at the end of a set time, even if the desired inflation pressure is not reached
- Inspiratory flow rate *must* be set at high enough level to reach desired pressure in the time allowed for inspiration
- Tidal volume delivered is affected by changes in lung compliance
- Examples include paediatric Babylog, Sechrist, Nuffield 200 with paediatric valve.

Time cycled, pressure generator
- Weighted bellows apply constant set pressure during inspiration
- Inspiratory flow is high initially and then declines (characteristic of a pressure generator)
- Delivered tidal volume will depend on the pressure in the bellows and the lung compliance
- Possible to set a desired tidal volume *only* if there is sufficient weight on bellows
- Examples include East-Radcliffe, Manley Blease.

Other ventilators
Ventilators can also be classified by how they work. The commonest types used in operating theatres are:

- *Minute volume dividers* – these use the power of the fresh gas flow from the anaesthetic machine and divide the delivered minute volume into preset tidal volumes.
- *T-tube occluders* – these occlude intermittently the expiratory limb of a T-piece; the constant gas flow into the circuit then inflates the patient's lungs
- *Bag squeezers* – these compress a bellows in the breathing circuit, usually by means of high pressure gas or an electric motor
- *Intermittent blowers* – these are powered by a high pressure driving gas which enters the breathing circuit in controlled 'bursts'.

CHECKING AND SETTING

Checking and setting the ventilatory breathing system before use is vital:

- Connect to electricity supply, high pressure gas, low pressure gas, etc.
- Set tidal volume to 10–15 ml kg^{-1} or inflation pressure to 20 cmH_2O
- Set respiratory rate to 10–16 breaths min^{-1}
- Set I/E ratio to 1:2 or 1:3, with an inspiratory time of not less than 1 s
- Switch on and see if pressure develops in the circuit
- Check that the pressure relief valve is functioning at correct value
- Check that gas monitoring is present and working
- Check that airway pressure monitor is working
- Check manual mode functioning (if fitted)
- Check that the emergency air intake is patent (if appropriate).

THE IDEAL VENTILATORY BREATHING SYSTEM

The ideal ventilatory breathing system should have the following characteristics:

- Wide range of tidal volumes and respiratory rates to encompass paediatric and adult use
- Adjustable inspiratory/expiratory timing (I/E ratio)
- Airway pressure display, with alarm limits
- Expired minute volume display, with alarm limits
- Adjustable, monitored inspired oxygen concentration
- Provision of PEEP/CPAP
- Sophisticated ventilatory modes (SIMV, pressure support, MMV, triggering)
- Humidification
- Adjustable inspiratory waveforms
- Adjustable pressure relief valve.

BIBLIOGRAPHY

Davey A, Moyle J, Ward C (eds). Ward's anaesthetic equipment, 3rd edn. W B Saunders, Philadelphia, 1992, p 197–241
Hayes B. Ventilators: a current assessment. In: Adams A P, Atkinson R S (eds) Recent advances in anaesthesia and analgesia. Churchill Livingstone, Edinburgh, 1993, vol 18, p 83–102
Ehrenwerth J, Eisenkraft J B. Anesthesia equipment, principles and applications. Mosby 1993

32

TECHNIQUES

J. C. Goldstone

AWAKE/BLIND NASAL INTUBATION

Q. Ainsworth

The procedure involves:

- Appropriate sedation ('awake' is a misnomer)
- Topical anaesthesia of the airway, sometimes with superior laryngeal nerve blocks and cricothyroid puncture.

INDICATIONS

- Anticipated difficulty for other techniques of intubation
- Severe risk of aspiration
- Severe risk of haemodynamic/respiratory instability on induction of general anaesthesia/paralysis.

If fibre-optic intubation is an option it should be performed first, as blood, secretions and oedema can make its use difficult later.

CONTRAINDICATIONS

- Airway tumours, abscesses or trauma
- Recent nasal surgery
- Coagulopathy
- Basal skull fracture.

PERIOPERATIVE MANAGEMENT

Thoroughly discuss the procedure and document this in the notes.

Premedication

Antisialogogue (e.g. glycopyrrolate 0.2 mg i.m., given 1 h before) to improve the mucosal contact of topical anaesthetics. Vasoconstrictor nose drops and sedatives may also be given.

Sedation

The patient should be able to speak and respond to commands. Intravenous sedatives should be given slowly in small increments, waiting each time for peak effect because of unpredictable effects on consciousness, respiration and haemodynamics. Opioids are the mainstay of sedation, supplemented after a moderate dose when necessary by butyrophenones and/or benzodiazepines. Popular drugs are fentanyl, droperidol and midazolam. Propofol is also effective in 10–20 mg boluses. Naloxone and flumazenil should be available.

Local anaesthesia

Local anaesthesia may worsen upper airway obstruction, and in the full stomach should be limited to above the glottis. The airway can be anaesthetized as a whole by the inhalation of nebulized local anaesthetic and/or in stages by a combination of methods. Recommended doses must not be exceeded. A vasoconstrictor should be applied to the nose.

Nebulized lignocaine

Lignocaine (4–10 ml, 4%) acts within 10 min and the vasoconstrictor phenylephrine (1 ml, 1%) can be included.

- *Nose*: use cocaine alone or lignocaine with a vasoconstrictor applied by pledgets, cotton-tipped applicators, sprays or catheters
- *Oropharynx/glottis*: lignocaine gargles/sprays, amethocaine lozenges, instillation down the tube, bilateral superior laryngeal nerve blocks (3 ml, 1–2% lignocaine, 1 cm inferomedial to the greater cornu of the hyoid after negative aspiration deep to the thyrohyoid membrane)
- *Trachea*: instillation down the tube, cricothyroid puncture (3–5 ml, 2–4% lignocaine rapidly after free aspiration of air, quickly removing the needle).

ANAESTHETIC PRINCIPLE

The tube is guided by increasing breath sounds heard at the end of the tube as it is advanced into the glottis. Other methods include tube whistles and capnography.

Preparation:

- In adults use a well-lubricated curved 7.0 or 7.5 tube cut (in the UK) to place the tip in the midtrachea; the lubricant must not obstruct the lumen

Table 1.
Tube placement

Position	Breath sounds	Voice	Resistance to tube	Neck bulge	Correction
Tracheal	Yes	No	No	No	–
Oesophagus	No	Yes	No	No	Extend atlanto-occipital joint. Backward pressure on thyroid cartilage. Reinsert
Anterior larynx	Yes	Yes	Yes	Midline or none	Flex neck with gentle presure on tube
Vallecula	No	Yes	Yes	Midline	Jaw thrust Protrude tongue Flex neck
Piriform fossa	No	Yes	Yes	Lateral	Rotate the tube and head to the opposite side Lateral pressure on thyroid cartilage

- The patient should be in the 'sniffing position', either supine or sitting
- If one nasal passage is obviously more patent this should be used, using the right passage will direct the tracheal tube bevel away from the turbinates
- A soft nasopharyngeal airway can be inserted first to determine the patency and dilate the nasal passage.

Technique:
- Intubate from above the patient's head or from the side
- Advance the endotracheal tube directly backwards into the nose and gently past the turbinates during inspiration
- Avoid excessive force at the posterior nasal aperture, because the tube may tear the nasopharyngeal mucosa and pass submucosally
- When the tube reaches the oropharynx breath sounds can be made louder by closing the mouth and occluding the opposite nostril
- Rotate the proximal end of the tube until its curve lies in the midline
- Breath sounds become louder and the patient may cough as the laryngeal inlet is approached
- Palpating superficial to the larynx quickly advances the tube 3–5 cm while the patient inspires deeply (or during the deep inspiration immediately after a cough).

Confirmation
See Table 1.

Further confirmation includes:

- Coughing if the trachea has not been anaesthetized
- Condensation on the tube
- Ausculating the chest and epigastrium while squeezing the bag
- Reservoir bag movement
- Capnography.

BIBLIOGRAPHY

Otto C W. Tracheal intubation. In: Nunn J F, Utting J E, Brown Jr B R (eds) General anaesthesia, 5th edn, Butterworth, Oxford, 1989, p 526–531

Stehling L C. Management of the airway. In: Barash P, Cullen B, Stoelting R (eds) Clinical anesthesia, 2nd edn. J B Lippincott, Philadelphia, 1992, p 695–698

Stone D J, Gal T J. Airway management. In: Miller R D (ed) Anesthesia, 3rd edn. Churchill Livingstone, Edinburgh, 1990, p 1282–1285

CLOSED CIRCLE ANAESTHESIA

Q. Ainsworth

32

DEFINITIONS

- *Totally closed system*: fresh gas inflow is adjusted to equal oxygen consumption plus anaesthetic uptake. The APL (spillover) valve is closed and exhaled gases are rebreathed after carbon dioxide absorption and mixing with fresh gases. Under such circumstances the reservoir bag distends if inflow is excessive, and collapses if inflow is deficient.
- *Low-flow system*: fresh gas flow is less than 3 l min^{-1} and, therefore, exceeds basal requirements. Fresh gas flow is not sufficient to prevent the return of some exhaled gas for carbon dioxide absorption and rebreathing. Excess gases vent to atmosphere during exhalation.

The use of the circle absorber allows the anaesthetist to consider the amount of anaesthetic agent required, and it is this quantitative approach which underlies the difference between closed circle and semiclosed breathing systems. In the semiclosed technique anaesthetic vapour is supplied in excess and dumped to the atmosphere via the spillover valve. When gas flow is reduced it is then possible to determine the amount of vapour (in millilitres) required to establish a constant blood and brain tension of agent.

In order to quantify the dose of anaesthetic agent we need to know:

- The fraction of MAC desired
- The amount of vapour needed to achieve this within the breathing system and lungs
- The amount of vapour required for uptake of agent into the circulation
- The amount of vapour needed for uptake of agent into the tissues.

THE DESIRED LEVEL OF ANAESTHETIC AGENT

The dose–response curves for anaesthetic agents is expressed in terms of MAC which is a measure of the ED_{50} dose. The ED_{95} dose of a volatile agent is achieved at concentrations of 1.3 MAC and above.

Agent	MAC (% v/v)	1.3 MAC
Halothane	0.75	>0.95
Enflurane	1.7	>2.21
Isoflurane	1.3	>1.69

MAC is remarkably stable but is affected by age, metabolic factors and other drugs. MAC is additive, and the target of 1.3 MAC can be made up of more than one inhaled agent.

The amount of anaesthetic agent needed to achieve this concentration in the breathing system and lungs is known as the *priming dose for ventilation*:

Ventilation priming dose = Desired concentration × (Volume of circuit + Volume of lungs)

Component required to be primed	Volume (ml)
Absorber (jumbo)	6000
Hoses (1 m)	1000
FRC	2500

The volume of the circuit + FRC is approximately 10 l, but this may be less in smaller absorbers.

Ventilation priming dose = 1.3 MAC × Volume of circuit and FRC/100
= millilitres of anaesthetic vapour

UPTAKE OF AGENT

Uptake into the circulation

To achieve the target level of anaesthetic agent in the blood we need to know:

- The target level (1.3 MAC) fMAC
- The solubility of the agent in blood $\lambda B/G$
- The cardiac output $\mathring{Q}$.

This is termed the *arterial prime*:

$$\text{Arterial prime} = f\text{MAC} \times \lambda BG \times \mathring{Q})$$

The arterial prime dose saturates the blood. Further anaesthetic agent is required to provide for uptake of the agent into the tissues.

Tissue uptake

The amount of anaesthetic agent taken up by the tissues reduces with time. A linear model of uptake of anaesthetic agent is achieved by expressing the amount of agent against the square root of time $\sqrt{t}$. This allows the same amount of agent (unit dose) to be given to the patient and the time periods will follow the sequence 1, 4, 9, 15 min. The unit dose is twice the arterial prime dose:

$$\text{Unit dose} = 2\ [f\text{MAC} \times \lambda B/G \times \mathring{Q}]$$

This amount of vapour is given for each time period (see Table 1).

Table 1.

	Halothane	Enflurane	Isoflurane
1.3 MAC	1.0	2.21	1.69
Ventilatory priming dose	100	221	169
Arterial prime	148	265	160
Total prime	248	486	329
Unit dose	296	531	321

At a flow rate of 1000 ml min^{-1}, a calibrated vaporizer set at 1% delivers 10 ml of vapour into the fresh gas flow.

PRACTICAL PROBLEMS

Initially, high levels of vapour need to be added to the circle in order to maintain a constant blood (arterial) level of anaesthetic agent. If the agent is introduced within the circle (direct injection or via a Goldman vaporizer), vapour delivery can be achieved. If the vaporizer is outside the circle, initial high flow rates are required over the first three time periods (9 min). It is possible to average the delivery over the first 9 min.

Nitrogen accumulation:

- A supine adult contains 2.5–3 l nitrogen (FRC: 1.5 l, tissues: 1–1.5 l)
- During inhalational anaesthesia nitrogen is washed out from the FRC and tissues; if it is rebreathed low partial pressures of inspired nitrous oxide/oxygen can result
- High initial flows (6–10 l min^{-1}) reduce the circuit and FRC nitrogen to 3–5% within 5 min
- Tissue nitrogen slowly accumulates in the circle thereafter.

Mechanical ventilation

The 'bag-in-bottle' ventilators are common. Ascending bellows are safer than descending bellows. Reservoir tube ventilators produce to-and-fro pulses of driving gas (oxygen/air) along tubing connected in place of the reservoir bag (N.B. *the tubing capacity must be greater than the tidal volume*). Driving gas enters the circle if the fresh gas flow is insufficient or if there is a significant leak.

EQUIPMENT CHECK

- Check that the tubing, circuit components and all connections are leak-free
- Measure the circuit compression volume (the ventilator 'tidal volume' which generates 'physiological' circuit pressures when the patient port is occluded); this is the volume not delivered during IPPV
- Ensure that rotameters rotate at low flows
- If oxygen consumption and derived variables need to be calculated, calibrate flowmeters by measuring the time taken to expand a known volume at flow rates of 50–300 ml min^{-1}
- Check absorber life and note the expected colour change of the indicator
- Check and alarm monitors for:
  - $P_{i}O_2$ (mandatory)
  - $P_{et}CO_2$ (mandatory)
  - $P_{et}N_2O$ (desirable)
  - P_{et}Vol (desirable)
- If the absorber has a water trap it should be below the level of the patient's airway, since this water may be strongly alkaline.

SUGGESTED TECHNIQUE USING NITROUS OXIDE

- Intravenous induction and cuffed endotracheal intubation/laryngeal mask anaesthesia
- Give high flows and the appropriate volatile

concentration for 9 min (first three time periods)
- High initial flows are needed to:
  - Provide sufficient dose during high uptake
  - Prevent excessive dilution of FGF
  - Remove nitrogen
- Close the circuit
- Adjust oxygen flow to the calculated VO_2 (3.5 ml kg^{-1} min^{-1})
- Keep the $P_{et}O_2$ and circuit volume constant by fine control of oxygen and nitrous oxide flow rates
- Give volatile percentage according to end-tidal values (or to unit dosage schedule) and clinical observations
- Maintain appropriate carbon dioxide levels by attention to ventilation and (where available) variable bypass of the absorber
- Give high flows for 5 min:
  - Every 1–3 h to wash out undesired gases and maintain the appropriate inspired concentrations
  - If the circuit is broken at any time
  - If there is a need to change composition rapidly.

Emergence:
- Open the system using high oxygen flows
- Exhaustion of soda lime is indicated by the presence of carbon dioxide in inspired gas.

BIBLIOGRAPHY

Andrews J J. Anesthesia systems. In: Barash P, Cullen B, Stoelting R (eds) Clinical anesthesia, 2nd edn. J B Lippincott, Philadelphia, 1992, p 675–679

Jones M J. Breathing systems and vaporizers. In: Nimmo W S, Smith G (eds) Anaesthesia. Blackwell, Oxford, 1989, p 331–341

Lowe H J, Ernst E A. The quantitative practice of anesthesia: use of the closed circuit. Williams and Wilkins, Baltimore, 1981

White D C. Closed circuit anaesthesia. In: Kaufman L (ed) Anaesthesia Review. Churchill Livingstone, Edinburgh, 1984, vol 2, p 189–199

White D C. Closed and low flow system anaesthesia. Current Anaesthesia and Critical Care 1992; 3: 98–107

EPIDURAL AND SPINAL ANAESTHESIA

R. Collis

INDICATIONS

Pre-emptive analgesia
The role of regional techniques in pre-emptive analgesia has stimulated recent research. Laboratory work shows an effect, but clinical studies have been less convincing. The use of axial blocks for the prevention of phantom limb pain has been established.

Modification of the perioperative stress response
Axial blocks reduce plasma concentration of the stress hormones. This may be of specific benefit in the management of high-risk surgical patients.

Benefit of awake patient
Surgery below T4 can be conducted with an axial block alone. This may be preferable where there is a risk of aspiration, difficult airway and respiratory impairment.

Postoperative pain management
Local anaesthetics and opioids in axial blocks reduce the requirement for other types of analgesics. Benefits are especially marked after major surgery and include shorter ITU stay, reduced episodes of postoperative hypoxaemia, myocardial ischaemia and deep vein thrombosis.

ABSOLUTE CONTRAINDICATIONS

- Patient refusal
- Severe clotting disorders

- Full anticoagulation
- Infection at sight of insertion; viral or bacterial
- Hypovolaemic shock
- Severe stenotic valvular heart disease
- Anaphylaxis to drug.

CONTROVERSIES

Increased risk of epidural haematoma formation

Aspirin
Bleeding time is not increased with 60 mg daily. Bleeding time increases with 600 mg daily, but thrombelastography, a measure of overall clotting function, is unchanged.

Low platelet count
The frequently quoted minimum count of 100×10^9 l^{-1} may be unnecessarily high. In immune-mediated thrombocytopenia platelet function is excellent, and in pre-eclampsia thrombelastography remains within normal limits with a count as low as 50×10^9 l^{-1}.

Prophylactic low-dose heparin and low-molecular-weight heparin (LMWH)
There is wide individual variability in the effect that heparin and LMWH has on clotting function. LMWH effect can be measured only by anti-Xa assay. Several large surveys have failed to show any increase in haematoma formation where epidurals were sited in patients on aspirin or low-dose heparin.

Full anticoagulation after establishing axial block
The risk of haematoma formation appears to be rare, but there are case reports in the literature. One must evaluate the potential benefits of the block in this situation.

Serious long-term neurological sequelae
A large prospective study has not been performed. In the obstetric population the incidence seems to be 0.0001% and that in the nonobstetric population 0.006%. Possible causes include spinal cord ischaemia, trauma, chemical contamination of the drug and direct neurotoxic effect of local anaesthetic solutions.

Pre-existing neurological deficit
There are no specific contraindications but patients should be carefully counselled. Patients with high spinal cord injuries may benefit during surgery and labour because of the reduction of autonomic hyperreflexia.

Pre-existing systemic infection
There is a definite association with CNS infection. Pretreatment with an appropriate antibiotic substantially reduces the risk.

EPIDURAL AND SPINAL OPIATES

Commonly used preservative-free drugs include morphine, pethidine, diamorphine, fentanyl and sufentanil. They offer a synergistic effect with local anaesthetic agents, with no associated motor, sensory or autonomic effects.

Side-effects

Pruritus:
This is very common after all opioids. It is not dose dependent and usually requires no treatment, although naloxone is effective.

Urinary retention
This is common, but not dose dependent.

Nausea and vomiting
This may be a problem associated with rostral spread of the drug. It is probably no more common than after opioid given by other routes.

Respiratory depression
This is more common after intrathecal than epidural administration, and the use of more water-soluble drugs such as morphine and pethidine. An incidence of 0.2–1% has been reported. Controlled studies comparing the incidence with other routes of opioid administration have not been conducted. Risk factors are old age, obesity, respiratory disease, and concurrent parental administration of opioids.

Epidural anaesthesia

Anatomy and technique
The epidural space runs continuously from the foramen magnum to the sacrococcygeal membrane. It may be accessed anywhere using the median or paramedian approach through the ligamentum flavum, or through the sacrococcygeal membrane as a caudal block. The spread of local anaesthetic agents is segmental and, therefore, the site of the epidural should be at the level that anaesthesia is required. Epidural opioids act at

spinal cord level, so the site of epidural cannulation is less important. Safety and ease has made the lumber approach most popular. Accidental dural puncture occurs more commonly with shallow epidural spaces (<4 cm), with the use of air rather than saline to identify loss of resistance, and in trainee rather than experienced hands. An overall rate of 1–3% can be expected.

Advantages:

- Level of analgesia can be controlled by site of epidural cannulation
- Slow rate of onset with accurate titration of fluid and vasopressors leading to increased cardiovascular stability
- Extension of anaesthesia and analgesia with top-ups via the epidural catheter.

Disadvantages:

- Time-consuming because of slow onset of anaesthesia
- Slow onset of sacral anaesthesia
- Use of potentially large toxic doses of local anaesthetic agents and accidental intravascular injection
- Catheter migration or catheter misplacement with part or all of the catheter in the subarachnoid or subdural space.

Differential sympathetic, sensory and motor blockade

The extent of the sympathetic block tends to be two dermatomes greater than the sensory block which is in turn two dermatomes greater than the motor block. The use of loss of cold sensation to map areas of anaesthesia correlates more accurately with sympathetic blockade and, therefore, sensory anaesthesia may be inadequate for surgery. The concept of differential blockade can also apply to sparing of large motor fibres to local anaesthetic blockade. Small sympathetic and pain fibres are easily penetrated by local anaesthetics. When using low dose, low concentration local anaesthetic solutions, motor power can be preserved whilst achieving analgesia.

Spinal anaesthesia

Anatomy and technique

Cerebrospinal fluid is contained within the dura from the cranium to the termination of the dura at S1. The spinal cord terminates between L1 and L2. Spinal anaesthesia can therefore be carried out safely below L2. The vertebral level at which spinal anaesthesia can be performed is limited therefore baricity, and the position of the patient will limit the upper extent of the block. Heavy bupivacaine, which contains 8% glucose, is hyperbaric to CSF, but most other drugs are slightly hypobaric at 37°C. If spinal anaesthesia is performed with heavy bupivacaine in the sitting position a saddle block results, but potentially there would be no limit to the upwards spread if a hypobaric solution is used. If a spinal block is performed in the lateral position and the patient then turned supine, the upper limit of the block rarely exceeds the upper thoracic dermatomes because of the upward concavity of the cervical spine.

Dose and volume

The volume of fluid in which a drug is suspended does not influence the spread of the drug within the CSF. The total dose of drug influences the density and length of the spinal block but not the height. A low intrathecal dose of bupivacaine can result in a differential block where sensory and sympathetic fibres are blocked whilst motor fibres are spared.

Advantages:

- Clear end-point of technique
- Rapid onset of block
- Small nontoxic dose of local anaesthetics
- Rapid sacral block
- Posture with heavy bupivacaine produces a reliable low haemodynamically stable block.

Disadvantages:

- Difficulty in controlling height of block above T10
- Rapid onset of block resulting in haemodynamic instability
- Increased incidence of postdural puncture spinal headache
- Usually no way of extending the length of anaesthesia or analgesia.

Postdural puncture headaches

There is an increased incidence with increased size of needle, cutting (quincke) rather than atraumatic (sprotte or whitacre) and young rather than old age. With 26 or 27 gauge atraumatic needles, the incidence is less than 1%.

Spinal catheters

These are introduced through a larger spinal needle into the CSF. Spinal catheters smaller than 25 gauge are associated with slow injection times, with poor mixing of the drug with CSF resulting in a high neurotoxic concentration of local anaesthetic at the caudal tip. 24 gauge spinal catheters do not exhibit this problem, but are introduced with an 18 gauge spinal needle which results in a high incidence of postdural puncture headache.

Combined spinal–epidural anaesthesia

- *Single-space technique:* a 12 cm spinal needle can be placed in the CSF by passing it through a 10 cm tuohy needle situated in the epidural space. On withdrawing the spinal needle the epidural catheter is passed into the epidural space.
- *Double-space technique:* a spinal injection is performed and an epidural catheter inserted in the space above.

The technique offers the reliable rapid onset of a spinal block with the flexibility of using the epidural catheter to extend anaesthesia or for postoperative analgesia.

BIBLIOGRAPHY

Bergqvist D, Lindlad B, Matzsch T. Low molecular weight heparin for thromboprophylaxis and epidural/spinal anaesthesia – is there a risk? Acta Anaesthesiologica Scandinavica 1992; 36: 605–609

Cousins M J, Mather L E. Intrathecal and epidural administration of opioids. Anesthesiology 1984; 61: 276–310

Etches R C, Sandler A N, Daley M D. Respiratory depression and spinal opioids. Canadian Journal of Anaesthesia 1989; 36: 165–185

Kane R E. Neurological deficits following epidural or spinal anesthesia. Anesthesia and Analgesia 1981; 60: 150–161

Owens E L, Kasten G W, Hessel E A. Spinal subarachnoid hematoma after lumbar puncture and heparinization. Anesthesia and Analgesia 1986; 65: 1201–1207

32

INDUCED HYPOTENSION DURING ANAESTHESIA

A. Dash and I. Verner

Intraoperative bleeding may be arterial in origin and is dependent on mean arterial pressure (MAP). Capillary bleeding is consequent on local flow in the capillary bed, and venous bleeding is related to venous tone and posture. The major factor in intraoperative bleeding is MAP, which is the product of cardiac output and total peripheral resistance.

PATHOPHYSIOLOGY

See Table 1.

INDICATIONS

- To improve operative conditions and surgical technique especially for plastic, maxillofacial and ENT surgery
- To reduce excessive blood loss and its sequelae
- To reduce the risk of vessel rupture, e.g. intracranial aneurysms, aortic dissection, arteriovenous malformations
- To minimize the need for homologous transfusion.

RELATIVE CONTRAINDICATIONS

- Cardiovascular instability, hypovolaemia, anaemia
- Severe peripheral or cerebral vascular disease
- Uncontrolled hypertension
- Severe renal, hepatic or respiratory disease
- Diabetes mellitus and narrow angle glaucoma, when using ganglion blockers.

32

Table 1.

	Physiology	Effect of hypotension and anaesthetic implications
Brain	CBF maintained at MAP 60–160 mmHg in normotensive patients. This autoregulation is shifted to a higher range of MAP in hypertension. Hypoxia, hypercarbia and acidosis produce cerebral vasodilatation Hypocarbia ($P_{a}co_2 < 35$ mmHg) produces cerebral vasoconstriction	Below 60 mmHg MAP, autoregulation is lost and cerebral perfusion becomes pressure dependent. Raised intracranial pressure (ICP) reduces cerebral perfusion pressure (CPP): CPP = MAP–ICP
Kidneys	Renal blood flow is maintained for a MAP of 60–150 mmHg. Glomerular filtration rate will fall at a systolic pressure of <70 mmHg	
Heart	Endocardial perfusion is dependent on diastolic blood pressure	Induced hypotension reduces coronary blood flow, reduces afterload, reduces myocardial work and oxygen consumption. Normally myocardial ischaemia will occur when the diastolic blood pressure is <30–40 mmHg; this threshold is higher in coronary artery disease, hypertension and cardiomyopathy
Lungs	Induced hypotension accentuates ventilation/perfusion mismatch leading to an increased physiological dead space	IPPV is indicated, with a raised inspired oxygen concentration

TECHNIQUE

General

Perioperatively, aim to keep the systolic pressure above the preoperative diastolic pressure.

Premedication

Adequate premedication will reduce circulating catecholamines. Avoid atropine.

Induction

Aim for a smooth, controlled anaesthetic. Intubate to prevent airway obstruction and carbon dioxide retention.

Maintenance

Use IPPV to produce moderate hyperventilation, with an inspired oxygen concentration of ≥50%. IPPV will also reduce venous return. Isoflurane, a peripheral vasodilator, is a suitable inhalational agent. At low inspired concentrations isoflurane, causes little myocardial depression; higher concentrations lead to CNS depression, marked vasodilatation and reduced reflex tachycardia. It has little effect on the CBF.

Specific

Posture:

- Positioning will reduce arterial bleeding if the operative site is above the level of the heart
- For each 2.5 cm vertical height above the heart, the local arterial pressure is reduced by 2 mmHg
- Venous pooling also aids hypotensive agents.

Hypotensive agents

Sympathetic ganglion blockade

Trimetaphan blocks both the sympathetic and parasympathetic ganglia, resulting in vasodilatation, mydriasis and tachycardia. It has a 10–15 min duration of action and is given either by intravenous bolus (5–15 mg) or by infusion (0.04–0.05 mg kg^{-1} min^{-1}). Problems associated with its use include tachycardia, tachyphylaxis and persistent mydriasis.

α-Receptor blockade

Phentolamine (5–10 mg i.v.) has a 20–40 min duration of action. Oxygen consumption and heart rate are increased due to direct myocardial stimulation.

Droperidol produces mild receptor blockade, and is useful when given preoperatively as an adjunct to other hypotensive agents.

β-Receptor blockade

Labetolol has alpha- as well as beta-blocking action. Its alpha-blocking action is weaker than its beta blockade and lasts for only 30 min compared with a beta-blocking duration of 90 min.

Propranolol can be given preoperatively (40 mg t.d.s.) or intraoperatively (0.5–1 mg i.v.). It reduces both cardiac output and heart rate, and is useful for treating the tachycardia associated with autonomic ganglion blockers and direct vasodilators.

Esmolol produces selective beta-1 blockade. It has a rapid onset and offset. Problems include profound myocardial depression.

Direct acting vasodilators

SNP has rapid onset and offset. It has a predictable hypotensive effect, and is predominantly an arterial dilator. Problems associated with its use include raised CBF and cyanide toxicity. The maximum safe total dose is 1.5 mg kg^{-1} and an infusion rate of 10 μg kg^{-1} min^{-1}. For prolonged use in the ITU, RBC cyanide levels should be measured.

Trinitroglycerine mainly acts on the venous system, with a consequent reduction in right atrial filling pressure. The systolic pressure is only moderately reduced, whilst the diastolic pressure is largely maintained and the coronary vasculature is dilated. Coronary perfusion pressure is therefore maintained or enhanced, making nitroglycerine of particular use in treating hypertension associated with cardiac surgery. Problems include raised ICP and resistance to its hypotensive effects.

Other

Spinal and extradural anaesthesia produce sympathetic blockade with arteriolar dilatation, hypotension and reduced venous tone. A block to T1–T4 affects the cardiac sympathetic fibres and minimizes any compensatory tachycardia.

Monitoring:

- ECG – ST depression and ectopics indicate inadequate myocardial perfusion
- BP – measure by using an arterial line, with a transducer at the level of the head if in the head-up position
- Oxygen saturation – low pressure may lead to loss of signal
- $ETCO_2$ – look for hypoventilation and air embolism
- Blood loss – careful observation is required, as normal compensatory mechanisms to hypovolaemia are lost.

Recovery:

- Maintain a clear airway and give oxygen
- Take care with posture
- Blood pressure should return to the preoperative level before the patient is discharged to the ward.

COMPLICATIONS

- Inadequate hypotension
- Reactive haemorrhage, haematoma
- Excessive hypotension leading to
  - Cerebral ischaemia, thrombosis, oedema
  - Acute renal failure
  - Myocardial infarction, cardiac failure, cardiac arrest.

BIBLIOGRAPHY

Blau W S, Kafer E R, Anderson J A. Esmolol is more effective than sodium nitroprusside in reducing blood loss during orthognathic surgery. Anaesthesia and Analgesia 1992; 75: 172–178

Simpson P J. Hypotensive anaesthesia. Current Anaesthesia and Critical Care 1992; 3: 90–97

Simpson P J. Perioperative blood loss and its reduction: the role of the anaesthetist. British Journal of Anaesthesia 1992; 69: 498–507

32

LOCAL ANAESTHETIC TECHNIQUES

A. Goodwin

32

INDICATIONS

Local anaesthetic blocks can be used:

- As the sole anaesthetic technique for an operative procedure
- In conjunction with either sedation or a general anaesthetic
- For providing analgesia.

CONTRAINDICATIONS

- Allergy to local anaesthetics (in practice this is rare and occurs more commonly with the ester type local anaesthetics, e.g. procaine)
- Infection at the site of intended block
- Coagulopathy.

PRACTICAL CONSIDERATIONS

Preoperative assessment

The patient should be assessed preoperatively as if they were to receive a general anaesthetic. There is always the small, but nonetheless serious possibility of local anaesthetic toxicity which may result in the patient being rendered unconscious and requiring support normally associated with a general anaesthetic. Similarly, in the event of failure of the local anaesthetic technique, conversion to a general anaesthetic may be required. The patient should therefore be starved, and particular attention paid to the assessment of airway and the history of any allergies or medication.

Perioperative management

Monitoring

This should be started prior to the local anaesthetic administration and include:

- ECG
- Noninvasive BP
- Sa_{O_2}.

Intravenous access must be established.

If the local anaesthesia block is to be combined with a general anaesthetic it can be performed either before or once the patient is asleep. It is obviously difficult to assess the block once the patient is asleep.

THE LOCAL ANAESTHETIC BLOCK

The patient should have been reassured and had the procedure explained, as their cooperation is often required. The patient should be accurately positioned for the block and the approach chosen. There are numerous books offering detailed technical information and illustrations to assist with this. The area to be blocked should be cleaned. It is not usually necessary to adopt a full sterile approach with gowns and gloves if a no-touch technique is used. However, for the inexperienced it is preferable to err on the side of caution.

Needles

In selecting a needle for the block the following should be considered:

- Short or long bevel
- Gauge
- Needle with or without catheter.

Standard needles have a 14° bevel. However, needles reground to a 45° bevel (i.e. a short bevel) have been shown to be associated with less fasicular damage.

A 22 gauge needle is suitable for most blocks. This minimizes the risk of trauma, whilst giving a rapid aspiration time.

Another useful practice, particularly in a block requiring large volumes of local anaesthetic to be injected, is to connect the syringe containing the local anaesthetic to the needle with a piece of short extension tubing and a three-way tap. This enables a second person to inject the solution while the first prevents the needle from moving.

To prolong the duration of a local anaesthetic block of a nerve lying within a sheath, e.g. the axillary nerve, it is possible to leave an intravenous cannula in situ lying within the nerve sheath, and use this to administer further doses of local anaesthetic or to provide local anaesthetic infusion.

Nerve stimulator

The use of a nerve stimulator can increase the accuracy and ease of performing a block and, by avoiding the need for paraesthesia, reduces the potential for nerve damage or patient cooperation. The nerve stimulator consists of a ground electrode, an exploring electrode and a power source. The nerve stimulator should have:

- Impulses at 0.5 or 1 s intervals
- Have variable voltage or current control
- The ability to stimulate at 0.5 mA
- A pulse width of 0.1–0.2 ms.

Technique

The ground electrode is attached to the patient at a site away from the block while the exploring electrode is attached to a conducting part of the needle to be used. A purpose-designed 'pole' needle is recommended. Initially, the settings are high and used to elicit a response from the nerve to be blocked. As the nerve is approached more accurately by the needle, far lower settings are required to achieve the same result.

CHOICE OF AGENT

The choice of local anaesthetic agent depends on:

- Potency
- Potential toxicity
- Duration of action.

The three local anaesthetic agents available in the UK are bupivacaine, lignocaine and prilocaine (see Table 1).

Bupivacaine is regarded as more cardiotoxic than the other agents, with ventricular fibrillation seen more commonly in overdose.

Prilocaine is the agent of choice for intravenous regional anaesthesia (IVRA). Its metabolite *o*-toluidine may cause methaemoglobinaemia. Methaemoglobinaemia appears as cyanosis when 1.5 g/100 ml of haemoglobin is in the reduced state. This is rapidly reversed with the intravenous injection of 1 mg kg^{-1} of methylene blue.

Table 1.
Comparison of local anaesthetic agents

Anaesthetic agent	Duration of action	Maximum safe dose (mg kg^{-1})	Maximum safe dose with adrenaline
Bupivacaine	+ + +	2	2
Lignocaine	+ +	3	6
Prilocaine	+	6	8 (with felypressin)

A study comparing equipotent doses of lignocaine to bupivacaine for a lumbar plexus block has shown that the time to onset of action of lignocaine and bupivacaine is comparable, but the recovery from motor and sensory block was more rapid with lignocaine.

	Lignocaine	Bupivacaine
Onset time (min)	20	20
Recovery time (min)	4–6	17–23

Vasopressors

Adrenaline and other vasoconstrictors are completely contraindicated in ring blocks and IVRA as they may cause ischaemia. It is preferable not to use concentrations of adrenaline greater than 1:200 000 due to the systemic side-effects of adrenaline, which are particularly undesirable in patients with cardiovascular disease. If given intravenously, 15 μg (3 ml of 1:200 000) of adrenaline will increase the heart rate by at least 30% within 1 min. Adrenaline is useful in combination with lignocaine, as it reduces the peak concentration in the blood. The addition of 1:200 000 adrenaline causes a 50% decrease in the peak plasma concentration when used for subcutaneous infiltration, but a 20–30% decrease when used for intercostal or brachial plexus blocks. Adrenaline decreases the blood concentration of bupivacaine significantly less than that of lignocaine, so that it is not usually worth using bupivacaine with adrenaline.

BIBLIOGRAPHY

Butterworth J F, Brownlow R C et al. Bupivacaine inhibits cyclic-3′,5′-adenosine monophosphate production. Anesthesiology 1993; 79: 88–95

Madej T H, Ellis F R, Halsall P J. Evaluation of '3 in 1' lumbar plexus block in patients having muscle biopsy. British Journal of Anaesthesia 1989; 62: 515–517

Moore D C, Batra M S. The components of an effective test dose prior to epidural block. Anesthesiology 1981; 55: 693–696

Raj P, Rosenblatt R, Montgomery S J. Use of the nerve stimulator for peripheral nerve blocks. Regional Anaesthesia 1980; April–June: 14–20

Rosen M A, Thigpen J W, Shnider S M, Foutz S E, Levinson G, Koike M. Bupivacaine-induced cardiotoxicity in hypoxic and acidotic sheep. Anesthesia and Analgesia 1983; 64: 802

Selander D, Dhuner K G, Lundborg G. Peripheral nerve injury due to injection needles used for regional anaesthesia. Acta Anaesthesiologica Scandinavica 1977; 21: 182–188

ONE-LUNG ANAESTHESIA

D. Higgins

INDICATIONS

One-lung anaesthesia involves the complete functional separation of the two lungs and is often the most important anaesthetic consideration for patients undergoing thoracic surgery. There are three absolute indications for one-lung anaesthesia:

- To prevent contamination of one lung by spillage of pus, secretions or blood from the other lung
- Where differential ventilation between the two lungs is required, e.g. in a bronchopleural fistula
- To perform unilateral bronchopulmonary lavage.

Relative indications are situations where surgical exposure may be facilitated, e.g. oesophageal surgery.

PHYSIOLOGY

During thoracotomy in the lateral position the compliance of the dependent lung is reduced and the upper lung is therefore ventilated preferentially during IPPV. The effect of gravity on the low pressure pulmonary circulation increases blood flow to the lower lung, and thus there is a mismatch between perfusion and ventilation. With the onset of one-lung ventilation the preferential distribution of ventilation to the upper lung is completely eliminated. Perfusion to this lung continues and this results in increased venous admixture. At this stage the dependent lung receives the entire minute volume and a high proportion of the cardiac output. An excess of perfusion relative to ventilation in areas of this lung may also contribute to the venous admixture which is in the range 30–40%. The resulting arterial hypoxaemia may be further increased by:

- A reduction in cardiac output
- Thoracotomy for disease not in the lung, or for disease in the dependent lung
- A misplaced double lumen tube with impaired ventilation to the dependent lung.

Three factors predict a significant fall in P_aO_2 during one-lung anaesthesia:

- Right (as opposed to left) sided thoracotomy
- Good preoperative FEV_1
- Low intraoperative P_aO_2 during two-lung ventilation.

PREOPERATIVE ASSESSMENT AND INVESTIGATIONS

- Full blood count; urea and electrolytes
- Chest X-ray – it is important to assess if endobronchial intubation is possible
- Arterial blood gases; spirometry
- ECG, if the patient is older than 50 years.

PERIOPERATIVE MANAGEMENT

Monitoring:

- ECG
- SaO_2
- $ETCO_2$
- Airway inflation pressure
- BP – this should be measured via arterial cannulation on the dependent side, which also allows for sampling for arterial blood gas analysis
- Fluid balance and blood loss
- Core temperature
- Central venous pressure.

Central venous cannulation should be performed on the same side as the thoracotomy.

Anaesthetic technique:

- Give generous premedication
- Give general anaesthesia with muscle relaxation and controlled ventilation through a double-lumen tube
- Use double-lumen tubes

Robertshaw double-lumen endobronchial tubes are the most common variety in use. The PVC derivative (Bronchocath) is associated with less trauma than the original red rubber form. In most cases of trauma, injury occurs from overdistension of the bronchial cuff. This may be avoided by using no more than 3 ml of air to seal the bronchial cuff.

The right main bronchus gives rise to the RUL bronchus after 2.5 cm. Right-sided endobronchial tube placement should be avoided where possible because of the high risk of RUL occlusion.

The correct positioning of a double-lumen tube is traditionally confirmed by observation of chest expansion and auscultation while each lumen in turn is occluded. This technique fails to detect suboptimal positioning in 48% of cases. The use of a flexible fibre-optic bronchoscope allows direct visual confirmation of tube position. Pressure and volume loop spirometry is an accurate alternative.

ARTERIAL HYPOXAEMIA

This is the most important problem encountered during one-lung anaesthesia. The degree of hypoxia may be reduced by the manoeuvres described below.

Manoeuvres for reducing hypoxaemia

- Reduce blood flow through the unventilated lung:
  - Ventilate both lungs for as long as possible to ensure that the time during which blood flows through the unventilated lung is kept to a minimum
  - During pulmonary resection the pulmonary vessels should be ligated at an early stage; the practice of temporarily interrupting pulmonary blood flow during thoracotomy for nonpulmonary surgery is considered unsafe.
- Reduce the mismatch between ventilation and perfusion in the dependent lung:
  - Increase the inspired oxygen concentration
  - Use a tidal volume of 12 ml kg^{-1} to reduce the tendency to atelectasis
  - Avoid the use of PEEP which tends to increase mean intra-alveolar pressure, reduce cardiac output, and redistribute blood flow in favour of the unventilated upper lung.
- Maintain cardiac output – avoid hypovolaemia, mediastinal manipulation, dysrhythmias, overventilation and depressant anaesthetic agents.

- Insufflate oxygen to the nonventilated lung.

The elimination of carbon dioxide during one-lung ventilation is not a problem if the minute volume is maintained at the amount previously delivered to the two lungs.

BIBLIOGRAPHY

Gothard J W W. Baillière's Clinical Anaesthesiology 1987; 1(1)
Gothard J W W, Branthwaite M A. Anaesthesia for thoracic surgery, Blackwell Scientific, Oxford
Vaughan R S. Double-lumen tubes (editorial). British Journal of Anaesthesia 1993; 70: 497–498

PROLONGED ANAESTHESIA

M. Nicol

Intraoperative, recovery room and major postoperative complications resulting in prolonged hospital stay have been shown to increase with an increase in anaesthetic time.

FACTORS ASSOCIATED WITH PROLONGED ANAESTHESIA

- Accumulation of anaesthetic agent (volatile or intravenous infusion) leading to slow elimination and delayed awakening
- Toxicity of administered agents:
  - Volatile agents – renal impairment due to elevated inorganic fluoride concentrations
- Nitrous oxide – bone marrow depression and expansion of air spaces
- Problems with accurate management of fluid and electrolyte balance
- Metabolic disturbances:
  - Decreased basal metabolic rate
  - Glucose metabolism
  - Liver enzyme changes
- Increased risk of infection – immunosuppression; depressed lymphocyte transformation; mucociliary depression leading to pooling of secretions
- Pressure area, care to avoid:
  - Nerve damage
  - Skin breakdown
  - Alopecia
  - Corneal damage
- Increased opportunity for human error.

Exposure to nitrous oxide

Continuous or repeated intermittent exposure to nitrous oxide has been related to bone marrow changes, leucopenia and agranulocytosis. Derangement in methionine metabolism may cause the neural injury resembling that of pernicious anaemia. Toxic manifestations may occur in susceptible individuals after shorter exposures.

Conditions predisposing to nitrous oxide toxicity:
- Exposure to DNA synthesis inhibitors (e.g. methotrexate)
- Pre-existing bone marrow depression
- Folate deficiency (e.g. alcoholism)
- Pernicious anaemia
- Diseases of the ileum (e.g. Crohn's disease).

THEATRE PREPARATION

- Manpower, patient supports and padding for pressure areas
- Adequate scavenging
- Low flow circuit
- Maintenance of body temperature (appropriate selection of theatre temperature, warming blanket, fluid warmers, humidification of inspired gases, clothing/limb wrapping, hat).

PERIOPERATIVE MANAGEMENT

Monitoring:
- ECG
- Sao_2
- Direct BP
- $ETco_2$
- Core temperature
- Blood loss
- Blood gases, electrolytes, glucose, coagulation
- Endotracheal tube cuff pressure
- Fluid balance (central venous pressure, hourly urine output via urinary catheter)
- Peripheral nerve stimulator
- Inspiratory concentration of oxygen and nitrous oxide
- End-tidal anaesthetic vapour concentration.

Anaesthetic technique
- Consider using oxygen/air technique, omitting nitrous oxide
- Consider using a low-flow circuit
- Limit F_Io2 to <50%, or the lowest tolerable fraction
- Isoflurane is the most suitable agent as it is the least metabolized
- Consider intravenous anaesthesia
- Pay careful attention to body positioning
- Reposition the head and available extremities frequently
- Cover exposed body surfaces
- Eye protection (lubrication, tapes, padding or eye shields)
- Frequent endotracheal tube suctioning
- Give muscle relaxants by infusion with guidance from train-of-four
- Deep vein thrombosis (DVT) prophylaxis (TED stockings/heparin/mechanical calf compression)
- Use a team of staff to avoid fatigue.

32

POSTOPERATIVE CARE

Consider:
- ITU stay for continued ventilation until warm and stable; awaken slowly
- Physiotherapy
- Maintenance of DVT prophylaxis
- Monitoring of marrow suppression and hepatic enzyme changes.

BIBLIOGRAPHY

Duncan P G, Cohen M M. Postoperative complications: factors of significance to anaesthetic practice. Canadian Journal of Anaesthesia 1987; 34: 2–8

Hogue C W, Perese D, Vacanti C A, Alston T A. Potential toxicity from prolonged anaesthesia: a case report of a thirty hour anaesthetic. Journal of Clinical Anesthesiology 1990; 2: 183–187

TOTAL INTRAVENOUS ANAESTHESIA

B. Al-Shaikh

32

A technique where a continuous intravenous infusion of one (or more) drugs is used to induce and maintain anaesthesia. Inhalational anaesthetic agents are not used.

CHARACTERISTICS OF THE IDEAL AGENT

- Soluble in water and stable for the duration of the infusion with no deterioration on exposure to light
- Long shelf-life
- No absorption into plastic
- Induces anaesthesia in one arm–brain circulation time
- Analgesic properties
- No side-effects on injection (pain, thrombophlebitis, anaphylactic/anaphylactoid reactions)
- Not irritant if injected extravascularly
- No adverse effects on major organ systems
- No epileptiform movements
- No major interaction with other anaesthetic drugs
- Rapid metabolism and elimination, through different pathways to ameliorate accumulation of drug or metabolites
- Rapid recovery without hangover or nausea.

At the present time, propofol is the only drug that is widely used for total intravenous anaesthesia (TIVA).

INDUCTION

Achieving and maintaining a constant level of effect by maintaining a constant plasma concentration is the objective of TIVA. This is generally achieved with a bolus dose. Many anaesthetists give the bolus from a syringe pump fitted with a rapid bolus facility. The size of the bolus dose required depends on the desired plasma concentration and the distribution volume.

Rapid infusion rates of propofol achieve unconsciousness sooner, but increase the incidence of cardiovascular and respiratory depression (see Table 1).

MAINTENANCE

This is achieved by a constant-rate infusion (about 6 mg kg^{-1} h^{-1}). If a constant rate of infusion is run from the start, multiple additional boluses will be required in the early stages to maintain anaesthesia. It is better to use a step-down sequence of infusion rates, the best known of which is 10 mg kg^{-1} h^{-1} for 10 min, 8 mg kg^{-1} h^{-1} for 10 min, and 6 mg kg^{-1} h^{-1} thereafter. Propofol is prepared as a 10 mg ml^{-1} solution and, therefore, a pump speed (ml h^{-1}) which is equal to the patient's body weight in kilograms gives 10 mg kg^{-1} h^{-1}, the starting rate. The step-down sequence is designed to overcome the low plasma concentrations which are often found initially with a

Table 1.
Infusion rate of propofol and the change in arterial pressure

Infusion rate (mg min^{-1})	**Propofol dose required for induction** (mg kg^{-1})	**Time to complete induction** (s)	**Mean % fall in arterial pressure at the end of induction**
200	2.52	51	20.3
100	1.60	67	19.7
50	1.24	103	8.8

constant rate infusion, although the total dose given is higher (Table 2).

Table 2.

Maintenance type	No. further doses required in first 30 min	Total dose given (mg kg^{-1} h^{-1})
Fixed rate (6 mg kg^{-1} h^{-1})	45	5.63
Step-down 10 mg kg^{-1} h^{-1} for 10 min 8 mg kg^{-1} h^{-1} for 10 min 6 mg kg^{-1} h^{-1} thereafter	23	6.08

A computer-controlled exponentially declining infusion rate is even better still.

Although it is possible to maintain anaesthesia with propofol alone, this requires high plasma levels during stimulating procedures. Recovery is subsequently delayed (time to respond to commands is 26 min, as compared with 8 min with propofol/fentanyl).

ANALGESIA

Although propofol may have some analgesic properties, TIVA is generally achieved by combining a propofol infusion with a regional local anaesthetic block or supplemental opioids.

The shorter acting opioids are often suggested as an ideal complement to propofol. Alfentanyl has been studied in several surgical environments and is given as a bolus followed by single-rate infusion (Table 3). As a rule, it is preferable to maintain the opioid infusion within the steep section of the dose–response curve and adjust anaesthetic depth by altering propofol infusion.

Table 3.
Example infusion rates of alfentanyl

	Alfentanyl bolus (μg kg^{-1})	Alfentanyl infusion (μg kg^{-1} h^{-1})
Major abdominal surgery	20	20
Cardiac surgery	50	50

The addition of nitrous oxide decreases hypnotic requirements during TIVA; 67% nitrous oxide decreases plasma concentrations of propofol by only 25%.

Propofol is cleared from the body mainly by metabolism. It has been successfully used in patients with liver cirrhosis, and the pharmacokinetics are not significantly affected by the disease. The pharmacokinetics of propofol may be influenced by age. Values for clearance and plasma concentration on awakening are higher in children than adults. Children require significantly higher doses of propofol than do adults.

The rapid recovery from propofol is due to its short distribution phase, high clearance rate and short elimination half-life.

DOSE–RESPONSE RELATIONSHIP

In order to compare TIVA with inhalational anaesthesia, the concept of minimum infusion rate (MIR), which is similar to the MAC, has been established. MIR is that rate of infusion which produces loss of motor responses to surgical stimulation in 50% of patients.

In monitoring the depth of anaesthesia during TIVA, the dose–response curve for spontaneous movement and for oesophageal contractility are close together.

Although children need higher doses than adults, the dose–response relationships are similar to those of the adults. A computer-controlled infusion has been developed using a pharmacokinetic model. It rapidly provides a fairly constant plasma concentration of propofol with stable anaesthesia. The anaesthetist is required to enter the patient's weight and the desired plasma concentration of propofol.

USES OF TIVA

TIVA has been used successfully in a wide range of surgical procedures, including cardiac, intracranial (propofol increases cerebral compliance) and obstetric surgery. For the latter, the placenta acts as a partial barrier to propofol. The neonate can rapidly clear propofol from its circulation. Negligible amounts of propofol were excreted with the breast milk in a small group of patients. TIVA is potentially useful when inhalational anaesthesia is difficult or contraindicated, e.g. rigid bronchoscopy, MH susceptibility.

ADVANTAGES OF TIVA

- Avoiding the use of nitrous oxide with its effect on air emboli and pneumothoraces, bone marrow suppression and intracranial suppression
- Elimination of volatile agents and their possible toxicity to the liver and kidney and their effect on the uterus
- Elimination of the need for accurately calibrated vaporizers
- Better quality recovery with less hangover.

DISADVANTAGES

- Pharmacokinetic and dynamic variability of response to the injected drug
- Variations in the haemodynamic state of the patient
- Intravenous access required
- Cost of equipment and drugs.

CARDIOVASCULAR SIDE-EFFECTS

- Pronounced falls in MAP in opioid premedicated patients or beta-blocked hypertensive patients
- The MAP is lower when nitrous oxide is administered
- Ameliorated by slow rate of induction
- Bradycardia occurs, and is accentuated by opioids (e.g. fentanyl); is vagally mediated and is prevented by atropine or glycopyrrolate.

In the compromised heart, propofol/nitrous oxide may cause a further decrement in function, although maintenance of filling pressure may offset this effect.

BIBLIOGRAPHY

Cockshott I D, Douglas E J, Prys Roberts C, Turtle M J, Coates D P. Pharmacokinetics of prolonged anaesthesia during and after i.v. infusions in man. Anaesthesiology 1990; 7: 265–276

Roberts F L, Dixon J, Lewis G T R, Tackley R M, Prys Roberts C. Induction and maintenance of propofol anaesthesia. A manual infusion scheme. Anaesthesia 1988; 43 (suppl): 14–17

Sear J W. Continuous infusions of hypnotic agents for maintenance of anaesthesia. In: Kay B (ed) Total intravenous anaesthesia. Elsevier, Amsterdam, 1991, p 15–55

32

33

MANAGEMENT PROBLEMS

T. E. J. Healy

ALLERGIC REACTION

T. Strang and
D. Tupper-Carey

Allergic reactions are unpredictable life-threatening events. Prompt recognition and treatment are essential.

The incidence is 1:6000 anaesthetics.

The estimated mortality is 5%.

The causative agent can be any drug, but in particular:

- Neuromuscular blockers (especially suxamethonium)
- Induction agents
- Antibiotics
- Plasma volume expanders
- Blood products
- Chymopapain
- Protamine
- Latex.

PATHOPHYSIOLOGY

Anaphylactic and anaphylactoid reactions are clinically indistinguishable (Figure 1). The terms refer to the triggering pathway responsible for the final common end-point, i.e. the release of potent circulating inflammatory mediators from degranulated mast cells.

Anaphylactic reactions involve cross-linking of two adjacent IgE antigen-specific antibodies to the mast-cell surface causing a type-I hypersensitivity reaction.

Reactions caused by any other triggering pathways are, therefore, anaphylactoid, as in anaesthetic drug mixtures causing 'aggregate anaphylaxis'.

In many cases, previous sensitization to the antigen or similar compound cannot be demonstrated.

SIGNIFICANT CLINICAL FEATURES

- Symptoms occur within 5 min in 98% of cases.
- Profound hypotension or cardiac arrest may be seen.
- Hypoxia:
  - Inability to ventilate
  - Bronchospasm
  - Laryngeal oedema
- Urticarial rash or erythema.

MANAGEMENT

Secure intravenous access and routine monitoring should already be established.

Immediate treatment

- Discontinue administration of suspected agent.
- *Call for help.*
- Discontinue surgery and anaesthesia, if possible.
- Administer 100% oxygen.
- Maintain airway – intubate if not already performed.
- Exclude:
  - Endotracheal tube malposition
  - Anaesthetic circuit malfunction.
- Start IPPV.
- Check carotid pulse – if absent start advanced life support. Give l-ml aliquots of 1:10 000 adrenaline i.v. simultaneously with rapid fluid infusion (e.g. 10 ml kg^{-1} colloid), titrating to response.
- Prolonged bronchospasm may require slow infusion of a bronchodilator, e.g. aminophyline, salbutamol, together with steroid and volatile inhalational therapy.
- Resistant cardiovascular collapse may require continued vasopressor therapy.
- Transfer to the ITU if necessary.

The above drill should be regularly rehearsed.

Further management

The anaesthetist must:

- Initiate investigations to identify the causative agent
- Inform the patient and issue an anaesthetic hazard card
- Inform the Committee on Safety of Medicines (CSM, Freepost, London SW8 5BR, UK).

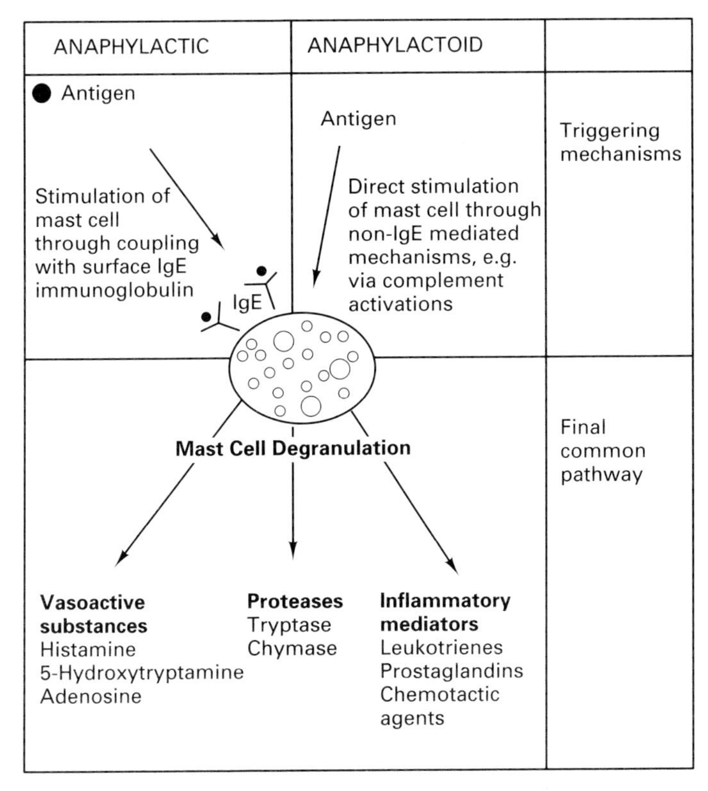

Figure 1
Immune mechanisms of anaphylactic and anaphylactoid reactions. The 'antigen' refers to the drug or substance responsible for activating the triggering mechanism. In some cases, for example penicillin, binding to a hapten (carrier protein) is necessary prior to coupling with surface membrane IgE antibody.

Immunological advice on the selection of tests varies. Anaesthetists should therefore confer with their local regional immunology laboratory or the Anaesthetic Reactions Advisory Service (Sheffield) to ensure that the correct samples can be meaningfully interpreted by the recipient immunologist.

Subsequent analysis of serum and urine collected shortly after the incident establish if an allergic reaction has taken place.

- Radioallergosorbent (RAST) tests are available for suxamethonium, alcuronium, thiopentone, protamine and morphine. False-positive results are common.
- Skin tests attempt to identify the causative agent. A wheal of 5 mm indicates a positive reaction. Operator expertise is essential.
- Cross-sensitivity occurs, so testing of drugs related to the suspected allergen is recommended. This is important when investigating bisquaternary ammonium compounds, e.g. muscle relaxants.
- Screening for anaphylaxis currently has no value.

Management of the patient with documented previous anaphylaxis:
- Identify severity of previous reaction
- Identify causative agent, if possible
- Consider using a regional technique
- Consider using an inhalational technique
- *Avoid causative agent*
- Avoid related agents, if possible.

If the above measures are not possible, or a reaction is thought possible:

- Premedicate with hydrocortisone, H_1 and H_2 antagonists and inhaled β agonists

Table 1.
Immunological identification of mast-cell degranulation

Test	Bottle	Time after event
Serum histamine	5 ml EDTA	Immediately
Serum mast cell tryptase	5 ml EDTA	1 and 3 h
Urine methylhistamine	5 ml	First voided sample
C_3 breakdown products	5 ml EDTA	1 and 3 h
Immunological identification of allergen		
Intradermal and prick test	–	4–6 weeks
RAST tests	–	Up to 8 weeks

- Ensure full monitoring and secure intravenous access with a cannula of at least 18 gauge in an adult
- Preoxygenate the patient
- Ensure that vasopressor therapy is immediately available
- The safest intravenous drug combination at present is etomidate, fentanyl and atracurium
- Volatile agents should all be safe
- Inject drugs slowly into freely flowing intravenous infusion
- Update the patient's hazard card for future information.

BIBLIOGRAPHY

Association of Anaesthetists of Great Britain and Ireland. Anaphylactic reactions associated with anaesthesia. 1990

Clarke R S J, Watkins J. Drugs responsible for anaphylactic reactions in anaesthesia in the United Kingdom. Annals Francais Anesthesie et Reamination 1993; 12: 105–108

Fisher M. Anaphylaxis to anaesthetic drugs: aetiology, recognition and management. Current Anaesthesia and Critical Care 1991; 2: 182–186

CROSS REFERENCES

Cardiopulmonary resuscitation
Anaesthetic Factors 34: 687

AMNIOTIC FLUID EMBOLISM

A. Corbett and E. L. Horsman

Amniotic fluid embolism (AFE) is the syndrome which occurs when amniotic fluid gains entry into the maternal circulation. It may be the composition of the amniotic fluid which determines whether the pathological events comprising the syndrome occur following entry. Primate models where clear autologous amniotic fluid was injected into the maternal circulation produced no clinical effect (Adamsons et al 1971).

AFE has an 80% mortality and featured as the fourth and fifth most common causes of maternal death in the 1982–84 and 1985–87 Triennial Maternal Mortality Reports (England and Wales 1982–84, United Kingdom 1985–87).

AFE occurs most commonly during labour, but has been associated with the list of events shown in Table 1.

Morgan (1979), in his review of AFE, effectively refuted the association between AFE and tumultuous labour, oxytocin augmentation of labour, traumatic delivery, large babies, and fetal death preceding AFE.

CLINICAL PRESENTATION

The two main features of AFE are:

- Cardiorespiratory problems
- Haematological problems.

Cardiorespiratory problems

The classical presentation is at or around delivery with the symptoms and signs of

Table 1.
Aetiological factors in AFE

Aetiological factors in AFE
Dilatation and curettage
Termination of pregnancy
Intra-amniotic saline
Amniocentesis
Amniotomy
Induction of labour
Insertion of prostaglandin gel
Vaginal/cervical tear
Caesarean section
Uterine rupture

severe cardiorespiratory collapse (Table 2). From case reports where patients have survived long enough to have a pulmonary flotation catheter inserted, the picture has been one of left ventricular heart failure with elevated left ventricular end diastolic pressure (LVEDP) and elevated pulmonary capillary wedge pressure (PCWP). These measurements validate the clinical and X-ray picture of pulmonary oedema which occurs in many of the 50–75% of patients who survive the initial cardiopulmonary collapse. Whether, as previously thought, severe intrapulmonary shunting, pulmonary hypertension and right heart failure precede, or even precipitate, the documented left heart failure, is unclear.

Table 2.
Cardiorespiratory symptoms and signs

Cardiorespiratory symptoms and signs
Dyspnoea
Hypoxia
Hypotension
Convulsions
Bronchospasm
Arrhythmias
Cardiac arrest

Haematological problems

Coagulopathy accompanying cardiorespiratory collapse, following cardiorespiratory collapse or occurring without cardiorespiratory symptoms or signs is the other main feature of AFE. The coagulopathy may be obvious as severe vaginal haemorrhage or as severe haemorrhage during Caesarean section and may be compounded by uterine atony. Occasionally, AFE has to be included in the differential diagnosis when abnormal bleeding occurs from wounds or intravenous access sites without preceding evidence of AFE. In 40% of cases of AFE there is evidence of coagulopathy, and this should be anticipated if the diagnosis of AFE has been made.

TREATMENT

Cardiac arrest

Commence cardiac arrest procedure.

Hypoxia or hypotension without cardiac arrest:

- Administer 100% oxygen; intubate and ventilate with 100% oxygen
- Site a large-bore cannula and give colloid rapidly if the patient is hypotensive
- Commence dopamine infusion if the patient is hypotensive
- Site a central venous pressure cannula or a pulmonary flotation catheter if available
- Manipulate fluids and cardiovascular drugs according to haemodynamic measurements
- Transfer to the ITU.

Coagulopathy:

- Take blood for a full coagulation screen, including platelets
- Inform the haematology laboratory of the problem
- Give fresh frozen plasma, platelets, cryoprecipitate and concentrated red cells, depending on clotting results and blood loss
- Give oxytocics if uterine atony is present, syntocinon (i.v.), ergometrine (i.v.), or prostaglandin $E_1\alpha$ by intramuscular or intrauterine injection.

CONFIRMATION OF DIAGNOSIS

Antemortem laboratory diagnosis of AFE

In 1947, Gross & Benz reported that centrifuged blood obtained from the right heart of AFE patients showed three strata rather than two, and that this was pathognomic AFE. They also advocated looking at sections of smears of this 'flocculent' layer for mucous and squames. In 1985, Masson & Ruggieri described a new diagnostic application of the pulmonary artery catheter to obtain microvascular blood and demonstrate the presence of fetal squames in suspected AFE. However, caution was advocated by Clark et al in 1986 when they showed that squames could be demonstrated in both pregnant and nonpregnant patients. Meticulous technique using the correct stain and evidence of other amniotic fluid debris such as mucin, hair and fat droplets should be obtained to validate the diagnosis of AFE. Recently, Japanese workers (Kobayashi et al 1993) have described a monoclonal antibody technique to detect mucin-like glycoproteins in maternal serum. A significantly elevated level of such antigens was found in four patients with symptoms suggestive of AFE.

Postmortem diagnosis of AFE

The presence of amniotic fluid debris, squames, lanugo hair and mucin on sectioning of lung specimens is the cornerstone of the diagnosis of AFE.

BIBLIOGRAPHY

Adamsons K, Mueller-Heubach E, Myer R E. The innocuousness of amniotic fluid infusion in the pregnant rhesus monkey. American Journal of Obstetrics and Gynaecology 1971; 109: 977

Clark S L. New concepts of amniotic fluid embolism: a review. Obstetrics and Gynaecology Survey 1990; 45: 360–368

Clark S L, Pavlova Z, Greenspoon J. Squamous cells in the maternal pulmonary circulation. American Journal of Obstetrics and Gynecology 1986; 154: 104–106

Gross P, Benz E J. Pulmonary embolism by amniotic fluid. Surgery, Gynecology and Obstetrics 1947; 85: 315–320

Kobayashi H, Ohi H, Terao T. A simple noninvasive sensitive method for diagnosis of amniotic fluid embolism by monoclonal antibody TKH2 that recognises Neu Ac alpha 2–6 Gal NAc. American Journal of Obstetrics and Gynecology 1993; 168: 848–853

Masson R G, Ruggieri J. Pulmonary microvascular cytology. A new diagnostic application of the pulmonary artery catheter. Chest 1985; 88: 908–914

Morgan M. Amniotic fluid embolism, Anaesthesia, 1979; 34: 20–32

CROSS REFERENCES

Obstetric anaesthesia
Surgical Procedures 20: 391

Caesarean section – general anaesthesia
Surgical Procedures 20: 402

Caesarian section – combined
Surgical Procedures 20: 404

Caesarian section – spinal anaesthesia
Surgical Procedures 20: 406

Epidural for caesarian section
Surgical Procedures 20: 412

Cardiopulmonary resuscitation
Anaesthetic Factors 34: 687

AWARENESS

C. J. D. Pomfrett

DEFINITION

- The patient remembers part or all of the anaesthetic or surgical procedure.
- Recall of specific words or sounds in the operating room will distinguish awareness from hallucination or dreaming.
- Awareness may be accompanied by unbearable pain, and give rise to postoperative psychological trauma, and litigation.
- Recall may be explicit, when the patient is capable of speaking of the event, or implicit, where subconscious learning during anaesthesia surfaces as a behavioral change. Implicit recall may be studied using postoperative hypnosis of the patient.

RECOLLECTION

Events recalled may be many if the patient is aware (Table 1). Auditory stimuli are most frequently recalled, especially negative comments regarding the patient's condition or appearance.

INCIDENCE

It is interesting to note that the incidence of awareness under anaesthesia has decreased over the last 30 years (Table 2). Estimates vary depending on the anaesthetic procedure and nature of postoperative interview.

Even with an incidence of 0.2%, 1:500 patients will be aware. It is not possible to determine the reason for this change. A number of factors are likely to be involved, including improved anaesthetic agents, improved monitoring and fear of litigation.

IDENTIFICATION

- Increased BP, heart rate, sweating, tear formation
- Advanced monitoring, e.g. electroencephalograph (EEG)
- Postoperative interview
- The hand-written anaesthetic record is limited as a method of determining why awareness and recall have occurred (Moerman et al 1993).

SEQUELAE

- Sleep disturbances, e.g. nightmares
- Flashbacks
- Anxiety, possibly bordering on psychosis
- Increased fear of anaesthesia.

Table 1.
Events recalled under anaesthesia*

Event	%	Sample size
Sounds	89	23
Paralysis	85	22
Visual perception	39	10
Intubation or tube	7	27
Anxiety or panic	92	24
Helplessness	46	12
Sequelae	69	18

*From Moerman et al (1993).

Table 2.
Incidence of awareness

Date of study	% Awareness	% Dreaming	Sample size
Structured interview (Liu et al 1991)			
1960	1.2	3	656
1971	1.6	26	120
1973	1.5	–	200
1975	0.8	7.7	490
1990	0.2	0.9	1000
No structured interview			
1983	13	–	91 (Caesarean)
1984	11	–	37 (Casualty)
1986	8	11	36 (Caesarean)
1988	0	19	120 (Paediatric)
1990	0	3	200 (Caesarean)

CAUSES

Induction:

- Intubation immediately after induction with an intravenous agent (i.e. too early) may lead to awareness of intubation
- Any delay before intubation (e.g. waiting for the relaxant to take effect, problems with intubation) may mean that the action of the intravenous induction agent will be wearing off.

Between induction and surgery

Any delay between induction and transfer into the operating room may allow the blood concentration of the intravenous agent to decay before an inhalational agent has reached anaesthetic levels, leading to awareness of incision.

During surgery:

- Anaesthetic machine incorrectly maintained
- Low minute-volume settings on some electrically driven ventilators may lead to dilution of the anaesthetic with air, leading to awareness during surgery
- Oxygen bypass tap left on
- Exhausted vapourizer
- Failure to eliminate air from a closed circuit
- Exhausted, disconnected or malfunctioning syringe driver.

PREVENTION

- Know exactly how your anaesthetic machine and associated equipment works and check it all before use
- Periodically check vapourizer levels and use an agent meter
- Flush circles with a high flow for the first 5 min
- Use a depth-of-anaesthesia monitor as soon as they are of proven reliability
- Remember that patients differ considerably in their anaesthetic requirements.

TREATMENT

- Postoperative interview
- Referral to psychologist for counselling.

BIBLIOGRAPHY

Couture L J, Edmonds H L. Monitoring responsiveness during anaesthesia. Baillière's Clinical Anaesthesiology 1989; 3: 547–558

Liu W H D, Thorp T A S, Graham S G, Aitkenhead A R. Incidence of awareness with recall during general anaesthesia. Anaesthesia 1991; 46: 435–437

Moerman N, Bonke B, Oosting J. Awareness and recall during general anaesthesia. Anesthesiology 1993; 79: 454–464

BLOOD TRANSFUSION

N. M. Tierney

Amongst other reasons, the advent of HIV has led to a more critical approach to the use of blood and blood products.

Two-thirds of all transfusions are given during the perioperative period.

INDICATIONS FOR TRANSFUSION

- *Blood*:
  - The treatment of acute life-threatening and on-going blood loss
  - Restoration of oxygen-carrying capacity
- *Platelets*: evidence of a clinical coagulopathy, and thrombocytopenia or platelet dysfunction
- *Fresh frozen plasma (FFP)*: a demonstrable deficiency of coagulation factors.

Blood transfusion remains the treatment of choice where there is severe blood loss, e.g. major trauma, ruptured aortic aneurysm. In extremis, group O Rhesus-negative packed cells or type-specific blood may be given. As a result, haemolysis will occur in 3% of these 'transfusion episodes'.

There is evidence that the treatment of continuing blood loss with coagulation factors and platelets leads to no reduction in blood loss. There is, however, evidence that in large volume blood transfusion continuing blood loss is exacerbated by hypotension, acidosis and hypothermia.

RISKS OF TRANSFUSION

The overall morbidity of blood transfusion is 1 in 30 transfusion episodes.

There are risks associated with all homologous transfusions:

Immunological
- Red cell antigen
  - Haemolysis
  - Immediate (ABO)
  - Delayed (non-ABO)
  - Alloimmunization
- White cell antigen
- Platelet antigen
- Plasma protein.

Transmitted infection
- Risk is <1 in 1000
- Hepatitis types A, B, non-A/non-B, C
- HIV1, HIV2
- Cytomegalovirus
- Bacterial contamination.

Immunosuppressive effects
- Increased transplant survival
- Increased incidence of recurrence of colorectal carcinoma
- Increased incidence of postoperative sepsis.

ABO incompatibility can be severe. It may be produced by only 30 ml of transfused blood. More than half of these events are due to clerical error. Their incidence is between 1 in 10 000 and 1 in 100 000. Of these, death from DIC occurs in 1 in 1000.

Blood can be demonstrated to reduce the immune competence of the recipient, and immunological mechanisms have been discovered which can explain these phenomena. No causal relationship has yet been proved, however.

There are particular problems associated with large volume transfusion (greater than one circulating volume):

- Fluid overload
- Dilutional thrombocytopenia

and further problems where blood is given at rates greater than 90 ml min^{-1}:

- Hyperkalaemia
- Hypothermia
- Hypocalcaemia.

METHODS FOR REDUCTION OF EXPOSURE TO HOMOLOGOUS BLOOD

- Intraoperative haemodilution
- Intraoperative controlled hypotension
- Autologous transfusion
- Intraoperative blood salvage
- Recombinant erythropoeitin
- Synthetic oxygen transport media.

Erythropoeitin may be used to increase preoperative haemoglobin concentration, and possibly increase the yield of autologous blood donation. Stroma-free haemoglobin and perfluorochemicals remain a potential method for avoiding homologous blood.

Intraoperative haemodilution represents the most widely available technique for avoiding homologous blood transfusion and its attendant problems. It is based on the premise that, whilst maintaining normovolaemia, the maximum oxygen delivery (Do_2) rises to 110% of normal at a haematocrit of 30% (Figure 1). This effect relies on a reduction in blood viscosity. The increase in Do_2 occurs without an increase in energy consumption. On the other hand, a haematocrit of 30% or below has been found to give an unacceptable risk of coronary ischaemia in patients with pre-existing ischaemic heart disease. In addition, it has been demonstrated that patients over 60 years of age are unable to increase their cardiac output to compensate for a haematocrit of less than 30% without an unacceptable rise in oxygen consumption.

- No clinical trials exist concerning the effects of moderate anaemia (6–9 g dl^{-1}) in the perioperative period

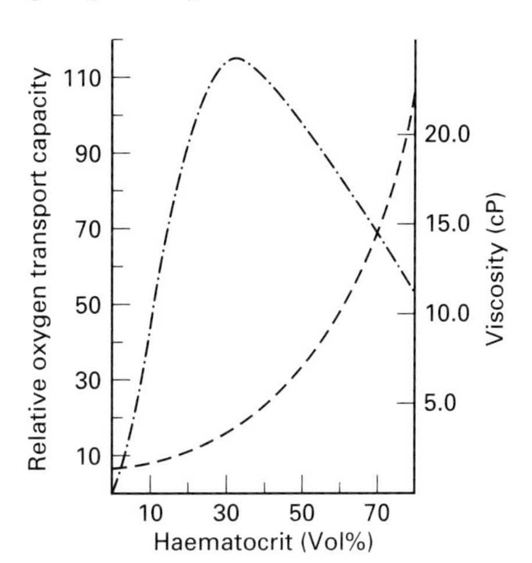

Figure 1
The influence of the haematocrit on viscosity (– – – – –) and relative oxygen transport capacity (– • – • – • –).

- In the absence of coexisting disease a postoperative haemoglobin of 8–9 g d^{-1} may be acceptable in reducing exposure to homologous blood
- Any decision regarding the patients' preoperative haemoglobin level should be linked to the potential surgical blood loss
- In patients over 60 years, those with coexisting medical disease and those with ischaemic heart disease, a haemoglobin level of no lower than 10 g dl^{-1} should be sought prior to operation.

BIBLIOGRAPHY

Crosby E T. Perioperative haemotherapy. I. Indications for blood component. Transfusion. Canadian Journal of Anaesthesia 1992; 39: 695–707

Crosby E T. Perioperative haemotherapy. II. Risks and complications of blood transfusion. Canadian Journal of Anaesthesia 1992; 39: 822–837

Nicholls M D. Transfusion: morbidity and mortality. Anaesthesia and Intensive Care 1993; 21: 15–19

CROSS REFERENCES

Massive transfusion
Patient Conditions 7: 180
Thoracic surgery
Surgical Procedures 17: 344
Obstetric haemorrhage
Surgical Procedures 20: 422
Valvular surgery
Surgical Procedures 22: 444
Transplantation
Surgical Procedures 23: 458
Total hip athroplasty
Surgical Procedures 24: 481
Cardiopulmonary bypass
Surgical Procedures 27: 506

COMPLICATIONS OF POSITION

J. M. Anderton

The dangers of failing to position the patient correctly can result in serious morbidity and even fatality. A knowledge of the reported complications together with a high standard of care and patient monitoring are necessary to reduce the risks.

Commonest causes of complications:
- Accidental trauma
- External pressure
- Inappropriate passive movement
- Physiological trespass

PREOPERATIVE ASSESSMENT

Check for:
- Head and neck mobility in patients where neck rotation is anticipated, e.g. for ENT or neurosurgical procedures, and in all cases of rheumatoid or ankylosing arthritis
- Intraocular lens prostheses
- Brachial neurovascular symptoms if the patient's arms are to be positioned above their head
- Symptoms of ulnar nerve entrapment syndrome
- Active and passive range of limb movement in elderly or arthritic patients where the anticipated position may cause problems
- Blood pressure changes or symptoms of supine hypotension in pregnant patients.

DANGERS OF THE POSITIONING PROCESS AND PATIENT TRANSFER

Complications may result from the following.

Failure to support the head adequately:
- A pillow unsupported by the stretcher canvas may fall away and cause whiplash injury to the neck
- Uncoordinated movement of assistants when turning the patient may damage the neck.

Failure to support the whole patient:
- Torn stretcher canvas
- Accidents where two stretcher canvases have one pole in each
- Accidents where the operating table transfer top fails to 'dock' correctly on its pedestal
- Failure to apply brakes on transfer trolley allows the patient to fall between the operating table and the trolley
- Inadequate physique of lifting attendants relative to the weight of the patient
- Failure to raise the side guard-rails on narrow transfer trolleys.

Failure to prevent localized damage:
- Fingers can be amputated by hinged sections of the operating table or by being caught between the carrier and pedestal sections
- The olecranon process can be fractured by forcible insertion of stretcher supporting poles
- Careless removal of the stretcher canvas can cause skin abrasions
- Accidental traction on infusion lines, drainage tubes and urethral catheters can cause internal damage
- The 'perineal post' of the orthopaedic traction table can cause genital damage and pudendal nerve trauma.

WELL-RECOGNIZED PROBLEMS ASSOCIATED WITH SPECIFIC POSITIONS

The supine position

Pressure necrosis of skin:
- Occipital – may be associated with alopecia
- Sacral – coincident thermal damage is also a risk with the use of warming blankets
- Heels – a special and serious risk in diabetic patients.

Postoperative backache

Use of a lumbar support is beneficial.

Nerve compression problems:
- The supraorbital nerve may be compressed by airway tubing
- The facial nerve can be compressed by a face-mask harness
- Brachial plexus neurapraxia can result from faulty armboard positioning
- The radial nerve can be trapped against a head-screen support
- The ulnar nerve may be damaged against the edge of the mattress.

33

The lithotomy position

Nervous system complications:
- Straight leg sling systems may cause sciatic and femoral nerve problems
- The common peroneal nerve may be trapped against the head of the fibula
- The saphenous nerve may be trapped against the supporting posts
- In extreme flexion of the thighs the femoral nerve can be kinked around the inguinal ligament.

Compartment syndrome

This can result from undue pressure on calf muscles and has been specifically implicated with use of the Bierhof system of leg supports (USA).

Skeletal damage:
- Ligamentous damage of the hip and knee joints ensue if passive movement exceeds the normal active range
- Sacroiliac joint strain is a risk if the legs are not raised symmetrically.

Physiological risks:
- The extent of surgically induced hypovolaemia may be masked by autotransfusion from the legs
- Increased intra-abdominal pressure enhances the possibility of gastric regurgitation – general anaesthesia should *never* be induced in this position.

The lateral position

Stability of position is essential. Evacuatable mattresses greatly enhance this.

Pressure problems:
- The skin below the iliac crest is at risk
- The underlying deltoid can suffer 'crush syndrome'

- The underlying sciatic nerve is at risk in emaciated patients
- The underlying common peroneal nerve is vulnerable around the neck of the fibula
- Axillary support is essential to protect the underlying brachial plexus.

The sitting position

Physiological problems:
- Venous air embolism – the classical risk
- Postural hypotension – can be exacerbated by bradycardia or surgical hypovolaemia
- Oedema and swelling of the tongue – can produce airway complications postoperatively if the neck has been too greatly flexed and rotated.

Nervous system complications:
- Quadriplegia has been reported following head flexion and cervical spine rotation
- Brachial plexus damage can occur if the arms are not properly supported
- The ulnar nerve can be compressed by misplaced arm supports
- The sciatic nerve can be stretched if the thighs are flexed and the knees extended
- Bilateral foot drop can result from compression of the common peroneal nerves.

Pressure problems:
- Sacral skin necrosis
- Haemarthrosis and dislocation of the elbow have been reported.

The prone position

- Very simple surgical procedures can be performed with the patient supported by a pillow beneath the chest and another beneath the pelvis. More complex procedures, e.g. spinal axis surgery, usually require that the groins and abdomen are completely free of external pressure.
- The Mohammedan prayer position should never be used; lower limb congestion can cause myoglobinuria and acute renal failure (Figure 1).
- Methods used to support the pelvis under the iliac crests are only satisfactory if the props are positioned so that the patient is unable to slip sideways (Figure 2). If this does occur, occlusion of one femoral neurovascular bundle is unavoidable, and

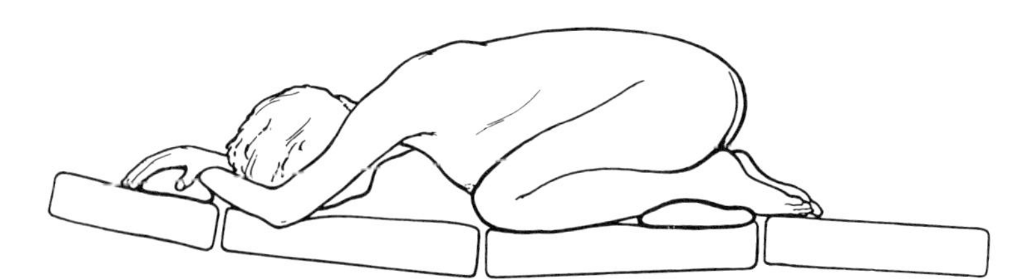

Figure 1
The Mohammedan prayer position. This position should never be used.

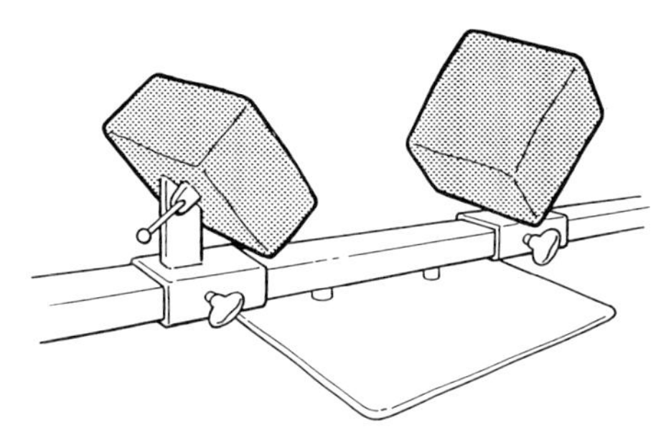

Figure 2
Positioning of props to support the pelvis under the iliac crests.

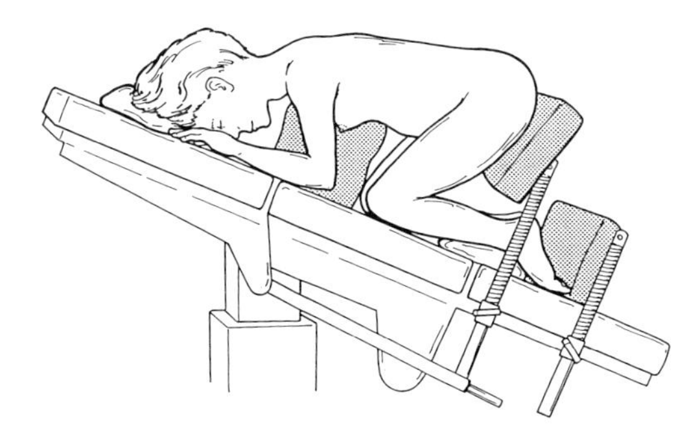

Figure 3
The safest position (Tarlov) for all lower thoracic and lumbar disc surgery.

back pressure transmitted to the epidural veins will cause troublesome surgical haemorrhage.
- The position originally described by Tarlov is the safest and most satisfactory for all lower thoracic and lumbar disc surgery (Figure 3). In some patients it can be used for operations on the cervical and upper thoracic spine. Although inferior vena cava pressures are known to be around 0–3 cmH_2O, venous air embolism is a very rare complication of surgery in this position.

OTHER DANGERS

Dangers resulting from the method of prone positioning:
- Pressure necrosis of weight-bearing skin areas
- Patients with previous coronary artery bypass graft surgery are at risk of graft occlusion
- Neurapraxia, both brachial and axillary, can occur if the arms are positioned above the head
- Meralgia paraesthetica

Table 1.
Potential eye damage

Dangers	Complications
Contamination by: • Surgical skin antiseptics • Gastric contents • Aerosol spray wound dressing	Corneal damage. Scarring
Surface drying and dehydration from failure to keep the eyelids closed	Infection. Corneal scarring. Secondary iridocyclitis
External pressure on the eye due to: • Misuse of the horseshoe headrest (especially for prone and laterally positioned patients) • Tightly applied, badly fitting face-mask • Prone positioning • Pressure by surgical assistants	Postoperative blindness. Earlier types of intraocular lenses may be dislodged. Acute glaucoma may precipitated

Action:
- Tape the eyelids closed and cover at all times
- Avoid any external pressure on the globe

Remember:
Any postoperative painful 'red-eye' needs skilled ophthalmological assessment to exclude iatrogenic or spontaneous acute glaucoma

- Blindness from external orbital pressure
- Malar skin burns from use of a Gigli saw at craniotomy.

Dangers arising from the surgery being performed

Damage to underlying abdominal major vessels or bowel perforation are well recorded when discectomy is being performed. Serious, hidden, intraperitoneal haemorrhage can rapidly cause acute hypovolaemic shock. Abandoning surgery and resuscitation in the supine position is the only action likely to avert disaster.

Complications of anaesthesia

The correct placement and securing of a nonkinking tracheal tube is the cornerstone of anaesthetic technique. Obesity and respiratory disease may necessitate the alternative use of the lateral position. Very poor-risk patients should have a Swan–Ganz catheter inserted.

VENOUS AIR EMBOLISM

This can be caused by any open vein or sinus above heart level.

Potentiating factors:

- Inability of the vein to collapse:
  - Intracranial venous sinuses and emissary veins
  - Self-retaining surgical retractors
  - Tracks formed around indwelling catheters, e.g. central venous pressure catheter.
- The level of venous pressure at the site:
  - Posture and positioning are important
  - Raising the adult patient's head to +25° lowers intracranial venous sinus pressure to zero, and at +90° produces a negative pressure of -12 ± 3 cmH_2O
  - Spontaneous ventilation causing negative intrathoracic pressure potentiates negative pressure at the operating site
  - In the prone position, the suction effect of a pendulous abdomen can potentiate negative venous pressure within the epidural veins.

Incidence:

- Posterior fossa surgery in the sitting position
- Head and neck surgery in the supine head-up position
- Caesarean section
- Intrauterine manipulations in the lithotomy position
- Major reconstructive spinal surgery in the prone position.

SUMMARY

- Look after the neck
- Do not drop the patient
- Avoid pressure on:
  - Major blood vessels
  - Main nerve trunks
- Do not strain arthritic joints or cause pressure sores.

BIBLIOGRAPHY

Albin M S, Newfield P, Paulter S et al. Atrial catheter and lumbar disc surgery (correspondence). Journal of the American Medical Association 1978; 239: 496

Alvine G F, Schurrer M E. Postoperative ulnar nerve palsy. Are there predisposing factors? The Journal of Bone and Joint Surgery 1987; 69A: 255–259

Anderton J M, Keen R I, Neave R. Positioning the surgical patient. Butterworths, London, 1988

Anderton J M. The prone position for the surgical patient: historical review of the principles and hazards. British Journal of Anaesthesia 1991; 67: 452–463

Connor H. Iatrogenic injuries in theatre. British Medical Journal 1992; 305: 956

Hickmott K C, Healy T E J, Roberts P, Faragher E B. Back pain following general anaesthesia and surgery. British Journal of Surgery 1990; 77: 571–575

Iwabuchi T, Sobata E, Susuki M, Susuki S, Yamashita M. Dural sinus pressure as related to neurosurgical positions. Neurosurgery 1983; 12: 203–207

Martin J T (ed). Positioning in anaesthesia and surgery, 2nd edn. Saunders, Philadelphia, 1987

Peters J L. Removal of central venous catheter and venous air embolism. British Medical Journal 1992; 305: 524–525

Vartikar J V, Johnson M D, Datta S. Precordial Doppler monitoring and pulse oximetry during Caesarean section delivery, detection of venous air embolism. Regional Anaesthesia 1989; 14: 145–148

Young J V I. The role of the evacuatable mattress. In: Anderton J M, Keen R I, Neave R (eds) Positioning the surgical patient. Butterworths, London, 1988, p 90

FAILURE TO BREATHE OR WAKE UP POSTOPERATIVELY

J. Barrie

NORMAL RESTORATION OF BREATHING

All anaesthetic agents and opioids are respiratory depressants and may cause apnoea. Failure to breathe postoperatively may also follow the use of intraoperative muscular relaxation. There may be more than one cause operating simultaneously, and these causes may be cumulative.

FAILURE TO BREATHE POSTOPERATIVELY

Causes

Nondepolarizing agents:

- Inadequate antagonism of neuromuscular block. The effects of nondepolarizing muscle relaxants are usually antagonized with neostigmine (50 μg kg^{-1}) (together with atropine (20 μg kg^{-1}) or glycopyrrolate (10 μg kg^{-1})), and this should have been given before 'failure to breathe' is noted.
- Concomitant drugs which themselves depress neuromuscular function or potentiate a neuromuscular blocking agent, e.g.
  - Aminoglycoside antibiotics
  - Verapamil
  - Phenytoin
  - Cyclosporin A.
- Cholinergic crisis secondary to excessive neostigmine (rare).

Depolarizing agents:

- Pseudocholinesterase deficiency (genetic or acquired)
- Dual block (type-II block).

Other factors:

- Respiratory depressants
- Opioids
- Volatile anaesthetic agents
- Benzodiazepines
- Pain, especially if thoracic or abdominal in origin
- Hypocapnia
- Severe hypercapnia
- Hypothermia, especially in children
- Metabolic disturbance
- Acidosis
- Hypokalaemia
- Hypomagnesaemia
- Coexisting neuromuscular disease
- Intraoperative cerebral event.

Management

The patient may be pink and display an acceptable Spo_2.

- Ensure the patient's safety.
- Ensure that the airway is protected and that adequate ventilation is maintained, by hand if necessary.
- If the patient is conscious, reassure them and consider sedation.
- Monitor vital signs:
  - ECG
  - Spo_2
  - Noninvasive BP
  - $ETco_2$, if possible.
- Determine cause:
  - Monitor neuromuscular function
  - Review doses of other agents which have been given
  - Check whether all anaesthetic agents are turned off
  - Consider the patient's metabolic status
  - Measure temperature.
- If residual paralysis is present and the post-tetanic count is 12 or more, give a further dose of neostigmine and an anticholinergic (up to 100 μg kg^{-1} total dose of neostigmine).
- If excessive narcotic is present, give increments of 0.1 mg naloxone
- If central respiratory depression is present, consider titrated doses of doxapram (1–1.5 mg kg^{-1} over 30 s).
- If excessive benzodiazepines have been used, give flumazenil (200 μg over 15 s, then 100 μg every 60 s, as required).
- Control pain with local techniques or carefully titrated doses of opioids.
- Optimize the patient's metabolic condition.
- If ventilation is still not adequate, transfer the patient to the ITU.

NORMAL AWAKENING

Awakening occurs when the concentration of anaesthetic agent in the brain falls to a level insufficient to maintain unconsciousness. This occurs due to the redistribution (usually) or metabolism of intravenous agents and the elimination of volatile agents. It is therefore a passive process, with specific antagonists existing only for opioids and benzodiazepines.

FAILURE TO WAKE UP

Causes

There may be more than one reason present, and effects are cumulative:

- Overdose (absolute or relative) of anaesthetic agent, premedication (including benzodiazepines), or opioid
- Hypothermia, particularly in children
- Hypercapnia
- Severe hypothyroidism
- Severe liver disease, in which anaesthesia may precipitate encephalopathy
- Cerebral hypoxia.

Management:

- Ensure the patient's safety.
- Ensure that the airway is protected and that ventilation is adequate.
- Continue monitoring:
  - ECG
  - Noninvasive BP
  - Spo_2.
- Assess cause:
  - Arterial blood gas analysis
  - Core temperature
  - Coexisting disease.
- Treat any treatable causes:
  - Correct any abnormalities in acid–base status
  - Rewarm if necessary
  - Administer a cautious dose of antagonists, if appropriate.
- Wait.
- Consider transfer to the ITU if awakening continues to be delayed.

The only cause of prolonged (hours or days) failure to recover from anaesthesia is a cardiorespiratory or cerebrovascular disaster with cerebral hypoxia. Thankfully, this is rare.

BIBLIOGRAPHY

Morris R W. Desaturation. Baillière's Clinical Anaesthesiology 1993; 7: 215–235

Ward D S, Temp J A. The role of hypoxia in the control of breathing. In: Kauffman L (ed) Anaesthesia review. Churchill Livingstone, London, 1991, vol 8, p 89–102

CROSS REFERENCES

Postoperative pain management
Anaesthetic Factors 33: 655
Pseudocholinesterase deficiency
Anaesthetic Factors 33: 660

FAT EMBOLISM

R. M. Slater

DEFINITION

Fat embolism is defined as the presence of fat globules within the lung parenchyma or peripheral microcirculation. The fat embolism syndrome (FES) is most commonly associated with:

- Fractures of long bones and pelvis
- Prosthetic joint replacement
- Lipectomy
- Bone marrow transplantation
- Acute haemorrhagic pancreatitis.

Three clinical forms of FES are described.

Subclinical FES

Seen in >50% of patients with long-bone fractures. Mild hypoxaemia and minor haematological abnormalities develop up to 3 days after injury.

Nonfulminant (subacute) FES

Seen in 1–5% of major trauma patients. Onset delayed by 1–6 days after injury. Classical syndrome of respiratory failure, petechiae, fever, tachycardia, CNS involvement and associated haematological abnormalities. A partial or incomplete picture is the commonest presentation.

Fulminant FES

Sudden onset, within a few hours of injury. Progresses rapidly, often with a fatal outcome.

PATHOPHYSIOLOGY

Fat emboli are thought to originate from exposed marrow at the site of injury. Fat globules enter the circulation, facilitated by movement of the fracture site. Subsequent pulmonary and neurological damage is thought to be partly due to vascular occlusion and partly to local effects of free fatty acids released from fat emboli. Respiratory insufficiency results from emboli entering the venous circulation and lodging in the pulmonary circulation. Cerebral involvement and petechial rash result from fat emboli entering the arterial circulation, either via the pulmonary alveolar capillaries or via precapillary pulmonary shunts which have opened as a result of pulmonary hypertension.

DIAGNOSIS

Respiratory insufficiency:

- Occurs in 75% of patients with FES
- Dyspnoea, tachypnoea and hypoxaemia associated with fine inspiratory crackles on auscultation, 2–3 days following injury
- Chest X-ray is normal at first, then shows bilateral fluffy shadowing
- In 10% of cases respiratory failure develops and progresses to the adult respiratory distress syndrome.

Cerebral features:

- Neurological signs exist in up to 80% of patients with FES
- Neurological signs can precede respiratory signs
- Encephalopathy produces an acute confusional state; a subgroup develop focal neurological signs.
- A CT scan is usually unhelpful.

Dermatological features:

- These occur in 60% of cases.
- A petechial rash develops within 36 h of the event. Found in conjunctivae, oral mucous membrane, neck and axillae. It is self-limiting, usually resolving within 7 days.

Other features:

- Pyrexia and tachycardia are common nonspecific findings
- ECG may show signs of right ventricular strain
- Retinal haemorrhages and exudates can occur
- Renal emboli may result in oliguria, lipuria, proteinuria or haematuria; these changes are short-lived and unrelated to any subsequent renal impairment
- Jaundice is rare and self-limiting.

Laboratory findings:

- Fall in haemoglobin, thrombocytopaenia and other coagulation abnormalities
- Fat macroglobulinaemia and elevated free fatty acids and triglyceride levels in serum.

Other investigations

Identification of fat droplets in cells recovered from bronchoalveolar lavage in trauma patients has shown promise as a rapid and specific method for diagnosing FES.

MANAGEMENT

- Maintain adequate oxygenation and ventilation
- Indications for respiratory support:
  - Sustained SaO_2 <90% and P_aO_2 <8 kPa on oxygen
  - Respiratory rate of >35 breaths min^{-1}
- Early immobilization of fractures
- Avoid hypovolaemia (increases mortality)
- Use of human albumin solution (thought to bind free fatty acids)
- Adequate analgesia.

A number of specific therapies have been tried, including alcohol, heparin, steroids, dextrans, and aprotinin. None have been shown to be of definite use in the treatment of FES.

OUTCOME

The overall mortality of FES is 5–15%. The condition is usually self-limiting with adequate supportive therapy. Long-term morbidity is related to focal neurological lesions.

BIBLIOGRAPHY

Bennier B, Poirier T et al. Bronchoalveolar lavage in fat embolism. Intensive Care Medicine 1992; 18: 59–60

Gurd A R. Fat embolism, an aid to diagnosis. Journal of Bone and Joint Surgery 1970; 52B: 732–737

Van Besouw J P, Hinds C J. Fat embolism syndrome. British Journal of Hospital Medicine 1989; 42: 304–311

CROSS REFERENCES

Orthopaedic surgery
Surgical Procedures 24: 474
Trauma
Anaesthetic Factors 33: 672

FLUID AND ELECTROLYTE BALANCE

J. Palmer and S. Varley

Disease processes can impair the complex homeostatic mechanisms which safeguard the *milieu interieur*. It is important to ensure that the stable chemical environment upon which normal cellular function depends is maintained during the perioperative period.

PHYSIOLOGY

Body water content varies with age and sex as a percentage of body weight (Table 1).

Table 1.
Body water composition in health as a percentage of TBW

	TBW	ICF (%)	ECF (%)
Neonate	75	40	35
Infant	70	40	30
Adult male	60	40	20
Adult female	55	35	20
Elderly female	45	30	15

Approximately two-thirds of the total body water (TBW) is intracellular fluid (ICF) and one-third is extracellular fluid (ECF). The ECF is further subdivided into interstitial fluid (ISF) and plasma.

The TBW and electrolytes in a 70-kg man are distributed between the various compartments as shown in Table 2.

Table 2.
Distribution of water and electrolytes in a normal 70-kg man

	ICF	ECF	
		ISF	Plasma
% of TBW	40	16	4
Volume (l)	28	11	3
Ions (mmol l^{-1}):			
Na^+	10	140	140
K^+	150	4	4
Ca^{2+}		2.5	2.5
Mg^{2+}	26	1.5	1.5
Cl^-	–	114	114
HCO_3^-	10	25	25
HPO_4^{2-}	38	1	1
SO_4^{2-}	–	0.5	0.5
$Prot^-$	74	2	16

OSMOTIC ACTIVITY

Water moves between compartments from areas of low solute concentration to areas of high concentration by osmosis. The number of osmotically active particles in solution is expressed in osmol (Osm). Osmolarity is the number of particles per litre of solvent (Osm l^{-1}), and osmolality is the number of particles per kilogram of solvent (Osm kg^{-1}). The density of water is 1 kg l^{-1}; osmolality and osmolarity are therefore equivalent in the body.

Osmolality can be estimated by adding the concentrations of osmotically active particles within compartments. ECF osmolality is usually calculated by adding the plasma concentrations (mmol l^{-1}) of sodium, potassium, chloride, urea and glucose. An alternative commonly used rule of thumb is to add twice the sodium plus urea plus glucose.

Osmotic pressure is calculated by multiplying osmolalities by 19.3 to give pressures (mmHg). Thus ICF has an osmolality of 281 mOsm l^{-1} and an osmotic pressure of 5430 mmHg, but plasma has an osmolality of 281 mOsm l^{-1} but an osmotic pressure of 5453 mmHg. This difference of 23 mmHg is due to the presence of plasma proteins.

THE FATE OF INTRAVENOUS FLUIDS

The redistribution of infused fluid within the body will depend on its composition relative to that of each compartment, as shown in Table 3. Salt solutions are excluded from the ICF by the cell membrane Na^+/K^+ pump. Dextrose (5%) behaves like water and is distributed throughout the TBW.

Table 3.
Approximate fractional distribution of infusions within compartments*

	ICF	ECF	
		ISF	Plasma
Saline (0.9%)	0	4/5	1/5
Dextrose (5%)	2/3	1/4	1/12

*These figures demonstrate why large volumes of crystalloids are required to expand plasma volume. To replace a given blood loss requires 3 times the volume as saline (0.9%) or 9 times the volume as dextrose (5%).

NORMAL REQUIREMENTS

Water

A normothermic 70-kg man with a normal metabolic rate loses approximately 2500 ml of water per day (urine 1500 ml, faeces 100 ml, sweat 500 ml, lungs 400 ml). Water is gained from ingested fluid (1300 ml), food (800 ml) and metabolism (400 ml). Maintenance requirements are therefore approximately 1.25–1.5 ml kg^{-1} h^{-1} for adult surgical patients.

Sodium

Loss in faeces and sweat is about 10 mmol day^{-1}, renal excretion being mainly dependent on dietary intake. Average requirements are 1 mmol kg^{-1} day^{-1}. This could be provided by:

- 2500 ml of 4% dextrose/0.18% saline over 24 h
- 2000 ml of 5% dextrose and 500 ml of 0.9% saline over 24 h.

Potassium

Loss is via the same routes as sodium, but renal retention is less efficient. The average requirement is 1 mmol kg^{-1} day^{-1}. This should be added to the infusion regime.

PERIOPERATIVE FLUID MANAGEMENT

The fluid status of a patient undergoing surgery will depend on the presenting complaint, the previous health of the individual and whether surgery is elective or urgent. Fluid and electrolyte depletion is a common problem faced by the anaesthetist.

The history and examination will point to decreased intake or increased loss:

- Note the duration of preoperative fasting
- Patients at the extremes of age are less likely to maintain fluid balance during illness
- Note the presence of diarrhoea and vomiting
- Pyrexia – insensible loss increases by 10% for each 1°C rise in body temperature
- Acute abdomen – large volumes of fluid may be sequestered in the abdomen.

Assessment of the deficit in TBW

- Up to 5%:
  - Dry mucous membranes
  - Skin turgor almost normal
  - Normal sensorium.
- Up to 10%:
  - Drowsiness
  - Decreased skin turgor
  - Decreased intraocular pressure
  - Increased heart rate and RR
  - Oliguria
  - Sunken fontanelle in infants.
- Up to 15%:
  - Stuporose
  - Parched mouth
  - Sunken eyes
  - Fast and thready pulse
  - Respiratory distress
  - Hypotension
  - Extreme oliguria.

Investigations

History and examination are the key to good assessment, although simple blood tests supply additional information:

- Look for elevated urea or creatinine
- Look for elevated haematocrit
- Check plasma levels of sodium and potassium.

PREOPERATIVE REQUIREMENTS

In general, healthy patients undergoing elective minor surgery do not need perioperative fluid replacement unless they are unable to drink normally in the early postoperative period. In other patients the following deficits should be considered:

Preoperative fasting

If there has been a fluid restriction of 1.5 ml kg^{-1} h^{-1}, replace with dextrose (4%)/saline (0.18%) or similar.

Abnormal losses

This is common in surgical patients. Replacement is based on an estimate of the composition and volume of loss. Losses from the gut are particularly important, and though the compositions of the various gastrointestinal secretions differ they are adequately replaced with equal volumes of saline (0.9%) and potassium chloride (10–20 mmol l^{-1}).

Severe hypovolaemia with signs of shock

Give colloid (10 ml kg^{-1}) as a bolus, with additional fluid given according to the patient's response.

INTRAOPERATIVE REQUIREMENTS

Maintenance

Give dextrose (4%, 1.5 ml kg^{-1} h^{-1}) with saline (0.18%).

Losses from skin, lungs, abdominal cavity and third-space sequestration

These losses can be replaced with 2–10 ml kg^{-1} h^{-1} of balanced salt solution. This should be judged according to the patient response: heart rate, BP, tissue perfusion, and urine output (not less than 0.5 ml kg^{-1} h^{-1}). Central venous pressure (CVP) monitoring may be necessary.

Blood loss

Consider transfusion when 10% of estimated blood volume has been lost (Table 4). Give blood when 15% or more has been lost. Take into account both pre- and intra-operative haemorrhage.

Table 4.
Estimated blood volumes

	Volume (ml kg^{-1})
Infant	90
Child	80
Adult male	70
Adult female	60

POSTOPERATIVE REQUIREMENTS

- Maintenance: 1.5 ml kg^{-1} h^{-1} of 4% dextrose with 0.18% saline
- Replace any further blood losses.

Opinions about the electrolyte requirements of postoperative patients differ widely in clinical practice. Though the stress response to surgery increases renal excretion of potassium, tissue trauma and catabolism release intracellular potassium, thus maintaining plasma levels. Potassium is not required for the first 24–48 h in most patients. Whatever fluid composition is chosen, all fluid replacement should be regularly reviewed according to the patient's response: heart rate, BP, RR, tissue perfusion, plasma electrolytes, urine output (at least 0.5 ml kg^{-1} h^{-1}) and CVP (if a central line is in situ).

BIBLIOGRAPHY

Ganong W F. Review of medical physiology, 13th edn. Lange, 1985
Guvton A C. Textbook of medical physiology, 6th edn. W B Saunders, Philadelphia, 1981
Shearer E S, Hunter J M. Perioperative fluid and electrolyte balance. Current Anaesthesia and Critical Care 1992; 3: 71–77

CROSS REFERENCES

Water and electrolyte disturbances
Patient Conditions 10: 244

INTRAOPERATIVE ARRHYTHMIAS

N. P. C. Randall

Over 60% of patients experience some form of arrhythmias perioperatively. This frequency must not obscure the association of rhythm disturbance with serious adverse outcomes. The significance of the arrhythmia has to be evaluated in the context of:

- Preoperative coexisting medical problems and drug treatment
- The surgical condition
- The operative procedure
- Anaesthetic drugs and technique
- Haemodynamic effect of the arrhythmias, and the risk of progression to a more serious arrhythmia.

For example, in a fit patient having a halothane anaesthetic for minor surgery, a nodal rhythm producing little fall in blood pressure can be observed and is unlikely to require treatment. The same rhythm in a patient with aortic stenosis, or in a fit patient about to have squint surgery, is likely to require intervention.

PREOPERATIVE EVALUATION

Conditions associated with arrhythmias are given in Table 1.

The following symptoms and signs may indicate an arrhythmia:

- Paroxysmal dyspnoea
- Palpitations
- Dizziness
- Syncope.

Table 1.
Preoperative conditions associated with arrhythmias

Ischaemic heart disease
Pre-existing arrhythmias
Hypertension
Congestive heart failure
Electrolyte disorders
Valvular heart disease
Medications:
– β_2 Agonists
– Theophylline
– Tricyclic antidepressants
Less common causes:
– Thyrotoxicosis
– Cardiomyopathies (including alcoholic)
– Myocarditis
– Trauma (myocardial and intracranial)
– Connective tissue disorders
– Drug and solvent abuse

Physical examination and a 12-lead ECG with rhythm strip may help little, and further evaluation requires 24-h ECG monitoring. The diagnosis and management of arrhythmias can be complex, particularly with the proarrhythmic potential of antiarrhythmic drugs. A cardiological opinion may be required.

Hypokalaemia

Hypokalaemia is a common electrolyte disturbance. It prolongs repolarization nonuniformly, which predisposes to arrhythmias. While a serum potassium as low as 3.0 mmol l^{-1} is usually acceptable, this may not be so in the presence of other risk factors (e.g. digoxin). The effect of ventilation should be remembered. A pH change of 0.1 will change the serum potassium 1.0 mmol l^{-1} in the opposite direction.

Hyperkalaemia, hypomagnesaemia and hypercalcaemia

These changes can all provoke arrhythmias. In contrast, extremes of sodium seem to have little effect.

MONITORING

V1 is the lead of choice for rhythm monitoring. In a three-lead system, MCL1 or II is best.

INTRAOPERATIVE FACTORS

Certain anaesthetic and surgical interventions may specifically induce arrhythmias. The development of arrhythmias, however, may indicate an adverse change to myocardial oxygen balance.

Anaesthetic factors

See Table 2.

Table 2.
Anaesthetic factors

Hypotension or hypertension (e.g. inadequate anaesthesia)
Oxygenation
Carbon dioxide
Laryngoscopy
Drugs:
– Volatile anaesthetic agents
– Suxamethonium
– Pancuronium
– Central venous pressure lines (microshock hazard)

The relationship between volatile agents and arrhythmias involves effects on:

- Action-potential duration
- Automaticity
- Calcium flux
- Interactions with adrenaline
- Myocardial oxygen balance.

Atrioventricular conduction is prolonged (least with isoflurane and sevoflurane). The direct volatile agent effect of decreased automaticity is countered by the potentiation of catecholamine arrhythmias. The significance of intercoronary steal in clinical practice is doubted.

Surgical factors

See Table 3.

Assessment

Intraoperatively, more than one factor is likely to be contributing to a new arrhythmia.

- Identify the rhythm and evaluate its significance
- Identify and remove any precipitating factors, which includes optimizing myocardial oxygen balance
- Only if the arrhythmia persists should specific treatment be given.

Management

The same management can be used for intraoperative dysrhythmias that is used for awake patients.

Table 3.
Surgical factors

Catecholamines
- Endogenous, from any surgical stimulus
- Exogenous – topical or infiltrated adrenaline

Autonomic stimulation
- Peritoneal and visceral traction
- Peritoneal insufflation
- Trigeminovagal reflexes (most notably the oculocardiac reflex, but seen throughout the trigeminal nerve distribution)
- Laryngoscopy, bronchoscopy, oesophagoscopy
- Carotid artery and thyroid surgery

Direct stimulation of the heart
In cardiac and thoracic surgery

Embolism
- Thrombus
- Fat
- Bone cement
- Air
- Carbon dioxide
- Amniotic fluid

Other
- Aortic cross-clamping
- Limb reperfusion
- Glycine intoxication

- Treat the whole patient and not just the ECG
- If the circulation is inadequate, external cardiac massage will be needed
- Synchronized d.c. shock is a more attractive treatment option in the already anaesthetized patient
- Consider an antiarrythmic drug.

The negative inotropic effect of many antiarrhythmic drugs should be remembered. Adenosine is a useful agent for supraventricular tachycardias. Its value in slowing supraventricular tachycardia but not ventricular tachycardia (see Table 4) is particularly valuable intraoperatively when a 12-lead ECG is difficult to record. Adenosine will also be effective in Wolff–Parkinson–White tachycardia. Alternatively, disopyramide or propranolol may be used, but verapamil and digoxin are contraindicated.

Table 4.
Distinguishing broad complex tachycardias*

Supraventricular tachycardia (SVT)
No axis change and same pattern of bundle branch block as pre-SVT ECG
Conforms to right or left bundle branch block pattern
Dominant R in V1 and Q in V6.

Ventricular tachycardia (VT)
Axis change from previous ECG
Deep S wave in V6
Fusion beats
Capture beats

*Haemodynamic stability is not a distinguishing factor. VT is much commoner than broad complex SVT, especially if a previous ECG shows narrow complexes.

BIBLIOGRAPHY

Atlee J L, Bosnjck Z J. Mechanisms for cardiac dysrhythmias during anaesthesia. Anesthesiology 1990; 72: 347–374
Singh B N, Opie L H, Marcus F I. Antiarrhythmic agents. In: Opie L H (ed) Drugs for the heart, 3rd edn. W B Saunders, Philadelphia, 1991, ch 8

CROSS REFERENCES

Conduction defects
Patient Conditions 4: 99
Coronary artery disease
Patient Conditions 4: 107
Water and electrolyte disturbances
Patient Conditions 10: 246
Fluid and electrolyte balance
Anaesthetic Factors 33: 626
Pacing and anaesthesia
Anaesthetic Factors 33: 651

INTRAOPERATIVE BRONCHOSPASM

J. Hammond

33

GENERAL FEATURES

- Lower airway obstruction due to bronchiolar constriction, characterized by an expiratory wheeze and elevated airway pressures
- Potentially fatal complication
- Rare in comparison to upper airway obstruction and occlusion of breathing circuit, both of which are to be excluded before the diagnosis of bronchospasm is made.

INCIDENCE

- Asthma, coronary artery disease, smoking and respiratory infection are recognized as risk factors. A majority of cases, however, including those leading to adverse outcomes (brain damage, death), will occur in those without such factors.
- One study revealed an overall incidence of 1.7 per 1000 anaesthetics, with a higher incidence at ages 0–9 years (4.0 per 1000) and 50–69 years (1.8 per 1000).

These subgroups were analysed according to a number of variables (Table 1). Interestingly, cardiac disease is associated with an increased frequency of bronchospasm. This may be due to abnormal cardiopulmonary reflexes.

Table 1.

Age group (years)	**Studied variable**	**Incidence of bronchospasm** (per 1000 cases)
0–9	Organic heart disease	15.3
	Abnormal ECG	24.3
	Respiratory infection	41.1
	Obstructive lung disease	21.9
	Tracheal intubation	9.1
50–69	Previous myocardial infarction	5.4
	Obstructive lung disease	7.7

CAUSES

Airway instrumentation:

- Instrumentation and irritation of the airway may produce reflex bronchospasm
- Tracheal intubation is the commonest trigger
- Carinal stimulation, e.g. by an endotracheal tube or suction catheter, is another common trigger
- More likely under light anaesthesia.

Surgical stimulation:

- Nociception may trigger reflex bronchoconstriction
- Patients undergoing upper abdominal, anal and cervical procedures are more prone to this reflex
- Inadequate anaesthesia may be a predisposing factor.

Bronchial aspiration:

- May present with unilateral bronchospasm
- Could account for the higher incidence in children and during abdominal surgery.

Anaphylactic and anaphylactoid reactions

Bronchospasm is the first sign in 25.5% of reactions and the sole feature in 8%.

Drugs

Various agents may predispose to bronchospasm:

- Beta blockers – inhibition of β_2 mediated bronchodilatation
- Neostigmine – muscarinic effect if inadequately blocked by anticholinergic drugs
- NSAIDs – contraindicated in patients with aspirin-induced asthma (beware of the 'aspirin triad' of asthma, nasal polyps and aspirin intolerance).

Overall it has been estimated that 1 in 10 adult asthmatics will react adversely to various drugs.

Regional techniques

These are not devoid of risk. Psychological factors may trigger spasm in asthmatics.

Reports of bronchospasm occurring during spinal and epidural anaesthesia exist. These were attributed to a fall in circulating catecholamines due to block of sympathetic outflow to the adrenals (T10–L1).

CLINICAL FEATURES

Spontaneous ventilation:

- Laboured respiration
- Intercostal recession
- Expiratory wheeze.

IPPV:

- Increased airway pressure
- Decreased compliance.

Depending on the severity, ventilation and oxygenation become increasingly difficult.

Air trapping occurs with hyperinflation of the chest.

Acute pulmonary hypertension and reduced venous return due to elevated intrathoracic pressure result in a fall in cardiac output in the severest cases.

Pneumothorax due to barotrauma may complicate the picture at any time. Suspect pneumothorax if there is a sudden deterioration.

MANAGEMENT

The action to be taken depends on the severity of the bronchospasm and the availability of equipment and agents. The majority of cases occur as a reflex response to airway instrumentation or surgery and are relatively mild. They are managed simply by temporarily interrupting surgery and deepening anaesthesia. Further methods are indicated if there is an inadequate response.

General management

It is vital to exclude a number of important differential diagnoses (Table 2).

Table 2.
Differential diagnosis of bronchospasm

Diagnosis	Notes
Upper airway obstruction	
Obstructed endotracheal tube	Verify patency. Pass suction catheter. Bronchoscope. If in doubt, remove
Breathing circuit malfunction or obstruction	Check equipment preanaesthesia
Tension pneumothorax	
Oesophageal intubation	Observe capnograph trace

Drug therapy

Volatile agents:

- All are effective bronchodilators
- Many cases respond to an increase in the inspired concentration
- Isoflurane is the least arrhythmogenic and is the agent of choice if using adrenaline.

β_2 Adrenoreceptor agonists:

- Salbutamol
  - 250 μg i.v. (4 μg kg^{-1})
  - Intravenous infusion (5–20 μg min^{-1})
  - Nebulize in circuit (2.5–5 mg)
- Terbutaline (250–500 μg i.v.).

Aminophylline:

- No additional bronchodilatation if volatile agents used
- Inferior to β_2 adrenoreceptor agonists
- Administer 5 mg kg^{-1} slowly intravenously.

Corticosteroids:

- Of benefit in acute bronchospasm
- Mechanism of action is unclear, but there is evidence that they are beneficial in the acute situation
- Hydrocortisone (200–500 mg i.v.) single dose *or* Methylprednisolone (1 g i.v.) single dose.

Adrenaline:

- First-line agent in severe reactions and in anaphylaxis
- Give 3–5 ml of 1:10 000 intravenously.

Ketamine:

- Powerful bronchodilator
- Consider if there is a poor response to other agents.

Ventilatory considerations

Aim to reduce any risk of barotrauma and maintain oxygenation:

- Give 100% oxygen
- Use a low frequency of ventilation with a long expiratory time; this minimizes pulmonary distension
- Use low tidal volumes to limit airway pressures.

A degree of hypercapnia is acceptable, provided that oxygenation is maintained. The minute volume can be increased as the bronchospasm resolves.

'Educated-hand' manual ventilation may produce better oxygenation with higher minute volumes and lower airway pressures than will mechanical ventilation.

In the most severe cases, expiration due to passive recoil of lung and thorax cannot occur – conventional ventilation is impossible. Manual deflation of the chest may buy time:

- Inflate with 100% oxygen
- Disconnect tracheal tube
- Squeeze lateral aspects of chest for 10–15 s
- Repeat this cycle.

Worst-case scenario: catastrophic bronchospasm with the risk of severe barotrauma; cardiac arrest is imminent. Consider cardiopulmonary bypass, if available.

BIBLIOGRAPHY

Entrup M H, Davis F G. Perioperative complications of anaesthesia. Surgical Clinics of North America 1991; 71: 1151–1173

Olsson G L. Bronchospasm during anaesthesia. A computer-aided incidence study of 136,929 patients. Acta Anaesthesiologica Scandinavica 1987; 31: 244–252

CROSS REFERENCES

Asthma
Patient Conditions 3: 68

INTRAOPERATIVE CYANOSIS

I. Banks and R. Hanley

Cyanosis is a clinical sign. It results from the dark blue coloration of reduced haemoglobin (*kyanos* (Greek) = blue). It occurs when the capillary concentration of reduced haemoglobin is greater than 5 g dl^{-1}.

Clinically there are two types of cyanosis:

- *Central*: results from imperfect oxygenation of blood in the general systemic circulation.
- *Peripheral*: results from extraction of oxygen from blood in peripheries where blood flow is very sluggish, e.g. extreme cold. If the patient is centrally cyanosed, then the patient will be peripherally cyanosed. However, a patient can be peripherally cyanosed without being centrally cyanosed.

Cyanosis results from:

- Hypoxic hypoxia (inadequate oxygenation)
- Stagnant hypoxia (inadequate circulation).

N.B. It is possible to be hypoxic without being cyanosed, e.g. anaemic hypoxia, carbon monoxide poisoning. The terms 'hypoxia' and 'cyanosis' are therefore not synonymous.

PREOPERATIVE CAUSES

- *Pulmonary disease*: e.g. severe chronic obstructive airways disease, lung collapse, trauma, restrictive lung disease, extreme obesity (Pickwickian syndrome)
- *Ventilatory inadequacy*: e.g. drugs, airway obstruction, neurological problems

- *Cardiac problems*: e.g. severe cardiac failure, right-to-left shunt (congenital cyanotic heart disease, Eisenmenger's syndrome).

INTRAOPERATIVE CAUSES

Respiratory

- Inadequate inspired fraction of oxygen (hypoxic mixture)
- Airway obstruction (e.g. foreign body, forgotten throat pack, tongue against posterior pharyngeal wall, incorrectly placed laryngeal mask airway, laryngospasm, endotracheal tube obstruction or kinking)
- Incorrect positioning of endotracheal tube; oesophageal intubation, inadvertent endobronchial intubation
- Inadequate ventilation:
  - Spontaneous ventilation (e.g. depressant drugs such as opioids, anaesthetic agents)
  - Mechanical ventilation (e.g. disconnection of breathing system, incorrect ventilator settings, inadequate flow, ventilator failure)
- Pulmonary problems (bronchospasm, collapse, pneumothorax, haemothorax, pre-existing lung disease, inhalation of gastric contents)
- Intentional one-lung ventilation.

Cardiovascular:

- Cardiac failure (e.g. from intraoperative fluid overload, myocardial infarction)
- Embolism (pulmonary, air, carbon dioxide, amniotic fluid, fat)
- Cardiac tamponade
- Tension pneumothorax
- Severe hypovolaemia
- Preferential right-to-left shunt after reduction of systemic vascular resistance (Fallot's tetralogy).

Other causes:

- Methaemoglobinaemia
- Transfusion reaction.

POSTOPERATIVE CAUSES

Almost all the above can also cause postoperative cyanosis. Other postoperative causes include:

- Inadequate inspired fraction of oxygen (diffusion hypoxia after use of nitrous oxide) (N.B. increased oxygen demand postoperatively).
- Airway obstruction (forgotten throat pack, blood clot, tongue against posterior pharyngeal wall, laryngospasm)
- Inadequate ventilation (residual depressant effect of anaesthetic drugs or opioids, inadequate reversal of neuromuscular blocking agents, pain, tight dressings, intraoperative intracerebral event, hypothermia).

DETECTION OF CYANOSIS

Patient observation may be difficult if the patient is completely draped, if the lights are turned off, or if the patient has dark skin. As cyanosis is a clinical sign, this is the only method of detecting cyanosis. Note that pulse oximetry will measure the percentage saturation of haemoglobin, which is helpful in the detection of hypoxia, but does not detect cyanosis itself.

TREATMENT OF THE CYANOSED PATIENT

- Administer a high concentration of oxygen.
- Assess airway patency. If obstructed consider manipulations of airway, e.g. jaw thrust, airway insertion, possibility of foreign body, laryngospasm.
- Assess ventilation (hand ventilation may aid assessment, as may auscultation):
  - If chest is not moving, consider disconnection of breathing system, bronchospasm, apnoea secondary to drug administration, endotracheal tube incorrectly positioned, endotracheal tube blocked or kinked, ventilator failure
  - If chest movement is unilateral, consider endobronchial intubation, pneumothorax, lung collapse.
- Assess cardiovascular status.
- Further treatment depends upon the underlying cause.

BIBLIOGRAPHY

Ganong W F. Review of medical physiology, 14th edn, 1989

CROSS REFERENCES

Adult congenital heart disease
Patient Conditions 4: 92
Children with CHD
Patient Conditions 4: 104
Tetrology of fallot
Patient Conditions 4: 127

INTRAOPERATIVE HYPERTENSION

M. J. Jones

33

Intraoperative hypertension is a common complication during anaesthesia. Whether it is ultimately harmful to the patient depends on its degree, cause and duration, and on the condition of the patient. These factors also govern how actively it is treated.

Definitions:
- An elevation of blood pressure over 15% of the patient's baseline (the baseline is determined by a series of recordings).
- A systolic BP greater than 160 mmHg and/or a diastolic BP greater than 95 mmHg.

HAEMODYNAMICS

$$\text{MAP} = \text{SVR} \times \text{CO}$$

where MAP is the mean arterial blood pressure, SVR is the systemic vascular resistance, and CO is the cardiac output.

The commonest cause of an increase in MAP is a raised SVR due to vasoconstriction. From the equation it can be seen that a raised BP does not imply a raised CO. Indeed, the increased afterload due to vasoconstriction often causes a reduced CO.

COMPLICATIONS

Cardiovascular
Hypertension may precipitate myocardial ischaemia (especially subendocardial), infarction or failure.

Haemorrhage
At operation site or from existing aneurysms.

Neurological
Cerebral encephalopathy, oedema or haemorrhage.

Renal
Severe hypertension may precipitate acute renal failure.

MANAGEMENT

If severe and life-threatening, aggressive immediate therapy is warranted (e.g. MAP >150 mmHg with signs of myocardial ischaemia). Confirmation of the diagnosis may require a trial of therapy. If there is no definite diagnosis, nonspecific therapy is instituted.

Inadequate anaesthesia/analgesia
This is the commonest cause. It usually accompanies a change in level of stimulation (e.g. movement of endotracheal tube) or a waning of drug effect. It is usually associated with tachycardia (bradycardia if vagal tone increased), lacrimation, tachypnoea, movement or laryngospasm.

Treatment:
- Increase anaesthesia and/or analgesia
- Consider reducing stimulation.

Anxiety during local anaesthetic techniques
Reassure the patient and give sedation, if necessary.

Inadequate ventilation
Carbon dioxide retention causes catecholamine release.

Treatment:
- Check equipment and correct fault
- Optimize airway/ventilation
- Institute IPPV.

Omission of regular antihypertensive medicine
This may cause rebound hypertension.

Treatment
Assess preoperative therapy and administer appropriate drug, or use nonspecific therapy.

Drug interaction
For example, monoamine oxygenase inhibitors + vasopressors or opioids (especially pethidine).

Treatment
May require drug therapy (e.g. beta blockers or sodium nitroprusside).

Drugs given by surgeon (for haemostasis)
For example, adrenaline infiltration.

Treatment
Beta blockers.

Drug error
The wrong drug, dose, or mode of administration (e.g. giving vasoactive drugs in variable carrier infusion).

Treatment:
- Careful handling and labelling of all drugs
- Use dedicated intravenous lines or locate connection close to patient to reduce risk of variable administration rate.

Artefact
This may be due to the use of the wrong size BP cuff, resonance in the arterial catheter, or an incorrect zero point.

Treatment:
- Use appropriate cuff
- Calibrate arterial line and compare to cuff BP
- Use correct tubing or clamping device
- Check zero point.

Tourniquet pain
Slow onset, often after 1 h.

Treatment:
- Consult with surgeon
- May need drug therapy.

Pre-eclampsia
Treatment is with a nonspecific hypotensive agent.

Phaeochromocytoma
This is a rare but important cause. Undiagnosed phaeochromocytoma is associated with a high perioperative mortality (*c.* 50%).

Treatment
- If suspected, a small bolus dose of phentolamine (2.5–5 mg) usually gives a significant fall in BP (if systolic BP falls more than 35 mmHg, phaeochromocytoma is likely)
- Give alpha blockers in addition to beta blockade (beta blockade alone may worsen vasoconstriction).

Rarer causes:
- Fluid overload
- Aortic cross-clamping
- Hyperthyroid storm
- Malignant hyperthermia
- Raised intracranial pressure
- Interference with carotid body or brainstem or spinal cord
- Bladder distension
- Alcohol or addictive drug withdrawal
- Autonomic hyperreflexia.

NONSPECIFIC TREATMENT

If the cause of hypertension cannot be removed or diagnosed, the following may be useful.

Vasodilators:
- Anaesthetic agents (e.g. isoflurane, propofol) – easy to control
- Hydralazine – arteriolar dilator, peak action after about 20 min following 5–10 mg i.v.
- Glyceryl trinitrate – arterial and venous dilator; dose 10–200 $\mu g\ min^{-1}$
- Nifedipine – sublingual or intranasal; onset 1–5 min following a 10 mg dose
- Labetalol – combined alpha and beta blockade; dose 5–20 mg i.v.
- Sodium nitroprusside – arteriolar dilator; very rapid response; administer by continuous intravenous infusion (0.5 $mg\ kg^{-1}\ min^{-1}$ starting dose); larger doses may cause cyanide poisoning.

Beta blockers
- Propranolol – nonselective; dose 0.5–1 mg i.v.
- Esmolol – rapid onset; short half-life (9 min); 500 $\mu g\ kg^{-1}$ loading dose; 50–780 $\mu g\ kg^{-1}\ min^{-1}$ infusion
- Metoprolol – cardioselective (β_1); 5–15 mg i.v.

Alpha blockers
Phentolamine (0.2–2 mg i.v.).

Ganglionic blockers
Trimetaphan (1–5 mg i.v.).

POSTOPERATIVE CARE

- Continue to monitor patient

- Provide adequate analgesia
- Consider face-mask oxygen (reduce myocardial ischaemia)
- May need continuing therapy
- May need investigations to exclude complications (e.g. myocardial infarctions) or to identify cause of hypertension.

CROSS REFERENCES

Hypertension
Patient Conditions 4: 111
Phaeochromocytoma
Surgical Procedures 25: 488
Awareness
Anaesthetic Factors 33: 614
Preoperative assessment of cardiovascular risk in noncardiac surgery
Anaesthetic Factors 34: 692

INTRAOPERATIVE HYPOTENSION

W. Wooldrige

Mild to moderate falls in blood pressure are ubiquitous under anaesthesia, but only very rarely result in any detriment to the patient. What is a dangerous level of hypotension? This depends on the duration of hypotension and the patient's preoperative medical condition. Full monitoring of patients gives essential guidance. Development of ectopic beats and ST segment depression are two vital signs of inadequate myocardial perfusion. Increased ventilation/perfusion mismatch secondary to pulmonary hypotension causes a fall in Sa_{O_2}. In awake patients receiving regional anaesthesia, nausea and dizziness are common symptoms of excessive hypotension. The lower limit of cerebral, renal and hepatic arterial autoregulation occurs at a mean arterial pressure of around 60 mmHg.

MECHANISMS

$$MAP = CO \times SVR$$
$$CO = HR \times SV$$

where MAP is the mean arterial pressure, HR is the heart rate, CO is the cardiac output, SV is the stroke volume, and SVR is the systemic vascular resistance.

Stroke volume depends on:

- Venous return
- Duration of ventricular diastole (which is affected by heart rate and rhythm)
- Cardiac contractility
- Proper functioning of heart valves and atria
- Afterload (SVR).

Heart rate is influenced by the cardiac rhythm (sinus rhythm or dysrhythmia) and the net effect of opposing vagal and sympathetic inputs.

Systemic vascular resistance is determined mainly by sympathetic vasoconstrictor tone. This is dictated by the brainstem vasomotor centre relaying via sympathetic ganglia to noradrenergic α_1 receptors on arteriolar and venous smooth muscle.

THE EFFECT OF GRAVITY

MAP is reduced by 2 mmHg for every 2.5 cm of vertical height above the heart. Hence in a head-up tilt position the cerebral perfusion pressure is significantly lower (40 mmHg lower in the complete upright position) than the MAP measured at heart level. Also venous return, and therefore cardiac output, fall with head-up tilt.

The beneficial effects on the cerebral perfusion pressure, cardiac output and MAP of putting the patient head-down, as an immediate treatment for excessive hypotension, should therefore be immediately apparent.

BARORECEPTOR COMPENSATION

Baroreceptors within the carotid sinus relay via the 9th cranial nerve to the brainstem. A reduced discharge in response to hypotension disinhibits the vasomotor centre, resulting in a compensatory tachycardia and vasoconstriction. The Valsalva manoeuvre tests the integrity of this reflex (Figure 1).

CAUSES OF HYPOTENSION UNDER GENERAL ANAESTHESIA

Cardiovascular disease:

- Ischaemic heart disease with diminished cardiac contractility (including recent myocardial infarction and unstable angina)
- Valvular heart disease (mitral or aortic stenosis and incompetence)
- Heart failure (including cor pulmonale)
- Dysrhythmias (rapid atrial fibrillation, third-degree heart block)
- Hypertension, especially if untreated or poorly controlled
- Other (cardiomyopathy, myocarditis, constrictive pericarditis, myocardial contusion, tamponade, congenital cardiac anomalies, aortic coarctation).

Cardiovascular medication

Especially beta blockers, but also ACE inhibitors, nitrates, calcium antagonists, α_1 antagonists (e.g. prazosin) and centrally acting α_2 agonists such as methyldopa and clonidine.

Autonomic neuropathy

This produces impaired baroreceptor response. For example:

- Diabetes mellitus (both insulin and noninsulin dependent); incidence and severity increase with duration of diabetes
- Spinal cord injury and postcerebrovascular accident states
- Parkinson's disease (in advanced cases)
- Guillain–Barré syndrome
- AIDS
- Amyloidosis
- Rare causes:
  - Familial dysautonomia (Riley–Day syndrome)
  - Shy–Drager syndrome.

ANAESTHETIC AGENTS

Induction agents

These cause a dose-related fall in blood pressure due to a complex combination of effects involving vasodilatation, myocardial depression, altered baroreceptor reflex and, especially with propofol, bradycardia. Ketamine is an exception due to its central sympathomimetic action.

Volatile agents

All volatile agents produce a dose-related fall in blood pressure, again due to a combination of vasodilatation, myocardial depression and impaired baroreceptor response. Myocardial depression and vagal stimulation resulting in bradycardia are features of halothane and higher doses of enflurane. Isoflurane at 1 MAC primarily produces peripheral vasodilatation.

Muscle relaxants (nondepolarizing)

Any hypotensive effect is principally secondary to histamine release. Tubocurarine is notable for its mild ganglion blocking action, but any fall in blood pressure is largely due to histamine-produced vasodilatation.

Opioids and antiemetics

Opioids, especially morphine, may precipitate histamine release, and hence vasodilatation. Bradycardia is also well recognized with larger

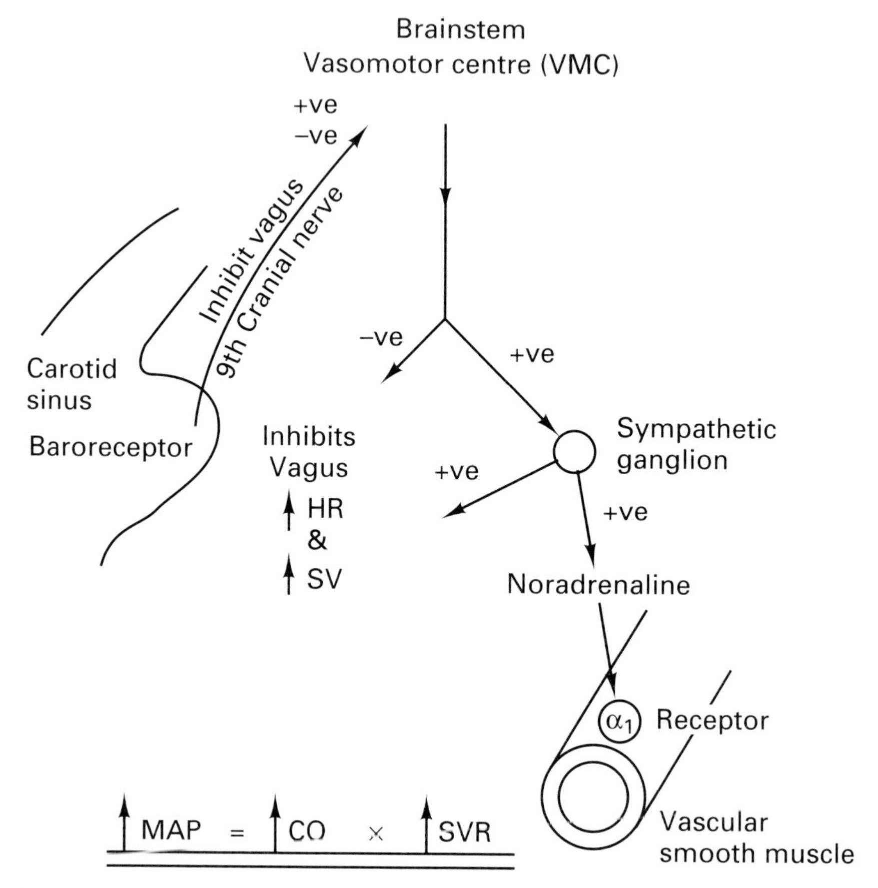

Figure 1
Baroreceptor reflex.

doses of opioids. The butyrophenones and phenothiazines are weak α_1 antagonists.

Drugs used in elective hypotensive anaesthesia

Interventions include sympathetic ganglion blockade with trimetaphan, and direct vasodilatation using GTN or sodium nitroprusside. Labetalol is notable for offering both α_1 and β blockade in a single agent (although much more β than α_1).

Positive pressure ventilation

The increased intrathoracic pressure that occurs with IPPV produces a decrease in venous return and, therefore, cardiac output. The effect is exacerbated with the application of PEEP. The baroreceptor response, although often partly obtunded under general anaesthesia, usually compensates for IPPV. However, this is not so in the presence of hypovolaemia, severe cardiac disease or autonomic neuropathy.

REGIONAL ANAESTHESIA

Epidural and spinal anaesthesia produce blockade of sympathetic as well as nociceptive fibres. The resulting vasodilatation reduces both venous return (and, therefore, cardiac output) and SVR. The height of the sympathectomy depends upon the site and dose used. Although reflex vasoconstriction occurs above the upper level of the block, blood pressure usually falls. With higher blocks (T4 or above) the cardiac sympathetics are obtunded, preventing a compensatory tachycardia. In obstetric cases, aortocaval compression must be prevented as this embarrasses venous return, and in combination with epidural or spinal anaesthesia may produce profound hypotension.

SURGICAL CAUSES

These include use of a head-up position, blood loss, aortic cross-clamping and use of lower limb tourniquets. Ischaemic tissues become maximally vasodilated. Release of the cross-clamp or tourniquet results in an acute fall in SVR and blood pressure. Inadvertent excessive intra-abdominal pressure during laparoscopic surgery may cause hypotension due to impaired venous return.

HYPOVOLAEMIA

Hypovolaemia, of whatever cause, is revealed under anaesthesia, producing hypotension. Examples include: dehydration from inadequate fluid intake, vomiting and diarrhoeal; haematemesis, melaena, small bowel obstruction or acute inflammatory bowel disease; trauma and burns. Additional causes include metabolic disorders such as diabetic ketoacidosis, hypercalcaemia and diabetes insipidus, and high output renal failure.

LESS COMMON CAUSES

Anaphylaxis

This may result in massive histamine mediated vasodilatation, producing cardiovascular collapse. In addition to resuscitation, adrenaline is the specific treatment. Pulmonary embolus (from a deep vein thrombosis), fat globules (from long-bone fractures), air bubbles (head and neck operations), or carbon dioxide emboli (laparoscopic surgery) may reduce cardiac output. Hypotension is accompanied by desaturation and alveolar hypocapnoea.

Intraoperative myocardial infarction

This is strongly associated with pre-existing cardiac disease, and is accompanied by ECG ischaemic changes.

TREATMENT

Principle

Remove the precipitating cause, e.g. correct hypovolaemia, and increase cardiac output and SVR.

Practice

A combination of actions increasing both cardiac output and SVR are most effective.

- Increase $F_{I}O_2$ to maintain SaO_2
- Place patient in head-down position
- Administer a rapid intravenous infusion (colloid gives a faster response than crystalloid)
- Vasopressors, e.g. ephedrine (mixed β and α_1 effects), methoxamine or phenylephrine (both α_1 agonists)
- If necessary, give an inotrope plus a vasoconstrictor, e.g. dobutamine and noradrenaline together.

BIBLIOGRAPHY

Little R C, Little W C. Physiology of the heart and circulation, 4th edn. Year Book Medical, Chicago

Simpson P J. Hypotensive anaesthesia. Current Anaesthesia and Critical Care 1992; 3: 90–97

CROSS REFERENCES

Induced hypotension
Anaesthetic Factors 32: 597
Epidural and spinal anaesthesia
Anaesthesia factors 32: 594

LOCAL ANAESTHETIC TOXICITY

I. McConachie

Considering the large numbers of local anaesthetics administered, the frequency of toxic reactions is very small. Here we concentrate on CNS and cardiac toxicity as manifestations of local anaesthetic toxicity. Causes of such toxicity are related to elevated plasma drug levels. This is due to:

- Accidental (or misinformed) overdosage
- Inadvertent intravenous injection.

There is a general relationship between plasma levels of local anaesthetics and symptoms and signs of toxicity (Table 1).

Table 1.
The effect of increasing plasma drug levels

Symptom/sign	Drug level
Tingling in tongue and perioral region	Low
Dizziness	↓
Blurred vision	↓
Tinnitus	↓
Twitching and signs of CNS irritability	Intermediate
Loss of consciousness	↓
Convulsions	↓
Deep coma	↓
Respiratory and cardiac depression	High

Initial excitation is due to selective inhibition of inhibitory pathways in the CNS. With increasing blood levels there is an inhibition of both inhibitory and facilitatory pathways, leading to generalized CNS depression.

However, although a general relationship between blood levels and toxicity exists, the rate of injection (if intravenous) or uptake also influences the chance of toxicity; for example, a faster rate of injection produces signs of toxicity at lower venous plasma levels.

METHODS OF REDUCING PLASMA LEVELS

Uptake is highest with concentrated solutions:

- Saturation of local binding sites
- Greater intrinsic vasodilating effects.

Uptake is highest from:

- Intercostal space
- Epidural space
- Peripheral nerve blocks
- Subcutaneous infiltration.

The principal technique for minimizing plasma levels is to reduce vascular uptake by the addition of adrenaline. Recent alternative methods studied include:

- Addition of octapressin or phenylephrine (less toxic than adrenaline)
- Addition of large molecules, e.g. dextran
- Low release formulations, e.g. those attached to lipid microspheres.

PHARMACOLOGY OF LOCAL ANAESTHETIC TOXICITY

- Potency varies directly with lipid solubility
- Cardiac depression varies directly with potency
- CNS excitability varies directly with potency.

The mechanism for cardiac depression is unclear, but some experiments suggest that it may be related to decreased intracellular calcium. In addition, at high plasma levels, there will be generalized vasodilation compounding the vascular collapse.

The relative potencies of bupivacaine and lignocaine are about 4:1, which is similar to their relative CNS toxicities. Both the blood levels required for cardiac toxicity and the ratio of the doses required for cardiac toxicity compared to doses required for CNS toxicity suggest that bupivacaine is considerably more cardiotoxic than lignocaine.

INFLUENCE OF ACIDOSIS

- The convulsive threshold is decreased
- An increase in $P_{a}CO_2$ leads to an increase in

CBF, thus allowing more drug to enter the brain
- A decrease in intracellular pH will increase the amount of ionized drug; this limits diffusion and prevents drug leaving the cell
- Decreased plasma protein binding results in more free drug.

Thus acidosis increases the chances of developing CNS toxicity and also prolongs the toxicity.

CLINICAL ASPECTS OF LOCAL ANAESTHETIC TOXICITY

Sensible precautions:
- All resuscitation facilities and drugs must be available
- Access to circulation should be secured before starting
- Trained assistance should be available
- Maintain dialogue with patient during performance of block.

Prevention
- Careful technique
- Aspirate before injection
- Choice of drug, e.g. do not use bupivacaine for intravenous regional anaesthesia.

Ester local anaesthetics are metabolized by plasma cholinesterase. Thus if toxic plasma levels are achieved the toxic reaction should be short lived (except in the rare case of atypical cholinesterase).

TREATMENT

Minor reactions:
- Stop injection
- Observe patient.

Major reactions
Resuscitate according to standard guidelines.

Convulsions
Convulsing patients rapidly become hypoxic and acidotic. Prompt treatment is therefore crucial. Convulsions should be quickly terminated.

- Thiopentone (50–100 mg) is likely to be effective
- Diazepam (5–10 mg) is also likely to be effective
- Cardiorespiratory effects should be closely monitored.

Suxamethonium may be required if the convulsions are severe or resistant to treatment, or if intubation is required. Clearly the patient will still require anticonvulsants.

Cardiac depression:
- Give oxygen – *this is of prime importance*
- Fluids
- Inotropes and vasopressors
- Defibrillation, if required (higher energy settings than usual may be required)
- Aggressive reversal of acidosis with bicarbonate is warranted, according to blood gas analysis
- If cardiac arrest supervenes, give cardiopulmonary resuscitation (CPR)
- Prolonged CPR and resuscitation may be required.

Arrhythmias

Lignocaine
- Is a potent antiarrhythmic agent itself
- Arrhythmias are uncommon after overdosage
- At high plasma levels, decreased cardiac conduction may be seen.

Bupivacaine
- The L isomer is mainly the toxic one
- May potentiate arrhythmias
- Exact mechanism is unknown
- Markedly depresses the rapid phase of depolarization of the cardiac action potential and prolongs the refractory period
- May cause one-way block leading to re-entrant arrhythmias
- Ventricular fibrillation is common in severe toxicity.

Bupivacaine seems to be significantly associated with cardiac toxicity compared to other local anaesthetics. CPR is very difficult in bupivacaine-induced cardiotoxicity because the drug binds to cardiac muscle (exacerbated by acidosis).

N.B. All amide type local anaesthetics have a similar mechanism for toxicity. The use of a lignocaine infusion for ventricular arrhythmias or after ventricular fibrillation may not therefore be as logical as originally believed. The present guidelines on CPR of the Resuscitation Council (UK) only suggest the use of lignocaine as a last resort. Animal studies differ in their implications for drug treatment of bupivacaine-induced arrhythmias. Amiodarone has been suggested.

Ropivicaine

This is a new amide drug intermediate in structure and potency to mepivacaine and bupivacaine. It is represented as the L isomer rather than a racemic mixture (less toxic than the L isomer of bupivacaine). Animal studies suggest much less cardiotoxicity than with bupivacaine, while of similar duration of action.

BIBLIOGRAPHY

Albright G A. Cardiac arrest following regional anaesthesia with etidocaine or bupivacaine. Anesthesiology 1979; 51: 285–287

Arthur G R, Covino B G. What's new in local anaesthetics? Anesthesiology Clinics of North America 1988; 6: 357–369

De La Coussaye J E, Eledjam J J. The pharmacology and toxicity of local anaesthetics. Current Opinion in Anaesthesiology 1991; 4: 665–669

Moore D C. Administer oxygen first in the treatment of local anaesthesia induced convulsions. Anesthesiology 1980; 53: 346–347

Scott D B. Maximum recommended doses of local anaesthetic drugs. British Journal of Anaesthesia 1989; 63: 373–374

CROSS REFERENCES

Postoperative analgesia for thoracic surgery patients
Surgical Procedures 17: 358
Analgesia for labour
Surgical Procedures 20: 397
Epidural and spinal anaesthesia
Anaesthetic Factors 32: 594
Local anaesthetic techniques
Anaesthetic Factors 32: 600
Cardiopulmonary resuscitation
Anaesthetic Factors 34: 687

MALIGNANT HYPERTHERMIA: CLINICAL PRESENTATION

P. M. Hopkins

Due to the reduction in major morbidity and mortality from other causes, malignant hyperthermia (MH) is now one of the major potential anaesthetic hazards for the otherwise healthy individual. This is despite the mortality from MH declining from above 70% prior to 1980 to below 5% over the past 5 years. It is argued by some that, with the use of modern monitoring equipment and the mandatory availability of intravenous dantrolene, mortality from MH should be zero.

The key to prevention of death from an MH reaction is undoubtedly recognition by the attending anaesthetist of the early signs of the reaction followed by an appropriate therapeutic response.

It is interesting to note that the rapid decline in mortality in the UK began before the introduction of intravenous dantrolene: this is attributed to increasing awareness of the condition amongst UK anaesthetists.

MH is now known to be a genetically heterogeneous disorder, but the precise molecular defects are yet to be determined. The result of each defect is, however, the same and that is to cause an uncontrollable rise in intracellular calcium ion concentration in skeletal muscle cells in the presence of the triggering drugs (any volatile anaesthetic drug or suxamethonium). This rise in myoplasmic calcium ion concentration is sufficient to explain all the clinical and biochemical features of MH, a knowledge of which is so crucial if an anaesthetist is to have the best chance of successfully managing a MH reaction.

The nature and course of MH reactions show considerable variation. The components of a reaction can be very crudely divided into metabolic and muscle activity, both of which lead to rhabdomyolysis. The balance and severity of metabolic and muscle activity components generally varies according to which triggering drugs have been used. This is assumed to be a reflection of the dynamics of the rise in intracellular calcium ion concentration.

THE RESPONSE TO SUXAMETHONIUM

Suxamethonium is thought to produce a rapid and marked rise in intracellular calcium, but its duration of effect is limited. The predominant feature is thus increased muscle activity evident as rigidity. This muscle rigidity is sometimes generalized, but may be limited to the jaw muscles (masseter muscle spasm is discussed in more detail in a separate section). Because of the limited duration of effect of suxamethonium, homeostatic mechanisms restore the intracellular calcium towards resting levels, usually within 10 min. The muscle activity leads to extrusion of potassium ions, creatine kinase and myoglobin. The hyperkalaemia due to suxamethonium alone is not life-threatening, but the myoglobinaemia may be sufficient to cause acute renal failure. Indeed, post-operative renal failure has been the only presenting feature in some MH-susceptible patients. Serum creatine kinase is an indicator of the degree of muscle damage, reaching a maximum (often >20 000 units) after about 24 h. Although metabolic processes will have been stimulated, the duration of the stimulus is so short that the resulting clinical features are mild and usually not noticed.

THE RESPONSE TO VOLATILE ANAESTHETICS

The nature of the response to volatile anaesthetics suggests that they cause a steadily increasing intracellular calcium ion concentration. Calcium, at concentrations lower than those required to activate the contractile apparatus, has other important intracellular functions. One of these is the regulation of the phosphorylation, and hence the activity, of various enzymes, including rate-limiting enzymes of the glycolytic pathway. During a gradually increasing intracellular calcium ion concentration, the first detectable features are due to this metabolic stimulation: the earliest clinical signs are due to increased carbon dioxide and lactate production. In the spontaneously breathing patient there will be an increasing respiratory rate, while where a circle system is in use the soda lime will be rapidly exhausted. Whatever mode of ventilation and breathing system is being used the increased carbon dioxide production will be detected as an increasing end-tidal partial pressure of carbon dioxide by capnography. Either simultaneously with, or shortly following, the hypercapnoea, a tachycardia develops due to the effects of acidaemia on the cardiovascular regulatory centre of the midbrain. By the same mechanism there is a tendency for the blood pressure to rise, although in some cases the blood pressure falls, presumably due to a predominant effect of local metabolites on the vascular smooth muscle. As well as an increase in lactate and carbon dioxide as by-products of metabolism, there is an increase in oxygen consumption which may lead to a fall in the saturation of haemoglobin with oxygen, detectable with pulse oximetry. Arterial blood gases taken at this stage will show acidaemia, hypercarbia, a base deficit and, usually, mild hypoxaemia.

The name, malignant hyperthermia, was originally coined because the most obvious clinical feature was that the patient would become excessively hot and then they invariably died. This was, of course, at a time when monitoring during routine anaesthesia was purely clinical. We now know that hyperthermia resulting from the hypermetabolic state is a relatively late manifestation and, whereas during the 1970s and early 1980s monitoring of body temperature was advised for every anaesthetic, capnography has now superseded it. However, when some doubt exists as to whether some metabolic signs are due to MH, the finding of a rapidly rising body temperature is very persuasive, although, as indicated above, in some cases there is a delay before the rate of temperature rise becomes remarkable.

It is commonly considered that there is a stage of a MH reaction beyond which death is almost inevitable: this is likely to relate to the integrity of the mitochondria. In the early stages of the reaction mitochondria respond to the increased production of pyruvate by increasing its utilization to produce more ATP. This is important in limiting the intracellular calcium ion concentration as ATP is required for the normal functioning of two of the most important mechanisms for removing calcium from the myoplasm: the calcium pumps of the sarcolemma, and the sarcoplasmic reticulum. The mitochondria themselves, however, also sequester calcium ions, the rate being entirely dependent on the myoplasmic calcium ion concentration. In the presence of continued release or influx of calcium into the myoplasm the intramitochondrial calcium ion concentration will continue to rise until the accumulated calcium disrupts the mitochondria. A situation is thus reached where glycolysis is stimulated and the only route for further metabolism of pyruvate is to lactate. Simultaneously, there is a rapid decline in ATP production, leading to a reduced rate of calcium removal from the myoplasm, and hence setting up a vicious cycle. It is at this stage that muscle rigidity will become apparent.

Calcium ions also stimulate activity of some intracellular phospholipases, leading to increased turnover of sarcolemmal phospholipid. Under these circumstances maintenance of the integrity of the sarcolemma is an ATP-dependent process, and when the demand for ATP exceeds the supply the membrane permeability increases. This will result in increased leakage of calcium into the cell and also leakage out of intracellular constituents such as potassium ions, creatine kinase and myoglobin. The resulting hyperkalaemia can be sufficient to cause cardiac arrest while, if the acute reaction is survived, the myoglobinaemia can result in renal failure.

The response to the volatile agents tends to be more rapid following suxamethonium, with some florid reactions occurring within 15 min. Halothane certainly seems to be the most potent trigger of the volatile agents, with responses to enflurane and, especially, isoflurane being more insidious. No cases of human MH triggered by desflurane have been reported as yet, although this drug does trigger porcine MH. The work on pigs suggests that desflurane is a less potent trigger than halothane.

CROSS REFERENCES

Malignant hyperthermia
Patient Conditions 2: 57

MASSETER MUSCLE SPASM

P. M. Hopkins

The major problem with masseter muscle spasm (MMS) is in defining what it means. The first common usage of the term arose when malignant hyperthermia (MH) reactions subsequently occurred in patients whose mouths had been difficult to open following the use of suxamethonium. This association was apparent in 70% of patients given suxamethonium who went on to develop MH. Awareness of this association between MMS and MH led to referral of many patients who developed MMS for investigation of their MH status. Of those with MMS as the only abnormal feature, 28% have proven to be susceptible to MH. This figure rises to 57% if there were accompanying metabolic features, or 76% if the MMS was followed by other features of muscle damage, such as myoglobinuria or severe incapacity from muscle pains. From this experience, which is similar amongst MH investigation centres, it seemed clear that patients developing MMS were at high risk from MH until proven otherwise. However, at that stage there was no definition of what was meant by MMS.

The situation really started to become confusing in the late 1980s with the publication of studies in which the tension developed by the jaw muscles following suxamethonium was found to rise in virtually all children and in a large proportion of adults. The unfortunate outcome of these studies was that some interpreted the results as meaning that most patients develop MMS following suxamethonium. The next stage in this trail of false logic was to extrapolate this interpretation for comparison with the incidence of MH in patients referred because of MMS. The result of this erroneous comparison could only be that the incidence of MH in the population was much higher than previously thought, or that the in vitro contracture tests used for MH diagnosis had a very high false-positive response rate.

A more consistent explanation can be realized by examining how patients came to be investigated for their MH status following an episode of 'MMS'. These cases were not those in which there was a measured increase in jaw muscle tension, rather they were cases in which the attending anaesthetist experienced a clinical problem in opening the mouth in order to achieve endotracheal intubation. Prior to the publications by van der Spek et al (1987) and Leary and Ellis (1990) the commonly encountered mild and transient resistance to mouth opening following injection of suxamethonium was probably attributed to a failure of relaxation rather than to muscle tension development. The cases referred for MH investigation were therefore outside the normal experience of the attending anaesthetist in terms of the severity and duration of the difficulty in mouth opening.

The term MMS is therefore of practical and clinical significance only if its use is restricted to severe and, perhaps more importantly, the prolonged (more than 2 min) episodes of resistance to mouth opening following suxamethonium.

Another misleading feature of the relationship between MMS and MH is the lack of metabolic response following MMS. This is a reflection of the disproportionate effect of suxamethonium as an MH triggering drug in terms of the balance between increased muscle activity and increased metabolic activity (see the section on malignant hyperthermia: clinical presentation). Also, a metabolic response may not be observed even if the anaesthetic is continued with volatile drugs, as we know that patients susceptible to MH do not have a reaction with every exposure to triggering drugs. The reasons for this are not clear.

MANAGEMENT OF MMS

Immediate

The patient who has been given suxamethonium will obviously be paralysed, so the first priority is ventilation of the lungs. Fortunately, upper airway muscle tone seems to be maintained, thereby making ventilation with a face-mask via the nose a viable proposition.

Differential diagnosis

Establish that the correct dose of suxamethonium has been given, intravenously; check the ampoule, syringe and injection site. It is, however, unusual for mouth opening to be a major problem even when no neuromuscular blocking drug has been given, unless the dose of induction agent was also inadequate: this would of course occur if a cannula had become dislodged from its intravenous site during induction.

Further anaesthetic management

This will depend on the urgency of the surgery and the feasibility of continuing nonurgent surgery without the use of volatile anaesthetic drugs. If the surgery is not urgent and continuation with a volatile-free technique potentially compromising, the patient should be allowed to wake up. Should the surgery need to proceed then ventilation should continue via the face-mask until the spasm has eased, when a nondepolarizing neuromuscular blocker can be given and intubation subsequently achieved. Anaesthesia should be maintained with intravenous drugs.

Recording of diagnostic predictors

Although the patient who develops MMS must be considered to be potentially susceptible to MH until proven otherwise, evidence of metabolic stimulation and other indicators of increased muscle activity increase the likelihood of MH. Therefore, the patient should be immediately observed for the presence of generalized muscle rigidity and the duration of MMS should be recorded. An accurate chart of heart rate, blood pressure, pulse oximeter, capnograph and central temperature readings should be made. Blood for arterial blood gas and serum potassium analysis should be sent. In the postoperative period, the first voided urine should be analysed for the presence of myoglobin and the serum creatine kinase should be estimated at 12 and 24 h.

Further investigations

The patient should be referred for determination of their MH status by muscle biopsy and in vitro contracture testing. They should he advised that they and all members of the family should be treated as potentially susceptible to MH until proven otherwise. In the interim, the reactor should undergo electromyographic studies to exclude congenital myotonia, some variants of which can be asymptomatic.

BIBLIOGRAPHY

Christian A S, Halsall P J, Ellis F R. Is there a relationship between masseter muscle spasm and malignant hyperthermia? British Journal of Anaesthesia 1989; 62: 540–544

Leary N P, Ellis F R. Masseteric muscle spasm as a normal response to suxamethonium. British Journal of Anaesthesia 1990; 64: 488–492

van der Spek A F L, Fang W B, Ashton-Miller J A, Stohler S, Coulson D S, Schork M A. The effect of succinylcholine on mouth opening. Anesthesiology 1987; 67: 459–465

CROSS REFERENCES

Malignant hyperthermia
Patient Conditions 2: 57

Malignant hyperthermia: clinical presentation
Anaesthetic Factors 33: 644

NEUROLEPTIC MALIGNANT SYNDROME

A. T. Hindle

Neuroleptic malignant syndrome (NMS) was first described in 1960 by Delay. It is a potentially fatal condition caused by either treatment with dopamine receptor antagonists or by withdrawal of dopamine receptor agonists.

PATHOGENESIS

Central mechanisms

There is acute dopaminergic transmission block in the:

- Nigrostriatum – which produces rigidity
- Hypothalamus – which produces hyperthermia
- Corticolimbic system – which produces an altered mental state.

Peripheral mechanisms

The clinical similarities between NMS and malignant hyperthermia (MH) suggest a common pathophysiological element. In vitro halothane–caffeine contracture tests carried out on NMS and MH patients have not, however, supported any intracellular association between the two syndromes.

The pathophysiological mechanism underlying the skeletal muscle rigidity in NMS is controversial. The current view leans towards this being central in origin. This is supported by the observation that neuromuscular blocking drugs produce flaccid paralysis in NMS, whereas in MH they have no effect.

Excitatory amino acids

There is now believed to be a relative glutaminergic transmission excess as a consequence of a dopaminergic block and it may be that drugs which antagonize glutamate have beneficial effects (see later).

INCIDENCE

Approximately 0.5–1%.

CLINICAL FEATURES AND DIAGNOSIS

NMS develops over a period of 24–72 h following exposure to neuroleptic agents. This exposure can have been over a period of days or months and may even follow a low dose of a neuroleptic agent. The features may continue for up to 10 days, even after stopping the triggering agent. (See Table 1.)

Table 1.
Criteria for diagnosis of NMS

Major criteria	Minor criteria
Fever	Tachycardia
Rigidity	Raised blood pressure
Elevated serum creatine kinase*	Tachypnoea
	Altered consciousness level
	Sweating

*No specific laboratory markers exist. Creatine kinase may be mildly or grossly elevated.

MORTALITY

Figures of 8–30% are frequently quoted, but the number of deaths has declined since 1984 (11.6% now, versus 25% before 1984). These figures are apparently independent of the use of dopamine agonists and dantrolene.

Mortality from NMS is due to:

- Respiratory failure (commonest cause)
- Renal failure secondary to myoglobinuria (a strong predictor of mortality, representing a risk of 50%)
- Cardiac arrest.

Other complications are outlined in Table 2.

Table 2.
Complications

Respiratory
Secondary infection
Aspiration pneumonia

Cardiovascular
Arrhythmias
Pulmonary embolism

Musculoskeletal
Peripheral neuropathy
Rhabdomyolysis
↓
Myoglobinuria

DIFFERENTIAL DIAGNOSIS

Early diagnosis and distinction from other conditions presenting in a similar fashion is crucial in order to prevent fatalities.

NMS versus lethal catatonia

Rigidity is intermittent in lethal catatonia. Lethal catatonia demonstrates severe psychotic excitement in the early stages.

MH versus NMS

Compared to MH, NMS demonstrates:

- Slow onset
- Rigidity of central origin (controversial)
- Latency of effect with dantrolene
- Uneventful anaesthesia with MH triggering agents
- Lack of familial tendency (MH is autosomal dominant).

Drugs of abuse

Ethanol withdrawal, sedative hypnotic withdrawal, cocaine and amphetamine intoxication or monoamine oxidase overdoses must be excluded before NMS is diagnosed. Some of these agents may also release central serotonin resulting in the central serotonin syndrome.

Neuroleptic heat-stroke

Flaccid muscle tone is the major distinguishing feature.

MANAGEMENT

Nonspecific therapy:

- Withdrawal of trigger agent
- Basic resuscitation measures
- Cooling.

Specific therapy

Dopamine agonists

Bromocriptine reduced death rates to 7.8%. Amantadine reduced death rates to 5.9%.

Dantrolene and bromocriptine

Dantrolene reduces the death rate to 8.6%. It may, however, cause hepatic damage (already altered liver enzymes are present in NMS).

The success of dantrolene supports the 'muscle hypothesis', but the time to clinical effect is slow (several days).

Bromocriptine may be the type of choice in patients with NMS associated with hepatic dysfunction.

The relative reduction in death rate holds up at all the levels of syndrome severity in both dantrolene and bromocriptine groups.

Anticholinergic agents

These drugs are best avoided when rigidity is associated with pyrexia.

Glutamate antagonists

Amantadine and memantine are antagonists at the *N*-methyl-D-aspartate (NMDA) type of glutamate receptor. They:

- Restore the balance between glutaminergic and dopaminergic systems when dopaminergic transmission has been antagonized by neuroleptic drugs
- Exhibit hypothermic and central muscle relaxant properties.

These drugs could therefore be effective in the reversal of NMS.

ELECTROCONVULSIVE THERAPY (ECT)

This is controversial, and may only be treating early psychosis following neuroleptic withdrawal rather than NMS.

RE-EXPOSURE TO TRIGGER AGENT

Withdrawal of a neuroleptic agent, when treatment is required for severely psychotic patients, is obviously hazardous.

Mortality following reintroduction is variable (17–87%). Mortality may be reduced by:

- Low potency neuroleptic agents
- Lowest possible dose of neuroleptic agent
- Monitoring of creatine kinase levels.

ANAESTHESIA

Anaesthetists need to be aware of this syndrome in the context of anaesthesia for ECT. It is important to note that the technique of anaesthesia must not aggravate the muscle disorder or produce the complications of NMS.

It is advisable to avoid suxamethonium in the presence of active muscle disease, as it may release potassium into the circulation and cause rhabdomyolysis. Propofol is best avoided in ECT as it shortens the duration of seizures and increase the frequency of treatment.

MAIN POINTS:

- The pathogenesis of NMS is still not fully understood
- Early diagnosis is crucial
- Differential diagnosis remains problematical in the absence of suitable animal models and biological markers for NMS
- Anaesthesia for NMS patients may continue safely in presence of MH trigger agents
- The cornerstones of management are withdrawal of the trigger agent and supportive therapy; pharmacological therapy is merely adjunctive
- Reintroduction of NMS trigger agents is possible, but must be done cautiously.

BIBLIOGRAPHY

Adne P J, Krivosic-Horber R M, Adamantidis M M et al. The association between the neuroleptic malignant syndrome and malignant hyperthermia (see comments).

Anderson W H. Lethal catatonia and the neuroleptic syndrome. Critical Care Medicine 1991; 19: 1333–1334

Dickey W. The neuroleptic malignant syndrome (review). Progress in Neurobiology 1991; 36: 425–436

Hard C. Neuroleptic malignant syndrome versus malignant hypothermia (letter; comment). American Journal of Medicine 1991; 91: 322–323

Weller M, Kornhuber J. A rationale for NMDA receptor antagonist therapy of the neuroleptic malignant syndrome (review). Medical Hypotheses 1992; 38: 329–333

CROSS REFERENCES

ECT
Anaesthetic Factors 28: 536
Malignant hyperthermia: clinical presentation
Anaesthetic Factors 33: 644

PACING AND ANAESTHESIA

A. Vohra

PATIENT CHARACTERISTICS

Most patients have a history of heart disease:

- Ischaemic
- Cardiomyopathy
- Idiopathic
- Congenital
- Following cardiac surgery.

There may be other associated conditions:

- Peripheral vascular disease
- Diabetes
- Hypertension.

PREOPERATIVE EVALUATION

History:
- Surgical operation, especially site
- Assessment of cardiac disease.

N.B. These patients cannot undergo nuclear magnetic imaging.

Pacemaker function:
- Reason for insertion
- Type of pacemaker:
  - Demand (synchronous)
  - Fixed (asynchronous)
  - Defibrillating
- When inserted – possibility of electrode displacement if within 4 weeks; possibility of battery failure if a long time ago
- History of vertigo or syncope (possible battery failure)
- Irregular heart rate (possible competition with intrinsic heart rate).

ECG:
- May indicate ischaemia or previous myocardial infarction
- Confirm pacing capture (if pacing rate > intrinsic rate)
- No intrinsic rhythm (patient is pacemaker dependent)
- Only intrinsic rhythm seen – test pacemaker function by converting it to fixed mode with magnet.

Chest X-ray
- Usual assessment of heart size and lung fields
- Continuity of pacing leads; distal tips within cardiac cavity (especially in patients with chest trauma).

Serum potassium
If high, pacing threshold is increased.

Acid–base balance
Changes may affect pacing threshold.

ADDITIONAL PREPARATION

Magnet
This is used to convert the pacemaker to a fixed rate if necessary.

Chronotropic drugs:
- Atropine (0.5–3.0 mg) – may not be effective
- Isoprenaline (10–100 μg bolus, or 1–10 μg min^{-1} infusion) – N.B. isoprenaline can decrease systemic vascular resistance
- Ephedrine (3–30 mg) – α and β effects
- Adrenaline (1:200 000; 0.5–1 ml boluses.)

Diathermy:
- Plate and current direction as far away from chest as possible
- No diathermy within 25 cm of pacing box
- Bipolar is safer than unipolar made
- TURP:
  - Cutting mode can interfere, use short bursts
  - Coagulation mode should not interfere
- Request surgeon to use short bursts
- May need to convert pacing state to fixed mode if diathermy around chest
- There is a possibility of phantom reprogramming due to electromagnetic induction.

PERIOPERATIVE MANAGEMENT

Premedication
Not essential. An opioid or benzodiazepine is suitable.

Monitoring:
- Routine minimal monitoring, especially peripheral pulse to confirm cardiac output
- Invasive monitoring if indicated for operation
- Caution: possibility of entanglement with pacing wires if inserting central venous or pulmonary artery catheters
- Nerve stimulators can interfere with pacing (caution when using for brachial plexus blocks).

Anaesthetic technique:
- Consider local anaesthesia
- Vasodilatation may be poorly tolerated with fixed heart rates
- Volatile anaesthetics may increase atrioventricular delay and pacing threshold; avoid halothane
- Total intravenous anaesthesia may be preferable
- Caution with suxamethonium:
  - Acute release of potassium may increase pacing threshold
  - Myopotentials during fasciculation may be abnormally sensed
- Avoid underhydration.

POSTOPERATIVE MANAGEMENT

- Continue with ECG monitoring
- Check that pacemaker programme is correct.

BIBLIOGRAPHY

Bloomfield P, Bowler G M R. Anaesthetic management of the patient with a permanent pacemaker. Anaesthesia 1989; 44: 42–46

Shapiro W A, Roizen M T, Singleton M A, Morady F, Bainton C R, Gaynor R L. Intraoperative pacemaker complications. Anaesthesiology 1985; 63: 319–322

Zaidan J R. Pacemakers. Anaesthesiology 1984; 60: 319–334

CROSS REFERENCES

Cardiomyopathy
Patient Conditions 4: 103
Coronary artery disease
Patient Conditions 4: 107
Patients with permanent pacemakers
Patient Conditions 4: 116
Preoperative assessment of cardiovascular risk in noncardiac surgery
Anaesthetic Factors 34: 692

POSTOPERATIVE OLIGURIA

P. Nightingale

Postoperatively the metabolic response to surgery produces sodium retention and decreased free water clearance for up to 3 days, so that a decreased urine output is common. The mean postoperative solute load is 600 mOsm day^{-1} (range 450–750 mOsm day^{-1}). The maximum renal concentrating ability is 1200 mOsm kg^{-1} water, so the minimum urine volume required is:

$$\frac{600 \text{ mOsm day}^{-1}}{1200 \text{ mOsm/kg } H_2O} = 0.5 \text{ kg } H_2O = 20 \text{ ml h}^{-1}$$

Oliguria is conveniently defined as a urine output of <20 ml h^{-1} for two consecutive hours.

PATHOPHYSIOLOGY

Postoperative oliguria implies one or, more commonly, more than one of the following.

Reduced renal blood flow:
- Hypovolaemia
- Poor cardiac output
- Hypotension
- Pre-existing renal damage
- Renal vascular disease (beware ACE inhibitors)
- Renal vasoconstriction (beware NSAIDs)
- Sepsis.

Intrinsic renal damage
- Hypoxia:
  - From pre-renal causes
  - Renal vein thrombosis.
- Nephrotoxins:
  - Aminoglycosides

- Amphotericin
- Chemotherapeutic agents
- NSAIDs
- Radiocontrast media
- (Beware diabetes/myeloma).

- Tissue injury:
  - Haemoglobinuria
  - Myoglobinuria
  - Uric acid (tumour lysis).
- Inflammatory nephritides:
  - Glomerulonephritis
  - Interstitial nephritis
  - Polyarteritis.
- Myeloma.

Obstruction to flow

- Renal or ureteric:
  - Calculi
  - Clots
  - Necrotic papillae
- Pelvic surgery
- Raised intra-abdominal pressure
- Prostatic enlargement
- Bladder neck obstruction
- Blocked drainage system.

Oliguria is most commonly due to renal hypoperfusion, and only rarely from withdrawal of diuretic therapy. Total anuria is usually mechanical in origin.

Renal hypoperfusion may not produce oliguria if the ability to concentrate is poor. This may be due to:

- Prior renal disease
- Diuretic therapy
- Old age.

INITIAL ASSESSMENT

History

Acute renal failure is associated with a number of factors (Table 1). Check anaesthetic and other charts for episodes of tachycardia and/or hypotension. From estimates of fluid loss, determine whether adequate volumes of appropriate fluids have been given.

Examination

A physical examination and chest X-ray alone are unreliable in assessing the haemodynamic and volume status in the seriously ill patient. Cardiac filling pressures bear little relation to blood volume. Note any of the following:

- Tachypnoea
- Tachycardia or hypotension (check for postural drop)
- Pyrexia
- Reduced skin turgor (assess on forehead or neck)
- Jugular venous pressure
- Tense abdomen
- Muscle damage or ischaemia
- Third heart sound or peripheral oedema
- Absent peripheral pulses or vascular bruits
- Palpable bladder or obstructed drainage system

Table 1.
Factors associated with acute renal failure

Patient factors	Perioperative factors
Advanced age	Hypotension
Aortic surgery	Hypovolaemia:
Atherosclerosis (especially aortic)	Diuretic therapy
Cardiac surgery	Preoperative starvation
Chronic renal disease	Gastric aspiration/vomiting
Cirrhosis	Ileus/obstruction
Diabetes	Diarrhoea/bowel preparation
Heart failure	Surgical oedema
Hepatobiliary surgery (jaundice)	Prolonged tissue exposure
Hypertension	Blood loss
Myeloma	Hypoxia
Nephrotoxic drugs	Tissue damage/inflammation:
Pre-eclampsia/eclampsia	Ischaemia and reperfusion
Sepsis	Major burns
	Pancreatitis
	Multiple fractures
	Muscle damage
	Transfusion reactions

- Evidence of renal disease or systemic disease associated with nephritis:
  - Cloudy urine
  - Fever
  - Vasculitic rash.

Investigations

Exclude obstruction if the cause of oliguria is not immediately obvious.

- Ultrasound:
  - Renal size and parenchymal pattern
  - Hydronephrosis
  - Thrombosis of renal veins.
- X-rays:
  - Calculi
  - Nephrocalcinosis.

Blood analysis

- Arterial blood gas and lactate
- Full blood count, urea and electrolytes, and blood sugar
- Coagulation studies
- Amylase
- Creatinine kinase and myoglobin
- Uric acid
- Haptoglobins, direct and indirect bilirubin if haemolysis suspected
- Immunoglobulin electrophoresis to exclude myeloma.

Estimate creatinine clearance on a 2 h urine collection, since plasma creatinine may not reflect the glomerular filtration rate, especially in the elderly with little muscle mass.

Isotope investigations, angiography and renal biopsy may occasionally be indicated.

Urinalysis

- Blood, protein and myoglobin
- Microscopy to detect crystals and casts in the urine and to assess red cell morphology:
  - Hyaline/granular casts suggest underperfusion or chronic renal damage
  - Tubular casts suggest acute intrinsic renal injury
  - Dysmorphic red cells or casts suggest glomerulonephritis
  - White cell casts suggest pyelonephritis or possible interstitial nephritis.

Urinary indices

These are relatively imprecise, and become inaccurate after mannitol and loop diuretics (see Table 2).

Table 2.
Common urinary indices

	Under-perfusion	Intrinsic renal failure
U/P osmolality	>1.5	<1.1
U/P creatinine	>40	<20
U_{Na} (mmol l^{-1})	<20	>40
FE_{Na} (%)	<1	>3

Urinary osmolality and sodium concentration are insensitive discriminators between pre-renal azotaemia and acute renal failure. The fractional excretion of sodium (FE_{Na}) is a more accurate guide to renal integrity:

$$FE_{Na} = \frac{U_{Na}}{P_{Na}} \div \frac{U_{Cr}}{P_{Cr}}$$

where U_{Na} and U_{Cr} are ...., P_{Na} and P_{Cr} are ....

MANAGEMENT

- Maintain adequate oxygenation and ventilation
- Catheterize the bladder
- Consider invasive monitoring early in high-risk groups
- Assess fluid deficits and correct accordingly; postoperative patients have an impaired ability to excrete a water load, so avoid excessive dextrose administration
- Maintain mean arterial blood pressure at >80 mmHg or higher if previously hypertensive
- Induce diuresis:
  - Mannitol (20 G; 100 ml of 20%)
  - Frusemide (up to 250 mg)
  - Dopamine (200 mg in 50 ml at 3 ml h^{-1}).

For myoglobinuria, alkalinize the urine (to maintain the pH at >7):

- Intravenous sodium bicarbonate
- Consider acetazolamide (250 mg b.d.)

For urate nephropathy, add allopurinol (200 mg t.d.s.).

Maintain intravascular volume, but restrict fluids if oliguric acute renal failure is established.

BIBLIOGRAPHY

Baek S-M, Makaball G G, Bryan-Brown C W, Kusek J M, Shoemaker W C. Plasma expansion in surgical patients with high central venous pressure (CVP); the relationship of blood volume to hematocrit, CVP, pulmonary wedge pressure, and cardiorespiratory changes. Surgery 1975; 78: 304–315

Connors A F, McCaffree D R, Gray B. Evaluation of right-heart catheterization in the critically ill patient without acute myocardial infarction. New England Journal of Medicine 1983; 308: 263–267

Sladen R N, Endo E, Harrison T. Two-hour versus 22-hour creatinine clearance in critically ill patients. Anesthesiology 1987; 67: 1013–1016

CROSS REFERENCES

Acute renal failure
Patient Conditions 6: 154
Prostatectomy
Surgical Procedures 21: 441
Vascular Surgery
Surgical Procedures 22: 444
Hypotension
Anaesthetic Factors 33: 638

POSTOPERATIVE PAIN MANAGEMENT

D. O'Malley

Good postoperative pain management is important not only from the humanitarian aspect, but also because it can result in earlier mobilization and shortened hospital stay.

PREOPERATIVE CONSIDERATIONS

During the preoperative assessment, the anaesthetist should consider the provision of adequate postoperative pain relief and factors which might affect it, including:

- Available resources
- Pain characteristics:
  - Site and origin
  - Intensity
  - Expected duration
- Patient's previous experience with pain relief
- Underlying medical conditions and current drug therapy
- Special needs (joint mobilization, deep breathing, coughing, ambulation, etc.)
- Risk–benefit ratio
- The method of pain assessment, and teaching the patient how to use it, if necessary.

MEASUREMENT OF ACUTE PAIN

In order to treat pain and to evaluate analgesia effectively, it is necessary to be able to assess the pain.

A number of different methods are available, but a simple pain scoring system, such as a verbal rating scale with measures between

0 and 10 (0 = no pain; 10 = the worst possible pain) given by the patient both at rest and on movement is easy and quick to use.

MANAGEMENT OPTIONS

The management of an individual patient can include one or more of a number of options. The provision of 'balanced analgesia' using a combination of techniques can provide optimal pain relief with the minimum of side-effects.

NSAIDs

- Useful for the management of mild to moderate postoperative pain
- Particularly useful for out-patient surgery, dental surgery and following a variety of orthopaedic procedures
- Can be used in conjunction with opioids for moderate to severe pain
- Consider prescribing regularly, not 'as required'
- Available in oral, rectal and parenteral preparations.

Contraindications

There are a number of situations where NSAIDs are not recommended. Their use may, however, be considered with appropriate prophylaxis and monitoring. Contra-indications include:

- Coagulopathies
- Risk of bleeding
- History of gastrointestinal bleeding or ulceration
- Poor renal function
- Caution with asthmatic patients.

OPIOID ANALGESICS

- These comprise the cornerstone of postoperative pain management
- Moderate to severe pain should normally be treated initially with an opioid analgesic
- When used in conjunction with NSAIDs, including paracetamol, there are significant opioid dose-sparing effects which can be useful in reducing opioid side-effects.

Intramuscular/subcutaneous injections

Analgesia can be provided using this method of intermittent injections. Opioid administration relying on the patient's demands for analgesia 'as needed' ('PRN'), however, produces delays in administration and intervals of inadequate pain control. If this method is to be used, choose an appropriate drug, dose and interval of administration, and consider using an intramuscular algorithm (see Figure 1)which can provide more effective administration.

Intravenous injections

Intravenous administration is the route of choice after major surgery. This route is suitable for bolus administration, patient-controlled analgesia (PCA) and continuous infusion. Consider giving a loading dose to achieve minimum effective analgesic concentration. Table 1 provides simple guidelines for the loading doses for the most commonly used drugs.

Continuous infusions

This is a relatively simple technique, but is rather inflexible and requires careful monitoring. It can lead to side-effects, including oversedation.

Patient-controlled analgesia

The opioid requirements of individual patients can vary by up to 400%. PCA allows self-administration of small boluses of opioid, as required. The bolus dose is set and the minimum length of time between boluses programmed (lockout interval). One standard programme can encompass the needs of most patients, e.g. for morphine a 1-mg bolus and a 5-min lockout is suitable. A 4 h dose limit is not normally recommended.

This approach is based on a negative feedback loop. When pain is reduced there will be no further demand for analgesia until the pain returns. Patients thus titrate the analgesia to their own needs within safe clinical parameters.

ORAL ANALGESIA

Oral administration of drugs is convenient and inexpensive. It is appropriate as soon as the patient can tolerate oral intake. Consider giving drugs regularly rather than 'as required'. There are a variety of oral analgesics available which are suitable for use in the postoperative period. Many combination analgesics are available, most of which consist of one or more of the following.

Paracetamol

This is a very useful analgesic and antipyretic. It may be used in conjunction with opioids

Morphine hourly dose intramuscularly	
Weight (kg)	Dose (mg)
40–65	7.5
66–100	10

Pethidine hourly dose intramuscularly	
Weight (kg)	Dose (mg)
40–65	50
66–100	75

Papaveretum hourly dose intramuscularly	
Weight (kg)	Dose (mg)
40–65	10
66–100	15

If weight less 40 kg or more than 100 kg, seek advice of an anaesthetist

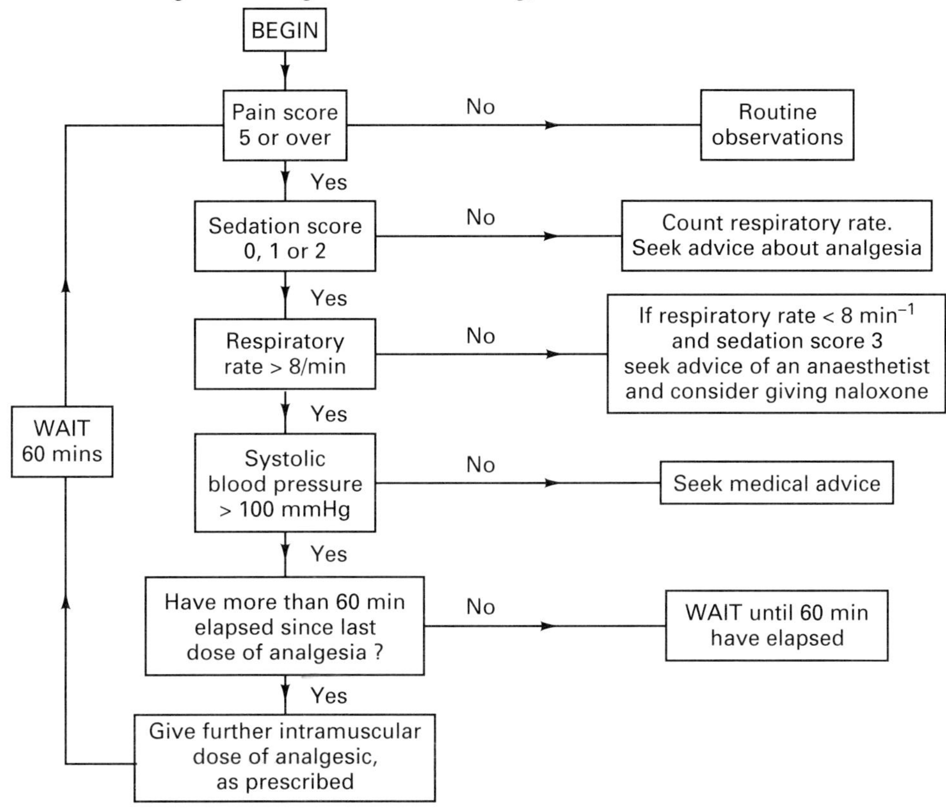

1. Respiratory rate: while patient is at rest, count respiratory rate for one minute.
2. Sedation score: Look at patient and decide which of the following apply.

Awake	0
Dozing intermittently	1
Mostly sleeping	2
Difficult to waken	3

3. Pain assessment score: 0 = no pain; 10 = worst pain imaginable.
   Measure pain score at rest and on movement.

Figure 1
Guidelines for postoperative intramuscular analgesia.

33

Table 1.
Dosing data for opioid analgesics*

Drug	Approximate equianalgesic dose (mg)		Recommended starting dose (adults >50 kg body weight)		Loading dose (mg kg^{-1}, i.v.)	Maintenance dose (mg kg^{-1}h^{-1}, i.v.)
	Oral	Parenteral	Oral	Parenteral		
Opioid agonists						
Morphine	30 (3–4 hourly)	10 (3–4 hourly)	30 (3–4 hourly)	10 (3–4 hourly)	0.15	0.01–0.04
Codeine	130 (3–4 hourly)	75 (3–4 hourly)	60 (3–4 hourly)	60 (2 hourly) (i.m./s.c.)		
Pethidine	300 (2–3 hourly)	100 (3 hourly)	Not recommended	100 (3 hourly)	1.5–2.0	0.3–0.6
Oxycodone	30 (3 hourly)	Not available	10 (3–4 hourly)	Not available		
Methadone	20 (6 hourly)	10 (6–8 hourly)	20 (6–8 hourly)	10 (6–8 hourly)	0.15	Unsuitable
Opioid agonist–antagonists and partial agonists						
Buprenorphine	Not available	0.3–0.4 6–8 hourly	Not available	0.4 6–8 hourly	0.004	0.002
Pentazocine	150 (3–4 hourly)	60 (3–4 hourly)	50 (4–6 hourly)	Not recommended	1.0	0.7–1.0

*Published tables vary in the suggested doses that are equianalgesic to morphine. Clinical response is the criterion that must be applied for each patient; titration to clinical response is necessary.

when NSAIDs are contraindicated. It is available in suppository form.

Codeine

This is a naturally occurring, weak opioid. The usual adult dose is 30–60 mg every 4 h. The small amount (8–10 mg) found in proprietary combination analgesics probably has little effect.

Dextropropoxyphene

This opioid is of similar potency to codeine, and is often combined with paracetamol in a dose of 65 mg of dextropropoxyphene with 500 mg of paracetamol (coproxamol).

Dihydrocodeine

This semisynthetic derivative of codeine is about one-third more potent than codeine. It may cause confusion in the elderly.

LOCAL ANAESTHETICS

A variety of neural blockade techniques may be continued into the postoperative period and can result in effective safe analgesia. They include the following.

Local wound infiltration

- Interscalene brachial plexus anaesthesia for shoulder surgery
- Sciatic and femoral nerve blocks for ankle and foot surgery
- Intercostal blocks for thoracic and upper abdominal surgery
- A catheter in the intrapleural space can produce analgesia with little or no evidence of sensory block following a number of procedures, in particular renal surgery, cholecystectomy and unilateral breast surgery
- Local anaesthetic infusions into the femoral sheath, lumbar plexus, and sciatic nerve have been used to maintain analgesia and sympathetic blockade after a variety of procedures; these may be particularly useful in patients in whom spinal or epidural blockade is contraindicated.

Spinal analgesia

A spinal block can provide analgesia for several hours after the completion of surgery. Continuous spinal techniques have been shown to provide effective treatment of acute postoperative pain.

Epidural analgesia
Local anaesthetic boluses or infusions can provide profound analgesia. The epidural catheter tip should be near the appropriate spinal cord segments which mediate sensation for the area around the surgical incision.

Spinal and epidural opioids
Intrathecal opioids are easy to administer either at the time of the spinal analgesic injection for surgical anaesthesia or as an accompanying technique when general anaesthesia is administered. Many patients will remain comfortable for 24 h or more after a single injection of intrathecal morphine.

Opioids alone produce good analgesia when put into the CSF or epidural space. A combination of low dose local anaesthetic and opioid work synergistically and can provide excellent analgesia over a prolonged period. Small doses can be effective, and allow early mobilization because there should be little motor blockade and good analgesia.

Side-effects of spinal opioids include:

- Hypotension
- Respiratory depression
- Nausea and vomiting
- Itching
- Urinary retention.

Patients with epidurals continuing into the postoperative period require careful monitoring. Routine monitoring should include sedation level, respiratory rate and blood pressure. An intravenous access should be maintained. Epidural infusions should be discontinued gradually and all monitoring continued for at least a further 12 h. Patients with epidurals are sometimes nursed on HDUs, but it has now been demonstrated that with good staff education and clear guidelines these patients can be safely managed in the general wards.

NONPHARMACOLOGICAL APPROACHES

Psychological factors are always present, and nonpharmacological therapy can be useful in helping to treat acute pain. It does not necessarily take more time to put some of these forms of therapy to use, but it does take awareness, sensitivity and willingness to approach pain management from a broad perspective. The techniques which seem to have the broadest application are those which increase the patient's sense of control, provide psychological support and permit relaxation.

BIBLIOGRAPHY

Allen H H, Ginsberg B, Preble L M. Acute pain mechanisms and management. Mosby, 1992
Bramley L. Improving the management of acute pain. British Journal of Hospital Medicine 1993; 50: 616–118
Ready B L, Edwards T W. Management of acute pain: a practical guide. ASP Publications, Seattle, 1992
Simpson K H. Primary analgesia. Current Anaesthesia and Critical Care 1993; 4: 70–76
US Department of Health and Human Services. Acute pain management: operative or medical procedures and trauma. Rockville, Maryland, 1992

CROSS REFERENCES

Local anaesthetic techniques
Anaesthetic Factors 32: 600
Local anaesthetic toxicity
Anaesthetic Factors 33: 642

PSEUDO-CHOLINESTERASE DEFICIENCY

D. Ostergaard and J. Viby-Mogenson

33

Pseudocholinesterase (PChe), also known as plasma cholinesterase (acylcholine acylhydrolase E.C.3.1.1.8.), is a soluble enzyme found in the plasma and manufactured in the liver.

IMPORTANCE FOR ANAESTHESIA

Decreased PChe activity may cause a reduction in the rate of hydrolysis and hence a prolonged duration of action of:

- Succinylcholine
- Mivacurium.

DETERMINATION OF PChe ACTIVITY AND PHENOTYPE

Biochemical analysis involves measuring:

- The rate of hydrolysis of a substrate catalysed by PChe
- The percentage inhibition of the hydrolysis in the presence of different inhibitor substances, often dibucaine.

Structural analysis is at the DNA level.

See Tables 1 and 2.

Table 1.
Aetiology of decreased PChe activity

Condition	Change in PChe activity
Physiological variation	
Sex	Males > females
Age	Newborns 50% of adults
Pregnancy	70–80% of pre-pregnancy level until 6–8 weeks after delivery
Disease	
Liver failure	40–70% decrease
Renal failure	10–50% decrease
Malignant tumours	25–50% decrease, depending on the localization
Burned patients	Lowest value 5–6 days after the injury. Depending on the degree of injury, the reduction may exceed 80%

Table 2.
Iatrogenic factors which decrease PChe activity

	Decrease in PChe activity (%)
Glucocorticoids, oestrogen	30–50
Cytotoxic compounds	35–70
Neostigmine	5–100
Ecothiopate eye drops	70–100
Bambuterol	30–90
Organophosphates	100
Plasmapheresis (removes PChe)	60–100

GENETICALLY DETERMINED CHANGES

- Seven different genetic variants and 28 different phenotypes are known.
- The cholinesterase activity of the different phenotypes differ qualitatively as well as quantitatively.
- Because of the above factors, it is not possible to estimate the clinical significance from the PChe activity alone. The phenotype must also be identified.

See table 3.

CLINICAL IMPLICATIONS OF DECREASED PChe ACTIVITY IN RELATION TO SUCCINYLCHOLINE

Normally 90% of an injected dose of succinylcholine is hydrolysed in plasma and only a small amount reaches the neuromuscular receptor. If PChe activity is decreased, more succinylcholine reaches the receptor.

Low activity in phenotypically normal patients

The duration of action of 1 mg kg^{-1} succinylcholine may be moderately prolonged (20–45 min).

Table 3.
Frequency and biochemical characteristics using benzoylcholine as a substrate of the clinically most important PChe variants in Caucasian populations

Phenotype	Frequency (%)	PChe activity (U l^{-1})	Dibucaine number
E^uE^u	95–97	690–1560	79–87
E^uE^a	2–4	320–1150	55–72
E^aE^a	0.04	140–730	14–27

Phenotypical abnormal patients

In patients that are heterozygous for the normal and the atypical genes:

- The duration of action is normal or slightly prolonged (10–15 min)
- More prolonged responses and a phase 2 block may be seen if the PChe activity is further decreased by other reasons (Tables 1 and 2).

In patients homozygous for two abnormal genes, a very prolonged response (120–180 min) and a phase 2 block are always seen.

MANAGEMENT OF PROLONGED RESPONSE TO SUCCINYLCHOLINE

Management depends on the PChe activity and the phenotype. Often the patient's phenotype is unknown. Therefore:

- Keep the patient ventilated and anaesthetized
- Evaluate the response to peripheral nerve stimulation.

THEORETICAL CONSIDERATIONS CONCERNING RECOVERY

In phenotypically normal patients and in heterozygous abnormal patients, a prolonged response can be antagonized with a cholinesterase inhibitor. In homozygous atypical patients, succinylcholine is not hydrolysed in plasma. The effect of a cholinesterase inhibitor is therefore unpredictable and may eventually potentiate the block. Administration of purified PChe, blood or plasma may antagonize the block. However, because of the risks associated with their use, infusion of banked blood or fresh frozen plasma cannot be recommended.

CLINICAL IMPLICATIONS OF DECREASED PChe ACTIVITY IN RELATION TO MIVACURIUM

The rate of hydrolysis of mivacurium is 70–80% of that of succinylcholine in vitro.

Low PChe activity in phenotypically normal patients:

- May cause a prolonged block
- A prolonged block has been seen in patients with renal and hepatic failure.

Phenotypically abnormal patients

In patients heterozygous for the normal and the atypical genes:

- The duration of action may be moderately prolonged (50%)
- The infusion rate is decreased (33%)
- Reversal with neostigmine is prompt when two responses to TOF stimulation are present.

In patients homozygous for two abnormal genes:

- A normal intubating dose causes a very prolonged duration of action (no signs of recovery for 40–180 min)
- Reversal with neostigmine should not be attempted before two responses to TOF stimulation are present
- Purified human PChe can be used, but the exact dose and optimal time are not yet known; fresh frozen plasma or blood should not be given.

PATIENT FOLLOW-UP

- The patient should be informed about the prolonged block. Has the patient been awake during the incident? If so, the patient might develop severe psychological problems and require counselling.
- Blood samples should be drawn for determination of PChe activity and phenotype.
- Warning cards should be issued to the patient.

BIBLIOGRAPHY

Basta S J. Clinical pharmacology of mivacurium chloride: a review. Journal of Clinical Anesthesia 1992; 4: 153–163

Jensen F S, Viby-Mogensen J, Ostergaard D. Significance of plasma cholinesterase for the anaesthetist. Current Anaesthesia and Critical Care 1991; 2: 232–237

Viby-Mogensen J. Interaction of other drugs with muscle relaxants. Seminars in Anesthesia 1985; 4: 52–64

Viby-Mogensen J. Cholinesterase and succinylcholine. Danish Medical Bulletin 1983; 30: 129–150

Whittaker M. In: Beckman L (ed) Cholinesterase. Exeter, 1986

CROSS REFERENCES

Liver failure
Patient Conditions 5: 135

Burns
Surgical Procedures 16: 331

Failure to breathe or wake up postoperatively
Anaesthetic Factors 33: 623

Awareness
Anaesthetic Fctors 33: 644

RAISED ICP/CBF CONTROL

M. Simpson

INTRACRANIAL PRESSURE

The principal constituents within the skull are brain, blood and cerebrospinal fluid (CSF). The Monroe Kellie doctrine describes how an increase in the volume of one component must be accompanied by an equal reduction in another to maintain the same pressure (Figure 1).

Initially, the volume increase is compensated for by extrusion of CSF into the spinal sac. When this mechanism is exhausted further volume increases result in a sudden large increase in intracranial pressure (ICP).

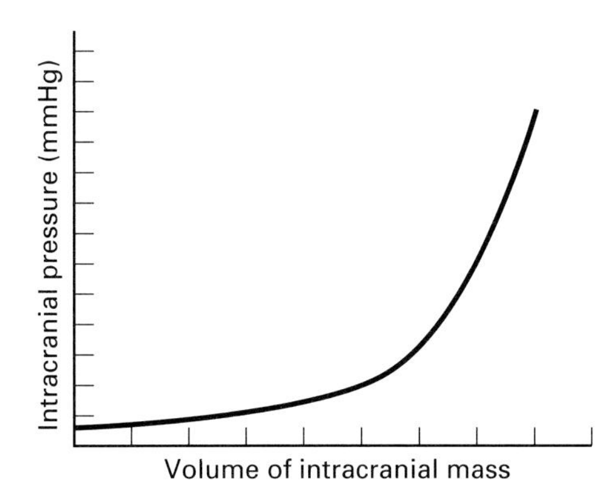

Figure 1
The effect of increasing intracranial mass on ICP. Small changes in ICP, initially, become much greater beyond a critical intracranial mass.

Further brain swelling causes:

- Herniation of the temporal lobe through the tentorium and of the cerebellar tonsils through the foramen magnum
- Brainstem torsion with reduced cerebral blood flow (CBF) and sudden obstruction of CSF flow with acute hydrocephalus.

Clinical signs of raised ICP:
- Nausea and vomiting
- Frontal headaches on waking
- Papilloedema
- Drowsiness
- Hypertension and bradycardia.

Causes of raised ICP:
- Severe head injury
- Space-occupying lesions (e.g. tumour, subarachnoid haemorrhage)
- Acute hydrocephalus.

Aggravating factors:
- Venous obstruction (e.g. from poor neck positioning)
- Raised intrathoracic pressure (e.g. from respiratory obstruction).

Ameliorating factors:
A head-up tilt of 30° gives maximal benefit from venous drainage, whilst minimizing the reduction in cerebral arterial pressure due to the hydrostatic pressure difference between the heart and brain level.

CEREBRAL BLOOD FLOW

Normal CBF is 50–65 ml/100 g min^{-1}.

Regulating factors:
- Cerebral perfusion pressure
- $P_{a}O_2$
- $P_{a}CO_2$
- Other (e.g. adenosine, neuropeptides, ions, neurogenic mechanisms).

CBF doubles as $P_{a}O_2$ declines from 50 to 30 mmHg.

For every 1 mmHg decrease in $P_{a}CO_2$ between 60 and 20 mmHg, the CBF decreases 1.1 ml/100 g min^{-1}. The reduction in CBF is maximal when $P_{a}CO_2$ <25 mmHg. If hypocapnia continues for more than 5 h the CBF returns to control values.

Cerebral perfusion pressure
CPP is defined as the difference between the systemic mean arterial pressure and the ICP.

Cerebral vascular resistance
This is proportional to the fourth power of the vessel radius.

Autoregulation
This is the coupling of blood flow to metabolic demand in normal brain by the dynamic interplay of vasoconstriction and vasodilation in the cerebral vascular bed.

Loss of autoregulation
This occurs:

- At CPP <50 mmHg
- In the traumatized or ischaemic brain
- With vasodilators (e.g. sodium nitroprusside)
- With high doses of volatile agents.

Pharmacological agents that affect CBF

Volatile agents
Halothane and enflurane increase CBF by a direct vasodilating effect on cerebral vasculature. Autoregulation is lost at high concentrations. Hypocapnia prevents the CBF rise.

Isoflurane has an indirect vasoconstricting effect secondary to reducing the metabolic rate and a direct vasodilating effect. Isoflurane provides cerebral protection and ischaemic changes do not develop until the CBF is reduced to 8–10 ml/100 g min^{-1} (compared with 18–20 ml/100 g min^{-1} for halothane or when awake). At >1.5 MAC or in damaged brain the vasodilating effect predominates.

Sevoflurane has similar effects to isoflurane.

Nitrous oxide causes significant global increase in CBF by direct vasodilatation.

Hypnotics
Barbiturates and midazolam produce a dose-dependent reduction in metabolic rate, CBF and cerebral blood volume.

Propofol causes a reduction in ICP and CPP (not less than 70 mmHg).

Narcotics
Unless ventilation is supported, narcotics increase ICP secondary to hypercapnia from respiratory depression. Injudicious use can reduce CPP by reducing systemic blood pressure.

Mannitol
The initial effect of a bolus of mannitol is haemodynamic, augmenting intravascular

volume and increasing systolic arterial pressure and CPP. With an intact autoregulation reflex, cerebral vasoconstriction and a decreased metabolic rate reduce ICP. With impaired autoregulation ICP falls by 5%, but CBF increases by 17%. The osmotic effect occurring 15 min later is less effective in damaged brain. Mannitol increases flow in the microcirculation improving oxygen delivery and clearance of vasodilating substances.

Other drugs

Dimethyl sulfoxide and hypertonic saline have beneficial effects on ICP.

Dexamethasone is used to reduce ICP.

Suxamethonium raises ICP.

Calcium channel blockers and magnesium sulphate improve blood flow to ischaemic brain areas.

BIBLIOGRAPHY

Fessler R D, Diaz F G. The management of cerebral perfusion pressure and intracranial pressure after severe head injury. Annals of Emergency Medicine 1993; 22: 998–1003

Walters F J M. Neuroanaesthesia – a review of the basic principles and current practices. Central African Journal of Medicine 1990; 36: 44–51

CROSS REFERENCES

Head injury
Patient Conditions 1: 11
Neuroanaesthesia
Surgical Procedures 12: 262

THROMBOTIC EMBOLISM

A. Devine

The effects of thromboembolism can be seen in both the systemic circulation, manifest as cerebral infarction or peripheral arterial occlusion, and also in the pulmonary circulation where it will present as pulmonary embolism. It is a major cause of morbidity and mortality, much of which can be prevented with simple prophylactic measures.

Factors important in the formation of thrombus can still be considered in terms of Virchow's triad:

- Abnormality of the blood vessel wall or heart
- Slowing or other disturbances of blood flow
- Changes in the composition of the blood, favouring platelet aggregation and fibrin formation.

DEEP VEIN THROMBOSIS AND PULMONARY EMBOLISM

Deep vein thrombosis (DVT) is a common event in hospital patients. Pulmonary embolism has been reported to account for 10% of hospital deaths (0.9% of all admissions). The risk is less than 3% for patients aged under 40 years undergoing surgery lasting less than 30 min. Surgical patients most at risk (Table 1) are those with a previous history of DVT or pulmonary embolism, those who are obese and those who have a malignant disease. Surgery involving the pelvis, hip and knee are most closely associated with DVT formation.

Diagnosis of DVT

Diagnosis on the clinical features of leg swelling, pain, warmth and positive Homan's sign has a sensitivity of only 30%. Diagnostic tests for DVT include:

- Venography – this is the most reliable technique; however, up to 2% of patients develop a DVT as a result
- Impedance plethysmography – this is sensitive and specific, but not for calf vein thrombi
- Doppler ultrasound scan
- Duplex venous scan
- Radiolabelled fibrinogen scan.

Treatment of DVT

Anticoagulation with heparin should be started with a bolus of 100 units kg^{-1} followed by an infusion of approximately 20 000–30 000 units daily, aiming to keep the partial thromboplastin time (PTT) between 1.5 and 2.5 times normal. PTT should be monitored daily. The use of low-molecular-weight heparin in the treatment of DVT is a recent development currently under review. Warfarin may be started on the first day, but heparin should be continued for 5 days while the warfarin becomes effective.

Perioperative prophylaxis of venous thromboembolism

The intensity of prophylaxis should be related to the degree of risk. Low-risk patients should be encouraged to mobilize early. Intermediate and high-risk patients should in addition receive prophylaxis. This should include either low-dose subcutaneous heparin (5000 units 8–12 hourly) or a low-molecular-weight heparin of proven efficacy. When heparin is contraindicated intermittent pneumatic compression or graduated compression stockings should be used. Their effect on prevention of pulmonary embolism is, however, unknown.

Three out of four patients dying from pulmonary embolism have not had recent surgery, emphasizing the importance of prophylaxis in medical patients at risk.

Table 1.
Risk factors for venous thromboembolism in in-patients

Patient factors
Age
Obesity
Varicose veins
Immobility (bed rest >4 days)
Pregnancy and puerperium
High-dose oestrogens
Previous DVT or pulmonary embolism
Thrombophilias
Disease or surgical procedure
Surgery or trauma, especially to the pelvis, hip or lower limb
Malignancy, especially pelvic, abdominal or metastatic
Heart failure
Recent myocardial infarction
Lower limb paralysis
Infection
Inflammatory bowel disease
Polycythaemia

DIAGNOSIS AND TREATMENT OF PULMONARY EMBOLISM

Clinical features will depend partly on the degree of obstruction and include tachypnoea, pleuritic or dull central chest pain, tachycardia, cyanosis, raised CVP and gallop rhythm. Massive acute pulmonary embolism usually presents with cardiac arrest. Electrical activity may continue without any cardiac output (electromechanical dissociation).

Investigations include: ECG (common changes include tachycardia, right bundle branch block, or S1:Q3:T3 in 25% of patients); chest X-ray, which may show pulmonary oligaemia or wedge shaped opacity; and blood gases, which may show hypoxaemia. Isotope ventilation–perfusion (V/Q) scanning is the most widely used specific investigation. These are reported as representing a low, moderate or high likelihood of pulmonary embolism. When compared with angiography, radionuclide scans underestimate the severity of pulmonary embolism.

The treatment of pulmonary embolism includes the supportive measures of oxygen, fluids and analgesia, depending on the severity of cardiopulmonary disturbance. Obstruction of the pulmonary veins greater than 25% produces raised right ventricular pressure, a fall in left heart filling pressure and displacement of the interventricular septum into the left ventricular cavity. This helps to explain why dyspnoea is eased by manoeuvres to raise left ventricular preload with fluid loading and supine position. Specific treatment options include anticoagulation, thrombolysis and pulmonary embolectomy. The place of pulmonary embolectomy is controversial; surgery can only be justified if the patient is thought to be unlikely to survive without operation.

Acute minor pulmonary embolism with no haemodynamic disturbance can be treated with heparin as described above, followed by warfarin for a period of 3–6 months.

Acute major pulmonary embolism presenting with haemodynamic disturbance will initially require resuscitation with oxygen and fluids and direct haemodynamic monitoring in a HDU. This should be followed by thrombolysis with streptokinase 250 000–600 000 IU over 20–30 min, with or without 100 mg hydrocortisone, followed by 100 000 IU h^{-1} for up to 72 h. Tissue plasminogen activator produces more rapid resolution of thrombus, but the results are similar after 12–24 h.

ARTERIAL THROMBOEMBOLISM

The source of arterial thromboembolism is often from the heart. Over half of all thromboemboli of cardiac origin are the result of atrial fibrillation, particularly when this is associated with mitral stenosis or thyrotoxicosis. Other predisposing conditions include valvular prostheses, recent myocardial infarction with mural thrombus formation and low cardiac output states. Resulting thromboemboli may take the form of peripheral emboli or, more commonly, cerebrovascular events producing a stroke. Studies have recently shown the benefits of anticoagulation in patients with atrial fibrillation.

BIBLIOGRAPHY

Dunn M, Blackburn T. Anticoagulant treatment of atrial fibrillation in the elderly. Postgrad Medical Journal 1992; 68 (suppl 1): S57–S60
Gray H H, Firoozan S. Management of pulmonary embolism. Thorax 1992; 47: 825–832
Hull R D, Pineo G F. Treatment of venous thromboembolism with low molecular weight heparins. Hematology and Oncology Clinics of North America 1992; 6: 1095–1103
Mammen E F. Pathogenesis of venous thrombosis. Chest 1992; 102 (suppl 6): 640S–644S
Thromboembolic Risk Factors (THRIFT) Consensus Group. Risk of and prophylaxis for venous thromboembolism in hospital patients. British Medical Journal 1992; 305: 567–574

CROSS REFERENCES

Obesity
Patient Conditions 5: 148
The elderly patient
Patient Conditions 11: 252
Abdominal surgery
Surgical Procedures 18: 364
Gynaecological surgery
Surgical Procedures 19: 380
Caesarean section
Surgical Procedures 20: 402
Urological surgery
Surgical Procedures 21: 432
Orthopaedic surgery
Surgical Procedures 24: 474

TOTAL SPINAL ANAESTHESIA

M. Y. Aglan

DEFINITION

- Spread of local anaesthetic to block all of the spinal nerves and/or intracranial extension
- Life-threatening extensive block results in severe hypotension which may progress to cardiac arrest, respiratory failure and unconsciousness
- High spinal anaesthesia includes profound hypotension without respiratory failure.

PHYSIOLOGICAL EFFECTS

See Figure 1.

Cardiovascular collapse:
- Total preganglionic efferent sympathetic block
- Peripheral sympathetic (T1–L2) block leads to loss of vasoconstrictor tone with profound reduction in systemic vascular resistance and venous return
- Block of cardiac sympathetic fibres (T1–T4) with unopposed vagal innervation results in severe bradycardia.

Respiratory failure:
- Diaphragmatic paralysis (C3–C5)
- Inhibition of respiratory centre due to direct effect of local anaesthetic or secondary to cerebral hypoperfusion.

Loss of consciousness:
- Direct action of local anaesthetic on the brain
- Secondary to cerebral hypoperfusion due to severe hypotension.

AETIOLOGY

Intentional

Total spinal anaesthesia (TSA), with respiratory and cardiovascular support, has been used as a means of deliberate hypotension:

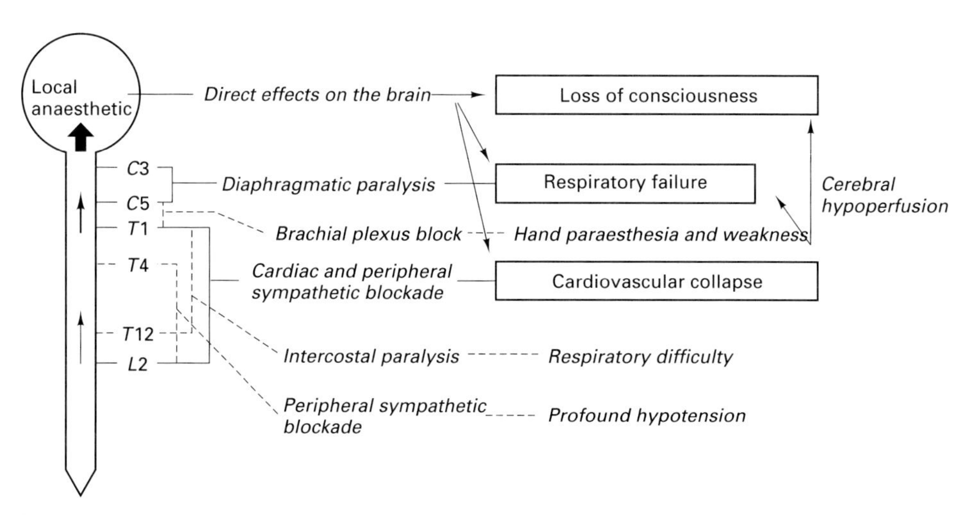

Figure 1
Physiological effects of total spinal anaesthesia.

- To provide a bloodless operative field (e.g. for ear surgery)
- To reduce intraoperative blood loss, e.g. for surgery in a patient who is a Jehovah's Witness.

Accidental:
- Has been reported as a complication of intentional spinal anaesthesia.
- Most commonly occurs when larger volumes of local anaesthetic are injected accidentally into the subarachnoid space (SAS):
  (a) Central block:
    - Extended epidural
    - False-negative aspiration and test dose
    - Subdural block
    - Increased risk following a dural tap
    - Catheter migrated into the subarachnoid space
  (b) Peripheral block:
    - Retrobulbar block
    - Brachial plexus (interscalene approach)
    - Stellate ganglion block
    - Paravertebral block
    - Intercostal block.
- Local anaesthetic spreads to the SAS along the dural cuff or via the perineural space in case of intraneural injection.

DIAGNOSIS

One or more of:

- Loss of consciousness
- Respiratory collapse
- Cardiovascular collapse or cardiac arrest.

PREVENTION

Pay close attention to details when performing blocks close to the spinal cord.

Factors which may lead to high spinal block are:

- Patient position
- Pregnancy (engorgement of epidural veins)
- Barbotage
- Straining or coughing
- Cephalad direction of a small lateral hole spinal needle combined with rapid injection.

Precautions that should be taken when using an epidural catheter are:

- Aspirate without a filter
- Use a test dose sufficient to produce a reliable subarachnoid block
- Wait sufficient time for the block to occur
- Titrate the injected local anaesthetic in incremental doses
- Avoid injection during uterine contractions
- Frequently assess both the sensory and the motor block.

Precautions to be taken with other blocks are:

- The shortest practicable needle should be used
- Careful aspiration.

Early recognition and treatment of potential TSA:
- Resuscitation equipment and anaesthetic help should be available before any regional block.
- Signs and symptoms:
  - Respiratory difficulty (weak voice, inability to cough)
  - Upper limb paraesthesia and weakness
  - Horner's syndrome (spinal or epidural)
  - Cerebral hypoperfusion (restlessness, nausea, vomiting, headache).
- Management directed at restricting spread of local anaesthetic:
  - Hyperbaric solution (spinal), antitrendelenberg
  - Solutions intended for nonsubarachnoid use are likely to be isobaric or hypobaric within CSF; the patient should be kept still; a slight head-down tilt will encourage caudal spread of hypobaric local anaesthetic and help to maintain venous return
  - Obstetric patients should be managed in a left lateral tilt to avoid aortocaval compression.

TREATMENT

Support the cardiorespiratory systems until the effects of high block recede.

- Give 100% oxygen to maximize oxygen supply.
- Cardiovascular support:
  - Maintain venous return (elevation of legs; left lateral tilt (obstetric patient); intravenous fluids (colloids or crystalloids))
  - Give atropine and vasopressor drugs if required (Table 1).
- Endotracheal intubation and assisted ventilation, which may require general anaesthetic or muscle relaxant.

Table 1.
Drugs used for the treatment of cardiovascular collapse*

Heart rate (beats min^{-1})	**Drug**	**Comments**
Asystole	Adrenaline	CPR guidelines
<60	Atropine	Vagolytic
60–90	α and β agonist, e.g. ephedrine	Increases SVR and cardiac output
>90	α agonist, e.g. phenylephrine or metaraminol	Reflex bradycardia

*In the obstetric patient, ephedrine is the drug of choice because it does not depress uterine blood flow.

- Cardiopulmonary resuscitation (CPR) if cardiac arrest occurs.

If a dural puncture is not recognized and a volume of local anaesthetic is injected into the CSF, an attempt could be made immediately to withdraw a volume of CSF equal to the volume of anaesthetic through the catheter. Some of the drug will theoretically be aspirated and the remainder will be diluted as the CSF is formed.

BIBLIOGRAPHY

Bonica J J. Regional anaesthesia: recent advances and current status. High or total spinal or epidural block. Blackwell Scientific, Oxford, 1971

Morgan B. Unexpectedly extensive conduction blcoks in obstetric epidural analgesia. Anaesthesia 1990; 45: 148–152

Morton C P J, Wildsmith J A W. Crises in regional anaesthesia. Baillière's Clinical Anaesthesiology 1993; 7: 367–375

Russell I F. Total spinal anaesthesia: the effect of spinal infusions. In: Reynolds F (ed) Epidural and spinal blockade in obstetrics. Baillière Tindall, London, 1990, p 107–120

CROSS REFERENCES

Spinal and epidural anaesthesia
Anaesthetic Factors 32: 594
Local anaesthetic toxicity
Anaesthetic Factors 33: 642
Cardiopulmonary resuscitation
Anaesthetic Factors 34: 687

TRANSPORTATION/ TRANSFER OF PATIENTS

R. S. Wheatly

33

In the UK, transportation of patients from the site of illness or injury to hospital (primary transport), or from one hospital to another (secondary transport), is primarily the responsibility of the Ambulance Service. Anaesthetists are rarely involved in primary transport, but are frequently involved in secondary transport. Anaesthetists may also be asked to accompany critically ill patients from one part of a hospital to another for specialist investigation or treatment.

Reasons for patient transfer include:

- Investigations not available in original hospital
- Specialist treatment not available in original hospital
- Need for admission to ITU and none available in original hospital.

Problems during patient transfer are mainly due to:

- Lack of thorough assessment of the patient
- Inadequate resuscitation and stabilization before transfer
- Inadequate equipment for transfer
- Inadequate monitoring during transfer
- Inexperienced personnel accompanying the patient
- Failure of communication between referring and recipient hospitals.

Such problems can be avoided either by having dedicated transfer teams or by following simple transfer guidelines.

REFERRAL

Full assessment must be done and resuscitation be in progress prior to referral:

- The senior referring doctor should speak to senior accepting doctor.
- When accepted, check:
  - Which hospital?
  - Which ward/department?
  - Any further tests/monitoring required?
- The transfer anaesthetist should speak to the receiving anaesthetist giving details of:
  - Initial and present vital signs
  - Whether patient will be intubated
  - Blood gas results
  - Any other relevant details.

Referrals should be succinct and informative – do not waste time.

PREPARATION FOR TRANSFER

- Anticipate 1 h for preparation
- Continue resuscitation/stabilization
- Organize transport
- Arrange further tests/monitoring requested by recipient hospital
- Determine whether the patient needs intubation (Table 1)
- Sedate, paralyse and ventilate all intubated patients
- Pass a nasogastric or orogastric tube in all intubated patients
- Catheterize all patients, unless urethral trauma likely
- Consider chest drains in chest trauma or barotrauma
- Organize and check equipment
- Ensure relatives have been informed of transfer, etc.
- Arrange cover for the doctor going with the patient

Table 1.
Indications for intubation prior to transfer

- Glasgow Coma Score <8 from any cause
- Tolerating an oral airway or pharyngeal suction with no gag reflex
- Risk of losing airway (e.g. facial trauma/smoke inhalation)
- Ventilatory failure (P_ao_2 <9 kPa on air, <13 kPa on oxygen and/or P_aco_2 >6 kPa)
- Potentially unstable or deteriorating
- Seizures
- If in doubt, intubate

- Inform the consultant and the switchboard
- Consider antiemetic for staff travelling with patient.

ORGANIZING TRANSPORT

The ambulance service needs to know:

- Urgency of transfer
- Location of patient
- Destination
- Number of people travelling in ambulance
- Equipment going with patient (drips, monitors, etc.)
- Anticipated problems with patient in ambulance (e.g. splints, back board, cervical immobilization).

You need to ask for:

- Paramedic-staffed ambulance, if available.
- Enough oxygen to last the journey (most ambulances carry size F (1360 l) or G (3400 l) cylinders).

Consider requesting a police escort if a smooth steady journey would not be possible otherwise, e.g. congested roads/difficult route.

EQUIPMENT FOR TRANSFER

Most hospitals have specific transfer packs, but all should be checked before use. The pack should include the following equipment.

Airway:
- Guedel and nasopharyngeal airways
- Laryngoscope with spare batteries/blade/bulb
- Endotracheal tubes
- 10-ml syringe (for cuff)
- Mouth pack
- Suction catheters (soft and rigid).

Breathing:
- Masks
- Self-inflating bag (essential if oxygen and/or ventilator fail)
- Portable ventilator and oxygen cylinder (check that connections are compatible)
- Catheter mount and angle piece.

Circulation:
- Selection of intravenous cannulae
- Intravenous giving sets
- Three-way taps
- Strong adhesive tape
- Intravenous fluid (take twice as much as anticipated)

- Sphygmomanometer
- Stethoscope.

Drugs:
- Cardiac resuscitation
- Sedation
- Analgesia
- Muscle relaxation (do not forget those in the fridge!)
- Inotropes
- Anticonvulsants
- Bronchodilators
- Mannitol.

Ensure that you have enough for a return journey if necessary.

Electrical equipment:
- Pulse oximeter
- ECG monitor and defibrillator
- Vital-signs monitor with invasive pressure monitoring facility (if available)
- Transducers for the above
- Capnography (if available)
- Syringe pumps
- Infusion pump/s (not those relying on a drip counter chamber).

Electrical equipment for transfer must be capable of running on a battery and the latter kept fully charged. If in doubt, or if the journey time is likely to exceed battery time, take a spare.

WHO SHOULD GO WITH THE PATIENT?

- A senior doctor, trained and experienced in airway management and patient transfer
- A trained nurse or operating-department assistant who has been looking after the patient
- A second doctor may be necessary in some circumstances
- A relative may only come if the doctor in charge agrees.

ON ARRIVAL OF THE AMBULANCE

- Simplify intravenous lines to the minimum necessary and secure well
- Cover the patient with a space blanket.
- Gather notes/X-rays/charts/test results/ blood (if cross-matched)
- Inform recipient hospital of vital signs and estimated time of arrival
- Connect patient to portable monitors and ventilator
- Do not begin unless you are happy with the patient's condition
- Do not remove a cervical collar in a trauma patient, even if the X-ray shows no abnormality.

IN THE AMBULANCE BEFORE DEPARTURE

- Check oxygen (is there enough?) and suction
- Connect ventilator to ambulance oxygen supply
- Secure patient/intravenous lines/monitors/ infusion pumps/catheter
- Check that the drip is running freely
- Ensure you have access to:
  - Pulse
  - Circulation, via injection port
  - The patient's head
  - Monitor screens
- Secure all other mobile equipment
- Ensure your own safety – wear a safety belt if possible
- Request a smooth, steady transfer rather than speed.

DURING THE JOURNEY

- The patient must be monitored with a minimum of:
  - Pulse oximeter
  - ECG monitor
  - Blood pressure – preferably invasive for all but the shortest journeys
- Continue documentation of vital signs and events
- If an untoward event occurs and intervention is needed, stop the ambulance first.

ON ARRIVAL AT RECIPIENT HOSPITAL

- Stay with the patient until they are handed over to an appropriate doctor
- Ensure that the receiving doctor knows of any changes during the journey.

RETURN JOURNEY

- Take all your own equipment back
- If the patient is to return with you ensure there are sufficient drugs, fluids and oxygen for the journey.

HELICOPTER TRANSFER

This is rarely needed in the UK, although some areas are covered by a medically staffed and equipped helicopter emergency service.

Helicopter transfer is useful for long-distance transfers where land transfer would be difficult and/or dangerous.

Problems include:

- Cost
- Lack of space
- Noise
- Vibration
- Restrictions due to weather/time of day
- Not available in all areas of the country.

The RAF at High Wycombe (Tel. 01494 461461) can provide a staffed and equipped helicopter to any part of the country at short notice for patient transfer, but only if:

- Helicopter transfer is clinically necessary
- All other means of transfer have been explored first
- The hospital or other agency are able to pay.

BIBLIOGRAPHY

Gentleman D, Dearden M, Midgley S, MacLean D. Guidelines for resuscitation and transfer of patients with serious head injury. British Medical Journal 1993; 307: 547–552

Hope A, Runcie C J. Inter-hospital transfer in the critically ill adult. British Journal of Intensive Care 1993; 187–192

Jeffries N J, Bristow A. Long distance inter-hospital transfers. British Journal of Intensive Care 1991; 197–204

Ridley S A, Wright I H, Royers P N. Secondary transport of critically ill patients. Hospital Update 1990; 289–299

CROSS REFERENCES

Trauma
Anaesthetic Factors 33: 672

TRAUMA

C. Gwinnutt

In the UK, trauma is the commonest cause of death between the ages of 1 and 35 years. Road traffic accidents alone account for 60 000 admissions annually, and trauma patients occupy more bed-days than cancer and cardiac patients combined. The cost to the nation is around 1% of the Gross National Product.

Most people suffer blunt trauma, with one system sustaining severe injuries and one or two other systems lesser injuries. The incidence of life-threatening injuries to different systems is:

- Head 50%
- Chest 20%
- Abdomen 10%
- Spine 5%.

Approximately 30% of emergency operating workload is trauma related (personal observation). All anaesthetists should have an understanding of the problems they may encounter and how to deal with them.

PREOPERATIVE ASSESSMENT

This is often limited due to the urgency of the situation or because the patient is unconscious. If possible, question paramedics, relatives, the patient's GP about:

- Allergies
- Medications (elderly in particular)
- Past medical and anaesthetic history
- Last meal
- Time, place and mechanism of injury

Limit investigations to those influencing management:

- X-rays (chest, pelvis, cervical spine)
- Arterial blood gases
- Urea, electrolytes, blood sugar
- ECG
- Blood group and cross-match.

THEATRE PREPARATION

Having assembled appropriate personnel, check:

- Anaesthetic machine, ventilator
- Intubation equipment, including cricothyroidotomy set
- Equipment for vascular access (pressure infusers)
- Monitors (check function and correct calibration)
- Drugs (anaesthetic, resuscitation)
- Patient-warming devices
- Equipment for positioning.

PERIOPERATIVE MANAGEMENT

Establish adequate venous access before surgery. Catheters, drains, etc., already in situ must be checked for position, function and security.

Anaesthetic technique

The technique used is determined by the physiological status of the patient, surgical plan, availability of equipment and drugs, and experience of the anaesthetist.

General anaesthesia

This is the most commonly used technique:

- Regard all patients as having a full stomach
- Use rapid sequence induction if not contraindicated
- Drugs used for induction and maintenance are dictated by haemodynamic status
- Consider avoiding nitrous oxide if pneumothorax or bowel obstruction is present
- Induce unstable patients in theatre to reduce movement, risk of intravenous lines being dislodged, and time to surgery; there is no need to disconnect the patient from the ventilator.

Regional anaesthesia:

- Sympathetic block may worsen hypotension
- Difficulty in positioning injured patients for epidural/subarachnoid block
- Delay in achieving adequate block
- Inadequate when surgery in different body areas
- May be appropriate for isolated peripheral surgery.

POINTS TO NOTE

Airway

An endotracheal tube may have already been inserted during resuscitation. Check:

- Position – (listen, chest X-ray, ETCO_2)
- Cuff integrity
- Security
- Diameter and length.

Anticipate difficult intubation if there is:

- Trauma to soft tissues of face and neck
- Midface fractures
- Actual or potential injury to the cervical spine
- Upper airway burns

Consider:

- Inhalation induction and direct laryngoscopy
- Blind nasal intubation
- Awake intubation with topical anaesthesia
- Fibre-optic intubation
- Surgical airway, cricothyroidotomy or tracheostomy
- Double-lumen tubes if thoracotomy planned.

Ventilation

IPPV in the presence of multiple rib fractures requires a chest drain to prevent a tension pneumothorax developing. In all ventilated patients:

- Check air entry bilaterally by listening in midaxillary lines
- Monitor end tidal CO_2 and O_2 saturation
- Measure expired tidal and minute volume, rate and pressure
- Adjust $F_{I}O_2$, I/E ratio and PEEP to optimize oxygenation.

Difficult ventilation may be due to:

- Gastric dilatation (pass a nasogastric or orogastric tube)
- Pneumothorax or haemothorax (insert chest drain)
- Diaphragmatic hernia.

A large air leak (e.g. bronchial tear) may require a double-lumen tube.

The final check of the adequacy of ventilation is by analysis of arterial blood gases.

Aim for normocapnia in order not to confuse interpretation of acid–base status (unless there is a head injury).

Circulation

Maintenance of circulating volume is more important than a normal haemoglobin.

- Intravenous access with short, wide cannulae (Poiseuille's law)
- Secure all intravenous lines
- Avoid intravenous line in limbs with fractures whenever possible
- Check that the cannula is in the vein before administering drugs/fluids
- Central venous access can cause pneumothorax or haemothorax
- Warm all fluids before administration
- Use cell-savers or autotransfusion where possible
- Urine output 50 ml h^{-1} minimum (excluding diuretics).

Measure blood pressure directly in an upper limb (when the aorta cross-clamped). This is more accurate at low pressures, allows repeat sampling of arterial blood, and is less subject to interference (e.g. surgeons).

In persistent hypotension:

- Ensure monitors are correctly calibrated
- Check for occult haemorrhage
- Correct profound acidosis (pH < 7.2)
- Adjust the ventilator to give the lowest mean intrathoracic pressure.

Then consider:

- *Cardiac tamponade*: low BP, pulsus paradoxus, increased central venous pressure (CVP).
  Use fluids and maintain heart rate to preserve cardiac output. Attempt pericardiocentesis if skills available. Maintain spontaneous ventilation as long as possible. Induce anaesthesia using rapid sequence induction with ketamine and suxamethonium.
- *Tension pneumothorax*: low BP, high inflation pressures, hyperresonant, deviated trachea, increased CVP.
  Emergency decompression by needle thoracentesis followed by chest drain. Have a high index of suspicion after central line insertion.
- *Neurogenic shock*: low BP, bradycardia, vasodilatation.
  Use volume expansion initially and institute early measurement of CVP to guide fluid replacement. Atropine and vasopressors may be required when CVP is adequate.
- *Septic shock*: low BP, tachycardia, vasodilatation.
  Uncommon early after injury and usually associated with abdominal injuries.
- *Myocardial infarction*: low BP, arrhythmias, pulmonary oedema, chest pain (if conscious).

Disability

Beware when moving or using fractured/injured limbs. Neurovascular injuries may be worsened or caused, especially around joints. Ensure adequate manpower for safe positioning of patients. A head injury is not a contraindication to general anaesthesia. Adequately protect peripheral nerves and pressure areas, particularly the eyes, when prone.

Exposure

Around 20% of patients arrive at hospital hypothermic. This will be worsened by administration of cold fluids and exposure of body cavities (e.g. abdomen, chest). Cooling predisposes to arrhythmias, decreases cardiac function, causing an acidosis, adversely affects coagulation and enhances anaesthetic drugs. On recovery, shivering increases oxygen consumption up to 700%. Therefore:

- Warm all fluids, especially blood
- Monitor core and peripheral temperature
- Warm and humidify all anaesthetic gases
- Cover all exposed parts, including head
- Raise theatre temperature when possible.

Monitoring

- ECG
- BP (direct)
- Sp_{O_2}
- ET_{CO_2}
- CVP (or pulmonary artery wedge pressure)
- Temperature (core and peripheral)
- Urine output
- Fluid balance
- Ventilatory parameters
- Coagulation.

POSTOPERATIVE MANAGEMENT

On completion of surgery, ensure the following before extubation:

- Hypovolaemia corrected
- pH normal
- P_aO_2 acceptable
- Temperature >34°C

- Reflexes intact
- Adequate analgesia.

Any instability requires transfer to an ITU/HDU until problems are resolved, or if there is a risk of the patient developing adult respiratory distress syndrome (ARDS) (Table 1).

Beware of problems of transfer, even over short distances.

Table 1.
Factors predisposing to ARDS

Aspiration
Multiple fractures
Pulmonary contusion
Blood transfusion >12 units
Hypotension >30 min (<90 mmHg)
Sepsis
Risk:
1 factor 18%
2 factors 42%
3 factors 85%

BIBLIOGRAPHY

American College of Surgeons Committee on Trauma. Advanced trauma life support, program for physicians. Chicago, American College of Surgeons, 1993

Cane R D. Haemoglobin: how much is enough? Critical Care Medicine 1990; 18: 1046–1047

Pepe P E, Potkin R T, Holtman Reus D, Hudson L D, Carrico C J. Clinical predictors of the adult respiratory distress syndrome. The American Journal of Surgery 1982; 144: 124–128

Trunkey D D (ed). The Surgical Clinics of North America 1982; 62:

CROSS REFERENCES

Cardiopulmonary resuscitation
Anaesthetic Factors 34: 687

Complications of position
Anaesthetic Factors 33: 618

Difficult airway – difficult intubation
Anaesthetic Factors 30: 558

Transportational transfer of patients
Anaesthetic Factors 33: 669

TUR SYNDROME

D. Nolan

The profound alterations in cardiovascular and nervous system functioning produced by absorption of electrolyte-free irrigating fluid, e.g. glycine, during transurethral resection of the prostate (TURP) is often described as the 'TUR syndrome'. It has also been described in connection with percutaneous ultrasonic lithotripsy, vesical ultrasonic lithotripsy and intrauterine laser endoscopy.

PATHOPHYSIOLOGY

Cardiovascular system:

- The syndrome is very likely to occur if uptake of fluid is greater than about 50 ml h^{-1} during the first 30 min of surgery
- There is hypervolaemia, raised central venous pressure (CVP) and diffusion of electrolytes from interstitial fluid to plasma
- If untreated, a 'shock-like' syndrome results with reduced blood volume and reduced CVP, producing hypotension.

Dilution effects of glycine

Irrigating fluids are electrolyte free in order to be nonconductive. Absorption of these fluids will therefore dilute protein and electrolyte concentrations in body fluids.

Protein

A reduction in oncotic pressure promotes fluid leakage from plasma to the interstitial compartment.

Sodium

True water intoxication produces a serum

sodium less than 120 mmol l^{-1}. There is cerebral oedema, nausea, muscle weakness, encephalopathy and grand mal seizures. The low serum sodium seen in the TUR syndrome is not usually associated with a change in serum osmolality and the contribution of cerebral oedema to the symptoms and signs is uncertain. A very low serum sodium is, however, associated with more severe symptoms and a poorer prognosis.

Potassium

Transient elevation of the serum potassium has been observed in the absence of haemolysis. Hyperkalaemia may be implicated in the production of cardiac arrest during uptake of irrigating fluid.

Osmolality

There is no fall in osmolality in response to the lower serum sodium because irrigating solutions contain osmotically active solutes. It may be the case that a decrease in osmolality, rather than a reduction in serum sodium, distinguishes asymptomatic from symptomatic patients. It has been suggested that the reason for the reduction in serum osmolality seen in some patients is a more rapid diffusion of glycine into the cells.

Direct adverse effects of glycine

Glycine itself may produce altered ocular retinal potentials, visual disturbances and release of vasopressin.

Renal function

In severe TUR syndrome renal function may be impaired due to acute tubular necrosis, which may be the result of the reduction in renal blood flow produced by hypotension or by renal swelling.

SIGNS AND SYMPTOMS

These are related to the volume of irrigant absorbed:

- 1–2 l: mild reduction in systemic BP; postoperative nausea and vomiting
- 2–3 l: more marked circulatory problems
- 3–4 l: more severe symptoms from dilution of body fluids.

Cardiovascular effects:

- Blood pressure – initial rise due to hypervolaemia.
- Heart rate and ECG:
  - Reduction in heart rate by 10–25 beats min^{-1} if plasma sodium is less than 120 mmol l^{-1}
  - Bradycardia
  - Loss of P waves
  - Nodal rhythm
  - Ventricular tachycardia
  - Widened QRS complexes
  - Depressed ST segment
  - T wave inversion.
- Chest pain may be observed after 20 min of absorption, and reflects hypervolaemia.

Respiratory effects:

- Dyspnoea
- Cyanosis
- Pulmonary oedema (associated with a poor prognosis)
- Metabolic acidosis.

Nervous system:

- Skin – prickly, burning sensation.
- Vision:
  - Blurred vision
  - Transient blindness.
- General:
  - Encephalopathy
  - Apprehension
  - Nausea
  - Erratic behaviour
  - Confusion
  - Twitching
  - Altered consciousness
  - Grand mal seizures.

MANAGEMENT

Early serum sodium measurement should be performed. Treatment should be directed towards management of hypotension, hyponatraemia, and anuria.

Hypotension:

- May be difficult to manage
- Liberal volume expansion does not appear to help
- Measurement of pulmonary capillary wedge pressure is useful.

Hyponatraemia

There are two approaches to management of a serum sodium of <120 mmol l^{-1}. Both are claimed to be effective!

- Do not give hypertonic saline because of the risk of vascular overload and pulmonary oedema. Await spontaneous diuresis or induce a diuresis using frusemide.

- Give 200–500 ml of hypertonic sodium chloride (3–5%) over 4 h to restore the serum sodium.

It seems to be accepted that hypertonic saline should be given when hyponatraemia coexists with hypo-osmolality.

Anuria:
- Induce diuresis when supportive measures have been instituted
- Hypertonic mannitol is more effective than loop diuretics, as it not only operates independently of the serum sodium level but also promotes a lower renal excretion of sodium.

BIBLIOGRAPHY

Hahn R G. Ethanol monitoring of irrigating fluid absorption in transurethral prostatic surgery. Anesthesiology 1988; 65: 867–873
Hahn R G. The transurethral resection syndrome. Acta Anaesthesiologica Scandinavica 1991; 35: 557–567

CROSS REFERENCES

Prostatectomy
Surgical Procedures 21: 441
Arrhythmias
Anaesthetic Factors 33: 629
Cyanosis
Anaesthetic Factors 33: 634
Hypotension
Anaesthetic Factors 33: 638

33

WEANING FROM MECHANICAL VENTILATION

J. C. Goldstone

INTRODUCTION

Of all patients receiving mechanical ventilation, 20% fail initial trials of spontaneous respiration, and further ventilation or re-intubation is required. Those patients in whom weaning is prolonged present complex respiratory problems. This group, some 2% of all ITU admissions, consists of patients with pre-existing lung disease as well as those patients surviving after severe multi-organ failure or neuromuscular disease.

PATHOPHYSIOLOGICAL PRINCIPLES INVOLVED IN WEANING

The ability of the patient to sustain spontaneous ventilation is dependent on the triad of central nervous system drive, the strength of the respiratory muscles and the load which is imposed on them.

Central drive

Pre-existing intrinsic lung disease is often characterized by a high resting drive. In order that weaning be successful, drive needs to be maintained above that seen in normal subjects. Optimization of drive may require the patient to be awake and alert and, in some cases, conscious level needs to be adjusted.

The capacity of the respiratory muscles

The respiratory muscles may already be weak before ITU admission or may deteriorate further during critical illness. Acute and chronic causes of weakness are:

- Hypophosphataemia
- Hypomagnesaemia
- Hypocalcaemia

- Hypoxia
- Hypercarbia
- Acidosis

- Infection

- Muscle atrophy
- Malnutrition.

When measured, most studies suggest that the respiratory muscles are severely weak in intubated patients recovering from critical illness.

The work performed by the respiratory muscles

Work is performed by the muscles each breath and this can be substantially affected by disease. Factors which increase respiratory work include:

- Bronchoconstriction
- Left ventricular failure
- Hyperinflation
- Intrinsic positive-end expiratory pressure
- Artificial airways
- Ventilator circuits.

Strength and load: a dynamic relationship

Ventilatory failure can occur if the strength of the respiratory muscles is reduced or if the load applied to them is excessive. When patients are weak, small increases in applied load, insufficient to affect ventilation in the fit, may precipitate respiratory failure, and weaning will not progress.

Initial assessment prior to weaning

The aim of assessment is to prevent patients undergoing trials of weaning which are unlikely to succeed and to set realistic goals to avoid repeated weaning attempts. The ideal patient to assess is an awake, stably oxygenated patient who is comfortable on the ventilator. Often this is not achieved.

A prerequisite of spontaneous breathing is the ability to oxygenate effectively, and this can be assessed by measuring PaO_2 during mechanical ventilation in the light of the inspired oxygen tension. Weaning is generally not attempted until there is:

- A stable inspired oxygen tension
- F_IO_2 of 0.40 or less
- PaO_2/F_IO_2 ratio of 250 or greater.

Occasionally patients are weaned when oxygenation is poor. This would include patients with congenital shunts and some chronic lung conditions.

Initial assessment of breathing: rapid shallow breathing

Ventilation is best assessed off the ventilator in the majority of patients. Care should be taken to support the patient during spontaneous ventilation, especially when assessment follows many days of intensive treatment. Rapid shallow breathing is frequently found in patients who will not sustain spontaneous breathing, and it occurs during the initial period off the ventilator. Rapid shallow breathing can be quantified as the f/Vt ratio where f is the breathing frequency and Vt the tidal volume *measured in litres*. In order to assess the patient it is suggested that:

- Use be made of CPAP via high-flow system
- CPAP be set at the level of PEEP required during mechanical ventilation
- Patient be sitting upright.

After 5 minutes, measure f/Vt by averaging breaths over the previous 30 seconds, measure Vt with a simple spirometer (Wrights), and take an average over five breaths. f/Vt should be 40 in health, and when it is greater than 105 spontaneous breathing is unlikely.

Some patients, especially those who have been ventilated for a few hours, will immediately revert to spontaneous breathing. When f/Vt is a borderline value (80–105) it is sometimes worth continuing with the spontaneous breathing trial for longer than 5 minutes and re-assessing f/Vt at half-hourly intervals.

If the patient responds to spontaneous breathing with hyperventilation and shallow breathing in the first 5 minutes (f/Vt >105) the likelihood of failure is high and the patient should receive ventilatory support. This should be of the form which allows the patient to continue to breathe spontaneously.

When the patient is back on the ventilator it is important that assessment be systematic to exclude severe disease or an obvious reversible cause.

Conscious level

If the patient is not conscious, respiratory drive may not be adequate for the increased respiratory demands that are common during weaning. The ventilatory parameters set may result in over-ventilation, and this is especially likely when the patient is not triggering the ventilator. This is seen by the absence of patient-initiated breaths and a measured minute ventilation similar to that set. Care should be taken to observe the patient during the assessment as it is often the case that patient efforts are present which are not sensed by the ventilator. Premorbid blood gases may well be abnormal, and this may be reflected by a high bicarbonate in the initial blood gases prior to mechanical ventilation.

CENTRAL DRIVE

Spontaneous breathing is unlikely if:

- The patient is not triggering when $Paco_2$ is adjusted to likely permission levels
- After a trial of spontaneous breathing, the patient sleeps during IPPV and is apnoeic.

Weaning should not continue in the face of a depressed conscious level; rather he should be fully ventilated until consciousness is lighter.

ASSESSMENT OF RESPIRATORY MUSCLE STRENGTH

Of central importance is to establish whether the patient is weak. If weakness is severe, repeated attempts at weaning are likely to fail, and this effort can be avoided by a simple bedside test. The maximum *negative* pressure generated at the bedside indicates how strong the inspiratory muscles are:

- Most adults can achieve -100 cmH_2O
- Severely weak patients achieve -20 cmH_2O
- Most patients can breathe spontaneously when PI max is > -30 cmH_2O *providing* their lungs are compliant.

Inspiratory muscle strength is measured by asking subjects and patients to perform a maximum inspiratory effort through a mouthpiece closed at one end. Marini describes the use of a one-way valve connected to the patient in order that expiration may occur but inspiration is occluded. With verbal encouragement a series of inspiratory gasps can be recorded and the most negative deflection measured. A suitable one-way valve can be found on ITU by connecting the patient to a CPAP valve via a catheter mount. In order to perform this test:

- The patient should be pre-oxygenated
- The patient should gasp for eight breaths or 20 seconds
- It is not mandatory for the patient to be awake.

If the patient is weak and has been able to make good efforts (i.e. the maximum strength recorded is likely to be accurate) during respiratory strength assessment, respiratory support should be continued.

If the patient is either strong or has a level of weakness which could be compatible with spontaneous breathing then the load applied to the muscles is crucial, and this should be assessed.

THE LOAD APPLIED TO THE RESPIRATORY MUSCLES

When the respiratory muscles contract, work is performed against the elastic recoil of the lung and chest wall and against the resistance offered to gas flowing along branching airways. As the load increases, weak patients are likely not to be able to breathe unassisted. Dynamic compliance (Cdyn) measures both elastic and flow-resistive components of load and can be assessed by the bedside during ventilated breaths. For this measurement to be accurate:

- The patient must receive constant flow ventilation
- The patient must be relaxed *or*
- a relaxed breath is selected during ventilated and spontaneous breathing.

Cdyn is calculated from the equation Cdyn = tidal volume/(peak airway pressure – PEEP).

WEANING MODES

Considerable debate has centred on whether synchronized intermittent mandatory ventilation (SIMV) enhances weaning. Few controlled prospective studies are available, and those that have been reported fail to support the initial hope that SIMV would enable patients to be weaned over a shorter time period. While the form of ventilation itself is unlikely to effect the major determinants of ventilation (drive, respiratory muscle strength and the applied load), work performed to initiate a breath can add a considerable load, especially when the respiratory muscles are compromised.

Pressure support ventilation (PSV) has some advantages when partial support of spontaneously breathing patients is required. Unlike SIMV, PSV has no mandatory minute ventilation set by the clinician; rather, each breath is initiated by the patient, and the timing and duration of each breath is also set by the patient, not the clinician. PSV has many advantages but is dependent on the patient's breathing effort. Furthermore, a preset tidal volume is not ensured, and Vt will change if lung compliance alters.

The technique used to wean patients from mechanical support has been the subject of great interest in order to select the best method used to wean. Recently, PSV, SIMV or a t-piece have been prospectively compared to wean 109 patients according to a defined protocol. The patients were randomly allocated into the three modes of ventilation and studied over a 21-day period. Many of the patients were unlikely to wean (f/Vt >80), and all the patients adhered to a rigorously controlled protocol-driven assessment. Patients ventilated with PSV were more likely to be weaned. PSV-ventilated patients were also less likely to remain on ventilation, weaning duration was shorter, and the total length of time on ITU was reduced. This contrasts with the findings in patients who were weaned over a shorter period of time (6 days). In this study, daily t-piece breathing was associated with less time spent on mechanical support. On the basis of this current research, patients who are likely to wean within a week would appear to be better breathing on a t-piece circuit whereas patients who wean over a number of weeks may be more effectively weaned with PSV.

BIBLIOGRAPHY

Brochard L, Rauss A, Benito S et al. Comparison of three methods of gradual withdrawal from ventilatory support during weaning from mechanical ventilation. American Journal of Respiratory and Critical Care Medicine 1994; 150: 896–903

Esteban A, Frutos F, Tobin M J et al. A comparison of four methods of weaning patients from mechanical ventilation. Spanish Lung Failure Collaborative Group. New England Journal of Medicine 1995; 332; 345–350

Marini J J, Smith T C, Lamb V. Estimation of inspiratory muscle strength in mechanically ventilated patients: measurement of maximum inspiratory pressure. Journal of Critical Care 1988; 1: 32–38

Yang K L, Tobin M J. A prospective study of indexes predicting the outcome of trials of weaning from mechanical ventilation. New England Journal of Medicine 1991; 324: 1445–1450

34

ASSESSMENT AND SCORING

J. F. Bion

AUDIT

J. F. Bion

34

DEFINITION

'Anaesthetic audit' means setting standards of anaesthetic practice, monitoring the application of those standards, measuring the process and outcome of care, identifying strengths and deficiencies, and implementing changes which improve clinical practice.

CURRENT STRUCTURES

National

The Royal College of Anaesthetists undertakes formal examination of anaesthetists in training and inspects hospitals for post-graduate training and accreditation. College tutors exercise an important pastoral role for the trainees.

The Association of Anaesthetists of Great Britain & Ireland together with the Royal College sets standards relating to the structure of anaesthetic departments and the work which they perform. They also provide educational activities.

The National Confidential Enquiry into Perioperative Deaths is an independent intercollegiate professional body which has had a major impact on the assessment of quality of care provided by anaesthetists and surgeons.

Local

Departments and divisions of anaesthesia organize morbidity and mortality meetings. Some are better structured, attended and funded than others. Joint meetings with surgeons and other disciplines should be held at regular intervals.

Audit committees may provide funding for specific projects, but the intention is that much of this will eventually be derived from quality assurance components of contracting.

HISTORY

Hospital quality assurance

1916: Dr Ernest Codman of the Massachusetts General Hospital.

1919: Survey of American hospitals by the American College of Surgeons.

1924: American College of Surgeons published five minimum standards.

1930: Committee on Maternal Morbidity and Mortality.

1952: The Confidential Enquiry into Maternal Deaths published triennially.

Anaesthesia

1949: Association of Anaesthetists commissioned a number of studies of mortality related to anaesthesia. The first collected 1000 voluntary reports of deaths occurring over 5.5 years, and stated that 'in the great majority of reports there were departures from ideal practice'.

1954: Beecher & Todd (1954) in the USA, surveyed prospectively nearly 600 000 anaesthetics over a 5-year period. They examined all deaths occurring in surgical patients, and separated anaesthetic causes of mortality from those attributable to surgery. Anaesthesia could be identified as a factor contributing to death in 1:1560 procedures, and causative in 1:2680.

1961: Dripps et al (1961) identified poor physical health as a risk factor.

1964: Dinnick reviewed 600 deaths. There was no denominator information. He demonstrated the presence of important surgical factors in high-risk patients whose deaths had been attributed to anaesthesia.

1977: The Association of Anaesthetists and Nuffield Provincial Hospitals Trust initiated a study of anaesthetic deaths in Britain. Surgical collaboration was not obtained, so it is difficult to interpret the results. Published in 1982 by Lunn & Mushin.

1987: Confidential Enquiry into Perioperative Deaths (CEPOD) was published in conjunction with Association of Surgeons. Factors were examined contributing to deaths within the first 30 days following surgery in the hospitals of three Regional Health Authorities. Ten recommendations concerning quality assurance, accountability, clinical decision-making and organizational issues were made that had direct relevance to the standards of practice of anaesthetists and surgeons.

1988: The College of Anaesthetists established an audit committee, which was subsequently expanded to become the Quality of Practice Committee. The first report provides guidance on audit to anaesthetic departments.

1990: The National Confidential Enquiry into Perioperative Deaths (NCEPOD 1990) produced its first report. The NCEPOD initiative was presented as an exemplar in the Government document entitled 'The Quality of Medical Care'.

STRUCTURE, PROCESS AND OUTCOME IN ANAESTHESIA

Structure

The structure of anaesthetic services refers to the type of clinical activities provided and their administration, the number of senior and junior medical staff, their organization and work patterns, the level of funding, postoperative-care units, anaesthetic equipment, secretarial and clerical support, and postgraduate and undergraduate education.

Poor organization has been identified as an important factor contributing to anaesthesia-related critical incidents and morbidity. The director of anaesthetic services may need to delegate specific administrative responsibilities, and the trainees' on-call rota should be prepared by the administrative senior registrar at least 2 weeks in advance. Fifty per cent of clinical time should be educational and supervised, and logbooks should be used to record this as well as case mix and anaesthetic practice.

Process

Standards of anaesthetic care:

- Preoperative visiting and risk assessment
- Supervision and assistance
- Anaesthetic technique
- Monitoring
- Management of emergencies
- Critical incidents
- Postoperative care.

The value of the preoperative visit is well known, but not always well practised. Clear protocols should be available (e.g. as wall posters) for managing uncommon life-threatening emergencies (failed intubation, cardiac arrest, malignant hyperthermia), and for equipment checks as part of a comprehensive system of risk minimization and critical-incident avoidance.

Around 11% of critical incidents may be attributed to incomplete preoperative assessment; 82% of preventable incidents have human error as a contributory cause, and only 14% are caused by equipment failure. Most critical incidents (42%) occur during the middle of anaesthesia, and 26% at induction. Patients graded ASA III–V have an increased risk of a critical incident resulting in a negative outcome. Trainees should be given explicit instructions about when to inform senior staff or seek assistance, and again the ASA grading could be used to audit this.

The anaesthetic operating department assistant (ODA) or nurse is one of the most important facilitators of quality of anaesthetic care in the UK, and no anaesthetist should be expected to provide a service without the ODA's assistance. Standards for monitoring should be known, agreed, and applied, but will not compensate for the ignorant, uncaring or absent practitioner.

Routine postoperative visiting of all patients may not be possible, but higher risk patients (e.g. ASA III–V) should be seen. Anaesthetic responsibilities are said to end with the return of the patient to the ward, a potentially short-sighted view when anaesthetic expertise in applied physiology and analgesia may contribute substantially to the quality of postoperative care, the relief of pain, and the image of the speciality. Postoperative assessment is especially important for day-case surgery.

Outcome

It is easier to identify the presence or absence of harm from anaesthesia than it is to attribute a beneficial outcome. This complicates outcome audit. Death is also an uncommon outcome, and is of limited value as the sole marker of quality of care because it identifies only the more gross departures from proper practice. The NCEPOD report (NCEPOD 1990) identified anaesthesia as wholly responsible for a fatal outcome in three of half a million procedures. Routine anaesthetic outcome audit should be based on morbidity and critical-incident monitoring, patient satisfaction, and cost–benefit analyses. Results should be related to predicted risk.

Complications are adverse events arising in part from pre-existing disease which, when combined with human error or equipment failure can result in major morbidity. They range from transient bradycardia in a patient receiving beta-blocking drugs, to failed intubation with cerebral damage. Many complications occur in the first 24 h postoperatively, and are avoidable. Renal impairment, thromboembolism, or myocardial infarction are important end-points which should be recorded. Anaesthetists are well placed to detect limited physiological reserve and prevent associated morbidity. For example, the lower mortality rates associated with immediate rather than delayed operative fracture fixation may be due to earlier anaesthetic involvement and hence better resuscitation.

Secker-Walker (1991) suggests a four-point scale for grading the severity of complications:

1 A transient complication not requiring treatment
2 A potentially harmful event successfully remedied
3 An event causing minor morbidity
4 An event causing serious harm to the patient.

Costs may be measured as an outcome, and should be related not only to throughput, but to case mix and postoperative morbidity. Anaesthetic costs are modest compared with those relating to surgery, and the major item is the salary component. Disputes about specific drugs should be resolved by consensus.

DATA COLLECTION

Anaesthetists are particularly adept at data collection and processing, but audit initiatives will fail if the volume of additional information required exceeds the immediate benefit to be gained from it. A minimum dataset should be agreed by the members of the department. Data collection should be contemporaneous with data generation, should not result in a substantial increase in work, and must not detract from patient care. It is possible in the future that hand-held computers will facilitate preoperative risk assessment and perioperative data collection, but at present more simple measures are required. ASA grading remains a simple method for stratifying patients as low-risk or high-risk, and therefore facilitates identifying unexpected outcomes.

Identifying those outcomes remains the responsibility of the anaesthetist. Anaesthetic records of patients graded ASA III–IV, all emergency cases, and all critical incidents, should be presented for monthly review. Carbon-copy anaesthetic records can be stored and processed at leisure by departmental secretaries. Smart cards and networked computing with keyboards at the anaesthetic machine may be the methods for the future.

CLOSING THE LOOP

The data which have been collected must be useful. They should have an impact on standards and quality of training and medical care. The trainees' log book should be inspected by the College Tutor at regular intervals. Records should be maintained of morbidity and mortality meetings and the conclusions reached. Analysis of audit data may form the basis for specific research projects for junior staff, for whom research time should be made available. When possible, hard end-points should be used to allow comparison. Failure to meet agreed standards must be addressed by the director of anaesthetic services. Time must be set aside for joint meetings, so that a consensus can be reached.

BIBLIOGRAPHY

Association of Anaesthetists of Great Britain & Ireland. Recommendations for standards of monitoring during anaesthesia and recovery. London, 1988

Beecher H K, Todd D P. A study of the deaths associated with anaesthesia and surgery. Annals of Surgery 1954; 140: 2–34

Cooper J B, Newbower R S, Kitz R J. An analysis of major errors and equipment failures in anaesthesia management: considerations for prevention and detection. Anesthesiology 1984; 60: 34–42

Cooper J B, Newbower R S, Long C D, McPeek B. Preventable anaesthetic mishaps: a study of human factors. Anesthesiology 1978; 49: 399–406

Dripps R D, Lamont A, Eckenhoff J E. The role of anaesthesia in surgical mortality. Journal of the American Medical Association 1961; 178: 261

Flanagan J C. The critical incident technique. Psychology Bulletin 1954; 51: 327–358

NCEPOD. National Confidential Enquiry into Perioperative Deaths Report 1989. NCEPOD, London, 1990 (and subsequent years 1990, 1991/1992)

Riddington D W, Bion J F. Audit in anaesthesia. In: Frostick et al (eds) Medical audit. Rationale and practicalities. Cambridge University Press, Cambridge, 1993

Secker-Walker J. Audit in anaesthesia. In: Kaufman L (ed) Anaesthesia review. Churchill Livingstone, Edinburgh, 1991, vol 8

Working Party. Report on Pain after Surgery. The Royal College of Surgeons of England and The College of Anaesthetists, London, 1990

CARDIOPULMONARY RESUSCITATION

J. M. Elliot

34

MECHANISMS OF CARDIORESPIRATORY ARREST

Cardiorespiratory arrest results from either primary cardiac or respiratory arrest.

Cardiac arrest may be:

- *Primary* – due to dysrhythmia or severe myocardial failure
- Secondary – due to hypoxaemia (respiratory arrest), electrolyte imbalance, etc.

There are three fundamental 'rhythms' of cardiac arrest:

- Ventricular fibrillation (VF), or pulseless ventricular tachycardia (VT)
- Asystole, or extreme bradycardia
- Electromechanical dissociation (EMD).

FACTORS AFFECTING SURVIVAL

Survival is most likely when:

- The rhythm is VF or VT
- The arrest is witnessed
- Basic life support is started immediately
- Defibrillation and advanced life support are given early.

BASIC LIFE SUPPORT

All medical, nursing and other hospital staff, as well as the general public, should be able to perform basic life support (BLS). An assessment algorithm is shown in Figure 1.

Important points:

- Check that there is no danger to yourself or to the casualty before starting resuscitation.

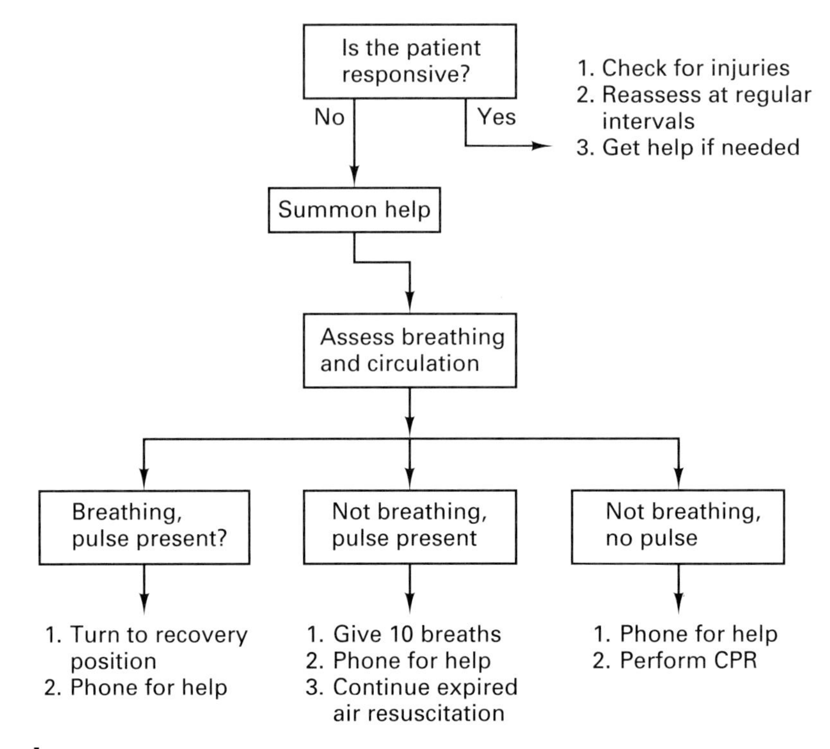

Figure 1
Basic assessment algorithm. (Adapted from the 1992 Resuscitation Council Guidelines.)

- If the casualty is unresponsive, first shout for help, then check airway, breathing and circulation.
- Airway foreign bodies may be removed under direct vision, or by finger sweeps, back blows or the Heimlich manoeuvre.
- If breathing and pulse are absent, get help *before* starting cardiopulmonary resuscitation (CPR). Survival is very unlikely without advanced life support and defibrillation.
- The ratio of chest compressions to ventilation should be 15:2 with one rescuer, and 5:1 with two rescuers.
- Ventilation can be performed either mouth to mouth or by using airway adjuncts. The original bag-and-mask equipment has been superseded by the pocket mask in many hospitals.
- Be aware of the possibility of neck trauma before considering extending the neck in order to open the airway.
- Lifting the jaw anteriorly (jaw thrust) may be required to open the airway.
- The technique of expired air resuscitation and external cardiac compression cannot be learnt from a book but only from a properly supervised training session.

ADVANCED LIFE SUPPORT

All medical staff and appropriate senior

nursing staff should be capable of performing advanced life support (ALS). The three principal algorithms are shown in Figures 2–4. Wall charts are available depicting all of these. All persons who may be called upon to perform ALS should be familiar with these algorithms. Regular refresher courses are recommended.

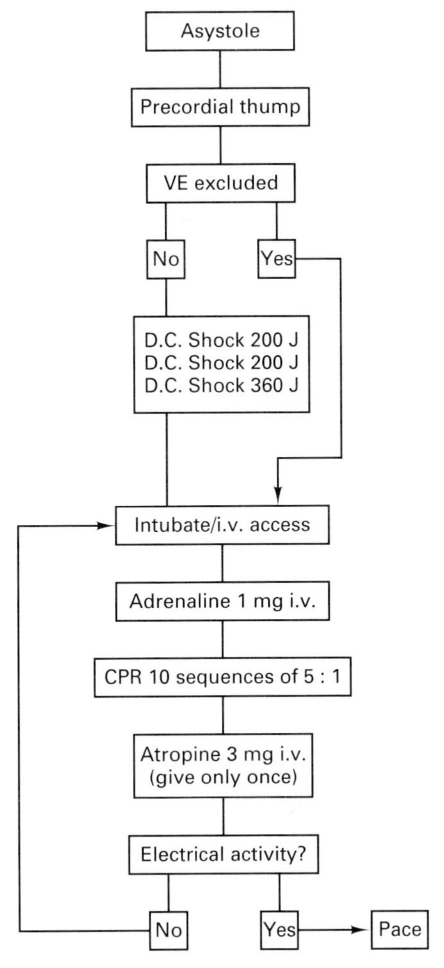

Notes:
1. Continue CPR between shocks if defibrillator slow charging or manual
2. If no i.v. access consider adrenaline (2 mg) via tracheal tube
3. Give adrenaline (1 mg) during each loop; give atropine only in first loop
4. After 3 loops consider adrenaline (5 mg i.v.); calcium; alkalinizing agent

Figure 2
Cardiac arrest algorithm for asystole. (Adapted from the Resuscitation Council Guidelines 1992.)

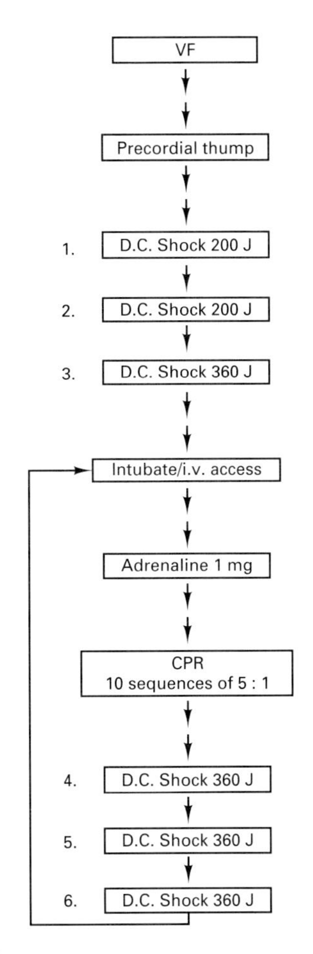

Notes:
1. Continue CPR between shocks if defibrillator is slow charging or manual
2. The interval between D.C. Shocks 3 and 4 should not be more than 2 min
3. Give adrenaline (1 mg i.v.) during each loop
4. If no i.v. access consider adrenaline (2 mg) via tracheal tube
5. After 3 loops consider alkalinizing agent, antiarrythmic (e.g. bretylium, amiodarone)
6. Consider change of paddle position

Figure 3
Cardiac arrest algorithm for VF. (Adapted from the Resuscitation Council Guidelines 1992.)

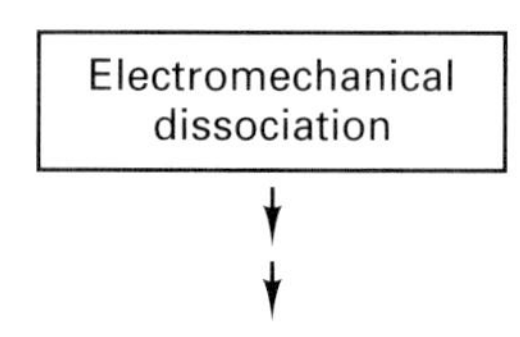

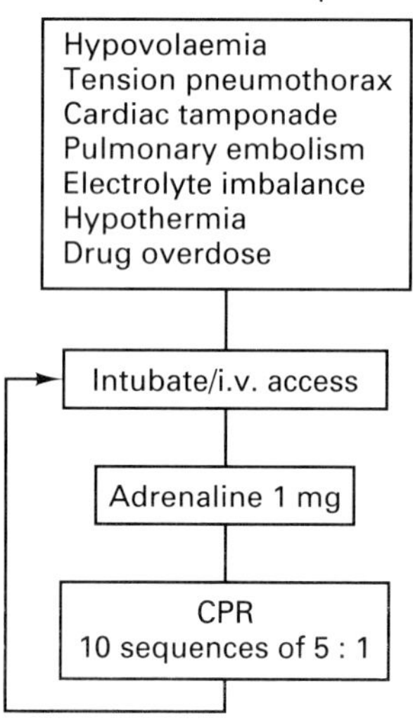

Notes:
1. If no i.v. access, consider adrenaline (2 mg) via tracheal tube
2. After 3 loops consider:
   - Adrenaline (5 mg i.v.)
   - Calcium chloride
   - Alkalinizing agents
   - Pressor agents

Figure 4
Cardiac arrest algorithm for EMD. (Adapted from the Resuscitation Council Guidelines 1992.)

Important points:
- A precordial thump may convert VF or VT to sinus rhythm, or stimulate a contraction in asystole. It is recommended in witnessed arrest situations.
- Defibrillation is the only cure for VF or VT, but must be given as soon as possible. Give the first three shocks without pausing for BLS in between shocks, if this can be done within 30–45 s.
- VF may masquerade as asystole on the ECG, so check leads, connections and gain. If in any doubt, defibrillate three times. (Automatic defibrillators may not allow this.)
- Adrenaline is given to improve cerebral and coronary blood flow, not to terminate VF or asystole.
- Sodium bicarbonate is no longer recommended at an early stage, as it may worsen intracellular acidosis. Up to 50 mmol intravenously may be given for severe metabolic acidosis later in the process of resuscitation, preferably guided by arterial blood gases.
- EMD is usually secondary, and CPR is unlikely to be successful unless the cause is treated.
- In EMD, calcium may be useful in hypocalcaemia, hyperkalaemia, or after use of calcium channel blockers.
- Bretylium, lignocaine or amiodarone may be considered in refractory VF. CPR must be continued for a further 20–30 min if bretylium is given, as its effect is delayed.
- Drugs are best given through a central line. Central line insertion during CPR is hazardous if done by the inexperienced. If intravenous access is not possible, the endotracheal route is an alternative for adrenaline, atropine and lignocaine, using 2–3 times the intravenous dose.

POSTRESUSCITATION CARE

The patient should be nursed in an ITU or HDU following successful resuscitation. The following points should be considered.

History:
- Previous medical history
- Events preceding the arrest
- Cause of the arrest.

Examination:
- Respiratory
  - Endotracheal tube position
  - Pneumothorax
  - Fractured ribs or sternum.
- Cardiovascular
  - Pulse
  - BP
  - Adequacy of perfusion
  - Jugular venous pressure
  - Urine output.
- Neurological
  - Glasgow Coma Score
  - Pupil size and reactivity
  - Neurological deficit.

Investigations:
- Arterial blood gases
- Chest X-ray

- 12-lead ECG
- Urea and electrolytes
- Consider invasive haemodynamic monitoring.

Treatment:
- Oxygen, according to arterial blood gases
- Continued ventilation
- Analgesia
- Antiarrhythmics
- Inotropes and/or vasodilators
- Specific organ system support, e.g. renal support.

PAEDIATRIC RESUSCITATION

The principles of CPR in children are very similar to those in adults, but the following differences apply.

Causes of arrest:
- Asystole or severe bradycardia are the commonest causes. They may be secondary to hypoxaemia or circulatory failure, and may be cured by BLS and oxygenation.
- Cardiac arrest may be due to sudden infant death syndrome, airway obstruction (foreign bodies, epiglottitis or croup), near-drowning, asthma, trauma or severe infections.

Airway and ventilation:
- Mouth to nose-and-mouth ventilation may be needed (remember the smaller tidal volumes required).
- The Heimlich manoeuvre, finger sweeps, and incisional cricothyrotomy are contraindicated in younger children. Back blows, chest thrusts and needle cricothyrotomy are alternatives.
- Endotracheal tube sizes (Table 1):
  Internal diameter = (4 + Age/4)
  Length = (12 + Age/2)
  Alternatively, choose the same diameter as the child's little finger or nostril.
- Uncuffed tracheal tubes should be used in children. Over the age of about 12 years, cuffed tubes may be used, depending upon the size and maturity of the child.

External cardiac massage
The compression rate should be 100–120 in infants, and 80–100 in older children. Remember to use less force.

Defibrillation
The initial charge is 2 J kg^{-1}, increasing to 4 J kg^{-1} if necessary.

Table 1.
Paediatric tracheal tube sizes

Age (years)	Approximate Weight (kg)	Tracheal tube: Internal diameter (mm)	Tracheal tube: Length (cm)
3 months	5	3.0–3.5	10
6 months	6–7	3.5	12
9 months	8–9	4.0	12
1	10	4.0–4.5	13
2	12	4.5–5.0	14
3	14	5.0	14
4	16	5.5	15
5	18	5.5	15
6	20	6.0	16
8	25	6.5	17
10	30	7.0	18
12*	40	7.0–7.5	18–20

*Cuffed tubes may be used in children over the age of about 12 years.

Drug doses
In children, drugs may be given by either the intravenous or the intraosseous routes.

- Adrenaline: 0.1 ml kg^{-1} of 1:10 000 adrenaline
- Atropine: 0.02 mg kg^{-1} (minimum 0.1 mg, maximum 0.6 mg)
- Calcium: 0.1 ml kg^{-1} of 10% calcium chloride
- Lignocaine: 0.1 ml kg^{-1} of 1% lignocaine
- Sodium bicarbonate: 1 mmol kg^{-1}.

BIBLIOGRAPHY

Advanced Life Support Group. Advanced paediatric life support – the practical approach. BMJ, London, 1993

Baskett P J F. Advances in cardiopulmonary resuscitation. British Journal of Anaesthesia 1992; 69: 182–193

Guidelines for advanced life support. A statement by the Advanced Life Support Working Party of the European Resuscitation Council. Resuscitation 1992; 24: 111–121

Guidelines for basic life support. A statement by the Basic Life Support Working Party of the European Resuscitation Council. Resuscitation 1992; 24: 103–110

Handley A J (ed) Advanced life support manual. Resuscitation Council (UK), 1992

34

PREOPERATIVE ASSESSMENT OF CARDIOVASCULAR RISK IN NONCARDIAC SURGERY

J. M. Hull and J. F. Bion

Perioperative cardiac morbidity (PCM) is a major cause of death following anaesthesia and surgery. It is generally defined as the occurrence of myocardial infarction, unstable angina, congestive heart failure (CHF), serious dysrhythmia or cardiac death during the intraoperative or postoperative period. Identification of populations at risk and preoperative assessment of their disease using routine and nonroutine tests is the basis of anaesthetic management.

Over the last 38 years, more than 100 outcome studies have examined perioperative cardiac morbidity. They differ in study design, method and analysis, making data interpretation difficult. The incidence of PCM may also vary according to the quality of the anaesthetic and surgical care, and this may explain some of the conflicting results of clinical studies. Most studies have focused on preoperative historical predictors. Predictors of PCM have been both supported and refuted by different studies. Data from recent prospective studies, using more sensitive investigative tools, suggest that outcome has improved and that intensive preoperative optimization (invasive monitoring, drug therapy, ITU or HDU care) may reduce PCM. However, the efficacy and cost-effectiveness of specialized preoperative investigation remains controversial.

PREOPERATIVE ASSESSMENT FOR CARDIOVASCULAR DISEASE

Routine:
- Clinical history
- Physical examination
- Laboratory tests
- Chest X-ray
- 12-lead ECG.

Nonroutine:
- Exercise stress testing
- Ambulatory ECG
- Echocardiography – assessment of regional wall motion, wall thickening, global ventricular function, valvular function, coronary anatomy and blood flow
- Nuclear imaging – assessment of myocardial perfusion, infarction, wall motion and ventricular function
- Cardiac catheterization
- Magnetic resonance imaging – ventricular function assessment.

HISTORICAL PREDICTORS

Age

Increasing chronological age does not appear to affect resting ejection fraction, left ventricular volume or regional wall motion, but is associated with a reduction in cardiac response to stress. As a predictor of PCM, age has been proposed (38% incidence of ischaemia, myocardial infarction or cardiac death in patients >70 years old versus 7% in those aged 40–49 years) and refuted. It is likely that age is only a predictor in the presence of other factors.

Previous myocardial infarction

These patients have a greater risk of perioperative infarction (5–8%) with an associated high mortality (36–70%). The more recent the infarction, the greater the risk. Recent studies indicate a lower risk with improved preoperative care (Table 1).

Angina

Angina is usually associated with angiographically significant (>70% stenosis) coronary

Table 1.
Incidence of reinfarction

Time of myocardial infarction (months)	**Without intensive preoperative optimization** (%)	**With intensive preoperative optimization** (%)
Within 3	>30	5.7
3–6	15	2.3 (4–6 months)
>6	6	–

artery disease (CAD). Most (75%) ischaemic episodes are painless ('silent ischaemia'), and 20–30% of postinfarct patients have silent ischaemia. Most perioperative ischaemia is silent and is more common during the first two postoperative days. Stable angina increases the risk of myocardial infarction or sudden death in CAD patients and has recently been found to be a predictor of PCM after noncardiac surgery. Unstable and variant (Prinzmetal) angina have not been adequately studied.

Congestive heart failure

CHF is associated with a poor prognosis in CAD patients and is a predictor of cardiac mortality after acute myocardial infarction. Although preoperative CHF is strongly predictive of PCM, the predictive value of specific signs is controversial. An ejection fraction of <40% (as measured by radionuclear imaging or ventriculography) is predictive of perioperative infarction, reinfarction and ventricular dysfunction.

Hypertension

Hypertension is a known risk factor for ischaemic heart disease, CHF and stroke. Risk is increased in the presence of other risk factors. Perioperative hypertension has not been found to predict PCM but may predict potentially reversible intermediates of cardiac outcome (e.g. intraoperative ischaemia). Withdrawal of antihypertensive drugs is associated with increased perioperative blood pressure lability.

Diabetes mellitus

Diabetics (especially those with autonomic neuropathy) are at higher risk of myocardial infarction (the leading cause of death in diabetics), myocardial ischaemia (which tends to be silent) and cardiomyopathy. Recently, diabetes has been shown to be a predictor of PCM in vascular and nonvascular surgery patients. Autonomic neuropathy confers greater risk of intraoperative blood pressure instability. The relative risks of type I and type II diabetes, and the effects of perioperative glucose control are unknown.

Dysrhythmias

Frequent preoperative premature ventricular beats or nonsinus rhythms are independent predictors of PCM. Bifascicular block, right bundle branch block and left anterior hemiblock appear not to increase the risk of PCM unless associated with more serious cardiac conditions.

Peripheral vascular disease

Significant coronary artery stenosis is present in 14–78% of patients with PVD, regardless of their CAD symptoms. Only 8% of patients with PVD have normal coronary angiograms. PVD patients undergoing vascular surgery have a high risk of PCM. Myocardial infarction occurs in 15% and accounts for 50% of perioperative mortality. For non-vascular surgery the risks are unknown.

Valvular heart disease

Aortic stenosis is probably a risk factor for PCM. The risk from other significant valvular lesions is difficult to assess, as they are usually associated with other cardiac abnormalities.

Cholesterol

Although there is a direct relationship between serum cholesterol and cardiovascular mortality, the risk of PCM is unknown.

Cigarette smoking

Smokers are at increased risk of myocardial infarction, but smoking has not been found to be a risk factor for PCM.

Previous coronary artery bypass graft surgery

CAD patients without a coronary artery bypass graft (CABG), undergoing noncardiac surgery, have a higher mortality than those who have had CABG surgery (1.1–6% versus 0–1.2%).

Percutaneous angioplasty

Following percutaneous angioplasty, coronary artery disease patients have a low risk of PCM.

Cardiovascular therapy

The preoperative withdrawal of nitrates, beta blockers and calcium-channel blockers is associated with a higher risk of perioperative ischaemia, dysrhythmia, myocardial infarction and cardiac death.

Risk indices

Several multivariate risk indices have been described. No consistently accurate and generally applicable risk index has been developed.

DIAGNOSTIC TESTS

Biochemical data

Preoperative laboratory data are usually normal in CAD patients.

12-lead ECG
ECG abnormalities are seen in 40–70% of CAD patients:

- ST–T wave changes 65–90%
- LVH signs 10–20%
- Q waves 0.5–8%.

PCM is often associated with preoperative ST–T wave ischaemia and intraventricular conduction defects, but the predictive value of these changes is not known.

Chest X-ray
In over 70% of CAD patients, cardiomegaly is associated with a low ejection fraction (<40%) and may predict PCM.

Exercise stress testing
This is highly predictive of subsequent cardiac events in CAD patients with ST abnormalities. It is more sensitive than clinical history or 12-lead ECG, but is an unproven predictor of PCM.

Ambulatory ECG monitoring
Successful in detecting silent myocardial ischaemia. Of patients with, or at-risk of, CAD, 18–40% have frequent ischaemic episodes (>75% are 'silent'). Preoperative ischaemia may predict PCM.

Precordial echocardiography
This is predictive of short- and long-term outcome after acute myocardial infarction, but the predictive value in the perioperative period is unknown. Since preoperative ventricular dysfunction or segmental wall motion abnormalities predict PCM, it is likely that echocardiography is also a predictor of PCM.

Transoesophageal echocardiography
Its value in noncardiac surgical patients has not been evaluated.

Radionuclear imaging
Gated-pool-determined ejection fraction is an independent predictor of PCM. Vascular surgery patients with a low ejection fraction (<35%) had a 75–85% incidence of perioperative myocardial infarction. Patients with an ejection fraction >35% had an infarction incidence of 19–20%. Dipyridamole/thallium imaging for myocardial perfusion defects may enable additional risk stratification within high-risk groups.

Magnetic resonance imaging
The perioperative predictive value of this technique in CAD patients has not been established.

Cardiac catheterization
This is the 'gold standard' for assessing ventricular function and coronary circulation. Ventricular function indices (ejection fraction, wall-motion abnormalities, end-diastolic volume, end-diastolic pressure) and significant left main vessel or multivessel disease are predictors of short- and long-term outcome in CABG patients. Cardiac catheterization is useful in determining which patients require CABG surgery before noncardiac surgery. It may be a predictor of PCM, though this has not been confirmed in noncardiac surgery patients.

SUMMARY

Recent myocardial infarction, current CHF and low ejection fraction are strong predictors of PCM. Preoperative dysrhythmias, myocardial ischaemia, aortic stenosis, peripheral vascular disease and diabetes are likely predictors of increased risk of perioperative cardiac morbidity.

BIBLIOGRAPHY

Coriat P, Reiz S. Cardiac outcome after non-cardiac surgery in patients with coronary artery disease. Baillière's Clinical Anaesthesiology 1992; 6(3): 491–513
Fleisher L A. Perioperative assessment of the patient with cardiovascular disease. Current Opinion in Anaesthesiology 1992; 5: 27–33
Mangano D T. Pre-operative assessment of the patient with cardiac disease. Baillière's Clinical Anaesthesiology 1989; 3(1): 47–102
Mangano D T. Perioperative cardiac morbidity. Anesthesiology 1990; 72: 153–184

CROSS REFERENCES

Diabetes mellitus (IDDM)
Patient Conditions 2: 42
Diabetes mellitus (NIDDM)
Patient Conditions 2: 44
Coronary artery disease
Patient Conditions 4: 107
Hypertension
Patient Conditions 4: 111
The elderly patient
Patient Conditions 11: 252

DIAGNOSIS OF BRAIN DEATH

P. D. Curry and J. F. Bion

The concept of brain death was first introduced by the French in 1959, and formally structured by Harvard Medical School in 1968. Subsequent memoranda have been produced by the Conference of Medical Royal Colleges in the UK which form the basis for guidelines published by the Health Department. The latest of these was in 1983. The diagnosis of brainstem death has only appeared as a clinical phenomenon because of the introduction of organ-system support and intensive care, in particular mechanical ventilation of apnoeic patients. Structured guidelines for diagnosis are required because of the emotional content and ethical implications of withdrawing life-support. The development of organ harvesting for transplantation adds to the importance of common criteria for the diagnosis of brainstem death. There is considerable variation in international practice in the diagnosis of brain death.

Recently, proposals have been made for the elective ('interventional') ventilation of patients with intracranial lesions who are expected to become brainstem dead in order to increase the supply of donors. This has important ethical and resource implications which require resolution.

Brainstem death should be distinguished from the persistent vegetative state in which there is preservation of brainstem function but irrecoverable damage to the cerebral cortex. The preservation of vegetative functions excludes such patients from inclusion as organ donors, but persistent coma allows them to be considered for withdrawal from life-support after an extended period of treatment and review. The law courts may be involved in such decisions.

UK CRITERIA FOR DIAGNOSING BRAINSTEM DEATH

There are three interdependent steps:

- Preconditions
- Exclusions
- Clinical tests.

All are essential.

Preconditions

The patient must be apnoeic, comatose, ventilator dependent and must have irreversible structural brain damage demonstrated, with a defined cause.

Exclusions

All factors which may produce actual or apparent depression of brain function must be excluded, in particular:

- Drugs – sedatives, hypnotics, analgesics, muscle relaxants
- Hypothermia – temperature less than 35°C
- Metabolic disorder – electrolytes, sugar and pH.

Drugs include alcohol and other intoxicating substances. Muscle relaxants, although not depressing brain function, produce apnoea and apparent unresponsiveness, and hence variable failure of the tests of brainstem function. Residual neuromuscular blockade should be excluded with a nerve stimulator. Particular care should be taken in patients with impaired renal or hepatic function in whom drug or metabolite accumulation may occur.

Tests:

- *The pupils are fixed in diameter and do not respond to sharp changes in the intensity of incident light.* The pupils must not respond either directly or consensually when a bright light is shone directly at them.
- *There is no corneal reflex.* There should be no response, usually blinking, to direct stimulation of the cornea.
- *The vestibulo-ocular reflexes are absent.* No eye movement occurs during or following the slow injection of 20 ml of ice-cold water into each external auditory meatus in turn,

clear access to the tympanic membrane having been established by direct inspection.

- *No motor responses within the cranial nerve distribution can be elicited by adequate stimulation of any somatic area.* This requires no grimacing in response to either cranial or peripheral stimulation of pain. Local reflex arcs may permit the appearance of spinal reflexes in response to pain, and these must be distinguished from responses mediated through the higher centres. Witnesses may need to be reassured that such reflexes do not represent brainstem function.
- *There is no gag reflex or reflex response to bronchial stimulation by a suction catheter passed down the trachea.*
- *Apnoea, despite hypercarbic oxygenation.* No respiratory movements occur when the patient is disconnected from the mechanical ventilator for long enough to ensure that the arterial carbon dioxide tension rises above the threshold for stimulation of respiration. This level is normally taken to be 6.65 kPa (50 mmHg), and must be confirmed by arterial blood gas analysis. Hypercarbia may take more than 20 min to reach this level, and if necessary initial ventilation with carbon dioxide in oxygen or the insertion of extra dead space may be required. Oxygen must be supplied through a tracheal catheter at a flow rate sufficient to maintain arterial saturations above 95%. Patients who normally have a hypoxic drive as a result of pre-existing chronic respiratory insufficiency should be expertly investigated.

The tests should be performed, either together or independently, by two practitioners with appropriate experience, one of whom should preferably have been qualified for more than 5 years. It is customary to perform the tests twice to exclude any possibility of observer error. The interval between tests is not stated, but may be used to give relatives time to cope with the initial shock of bereavement. The family should be given the opportunity to observe the performance of the second set of tests. At the conclusion of the second set of tests, the patient is diagnosed as dead. At this stage medical support may be withdrawn. Patients considered for organ donation will require expert physiological support until harvesting. The electroencephalography does not form part of the UK criteria because cortical activity can occur despite brainstem disruption, and an isoelectric electroencephalogram does not exclude cortical recovery following cerebral ischaemia.

SUMMARY

The formal diagnosis of brainstem death is not a legal requirement. Indeed, in intensive-care practice, when organ-system support is withdrawn it is usually from patients with irrecoverable multiple organ failure who have an intact brainstem. However, when complete brainstem destruction is present, the demonstration of the UK criteria is both expected and good practice. It is regarded as mandatory before organ harvesting can be considered. It is of great importance that the relatives are handled with tact and patience at what is a very painful time.

BIBLIOGRAPHY

BMA guidelines on treatment decisions for patients in persistent vegetative state. In: BMA Annual Report 1993. British Medical Association, London, 1993, Appendix VII

Health Departments of Great Britain & Northern Ireland. Cadaveric organs for transplantation: a code of practice including the diagnosis of brain death. HMSO, London, 1983

Pallas C. ABC of brain stem death. In: Articles from the British Medical Journal. British Medical Association, London, 1983

CROSS REFERENCES

Heart transplantation
Surgical Procedures 23: 460
Kidney transplantation
Surgical Procedures 23: 462
Liver transplantation
Surgical Procedures 23: 464
Lung and heart–lung transplantation
Surgical Procedures 23: 467
Management of the organ donor
Surgical Procedures 23: 470

PREOPERATIVE ASSESSMENT OF PULMONARY RISK

H. E. Brunner and J. F. Bion

The development of postoperative pulmonary complications is determined by the risk factors listed below. It is difficult to assess the influence which individual variables have on outcome, particularly with improvements in perioperative care, anaesthetic and surgical techniques, and the health of the population.

- The severity of pre-existing pulmonary disease
- The patient's general state of health
- The nature and extent of surgery
- The anaesthetic technique
- Prophylactic pre- and postoperative care.

Risk from pre-existing pulmonary disease should be determined by history and examination. Additional risk factors (surgical, anaesthetic, age, etc.) should then be considered.

PRE-EXISTING PULMONARY DISEASE

History

Dyspnoea

Undue awareness of breathing or awareness of difficulty in breathing. Graded using Roizen's classification (Table 1). Dyspnoea at rest (grade IV) with low $Pa\text{O}_2$ (<7 kPa, 55 mmHg) is associated with an increased likelihood of requiring assisted ventilation after abdominal surgery.

Determine the aetiology
- Asthma
- Chronic bronchitis
- Emphysema
- Fibrosing alveolitis.

Table 1.
Roizen's classification of dyspnoea

Grade 0	No dyspnoea while walking on the level at a normal pace
Grade I	'I am able to walk as far as I like provided I take my time'
Grade II	Specific limitation: 'I have to stop for a while after walking one or two blocks' (100–200 m)
Grade III	Dyspnoea on mild exertion: 'I have to stop while going from the kitchen to the bathroom'
Grade IV	Dyspnoea at rest

Hypoventilation due to failure of neural input or muscle weakness may not cause dyspnoea.

Cough

May indicate acute infection or, if productive of sputum on most days, suggests chronic bronchitis. Complications of excess sputum include airway plugging, atelectasis and respiratory infection. Loss of response to carbon dioxide and dependence on hypoxaemic respiratory drive need to be taken into account when planning the anaesthetic technique. Preoperative physiotherapy or bronchodilators may be required. Psychological preparation and training in breathing exercises can be invaluable. Sputum should be sent for culture.

Haemoptysis may be due to carcinoma, tuberculosis, pulmonary infarction or pneumonia, and must be distinguished from nasal bleeding.

Wheeze

May indicate asthma, chronic bronchitis, emphysema or acute foreign body inhalation. Asthma should be assessed by frequency of attacks, current drug therapy, and history of hospitalization and ventilation. Steroid treatment contributes to muscle weakness and immunoincompetence, both of which may result in prolonged ventilation and respiratory colonization. Bronchospasm may occur with laryngoscopy, tracheal intubation and anaesthetic drugs that release histamine, particularly when given rapidly intravenously.

Other factors

Cardiovascular disease, drugs, allergies, smoking.

34

Examination

Observation:

- Rate and pattern of breathing
- Ease of talking
- Use of accessory muscles
- Nicotine staining
- Clubbing (intrapulmonary shunting)
- Colour (cyanosis, anaemia)
- Deformity (kyphoscoliosis)
- Nutritional (obesity, malnutrition, muscle wasting).

Percussion:

- Pleural effusion
- Consolidation.

Auscultation:

- Reduced breath sounds
- Wheeze
- Bronchial breathing
- Pleural rub.

Investigation

Tests of pulmonary function will rarely be abnormal in the absence of physical symptoms and signs. They should be used to quantify risk.

Chest X-ray

Over 40 years of age, 4% of routine preoperative chest X-rays will detect an abnormality. The indications for a preoperative chest X-ray are:

- Symptoms or signs of active lung disease.
- Patients with possible lung metastases
- Symptoms and signs of heart disease
- Recent immigrants from countries where tuberculosis is endemic and who have not had a chest X-ray in the previous year.

Emphysematous bullae increase the risk of pneumothorax with positive pressure ventilation. Collapse, consolidation, pleural effusion or pneumothorax require preoperative treatment. Cardiomegaly and pulmonary oedema also indicate high risk and require specialist management. Unstable patients should be transferred to an ITU or HDU for appropriate monitoring in order to maximize physiological reserve before surgery.

Spirometry

Although peak flow, FEV_1 and vital capacity may be useful to follow the progression of pulmonary dysfunction, numerous studies have failed to demonstrate their predictive value for individual patient outcome. Even patients with an FEV_1 of <0.5 l may cope without requiring postoperative ventilation.

Maximum breathing capacity (MBC) calculated as $FEV_1 \times 35$ or Peak flow $\times$ 0.25, may be used to assess respiratory reserve. MBC greater than 60 l min^{-1} is normal, and less than 25 l min^{-1} indicates severe pulmonary impairment.

Arterial blood gas tensions

A P_aO_2 of less than 7.1 kPa or less than 70% of normal for age, in combination with dyspnoea at rest, has been shown to predict dependence on postoperative respiratory support in patients undergoing upper abdominal surgery. P_aO_2 may be used with a graph of isoshunt lines to assess pulmonary shunting and to estimate oxygen requirements.

However, P_aCO_2 is of little predictive value for postoperative ventilation, but may be useful for detection of those with a hypoxic respiratory drive in whom postoperative administration of oxygen will need careful monitoring. Detection of metabolic acidosis in the critically ill patient may indicate demands on respiratory work which cannot be met by spontaneous ventilation.

ADDITIONAL CONSIDERATIONS

Surgical factors

Thoracic and upper abdominal surgery, by interfering with diaphragmatic movement, cause a reduction in functional residual capacity (FRC) postoperatively. In addition, as FRC falls below closing capacity, dependent airways close leading to increased $\dot{V}/\dot{Q}$ mismatch, shunt and atelectasis. Pain and the supine position further contribute to a reduction in FRC.

Anaesthetic factors

Anaesthesia causes a reduction in FRC and lung volume, leading to reduced compliance and increased shunting. Gas trapping of oxygen and nitrous oxide, which are soluble, may lead to alveolar collapse. General anaesthesia in excess of 2 h increases risk of atelectasis and infection. The incidence of pneumonia in one study was 40% in patients following thoracic or abdominal surgery lasting >4 h (8% when <2 h).

Anaesthesia and surgery are associated with a reduced humoral immune response, impaired neutrophil chemotaxis and phagocytosis, and depressed mucociliary transport.

Age

Muscle weakness, a stiff rib cage, and loss of elastic recoil in the elderly results in airway closure at higher lung volumes. After approximately 45 years of age closing capacity exceeds FRC when lying supine, which may contribute to risk of atelectasis. The incidence of pneumonia in one study was 18% over 30 years compared with 9% under 30 years, following thoracic or abdominal surgery.

Nutritional state

Obesity reduces chest compliance and FRC, and increases closing capacity. These are worsened by supine or head-down position. Postoperatively, the semierect position is preferred in order to limit hypoxaemia. Epidural analgesia reduces pulmonary complications, but the benefit is less in the very obese patient. In those heavier than 115 kg, the incidence of postoperative pneumonia was reported to be doubled. Systemic illness, chronic disease and steroids cause muscle weakness which may increase risk of pulmonary complications. Low serum albumin levels have been linked with increased risk of postoperative pneumonia.

Smoking

Smoking causes impaired mucociliary transport, reduced neutrophil activity, raised closing capacity and increased V/Q mismatch. The tracheobronchial tree is hyperactive and there is an increased risk of bronchospasm following airway manipulation. The risk of postoperative pneumonia is doubled in smokers. Carboxyhaemoglobin levels are reduced by stopping smoking for 12 h, but 6 weeks is required for maximum benefit.

Sleep apnoea syndromes

Approximately 1 in 50 men develop obstructive sleep apnoea in the supine position, leading to hypoxaemia, hypercapnia and haemodynamic instability. Patients at risk may be identified by a history of snoring and daytime sleepiness. Sleep deprivation worsens the risk, as do hypnotic, analgesic and sedative drugs. Obstruction may occur following premedication, and airway maintenance may be difficult. Oxygen therapy alone may be inadequate, and nasal CPAP may be needed.

Upper respiratory tract infection

In a child with an upper respiratory tract infection (URTI) who receives a general anaesthetic, there is up to seven times the risk of a perioperative respiratory complication. Children under 1 year of age with an URTI should have elective surgery postponed. Risks increase if intubation is performed. In otherwise healthy children over 5 years and in adults, where there is no reduction in physical activity, no pyrexia and the chest examination is normal, there appears to be no increased risk from minor surgery of further respiratory complications. However, airways are often hyperactive with increased risk of bronchospasm, and lung defence mechanisms, particularly mucociliary clearance, may be impaired. For major surgery few data are available of the effect on pulmonary risk, but in combination with other risk factors, a cautious approach is wise.

Other factors

Other risk factors leading to respiratory failure should be identified. Prophylaxis may be needed for deep vein thrombosis leading to pulmonary embolus, particularly in the obese and patients with prolonged immobilization. Preoperative hospitalization of more than 2 days doubles the risk of postoperative pneumonia.

BIBLIOGRAPHY

Barrowcliffe M P, Jones J G. Respiratory function and the safety of anaesthesia. In: Taylor T H, Major E (eds) Hazards and complications of anaesthesia. Churchill Livingstone, Edinburgh

Garibaldi R A, Britt M R, Coleman M L, Reading J C, Page N L. Risk factors of postoperative pneumonia. The American Journal of Medicine 1981; 70: 677–680

Lawrence V A, Page C P, Harris G D. Preoperative spirometry before operations. A critical appraisal of its predictive value. Archives of Internal Medicine 1989; 149: 280–283

Nunn J F. Applied respiratory physiology, 3rd edn. Butterworths, Oxford

Nunn J F, Milledge J S, Chen D, Dore C. Respiratory criteria of fitness for surgery and anaesthesia. Anaesthesia 1988; 43: 543–551

CROSS REFERENCES

Asthma
Patient Conditions 3: 68
COPD and anaesthesia
Patient Conditions 3: 75
Smoking and anaesthesia
Patient Conditions 3: 85
Obesity
Patient Conditions 5: 148
The elderly patient
Patient Conditions 11: 252
Failure to breathe or wake up postoperatively
Anaesthetic Factors 33: 623

SCORING SYSTEMS RELEVANT TO ANAESTHESIA

J. F Bion

Scoring systems measure case mix, severity of illness, workload, or cost. Their accuracy is assessed by the ability to predict a given outcome, such as death, disability, or expenditure. Scoring systems are increasingly being used to correct for variations in case mix in order to examine differences in outcome which may be attributable to different treatments or quality of care. Anaesthesia may need objective measures of case mix relevant to anaesthetic practice, in order to explain variations in throughput and outcome which might be attributable to anaesthetic practice.

CLASSIFICATION

Scoring systems use physiological, clinical or anatomical variables, in varying combinations. Physiological methods are powerful and have been widely validated, but are sensitive to timing of data collection and to the effects of treatment. Methods using clinical variables (presence or absence of cancer, organ-system failures, symptoms) are often simple to apply and may be treatment independent, but require rigid definitions and may be unduly dependent on population characteristics. Anatomical methods are used mainly for trauma, but data can only be acquired once the full extent of injuries is known; these methods therefore tend to be applied retrospectively.

RISK PREDICTION IN ANAESTHESIA

Many intensive-care scoring systems predict mortality with overall correct classification rates of 75–85%. The problem for anaesthesia is usually different: how to quantify the prior risk of a given procedure on a stable patient with limited physiological reserve.

There are two difficulties. First, reserve is not easy to measure because detection may require a standardized stress, and there are few equivalents to the cardiac treadmill for other organ systems. Second, the independent impact of surgical and anaesthetic skills on outcome must also be taken into account. These difficulties may explain the absence of an objectively derived, universally applicable, scoring system to determine anaesthetic risk. Important factors are given in Table 1.

Table 1.
Factors increasing anaesthetic risk

- Ischaemic heart disease
- Impaired myocardial function
- Pulmonary hypertension
- Obstructive airways disease
- Impaired renal function
- Co-morbidities
- ASA status IV–V
- Emergency surgery
- Complex surgery
- Male sex
- Increasing age
- Diabetes

SCORING SYSTEMS

ASA

The American Society of Anesthesiologists' classification (Table 2) originally consisted of six categories (subsequently reduced to five) which described physical status in order to facilitate charging for services, a concept now being reintroduced in the UK. Although its simplicity may explain its continuing use, there is considerable variability between different anaesthetists in assessments made using the ASA system. It does not correlate linearly with mortality, but it was not intended as a prognostic system, more as a method of finding a common language to describe complexity and potential therapeutic effort. For audit, morbidity or mortality occurring in ASA classes I or II would be worthy of inspection.

Table 2.
ASA classification of physical status

I	Healthy patient
II	Mild systemic disease, no functional limitations
III	Severe systemic disease with functional limitation
IV	Severe systemic disease which constantly threatens survival
V	Moribund, not expected to survive 24 h without surgery
E	Additional code for emergency surgery

Cardiac Risk Index (Goldman)

The Cardiac Risk Index examined cardiovascular predictors retrospectively in over 1000 patients. It confirmed that ischaemic heart disease was a risk factor, but despite the initial enthusiasm generated by what was then a novel approach, others have been unable to validate the index as a whole, and it is now of historical interest rather than practical value.

POSSUM

This perioperative general surgical score uses multivariant analysis to identify 12 preoperative physiological variables and 6 grades of operative and diagnostic complexity to predict morbidity and mortality. It is probably too complex for routine use, but may have a role in audit or research projects. This type of approach needs development within single diagnostic categories in order to direct attention to those patients who might need postoperative HDU care.

Parsonnet Score

This is a good example of a well-designed system for predicting risk in a single diagnostic category: adult patients undergoing cardiac surgery. It uses routine preoperative data and is easy to apply. It has the two advantages that 'noise' is reduced by examining an homogenous patient group undergoing a standardized procedure, and many of the variables are objective and verifiable (e.g. ejection fraction, blood pressure, intra-aortic balloon pump).

Acute Physiology and Chronic Health Evaluation (APACHE) III

The APACHE method is one of the most widely used of all scoring systems for intensive care. The 34 variables and weights in the original version were selected by clinical consensus, and then refined by statistical techniques to 12 physiological variables, with additional weighting for previous health related to urgency of admission, and age. The sum of the weighted values provides the score, which is converted to a risk of death using logistic regression for specific weighted diagnostic categories. Version III employs 17 physiological variables, and has some improvement in predictive power over version II. The system uses the worst values recorded within the first 24 h of ITU admission. It is not designed to assess preoperative risk, but performs well when stratifying critically ill operative and nonoperative patients with their greater range of physiological derangements.

Mortality Probability Model (MPM)

The MPM employs binary variables, including emergency or previous ITU admission, age, coma, previous cardio-respiratory arrest, chronic renal failure, cancer, infection, systolic blood pressure, heart rate and surgery. It provides risk estimates at the time of ITU admission and, being treatment independent, can be used for prior stratification. It might therefore be of use for intensive care triage.

Organ-system failures

The advantage of simplicity is offset by the lack of formally agreed definitions, these being dependent on understanding the pathophysiology involved. The greater the number of organ-system failures and the longer their duration, the worse the outcome.

Glasgow Coma Scale (GCS)

This scale was developed to standardize terminology and facilitate communication in neurosurgical intensive care. It uses simple neurological responses to stratify patients who have been in a coma for 6 h or more from the time of head injury. Interobserver variation is low, and the system has been validated internationally for many thousands of patients. The scale has become converted to a score (3 = worst, 15 = best), thereby treating ordinal data as continuous data. This is not strictly valid; nevertheless, the system works. Care should be taken if the GCS is applied to patients with nontraumatic coma, as it was not designed for that purpose. As part of the APACHE system, it appears best to categorize the score, with values of 7 or less giving the worst outcome. Alternatives to the GCS are required for small children and infants, and two based on the adult version have been described.

Therapeutic Intervention Scoring System (TISS)

This system categorizes therapeutic intensity or workload. A score of 1–4 points are awarded to each of 70 nursing and medical procedures. At the end of the patient's stay all the daily TISS points are summed for the total score. TISS is used as a surrogate for measuring costs, and performs well for this purpose. Yearly recalibration will be needed. Nurses can collect the data, but training is required to ensure consistency. In the UK one TISS point is worth approximately £30.

Injury Severity Score (ISS), Trauma Score (TS) and TRISS

The ISS converts the gradings of the Abbreviated Injury Scale into a score by summing the squared values for each of six anatomical areas; this converts a quadratic relationship into one which is near-linear. It is calculated at death or discharge, in order to ensure accurate information. The revised form of the TS is a simple physiological system which sums coded values for three intervals of the GCS, and five intervals of systolic blood pressure and respiratory rate. Both systems perform well when used for outcome prediction of groups of patients. Combination of the two scores gives an anatomical and physiological index of severity of injury, the TRISS system, which is being used as the comparative index in the multiple trauma outcome study in the USA and the UK to examine the effect on mortality of differences in case mix and quality of care.

BIBLIOGRAPHY

Baker S P, O'Neil B, Haddon W, Long W. The injury severity score: a method for describing patients with multiple injuries and evaluating emergency care. Journal of Trauma 1974; 14: 187–196

Boyd C R, Tolson M A, Copes W S. Evaluating trauma care: the TRISS method. Journal of Trauma 1987; 27: 370–378

Champion H R, Sacco W J, Carnazzo A J, Copes W, Fouty W J. Trauma score. Critical Care Medicine 1981; 9: 672–676

Cullen D J. Results and costs of intensive care. Anesthesiology 1977; 47: 203–216

Dripps R D, Lamont A, Eckenhoff J E. The role of anaesthesia in surgical mortality. Journal of the American Medical Association 1961; 178: 261

Farrow S C, Fowkes F G R, Lunn J N, Robertson I B, Sweetnam P. Epidemiology in anaesthesia: a method for predicting hospital mortality. European Journal of Anaesthesiology 1984; 1: 77–84

Goldman L, Caldera D L, Nussbaum S R et al. Multifactorial index on cardiac risk in noncardiac surgical procedures. New England Journal of Medicine 1977; 297: 845

Jennett B, Teasdale G, Braakman R, Minderhoud J, Knill-Jones R. Predicting outcome in individual patients after severe head injury. Lancet 1976; i: 1031–1034

Knaus W A, Draper E A, Wagner D P et al. Prognosis in acute organ-system failure. Annals of Surgery 1985; 202: 685–693

Knaus W A, Draper E A, Wagner D P, Zimmerman J E. APACHE II: a severity of disease classification system. Critical Care Medicine 1985; 10: 818–829

Lemeshow S, Teres D, Klar J, et al. Mortality Probability Models (MPM II) Based on an International Cohort of Intensive Care Unit Patients. JAMA 1993; 270: 2478–2486

Owens W D. ASA physical status classifications: a study of consistency of ratings. Anesthesiology 1978; 49: 239

Parsonnet V, Dean D, Bernstein A D. A method of uniform stratification of risk for evaluating the results of surgery in acquired adult heart disease. Circulation 1989; 79: 3–12

Pine R W, Wertz, Lennard E S, Dellinger E P, Carrico C J, Minshew B H. Determinants of organ malfunction or death in patients with intra-abdominal sepsis. Archives of Surgery 1983; 118: 242–249

Reilly P L, Simpson D A, Thomas L. Assessing the conscious level in infants and young children: a paediatric version of the Glasgow Coma Scale. Child's Nervous System 1988; 4: 30–33

Ross A F, Tinker J H. Anaesthesia risk. In: Miller R D (ed) Anaesthesia, 3rd edn. Churchill Livingstone, New York, 1990

Teasdale G, Jennett B. Assessment of coma and impaired consciousness. A practical scale. Lancet 1974; ii: 81–84

INDEX